10th
Edition

Quick & Easy

MEDICAL TERMINOLOGY

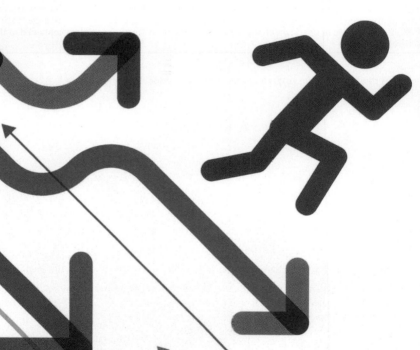

ELSEVIER

Peggy C. Leonard, MT, MEd

3251 Riverport Lane
St. Louis, Missouri 63043

QUICK & EASY MEDICAL TERMINOLOGY, TENTH EDITION

ISBN: 978-0-323-88395-5

Notices

Previous editions copyrighted 2020, 2017, 2014, 2011, 2007, 2003, 2000, 1995, 1990.

Senior Content Strategist: Luke Held
Director, Content Development: Laurie Gower
Senior Content Development Specialist: Betsy McCormick
Publishing Services Manager: Julie Eddy
Project Manager: Becky Langdon
Text Designer: Bridget Hoette

Printed in Canada

Last digit is the print number: 9   8   7   6   5   4   3   2   1

Working together
to grow libraries in
developing countries

www.elsevier.com • www.bookaid.org

Contents

Reviewers and Contributors

Preface

Make Learning Quick & Easy by This Proven Method

Jump right into using medical terms in the first chapter. *Quick & Easy Medical Terminology* simplifies difficult medical terms and concepts by teaching the meaning of word parts and how terms are put together!

The tenth edition of *Quick & Easy Medical Terminology* has made learning easier for students, but has retained what you liked about the ninth edition.

You will notice these new features:

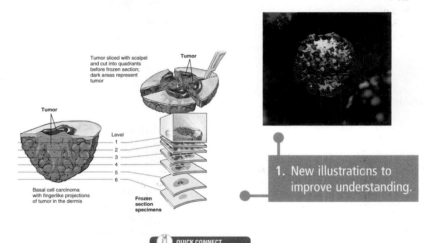

Tumor sliced with scalpel and cut into quadrants before frozen section; dark areas represent tumor

Tumor

Tumor

Level
1
2
3
4
5
6

Basal cell carcinoma with fingerlike projections of tumor in the dermis

Frozen section specimens

1. New illustrations to improve understanding.

2. New! Quick Connect!

> **QUICK CONNECT**
>
> *Review all lists of word parts and their meanings for Chapter 3 using the flashcards you prepared or the flashcards on the Evolve site.*
>
> A prefix is placed before a word to modify its meaning. Most prefixes, including those ending with a vowel, can be added to the remainder of the word without change.
>   Prefixes for numbers or quantities:
>
> ½ = hemi-, semi-
> 1 = mono-, uni-
> 2 = bi-, di-
> 3 = tri-
> 4 = quad-, quadri-, tetra-

I. READING HEALTH CARE REPORTS *Read the health report; then select one-word answers to complete the sentences.*

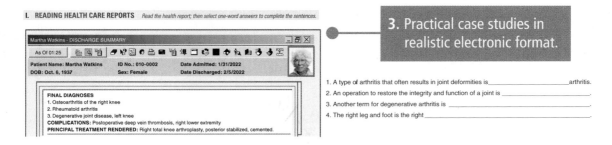

3. Practical case studies in realistic electronic format.

1. A type of arthritis that often results in joint deformities is_____arthritis.
2. An operation to restore the integrity and function of a joint is _____.
3. Another term for degenerative arthritis is _____.
4. The right leg and foot is the right _____.

More Features!

We have retained features students and instructors love.

4. Top-notch photos and illustrations of the body systems.

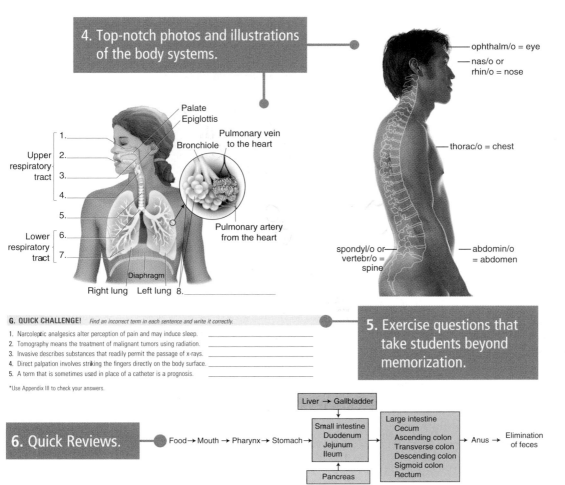

ophthalm/o = eye

nas/o or rhin/o = nose

thorac/o = chest

spondyl/o or vertebr/o = spine

abdomin/o = abdomen

Palate
Epiglottis

Upper respiratory tract
1. _____
2. _____
3. _____
4. _____

Pulmonary vein to the heart
Bronchiole

Pulmonary artery from the heart

Lower respiratory tract
5. _____
6. _____
7. _____

Diaphragm
Right lung   Left lung   8. _____

G. QUICK CHALLENGE! *Find an incorrect term in each sentence and write it correctly.*

1. Narcoleptic analgesics alter perception of pain and may induce sleep.   _____
2. Tomography means the treatment of malignant tumors using radiation.   _____
3. Invasive describes substances that readily permit the passage of x-rays.   _____
4. Direct palpation involves striking the fingers directly on the body surface.   _____
5. A term that is sometimes used in place of a catheter is a prognosis.   _____

*Use Appendix III to check your answers.

5. Exercise questions that take students beyond memorization.

6. Quick Reviews.

Liver → Gallbladder

Food → Mouth → Pharynx → Stomach →

Small intestine
Duodenum
Jejunum
Ileum

Pancreas

Large intestine
Cecum
Ascending colon
Transverse colon
Descending colon
Sigmoid colon
Rectum

→ Anus → Elimination of feces

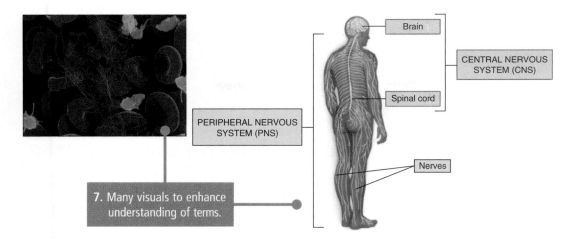

Brain

CENTRAL NERVOUS SYSTEM (CNS)

Spinal cord

PERIPHERAL NERVOUS SYSTEM (PNS)

Nerves

7. Many visuals to enhance understanding of terms.

A Career as an Ultrasonographer

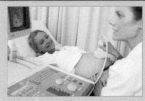

Chelsey Jones is really proud of her decision to study sonography. She had always wanted a career helping people directly. She works mostly with obstetric patients and truly feels that her talents are being used for an important purpose. Chelsey almost studied architecture because she knew she had a talent for visualizing objects in three dimensions, but that talent also applies to sonography. A bachelor's degree is not always required for ultrasonographers, but most employers prefer individuals registered through the American Registry for Diagnostic Medical Sonography or the American Registry of Radiologic Technologists. For more information, visit www.sdms.org, and click on the resources tab or www.arrt.org.

8. Professional career profiles.

QUICK CASE STUDY | EXERCISE 12

Write a term from the report to complete each sentence.

Emily's physician ordered chest x-rays. In the first image, she was positioned with her chest nearest the image receptor. In the second image, she was standing with her left side against the image receptor. Choose from the following directional terms to describe the projections: anteroposterior, posteroanterior, left lateral, right lateral

1. Which term is correct for the first position? _____
2. Which term is correct for the second position? _____

9. Quick case studies for immediate application.

QUICK & EASY (Q&E) LIST—cont'd

coronary heart disease (*kor*-uh-nar-ē hahrt di-*zē z*)
cuspid (*kus*-pid)
defibrillation (dē-fib-ri-*lā*-shun)
defibrillator (dē-*fib*-ri-lā-tur)
digoxin (di-*jok*-sin)
diuretic (di-ū-*ret*-ik)
dysrhythmia (dis-*rith*-mē-uh)
echocardiogram (ek-ō-*kahr*-dē-ō-gram)
echocardiography (ek-ō-kahr-dē-*og*-ruh-fē)
electrocardiogram (ē-lek-trō-*kahr*-dē-ō-gram)
electrocardiograph (ē-lek-trō-*kahr*-dē-ō-graf)
electrocardiography (ē-lek-trō-kahr-dē-*og*-ruh-fē)
elephantiasis (el-uh-fun-*tī*-uh-sis)
embolism (*em*-buh-liz-um)
embolus (*em*-bō-lus)
endocarditis (en-dō-kahr-*di*-tis)
endocardium (en-dō-*kahr*-dē-um)
epicardium (ep-i-*kahr*-dē-um)
fibrillation (fib-ri-*lā*-shun)
heart failure (hahrt *fā* lyur)
heart murmur (hahrt *mur*-mur)

myocarditis (mī-ō-kahr-*di*-tis)
myocardium (mī-ō-*kahr*-dē-um)
nitroglycerin (nī-trō-*glis*-ur-in)
occlusion (ō-*kloo*-zhun)
palatine tonsil (*pal*-uh-tīn *ton*-sil)
pericarditis (per-i-kahr-*di*-tis)
pericardium (per-i-*kahr*-dē-um)
pharyngeal (fuh-*rin*-jē-ul)
phlebectomy (fluh-*bek*-tuh-mē)
phlebitis (fluh-*bī*-tis)
polyarteritis (pol-ē-ahr-tuh-*rī*-tis)
pulse (puls)
semilunar (sem-ē-*loo*-nur)
septal defect (*sep*-tul *dē*-fekt)
shock (shok)
sinoatrial node (sī-nō-ā-trē-ul nōd)
spleen (splēn)
splenectomy (splē-*nek*-tuh-mē)
splenomegaly (splē-nō-*meg*-uh-lē)
stenosis (stuh-*nō*-sis)
tachycardia (tak-i-*kahr*-dē-uh)

10. Easy-to-understand pronunciations. Students listen to pronunciations on the Evolve site, which correspond with the pronunciation lists at the end of each chapter.

QUICK TIP

*A*xon *a*way; *d*endrites towar*d*

11. More Quick Tips and Word Origins.

WORD ORIGIN

obsession *obsidere* (L.), to haunt

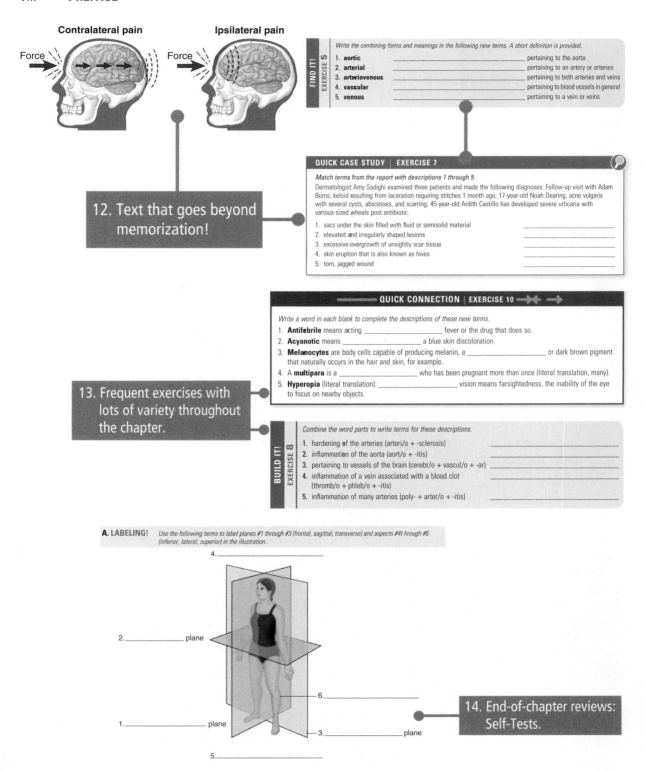

Contralateral pain

Force

Ipsilateral pain

Force

FIND IT! EXERCISE 5

Write the combining forms and meanings in the following new terms. A short definition is provided.

1. **aortic** _____ pertaining to the aorta
2. **arterial** _____ pertaining to an artery or arteries
3. **arteriovenous** _____ pertaining to both arteries and veins
4. **vascular** _____ pertaining to blood vessels in general
5. **venous** _____ pertaining to a vein or veins

12. Text that goes beyond memorization!

QUICK CASE STUDY | EXERCISE 7

Match terms from the report with descriptions 1 through 5.

Dermatologist Amy Sadighi examined three patients and made the following diagnoses: Follow-up visit with Adam Burns, keloid resulting from laceration requiring stitches 1 month ago; 17-year-old Noah Dearing, acne vulgaris with several cysts, abscesses, and scarring; 45-year-old Ardith Castillo has developed severe urticaria with various-sized wheals post antibiotic.

1. sacs under the skin filled with fluid or semisolid material _____
2. elevated and irregularly shaped lesions _____
3. excessive overgrowth of unsightly scar tissue _____
4. skin eruption that is also known as hives _____
5. torn, jagged wound _____

QUICK CONNECTION | EXERCISE 10

Write a word in each blank to complete the descriptions of these new terms.

1. **Antifebrile** means acting _____ fever or the drug that does so.
2. **Acyanotic** means _____ a blue skin discoloration.
3. **Melanocytes** are body cells capable of producing melanin, a _____ or dark brown pigment that naturally occurs in the hair and skin, for example.
4. A **multipara** is a _____ who has been pregnant more than once (literal translation, many).
5. **Hyperopia** (literal translation): _____ vision means farsightedness, the inability of the eye to focus on nearby objects.

13. Frequent exercises with lots of variety throughout the chapter.

BUILD IT! EXERCISE 8

Combine the word parts to write terms for these descriptions.

1. hardening of the arteries (arteri/o + -sclerosis) _____
2. inflammation of the aorta (aort/o + -itis) _____
3. pertaining to vessels of the brain (cerebr/o + vascul/o + -ar) _____
4. inflammation of a vein associated with a blood clot (thromb/o + phleb/o + -itis) _____
5. inflammation of many arteries (poly- + arter/o + -itis) _____

A. LABELING!   Use the following terms to label planes #1 through #3 (frontal, sagittal, transverse) and aspects #4t hrough #6 (inferior, lateral, superior) in the illustration.

4. _____

2. _____ plane

6. _____

1. _____ plane

3. _____ plane

5. _____

14. End-of-chapter reviews: Self-Tests.

Instructors Will Love These Extra Resources

The Evolve companion site provides a course management platform for instructors. Elsevier provides hosting and technical support. See the inside back cover for the listing of abundant resources available for students. The Practice Exam can be assigned by instructors, and results will be posted to the gradebook. The rest of the assets provide valuable practice in learning and retaining medical terms.

Your Job Is Simpler With Evolve Instructor Resources

Classroom Activities and Test Bank

Instructors have loved the wealth of materials provided on the Evolve Resources site. Classroom activities and exercises that require students to write and spell terms correctly are included in easy-to-use handouts or homework assignments. The ExamView Test Bank that includes multiple question formats is available for you to use directly or to alter to suit your needs.

TEACH Instructor Resources

TEACH links all parts of the education package by providing you with customizable lesson plans and lecture outlines based on learning objectives.

Each Lesson Plan Features:

- A format that correlates chapter objectives to content and teaching resources
- Lesson preparation checklists that make planning your class quick and easy
- Critical-thinking questions to focus and motivate students
- Teaching resources that cross-reference all of TEACH and Elsevier's curriculum solutions
- PowerPoint slides that present a compelling visual summary of the chapter's main points and key terms
- Practical, concise talking points that complement the PowerPoint slides
- Thought-provoking questions to stimulate classroom discussions
- Unique ideas for moving beyond traditional lectures and getting students involved

For more information on the benefits of TEACH, call Faculty Support at 1–800–222–9570.

This Text Adapts Perfectly to a Variety of Classroom Needs

The book is useful in a short medical terminology course or as self-paced material for anyone pursuing a career in the allied health professions. *Quick & Easy Medical Terminology* can be studied in conjunction with courses in anatomy, physiology, or introductory medical science, or in foundation programs for careers in health or medicine. After the first five chapters are completed, you have the advantage of being able to teach Chapters 6 to 15 in the order that complements the particular body system being studied.

Text Illustrations Enhance Classroom Discussion

The tenth edition provides more full-color illustrations to emphasize key terms and to help students understand difficult concepts. Students interact and learn more quickly as they complete the labeling of illustrations.

Contents

Basic Chapters

Body Systems

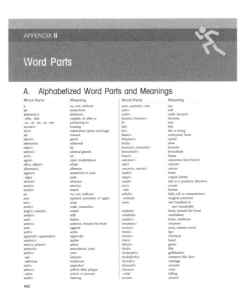

Resources in the Appendixes That Your Students Love

An alphabetized glossary of word parts, answers to exercises, and medical abbreviations are available in the appendixes. Abbreviations are presented by chapter. A pharmacology appendix, with drug classes and uses, is available online. Placement of the material in the appendixes is for your convenience and that of your students, whether or not you choose to use the material for a particular class.

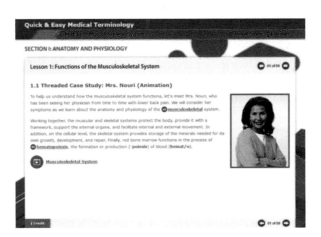

Online course!

Online course provides even more opportunity for students to use electronics and learn medical terms the QUICK & EASY way—Now with audio reviews and adaptive learning!

Pacing is FAST

With *Quick & Easy Medical Terminology*, **students start reading and writing medical terms the first day!**

Students set the pace! They can work on part of a chapter, all of a chapter, or several chapters in one study session. It is important that Chapters 1 through 5 are studied in the order in which they are presented, because these chapters build on the previous material learned. After completing the first five chapters, students may complete Chapters 6 through 15 in any order or as assigned by the instructor.

Helpful Hints Show How to Distinguish Between Confusing Terms

Caution boxes help differentiate terms that look alike, sound alike, or are easily mistaken for something else.

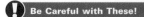

Be Careful with These!

catheter (instrument) versus *catheterize* (verb) versus *catheterization* (the process)
diagnosis (disease ID) versus *prognosis* (predicted outcome)
palpation (part of physical exam) versus *palpitation* (heart flutter)
radiograph (same as radiogram, x-ray record) produced in *radiography*
sonogram or *echogram* (the record produced in *sonography*, the process)
tomogram (the tomographic record) versus *tomography* (the process)

Opposites
acute versus *chronic*
diastolic pressure versus *systolic* pressure
radiopaque versus *radiolucent*
signs (objective) versus *symptoms* (subjective)

End-of-Chapter Review Helps Students Measure How They Are Doing Before the Test

Review materials are provided within the chapter, self-tests help students know if they're ready for the exam, and answers can be checked using Appendix III.

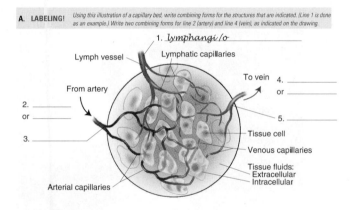

A. LABELING! *Using this illustration of a capillary bed, write combining forms for the structures that are indicated. (Line 1 is done as an example.) Write two combining forms for line 2 (artery) and line 4 (vein), as indicated on the drawing.*

1. *lymphangi/o*

Lymph vessel
Lymphatic capillaries
To vein   4. _____
or _____
From artery
2. _____
or _____
5. _____
3. _____
Tissue cell
Venous capillaries
Tissue fluids:
  Extracellular
  Intracellular
Arterial capillaries

Students Have Fun as They Take Charge of Their Learning!

This book provides an easy way to learn medical terms and allows students to move at their own pace.

You have EVERYTHING YOU NEED for a FABULOUS Quick & Easy Medical Terminology COURSE!

Peggy C. Leonard

Acknowledgments

A book that endures the test of time can be traced back to a group of dedicated individuals who have contributed their expertise to ensuring that the book retains what makes it stand out from the rest, while updating and adding features that improve it. New persons brought on board with each edition contribute the imagination and talent for developing novel ideas in teaching medical terminology.

I am blessed to have worked with Senior Content Strategist Linda Woodard and artist Jeanne Robertson for several editions of both *Quick & Easy Medical Terminology*, and *Building a Medical Vocabulary*. I greatly appreciate the efforts of the designer, proofreaders, production manager, and companies who allowed use of their illustrations to enhance the written word.

Suggestions from instructors have been incorporated, as well as analyses by reviewers. In addition, an outstanding group of contributors have added knowledge in their chosen fields, as well as their years of experience teaching medical terminology.

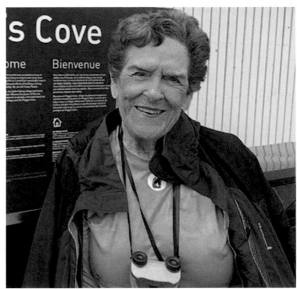

Peggy C. Leonard, MT, MEd
On vacation in Nova Scotia

Dedicated to the instructors and students whose enthusiasm and influence have helped shape this book, and to my family who support me in so many ways.

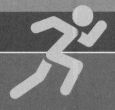

CHAPTER **1**

Simplified Medical Language

Medical terms are used by all medical professionals: physicians, nurses, medical laboratory personnel, respiratory therapists, pharmacists, and many others. You will quickly learn to recognize these new terms!

OBJECTIVES

After completing Chapter 1, you will be able to:

1. Recognize prefixes, suffixes, word roots, and combining forms.
2. Demonstrate understanding of the rules for combining word parts to write medical terms correctly.
3. Identify and distinguish abbreviations from eponyms.
4. Use the rules learned in this chapter to write the singular or plural forms of medical terms.
5. Demonstrate understanding of the primary accent used in pronunciation.

Simplifying Medical Terms

The great size of a medical dictionary is evidence of the vast number of words in the medical language.

The material in Chapters 1 through 5 is essential for learning medical terms because it explains *word building*, teaches you how to divide words into their component parts, and provides a foundation on which you can understand and write many terms. Chapters 6 through 15 do not have to be studied in the sequence in which they appear in this book, but they are presented with the assumption that you have learned the material in the first five chapters.

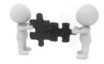

WHY MEDICAL TERMS LOOK DIFFERENT FROM ORDINARY ENGLISH WORDS

Extensive borrowing of medical words from Latin and Greek began about A.D.1500. As new diseases or treatments were recognized, scientists and physicians often used Latin or Greek to describe the new discoveries, so now the two languages are the origin of more than 90% of the medical terms. Experience has shown that learning Greek and Latin is not necessary if you learn word parts, as you'll do in this book.

WORD ORIGIN

Watch for this clue to tell you the origin of words:
(D.), German (Deutsch)
(G.), Greek
(I.), Italian
(L.), Latin

Many word parts are used to form medical terms that pertain to various body systems. For example, *-itis* is a suffix that means "inflammation." Therefore, you will see this word part used in describing various inflammatory conditions throughout the body.

No matter how eager you are to learn medical terminology pertaining to a particular body system, don't skip any of the material in the first five chapters of this book! It is the foundation on which you will base speaking, reading, and writing medical terms correctly.

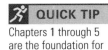

QUICK TIP

Chapters 1 through 5 are the foundation for the rest of the book.

Writing Is Key

Correct spelling is essential because a misspelled word may have an entirely different meaning. In many cases, correct spelling can also help with pronunciation. (You are not required to learn specific medical terms in Chapter 1.) Starting with Chapter 2, the correct pronunciations are provided at the end of each chapter. Also, use the Evolve website to listen to pronunciations.*

QUICK TIP

Learning to pronounce terms can improve your spelling.

WRITING WORDS HELPS YOU LEARN FASTER THAN SIMPLY READING THEM

You will often be asked to write answers. Write an answer whenever you see a blank or a question, and check every answer that you write to see if it is correct. Even when you are sure you know the answer, check your answer anyway. Sometimes you might misinterpret what you read, and this is an excellent way to check your understanding.

Variety Makes It Fun

Written exercises throughout each chapter get you actively involved. The Self-Test at the end of each chapter helps you know if you have learned the material.

As you study Chapter 1, word parts that make up medical terms are explained first, followed by other forms of communication, such as abbreviations. Plurals and pronunciations are also introduced.

Word Parts

Word Roots and Combining Forms

The *word root* is the main body of a word. All words have a word root, even ordinary words. Word roots are the building blocks for most medical terms. Compound words are sometimes composed of two word roots, as in collarbone (collar and bone). Most medical dictionaries show the origin of terms. If you study these, you will see that many are derived from Greek and Latin words. Look at the examples of word roots and their Greek or Latin origin in Table 1.1.

TABLE 1.1	ORIGIN OF WORD ROOTS	
Word Root	**Greek or Latin Origin**	**Use in a Word**
lith	*lithos* (G., stone)	lithiasis
psych	*psyche* (G., mind)	psychology
caud	*cauda* (L., tail)	caudal
or	*oris* (L., mouth)	oral

---

* A pronunciation guide is presented inside the back cover and on the bookmark included with the text.

A vowel called a *combining vowel* is often inserted between word roots to make the word easier to pronounce. In the word speed/o/meter, speed/o is a *combining form* that is simply the word root "speed" plus the vowel *o*. A combining form can be recognized in this book by the diagonal slash mark before an ending vowel. (The most frequently used vowel is *o*.) Cardi/o, gastr/o, and oste/o are all combining forms, but so is chol/e. In this book, you will learn the combining forms for word roots.

You will sometimes learn two word roots that have the same meaning. For example, both *dermal* and *cutaneous* mean "pertaining to the skin" (Fig. 1.1). As a general rule, Latin roots are used to write words naming and describing structures of the body, whereas Greek roots are used to write words naming and describing diseases, conditions, diagnosis, and treatment. As with most rules, however, there are exceptions.

> **QUICK TIP**
>
> A word root + a combining vowel = a combining form.

WRITE IT!* · **EXERCISE 1**

Write either WR (for "word root") or CF (for "combining form") in the blanks to identify these word parts.

_____ 1. aden/o	_____ 3. chol/e	_____ 5. or/o
_____ 2. carcin/o	_____ 4. lith	_____ 6. psych

*Use Appendix III, Answers, to check your answers to all the exercises in Chapter 1.

YOU CAN'T BREAK ALL WORDS INTO THEIR COMPONENT PARTS

Occasionally you will encounter a word that doesn't seem to fit the rules because it isn't composed of word roots that make sense or sometimes is formed from another language (Fig. 1.2). However, most medical words are composed of word parts you will learn to recognize.

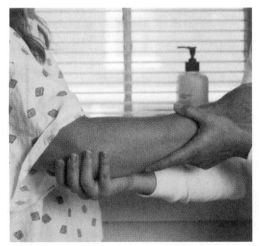

Fig. 1.1 Examination of the Skin. A patient's skin, the body's largest and most visible organ, can provide valuable information about the patient's health. The scientific name of the skin is *dermis,* from the Greek term *derma.* The Latin *cutis* also means skin. Both *dermal* and *cutaneous* mean pertaining to the skin. Inflammation of the skin is *dermatitis.*
derm/a = skin; **cutane/o** = skin; **-al, -ous** = pertaining to

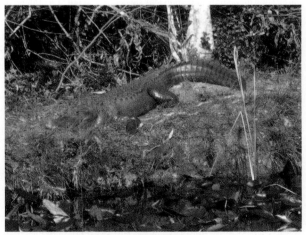

Fig. 1.2 Be Aware That Some Words Cannot Be Broken Into Component Parts. The alligator, for example, is so named because Spanish explorers mistook the nature of the reptile and named it "el lagarto" (the lizard). Perhaps after several years, "el lagarto" began to sound like *alligator.*

QUICK TIP

Prefixes **pre**cede (**c**ome be**f**ore) **c**ombining **f**orms.

Prefixes and Suffixes

A word root is usually accompanied by a prefix or a suffix, or sometimes by both. A *prefix* is placed before a word or word part to modify its meaning. When written alone, a prefix is usually followed by a hyphen (e.g., anti-), indicating that another word part follows the prefix to form a complete word.

Example: The prefix a- (meaning "without") joined with febrile (which refers to "fever") yields the term *afebrile*, which means "without fever."

A *suffix* is attached to the end of a word or word root to modify its meaning. Suffixes are joined to combining forms to write nouns (persons, places, or things), adjectives (descriptive words), and verbs (action words). A suffix is usually preceded by a hyphen when the suffix is written alone (e.g., -cyte), indicating that another word part generally precedes it before a complete word can be formed.

Example: The combining form erythr/o (meaning red) can be joined with the suffix -cyte (meaning cell) to write the term *erythrocyte*, which means a red blood cell (often shortened to red cell).

Occasionally a word is composed of only a prefix and a suffix (e.g., combining dys- and -pnea). Visualize the relationship of prefixes, combining forms, and suffixes as you study Fig. 1.4.

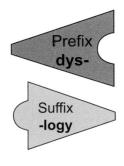

Prefix
dys-

Suffix
-logy

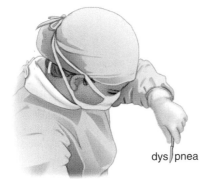

dys/pnea

Fig. 1.3 Dissect words into component parts. Look for a suffix first, then look for other recognizable word parts.

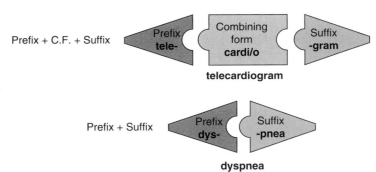

Prefix + C.F. + Suffix

Prefix **tele-**   Combining form **cardi/o**   Suffix **-gram**

telecardiogram

Prefix + Suffix

Prefix **dys-**   Suffix **-pnea**

dyspnea

Fig. 1.4 The Relationship of Prefixes, Combining Forms, and Suffixes.

WRITE IT! EXERCISE 2

Write CF (for combining form), P (for prefix), or S (for suffix) for each of the following word parts:

1. brady- _____
2. -cele _____
3. eu- _____

4. -graphy _____
5. hydr/o _____
6. -iasis _____

7. mal- _____
8. phon/o _____
9. -pathy _____

WRITE IT! EXERCISE 3

A prefix or suffix is underlined in each of the following terms. Write either P (for prefix) or S (for suffix) after each term:

1. <u>ad</u>hesion _____
2. adeno<u>pathy</u> _____
3. bili<u>ary</u> _____

4. derm<u>al</u> _____
5. <u>endo</u>cardial _____
6. hemato<u>logy</u> _____

7. <u>hypo</u>glossal _____
8. <u>micro</u>scope _____
9. <u>pre</u>natal _____

Check your answers with Appendix III, Answers.

Word roots, combining forms, prefixes, and suffixes are *word parts*. Learning the meaning of these word parts eliminates the necessity of memorizing each new term you encounter. Do not be concerned with the meanings of the word parts in Chapter 1; you will learn them in subsequent chapters. After writing answers in the blanks, check your answers against those shown in Appendix III. It is best to work all of a particular exercise before checking your answers. It is also important to confirm your answers before going on to the next exercise. (If you have made a mistake, you do not want to keep repeating it throughout the chapter!)

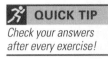

QUICK TIP

*Check your answers
after every exercise!*

WRITE IT!

EXERCISE 4

Combining forms for five body structures are shown. For each body structure that is labeled, write the corresponding combining forms. (#1 is done as an example.)

1. hair: trich/o, pil/o
2. eye: _____
3. nose: _____
4. mouth: _____
5. chest: _____

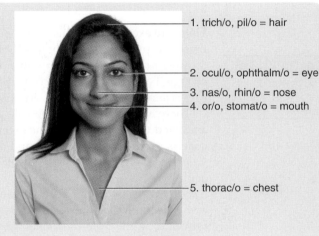

1. trich/o, pil/o = hair

2. ocul/o, ophthalm/o = eye
3. nas/o, rhin/o = nose
4. or/o, stomat/o = mouth

5. thorac/o = chest

Check your answers with Appendix III, Answers.

Combining Word Parts to Write Terms

Remember that when combining forms are written alone, they contain a combining vowel, often an *o*, as in hepat/o. When medical terms are written, the vowel at the end of a combining form is not always used.

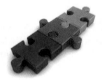

THIS RULE HELPS YOU DECIDE WHEN TO USE THE COMBINING VOWEL

The combining vowel is used before suffixes that begin with a consonant and before another word root. In other words, drop the combining vowel if the suffix also begins with a vowel (*a, e, i, o,* or *u*).

Example 1: When the combining form hepat/o is joined with the suffix -megaly, the combining vowel is used and results in the term *hepatomegaly*. Notice that -megaly begins with a consonant: hepat/o + -megaly = hepatomegaly.
Example 2: When the combining form hepat/o is joined with the suffix -itis, the combining vowel is not used and results in the term *hepatitis*. Notice that the *o* is dropped from hepat/o because -itis begins with a vowel: hepat/o + -itis = hepatitis.

BUILD IT!
EXERCISE 5

Use the rule you just learned to build terms, knowing that ot/o means ear.

1. ot/o + -ic = _____, pertaining to the ear
2. ot/o + -itis = _____, inflammation of the ear
3. ot/o + -logy = _____, study of the ear
4. ot/o + -plasty = _____, plastic surgery of the ear
5. ot/o + -rrhea = _____, discharge from the ear
6. ot/o + -tomy = _____, incision of the ear

Check your answers with Appendix III, Answers.

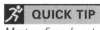 **QUICK TIP**

Most prefixes do not change when added to a word.

There are exceptions to this rule about using the combining vowel, and you will learn these exceptions as you progress through the material.

Most prefixes end with a vowel and may be added to other word parts without change. For example, *precancerous, preeruptive,* and *preoperative* result when the prefix pre- is joined with cancerous, eruptive, and operative.

There are exceptions to the rule concerning the use of prefixes. These exceptions are noted when they occur. One exception is *anti-*. When anti- is joined with biotic and coagulant, the terms *antibiotic* and *anticoagulant* result. Often, however, ant- is used when the prefix is joined to a vowel. The term *antacid* results when anti- is joined with acid.

Sometimes two terms are acceptable when a prefix is used to form a new word. *End-* and *endo-* both mean inside. End- is usually joined with word parts beginning with a vowel, as in the term *endarterial*. Common usage, however, has determined whether end- or endo- is used in certain cases. Some terms accept either prefix, as in *endaortitis* and *endoaortitis*. Both terms are acceptable, and the two have identical meanings. The word-building rules are summarized in Table 1.2.

As you learn word parts, you will begin to recognize them within medical terms. You will even be able to determine the meaning of many terms by breaking them down into their component parts.

TABLE 1.2   RULES FOR CONSTRUCTING TERMS
Joining Combining Forms
The combining vowel is usually retained between two combining forms.
Example: gastr/o + enterology = gastroenterology
Joining Combining Forms and Suffixes
The combining vowel is usually retained when a combining form is joined with a suffix that begins with a consonant.
Example: enter/o + -logy = enterology
The combining vowel is usually omitted when a combining form is joined with a suffix that begins with a vowel.
Example: enter/o + -ic = enteric
Joining Other Word Parts and Prefixes
Most prefixes require no change when they are joined with other word parts.
Examples: peri- + appendicitis = periappendicitis; dys- + -pnea = dyspnea

WORD DIVISION

Word division is used frequently throughout this book to help you recognize the parts that are used to build a term. For example, the first time you see appendicitis, it may be written as appendic+itis to emphasize its two component parts.

Fig. 1.5 summarizes examples of using word parts to write and interpret medical terms. Be aware that some terms do not follow the rules you have learned. As you progress through the material, you will find such exceptions noted.

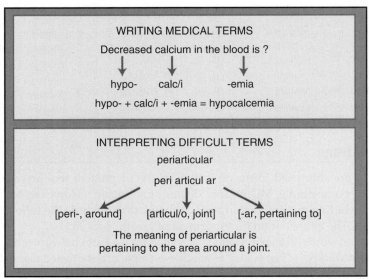

Fig. 1.5 Examples of Using Prefixes, Suffixes, and Combining Forms to Write and Interpret Medical Terms.

BUILD IT!

EXERCISE 6

Write terms from these word parts, deciding if you use or drop the combining vowel when present.

1. dys- + -pnea   _____
2. enter/o + -ic   _____
3. eu- + -pepsia   _____
4. tonsill/o + -itis   _____
5. ur/o + -emia   _____
6. anti- + anxiety   _____
7. leuk/o + -cyte   _____
8. appendic/o + -itis   _____
9. hyper- + -emia   _____
10. endo- + cardi/o + -al _____

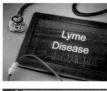
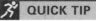

Proper Names are Special

Eponyms are names for diseases, organs, procedures, or body functions that are derived from the name of a person. Cesarean section, a surgical procedure in which the abdomen and uterus are surgically opened to deliver the infant, is an eponym that reflects the manner in which Julius Caesar supposedly was born. Parkinson disease and Alzheimer disease are also eponyms.

Eponyms are usually capitalized; however, some eponyms used as adjectives are written in lower case (*example:* cesarean section).

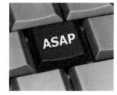

CHOOSE IT!   EXERCISE 7

Circle the eponyms in the following list.

1. Alzheimer disease vs. wasting disease
2. Beckman thermometer vs. oral thermometer
3. cesarean section vs. frozen section
4. cardiac catheter vs. Foley catheter
5. electronic fetal monitor vs. Holter monitor

6. forceps delivery vs. Alzheimer disease
7. Heimlich maneuver vs. horizontal plane
8. hormonal replacement vs. chronic disease
9. Parkinson syndrome vs. chronic disease
10. urinary system vs. Wilms' tumor

Abbreviations

Abbreviations are shortened forms of written words or phrases that are used in place of the whole. For example, MD means "doctor of medicine." However, MD has other meanings, including medical department. Abbreviations include the following:

- Letters (The abbreviation for "shortness of breath" is SOB.)
- Shortened words (The abbreviation *stat* is short for the Latin *statim,* meaning "at once" or "immediately.") "Pap smear" is another example of a shortened name (Fig. 1.6).
- *Acronyms* are pronounceable names made up of a series of letters or parts of words. (The acronym CABG, pronounced like the vegetable, stands for coronary artery bypass graft.)

Using abbreviations and symbols can be dangerous when medications are involved. The Institute for Safe Medication Practices (ISMP) publishes lists of what are considered dangerous abbreviations and recommends that certain terms be written in full

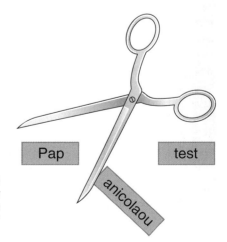

Fig. 1.6 Shortening of a Name. George N. Papanicolaou, a Greek physician practicing in the United States, found a simple smear method of staining and examining cells that are sloughed off by an organ (e.g., the cervix). This test is most often used to detect cancers of the cervix, but it may be used for tissue specimens from other organs. The name is often shortened to the simple word "Pap" smear, or Pap test.

because they are easily mistaken for other meanings. For example (especially when written by hand), qn, meaning "nightly" or "at bedtime," can be misinterpreted as qh, which means "every hour." Common abbreviations are presented in this book, but particular caution is required in both using and reading abbreviations. Appendix I has alphabetical listings of abbreviations and their meanings. If a common abbreviation is missing, you may consider checking whether its use is discouraged by the ISMP (*www .ismp.org*).

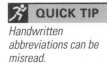
QUICK TIP

Handwritten abbreviations can be misread.

CHECK THE "DO NOT USE" LIST OF ABBREVIATIONS

The Joint Commission (formerly the Joint Commission on Accreditation of Healthcare Organizations), recognized nationwide as a symbol of quality, also publishes an official "Do Not Use" list of abbreviations and symbols. The Joint Commission is an independent, not-for-profit organization that accredits and certifies subscriber hospitals and other health care organizations. Look for their "Do Not Use" list of abbreviations under the "Patient Safety" tab at: *www.jointco mmission.org.*

MATCH IT!
EXERCISE 8

Choose A or B from the right column to classify the terms in the two left columns.

_____ 1. CAD   _____ 4. OSHA   A. abbreviation
_____ 2. D&C   _____ 5. Raynaud sign   B. eponym
_____ 3. Foley catheter

Pharmacology

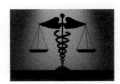

Pharmacology is the study of the preparation, properties, uses, and actions of drugs. Drugs are used in health care to prevent, diagnose, and treat disease and to relieve pain. Another term for medicines is *pharmaceuticals*. See the online appendix on the Evolve site (*http://evolve.elsevier.com/Leonard/quick/*) for the grouping of drugs into classes (e.g., anesthetics) based on their major effects.

Plurals

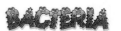

Plurals of many medical terms are formed using the rules you may already know, such as simply adding an s to the singular term. For example, the plural of abrasion is *abrasions*. Many nouns that end in *s, ch,* or *sh* form their plurals by adding *-es*. For example, the plural of sinus is *sinuses*. Singular nouns that end in *y* preceded by a consonant form their plurals by changing the *y* to *i* and adding *-es*. For example, the plural of allergy is *allergies*.

Use Table 1.3 to learn the rules for forming other plurals of medical terms, but be aware that a few exceptions exist and that only major rules are included. Also, note that some terms have more than one acceptable plural. Many dictionaries show the plural forms of nouns and can be used as a reference.

You'll see many of the singular endings (for example, us, ix, and on) are used as word endings (like suffixes) and simply mean a singular structure, thing, or unit. Plural endings are used in the same way, except they mean more than one structure, thing, or unit.

TABLE 1.3   FORMING PLURALS OF NOUNS WITH SPECIAL ENDINGS

If the Singular Ending Is	The Plural Ending Is	Examples (Singular)	Examples (Plural)
is	es	diagnosis, prognosis, psychosis	diagnoses, prognoses, psychoses
(Some words ending in *is* form plurals by dropping the *is* and adding *ides*, as in epididymis and epididymides.)			
um	a	atrium, ileum, septum, bacterium	atria, ilea, septa, bacteria
us	i	alveolus, bacillus, bronchus	alveoli, bacilli, bronchi
(Some singular terms ending in *us* form plurals by dropping the *us* and adding either *era* or *ora*, for example, *viscus* and *viscera* and *corpus* and *corpora*. Others form plurals by simply adding *es*, for example, virus becomes *viruses*.)			
a	ae	vertebra, patella, petechia	vertebrae, patellae, petechiae
ix	ices	appendix, varix, cervix	appendices, varices, cervices
(Through common use, appendixes and cervixes have become acceptable plural forms.)			
ex	ices	cortex	cortices
ax	aces	thorax	thoraces (thoraxes is also acceptable)
ma	s or mata	carcinoma, sarcoma	carcinomas or carcinomata, sarcomas or sarcomata
on	a	protozoon, spermatozoon	protozoa, spermatozoa
(Some singular forms ending in *on* form plurals by adding s, for example, chorion becomes *chorions*.)			
nx	nges	phalanx, larynx	phalanges, larynges

CHOOSE IT! **EXERCISE 9**

Circle the correct plural for these singular terms.

1. alveolus (alveoli, alveolus, alveoluses).
2. appendix (appendi, appendices, appendixs)
3. atrium (atria, atrion, atriums)
4. bacillus (bacilla, bacilli, bacilluses)
5. carcinoma (carcinoma, carcinomi, carcinomas)

6. diagnosis (diagnoses, diagnosi, diagnosus)
7. larynx (larynges, laryngi, laryngxes)
8. prognosis (prognoses, prognosi, prognosis)
9. protozoon (protozoa, protozoas, protozoces)
10. varix (varices, varixes, varixs)

QUICK CASE STUDY | EXERCISE 10 →✕← →

After reading part of a health care report, answer questions about the underlined terms.

This 68-year-old woman takes medication for <u>hypertension</u> and has presented at the <u>ED</u> frequently, complaining of <u>cardiac</u> pain, although extensive testing does not indicate heart problems. She is shown how to use a <u>Holter monitor</u> for the next 24 hours and has an appointment to see Dr. Sadighi, <u>OP</u> department, tomorrow.

1. Which word part is "hyper" in hypertension? _____
2. Which word part is "ac" in cardiac? _____
3. Which of the underlined terms is an eponym? _____
4. Which are abbreviations? _____ and _____ .

Pronunciation of Medical Terms

Beginning in Chapter 2, an alphabetical listing near the end of each chapter—the Quick & Easy (Q&E) List—shows the correct spelling of medical terms for each chapter, followed by the phonetic spelling to indicate their pronunciations. The primary accented syllable in a term is indicated by bold type. It is helpful to look at the term while listening to its pronunciation on the Evolve site.

Pronunciation of most medical terms follows the same rules that govern the pronunciation of all English words. Some general rules and examples to assist you in pronunciation are given in the Pronunciation Guide on the included bookmark and inside the back cover.

Remember that there are exceptions to these rules, and certain terms can have more than one acceptable pronunciation. Also, different pronunciations are often used in different parts of the United States, and certain diseases, disorders, and procedures incorporate proper names, which may be exceptions to English pronunciation.

WRITE IT!
EXERCISE 11

Write answers in the blanks.

1. How many syllables does the term ectasis (**ek**-tuh-sis) have? _____

2. Using the pronunciation of ectasis in Question 1, which syllable has a primary accent?

   _____

3. Which syllable has a primary accent in choledochostomy (kō-led-uh-**kos**-tuh-mē)?

   _____

4. How many syllables are in antibacterials (an-tē-bak-**tēr**-ē-ulz)? _____

5. Which syllable has the primary accent in cardiokinetic (kahr-dē-ō-ki-**net**-ik)? _____

Chapter 1 Career Highlight

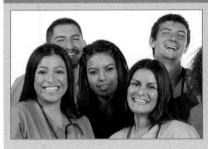

You'll find a career highlight in every chapter, introducing you to professions in which you would use medical terminology. There are so many possibilities! Have you decided on your chosen work? If not, review these highlights and picture yourself in each field. When one appeals to you, go to the website that is listed for more information. You're off to a splendid start!

! Be Careful With These!

- Drop combining vowels if the suffix begins with a vowel (*example:* ot/o + -itis = otitis).
- Singular words that end in *um* or *on* become *a* when plural. However, words that have the plural ending *ae* use *a* for the singular form. Study the medical terms in Table 1.3 until you can tell the difference.

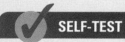

SELF-TEST

Work the following exercises to test your understanding of the material in Chapter 1. It is best to do all the exercises before checking your answers against the answers in Appendix III. Pay particular attention to spelling. If most of your answers are correct, you are ready to move on to Chapter 2.

Don't be concerned about learning the meanings of the word parts for Chapter 1, because all of them are included in subsequent chapters.

A MATCHING! *Choose A, B, or C from the right column to classify the word parts.*

_____ 1. bil/i   _____ 11. -lysis   A. prefix
_____ 2. crani/o   _____ 12. lip/o   B. suffix
_____ 3. -ectomy   _____ 13. -logist   C. combining form
_____ 4. gigant/o   _____ 14. mast/o
_____ 5. -iatrics   _____ 15. -meter
_____ 6. ili/o   _____ 16. noc/i
_____ 7. inter-   _____ 17. ocul/o
_____ 8. intra-   _____ 18. ne/o
_____ 9. -ist   _____ 19. -osis
_____ 10. kerat/o   _____ 20. peri-

B MATCHING! *Select A, B, or C from the right column to classify these descriptions (A and B may be used more than once).*

_____ 1. contains a slash before a vowel when written alone   A. prefix
_____ 2. is attached to the end of a word root to modify its meaning   B. suffix
_____ 3. is followed by a hyphen when written alone   C. combining form
_____ 4. is preceded by a hyphen when written alone
_____ 5. generally requires no change when joined with other word parts

C MATCHING! *Match the examples in the left column with the type of term in the right column.*

_____ 1. CPR   A. abbreviation
_____ 2. D&C   B. eponym
_____ 3. Gram stain
_____ 4. Foley catheter
_____ 5. lig.
_____ 6. PFT
_____ 7. Raynaud disease
_____ 8. stat

D   BUILDING!   *Using the rules you have learned in Chapter 1, combine the words or the word parts to write terms.*

1. hypo- + derm/o + -ic   _____
2. leuk/o + -emia   _____
3. melan/o + -oid   _____
4. my/o + cardi/o + -al   _____
5. thromb/o + -osis   _____
6. dys- + -pnea   _____
7. anti- + serum   _____
8. hyper- + -emia   _____
9. hyper- + -pnea   _____
10. psych/o + -osis   _____

E   WRITING!   *Write the plural of these terms.*

1. appendix (two acceptable plurals)   _____
2. bronchus   _____
3. ileum   _____
4. pharynx   _____
5. prognosis   _____
6. alveolus   _____
7. bacterium   _____
8. psychosis   _____
9. vertebra   _____
10. varix   _____

F   WRITING!   *Write the singular terms for these plurals.*

1. alveoli   _____
2. appendices   _____
3. atria   _____
4. bacilli   _____
5. cortices   _____
6. diagnoses   _____
7. phalanges   _____
8. protozoa   _____
9. septa   _____
10. vertebrae   _____

G   WRITING!   *Using the rules you learned for writing singular and plural forms, find one improper use of either a singular or plural form, underline it, and write the correct term.*

1. Randy's diagnosis differed from Gary's diagnosis; however, their prognosis were the same. _____

2. In looking through the microscope, Charla found 1 erythrocyte, 10 leukocytes, and numerous bacterium per high-power field of vision. _____

3. The anatomy class learned that the right side of the heart has a right atrium and a right ventricle; the left side of the heart has a left atrium and a left ventricle. Therefore, each human heart has two atrium and two ventricles. _____

4. An ejaculation of semen contains many spermatozoa; however, it takes only one spermatozoa to fertilize an ovum. _____

5. The thumb has one fewer phalanx than the other digits, which have three phalanx each. _____

6. Bones of the fingers and toes are called phalanges. There are two phalanx in the thumb; the remaining fingers have three. _____

7. The patella is commonly called the kneecap. Most persons are born with two patella. _____

8. The vertebral column is composed of 33 vertebra. _____

9. Cesarean section is an example of an eponyms. _____

10. Numerous tiny purple or red spots appearing on the skin may be petechae. _____

H   PRONOUNCING!   *Practice saying each of the following terms. Check to see if you are correct by listening to the pronunciations in Q&E glossary of audio files at* http://evolve.elsevier.com/leonard/quick/

1. adenopathy (ad-uh-**nop**-uh-thē)
2. cephalometer (sef-uh-**lom**-uh-tur)
3. cutaneous (kū-**tā**-nē-us)
4. dermal (**dur**-mul)
5. endocardial (en-dō-**kahr**-dē-ul)
6. hematology (hē-muh-**tol**-uh-jē)
7. hypoglossal (hī-pō-**glos**-ul)
8. otoplasty (**ō**-tō-plas-tē)
9. tonsillitis (ton-si-**lī**-tis)

I   QUICK CHALLENGE!   *Find one incorrect term in each sentence and write it correctly.*

1. Alzheimer disease is an example of an acronym, and stat is an abbreviation meaning "at once." _____

2. The chambers of the heart include two ventricles and two atrium. _____

3. Bacteria are classified as cocci, bacillus, spirochetes, and vibrios. _____

4. Mr. Gomez and Mrs. Clark had different diagnosis, but both were referred to the orthopedist. _____

5. A carcinomata is a malignancy that tends to metastasize to other parts of the body. _____

*See **QUICK CONNECT** for a review of what you learned in Chapter 1 on page 16. There is no expectation of remembering the pronunciation of medical terms in this chapter, only the rules for pronunciation.*

*Use Appendix III to check your answers.

Games and activities on the Evolve site (*http://evolve.elsevier.com/Leonard/quick/*) provide a fun way to review, but remember that the quick quizzes do not replace the Self-Test at the end of each chapter.*

- Two games help reassure you that you have learned each chapter's material. Play to "win" a million dollars, or rack up as many points as possible!
- Use the audio glossary of terms from Chapters 2 through 15 to check your pronunciation and spelling. The audio terms correspond to the Quick & Easy (Q&E) lists at the end of each chapter, beginning with Chapter 2. You can listen, speak the terms, and check the pronunciations while reading the written pronunciations from the list. Or listen, write the terms, and then check your spelling against the chapter Q&E list. The more senses you can use, the easier it will be to learn!
- Quizzes that simulate chapter tests help you determine whether you're prepared for the test.
- Health Reports for Chapters 6 through 15 build your confidence for recognizing and understanding terms from actual health care reports. To check your understanding, answer the quick questions with each case study.
- A variety of other activities help you review and learn the material in each chapter.

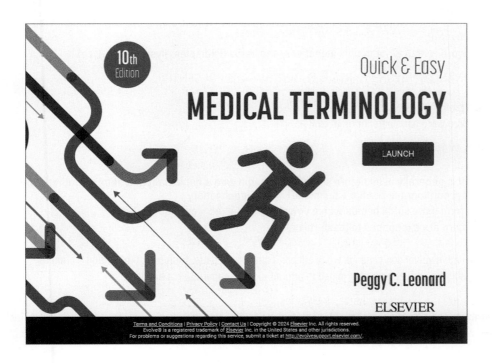

---

*Visit the website *http://evolve.elsevier.com/Leonard/quick/* for additional review activities.

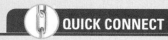

Construction of terms: Most terms consist of word parts.

Greek and Latin are the origin of most medical terms. Word parts are used to form many medical terms pertaining to body systems. Body systems studied include:

Musculoskeletal System   Reproductive System
Circulatory System   Integumentary System
Respiratory System   Nervous System
Digestive System   Special Sense Organs
Urinary System   Endocrine System

WORD PARTS: WORD ROOTS, COMBINING FORMS, PREFIXES, AND SUFFIXES

Medical terms need not be daunting if you learn the meaning of word parts and how a word is constructed. Word roots are the building blocks for most medical terms *(Example: derm and caud)*. A combining vowel (most commonly o) is often inserted between word roots.

Two terms, often derived from Latin and Greek, look different but have the same meaning. For example, *dermal* and *cutaneous* both mean "pertaining to the skin."

General rule for naming and describing:

Body structures (Latin)
Diseases/conditions, diagnosis, and treatment (Greek)

Combining form: word root plus a vowel (Example: tox/o)
Prefix: Modifies the meaning of word/word part (Example: *a*febrile). When written alone, prefixes are followed by a hyphen (Examples: a-, anti-, hypo-).
Suffix: Attached to word or word root to write nouns, adjectives, and verbs (Examples: -lysis, -lytic, -lyze).

BE ABLE TO RECOGNIZE UNKNOWN WORD PARTS BY HOW THEY ARE PRESENTED:

• Are they followed by "/o"?
• How do you differentiate a prefix from a suffix?
• You should recognize the three word parts here (bi/o, -ol, and pro-)

Combining word parts to write terms:

1. Writing with Word Roots:

   • The combining vowel is generally used before suffixes that begin with a consonant and before another word root: cardi/o + -gram = cardiogram; cardi/o + pulmonary = cardiopulmonary
   • Drop the combining form if the suffix begins with a vowel: cardi/o + -ac = cardiac
   • (You will learn that there are exceptions to these rules.)

2. Writing with Prefixes:

   • Many prefixes ending with a vowel don't change when added to other word parts. Examples: pre- + natal = prenatal.
   • There are exceptions, such as end- or endo- are joined to arterial to write endarterial or endoarterial.

Proper names:

Eponyms are names of diseases, organs, procedures, or body functions that are derived from the name of a person and usually capitalized (Holter monitor). An exception: cesarean section (named for Julius Caesar).

Abbreviations:

(Use with caution!) are shortened forms of written words or phrases that are used in place of the whole. Letters, shortened words, and acronyms (pronounceable names).

Plurals

Memorize the rules for forming 10 plural endings in Table 1.3.
   Primary accented syllable is in bold typeface. Example: gastric (*gas*-trik).

Pronunciation of Medical Terms

Primary accented syllable is in bold typeface. Example: gastric (*gas*-trik).

CHAPTER 2

Suffixes and Combining Forms Made Easy

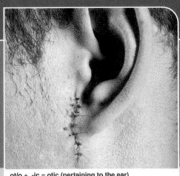

Learning one new word part will often help you write many new words.

ot/o + -ic = otic (pertaining to the ear)
ot/o + -itis = otitis (inflammation of the ear)
ot/o + -logy = otology (study of the ear)
ot/o + -plasty = otoplasty (plastic surgery of the ear)
ot/o + -tomy = ototomy (incision of the ear)

CONTENTS

Using Suffixes to Write Words
Suffixes: Medical Specialties and Specialists
Suffixes: Surgical Procedures
Combining Forms for Selected Body Structures
Suffixes: Symptoms and Diagnosis
Miscellaneous Suffixes
Miscellaneous Word Parts
Abbreviations
Pharmacology

Preparing for a Q&E Test
 Study the Word Parts
 Practice With the Self-Test
 Review With Quick Connect
 Practice With the Q&E List of Terms
✓ **SELF-TEST**
QUICK & EASY (Q&E) LIST
QUICK CONNECT

OBJECTIVES

After completing Chapter 2, you will be able to:

1. Write the meanings of Chapter 2 word parts or match word parts with their meanings.
2. Match medical specialists with the areas in which they specialize.
3. Identify selected medical conditions associated with each specialty.
4. Identify the suffixes for surgical procedures, symptoms, and diagnoses.

5. Identify combining forms for select body structures.
6. Build and analyze medical terms with combining forms and suffixes.
7. Write the correct term when presented with its definition or match terms with their definitions.
8. Spell medical terms correctly.

Using Suffixes to Write Words

The combining of suffixes with other word parts forms nouns, adjectives, and verbs. You learned in Chapter 1 that when a combining form is joined with a suffix that begins with a vowel, the combining vowel is almost always dropped from the combining form (*example:* append/o + -ectomy = appendectomy). To help you easily recognize word parts in new terms, word division (*example:* append+ectomy) will often be used in this text. Dividing words in this manner will help you recognize word parts.

Suffix
-logy

QUICK TIP

Written alone, a suffix follows the hyphen.

BOLD TYPE

Important! **Bold type** indicates that a term is included in the Quick & Easy (Q&E) list near the end of each chapter and is pronounced in the audio glossary on the Evolve site at: http://evolve.else vier.com/Leonard/quick.

Because it is helpful to know the types of words formed by the use of various suffixes, information on word usage is provided. It is logical that a suffix coincides with how its meaning is used in speech. For example, append+ectomy means surgical removal (-ectomy) of the appendix (append/o). **Appendectomy** is a surgical procedure, and thus it is a noun. From this, we see that the suffix -*ectomy* is used to write nouns.

INTERPRETING TERMS

To interpret a new word, begin by looking at its ending (Fig. 2.1). If the ending is a suffix, decide its meaning, then go to the beginning of the word and read from left to right, interpreting the remaining elements to develop the full sense of the term.

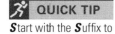

append/o = appendix
-ectomy = surgical removal

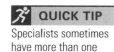
QUICK TIP
*S*tart with the *S*uffix to interpret a term.

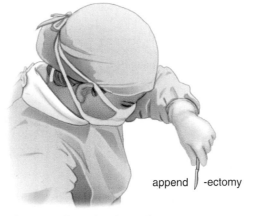

append | -ectomy

Fig. 2.1 Dissect Words Into Component Parts.   Look for a suffix first, then look for other word parts you recognize.

For example, in *appendectomy*, determine the meaning of the suffix -ectomy, then the meaning of the combining form at the beginning of the term, append/o. This method yields surgical removal, appendix. The full meaning of the term is "surgical removal of the appendix."

You will learn many suffixes in this chapter. Although suffixes are emphasized, a limited number of combining forms are also presented. As introduced in Chapter 1, *combining forms* are the foundation of most terms (Fig. 2.2), and learning terms is easier and more interesting than only memorizing suffixes. Also, to make it easier, Chapter 2 suffixes are divided into four categories: (1) suffixes used in naming medical specialties and specialists, (2) suffixes used in surgical procedures, (3) suffixes used in symptoms and diagnosis, and (4) miscellaneous suffixes.

Suffixes: Medical Specialties and Specialists

QUICK TIP
Specialists sometimes have more than one specialty.

This section introduces several combining forms, in addition to a few prefixes and suffixes that are used in naming medical specialties and specialists. Study the following suffixes, think of words that you already know that use these suffixes, and mentally prepare a definition of each term using the meaning. For example, the suffix -er may cause you to think of a "doodler." A shortened definition is "one who doodles." The funnier the association, the more likely you are to remember the meaning of the word part.

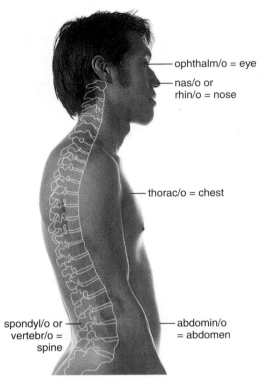

ophthalm/o = eye

nas/o or
rhin/o = nose

thorac/o = chest

spondyl/o or
vertebr/o =
spine

abdomin/o
= abdomen

Fig. 2.2 Combining Forms. You'll learn combining forms for both internal and external structures, the foundations of most terms.

SUFFIXES: MEDICAL SPECIALISTS AND THEIR SPECIALTIES

Suffix	Meaning	Suffix	Meaning
TERMS ABOUT SPECIALISTS		**TERMS ABOUT SPECIALTIES**	
-er, -ist	one who	-ac, -al, -ic, -ical	pertaining to
-iatrician	practitioner	-logic, -logical	pertaining to the study of
-logist	one who studies; specialist	-iatrics, -iatry	medical profession or treatment
		-logy	study or science of

Use the electronic flashcards on the Evolve site or make your own set of flashcards using the above list. Select the word parts just presented and study them until you know their meanings. Do this each time a set of word parts is presented.

MATCH IT!*

EXERCISE 1

Match the suffixes in the left column with their meaning in the right column (a choice may be used more than once).

_____ 1. -ac

_____ 2. -er

_____ 3. -iatrician

_____ 4. -iatry

_____ 5. -ic

_____ 6. -ist

_____ 7. -logist

_____ 8. -logy

A. medical profession or treatment

B. one who

C. one who studies; specialist

D. practitioner

E. pertaining to

F. study or science of

*Use Appendix III, Answers, to check your answers to all the exercises in Chapter 2.

QUICK TIP

Family practice and
family medicine
are often used
interchangeably.

The term *medicine* has several meanings, including "a drug" or "a remedy for illness"; and "the art and science of diagnosis, treatment, and prevention of disease." In addition, it sometimes is used to mean treating disease without surgery. The official symbol of medicine is represented by the caduceus (Fig. 2.3).

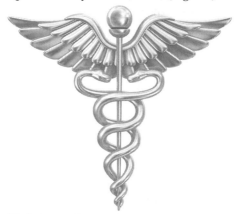

Fig. 2.3 Caduceus. The official symbol of the medical profession.

COMBINING FORMS FOR SELECTED MEDICAL SPECIALTIES

Combining Form	Meaning	Medical Specialty	Medical Specialist
cardi/o	heart	cardiology	cardiologist
crin/o	to secrete	endocrinology	endocrinologist
dermat/o	skin	dermatology	dermatologist
esthesi/o	feeling or sensation	anesthesiology	anesthesiologist
gastr/o, enter/o	stomach, intestines*	gastroenterology	gastroenterologist
ger/a, ger/o, geront/o	elderly	geriatrics	geriatrician
gynec/o	female	gynecology	gynecologist
immun/o	immune	immunology	immunologist
ne/o, nat/o	new, birth	neonatology	neonatologist
neur/o	nerve	neurology	neurologist
obstetr/o	midwife	obstetrics	obstetrician
onc/o	tumor	oncology	oncologist
ophthalm/o	eye	ophthalmology	ophthalmologist
orth/o, ped/o	straight, child[†]	orthopedics	orthopedist, orthopedic surgeon
ot/o, laryng/o	ear, larynx	otolaryngology	otolaryngologist
path/o	disease	pathology	pathologist
ped/o	child[†]	pediatrics	pediatrician
psych/o	mind	psychiatry	psychiatrist
radi/o	radiation (or radius)	radiology	radiologist
rheumat/o	rheumatism	rheumatology	rheumatologist
rhin/o	nose	rhinology	rhinologist
ur/o	urinary tract (or urine)	urology	urologist

Use the electronic flashcards on the Evolve site or make your own set of flashcards using the above list. Select the word parts just presented and study them until you know their meanings.

*enter/o sometimes refers specifically to the small intestine.
[†]ped/o sometimes means "foot."

Family practice is a medical specialty that encompasses several branches of medicine and coordinates health care for all members of a family. A family practice physician often acts as the primary health care provider, referring complex disorders to other specialists. The family practice physician has largely replaced the concept of a general practitioner (GP).

Internal medicine is a nonsurgical specialty of medicine that deals specifically with the diagnosis and treatment of diseases of the internal structures of the body. The specialist is called an **internist**.

-ist = one who
Think of "florist" or "balloonist."

It is important not to confuse *internist* with the term *intern*. An intern in many clinical programs is any immediate postgraduate trainee. A physician intern is in postgraduate training, learning medical practice under supervision before being licensed as a physician. An internist, however, is a licensed medical specialist.

FIND IT! EXERCISE 2

Find the combining form in each of these terms. Write the combining form as well as its meaning.

Term	Combining Form	Meaning
1. cardiology	_____	_____
2. dermatology	_____	_____
3. gynecology	_____	_____
4. immunology	_____	_____
5. neurology	_____	_____
6. oncology	_____	_____
7. ophthalmology	_____	_____
8. pathology	_____	_____
9. psychiatry	_____	_____
10. radiology	_____	_____
11. rhinology	_____	_____
12. urology	_____	_____

WRITE IT! EXERCISE 3

Write the meaning of these combining forms.

1. crin/o	_____	7. nat/o	_____
2. enter/o	_____	8. ne/o	_____
3. esthesi/o	_____	9. obstetr/o	_____
4. gastr/o	_____	10. orth/o	_____
5. ger/o	_____	11. ot/o	_____
6. laryng/o	_____	12. ped/o	_____

Study the following combining forms associated with the medical specialties and also learn the titles of the specialists. Think of people you know who either see or need to see each specialist, and you will remember the terms better.

Combining form **cardi/o**

Now use these combining forms with the suffixes you learned earlier to explore some new medical terms. One of the learning methods you will be using in this book is known as *programmed learning*. Programmed learning begins with what you already know and teaches new concepts by the progressive introduction of new information

PROGRAMMED LEARNING

Write down the answers as you work through the following programmed learning section. Details about how to use programmed learning are presented in the information below.

1. The left column is the answer column, which should be covered. Use the bookmark provided on the side cover or fold a piece of paper lengthwise and position it so that it covers only the answer column.

   In programmed learning, each block of information preceded by a number is called a *frame.* This is the first frame of this chapter. Within most frames, there will be a blank in which to write an answer. After writing your answer in the blank, check to see if it is correct by sliding the bookmark down so that the answer column is uncovered.

   By the information presented here, you know that the answer is located in the **left** _____ column of each frame. (Write an answer in the blank.)

2. You are using the programmed learning method. A block of information with a number is called a **frame** _____. Whenever you see frames, you will recognize that you are learning by the programmed method.

   Always check your answer immediately. If your answer is incorrect, look back at previous frames to determine where you went wrong. You are now ready to put this information to use.

3. You may already know some of the terms that are associated with the medical specialties. If you do not recognize the combining forms used in the following frames, look back at the listing that you just studied. For example, the study of the heart and its function is **cardio+logy**. A physician who specializes in diseases of the heart is a **cardiologist** _____ (Fig. 2.4).

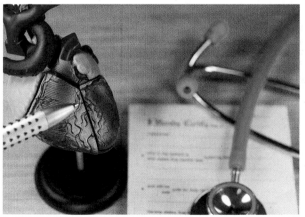

Fig. 2.4 Cardiologists often use models of the heart to explain heart disorders.
cardi/o = heart;   **-logist** = specialist

skin

4. A person with acne problems or skin allergies would be treated by a **dermatologist**. **Dermatology** is the medical specialty concerned with the diagnosis and treatment of diseases of the _____.

gynecologist

5. **Gyneco+logy** (GYN, Gyn, gyn) is devoted to treating diseases of the female reproductive organs, including the breasts. A physician who specializes in the treatment of females is a _____.

midwife

6. Many gynecologists also specialize in obstetrics. **Obstetrics** (OB) deals with pregnancy, labor, delivery, and immediate care after childbirth; however, obstetr/o means _____. Midwives assisted women during childbirth before obstetrics developed as a medical specialty. Physicians who specialize in obstetrics are **obstetricians**.

neonatologist

7. **Neo+nato+logy** is the branch of medicine that specializes in the care of newborns, infants from birth to 28 days of age. A physician who specializes in neonatology is a _____. Newborn infants, commonly called newborns, are generally assessed and cared for in the neonatal unit in the hospital when they are not with their mothers (Fig. 2.5).

practitioner

8. **Ped+iatrics** is devoted to the treatment of children. Diseases of children are often quite different from diseases encountered later in life. The combining form for child is ped/o. The suffix -iatrician, which means _____, is used to write the name of the physician who specializes in pediatrics. A **pediatrician** specializes in the development and care of infants and children and in the treatment of their diseases (Fig. 2.6).

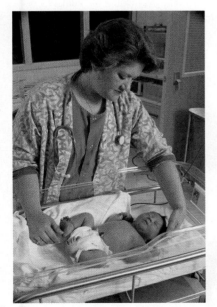

Fig. 2.5 Nurse Caring for a Newborn in the Neonatal Unit.
ne/o = new;   **nat/o** = birth

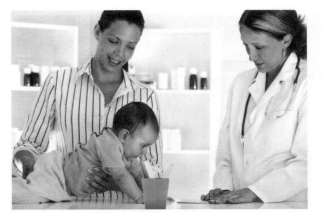

Fig. 2.6 Pediatrician With Young Child. Skill levels and much information is gained while watching and talking to a child.
ped/o = child;   **-iatrician** = practitioner

ophthalmologist	9. **Ophthalmo+logy** is the branch of medicine that specializes in the study, diagnosis, and treatment of disorders of the eye. Write the name of the specialist in ophthalmology by combining ophthalm/o and -logist: _____ (Fig. 2.7).
otolaryngology	10. An **oto+logist** specializes in **otology**, the study of the ear, including the diagnosis and treatment of its diseases and disorders. Physicians who specialize in ear, nose, and throat disorders are ear, nose, and throat (ENT) specialists. The combining form ot/o means ear, and laryng/o means larynx (voice box). **Oto+laryngo+logy** refers to the branch of medicine dealing with diseases and disorders of the ears, nose, throat, and nearby structures (Fig. 2.8). An **otolaryngologist** is a physician who practices _____.
rhinologist	11. **Rhino+logy** specializes in the diagnosis and treatment of disorders involving the nose. Write the name of the physician who specializes in rhinology: _____.
urologist	12. The combining form ur/o means urine or urinary tract. Urology is concerned with the urinary tract in both genders, as well as the male reproductive system. A specialist in **urology** is a _____.
neurology	13. A **neuro+logist** is a physician who specializes in _____, the field of medicine that deals with the nervous system and its disorders. In many words, neur/o refers to the nervous system, which comprises the brain, spinal cord, and nerves.
rheumatologist	14. **Rheumato+logy** is the branch of medicine that deals with rheumatic disorders. A specialist in rheumatology is a _____. Almost all words that contain the combining form rheumat/o pertain to **rheumatism**. Rather than just one disease, rheumatism is any of a variety of disorders marked by inflammation, degeneration, and other problems of the connective tissues, especially the joints and related structures.

WORD ORIGIN
rheum (G.), flow

Ancient Greeks believed that health was determined by the mixture of "humors," or certain fluids within the body. Rheumatism was thought to be caused by a flowing of humors in the body and was thus named.

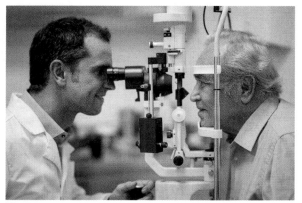

Fig. 2.7 Ophthalmologist. A senior patient should visit an ophthalmologist at least once a year.
ophthalm/o = eye;   **-logist** = specialist

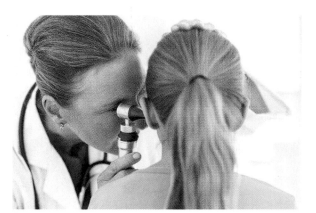

Fig. 2.8 An otolaryngologist specializes in ear, nose, and throat disorders.
ot/o = ear;   **laryng/o** = larynx;   **-logy** = science of

15. **Immuno+logy** represents one of the most rapidly expanding areas of science, and immun/o is the combining form for immune. This branch of medicine involves assessment of the patient's immune defense mechanism against disease. The immune mechanism includes the natural defenses that protect the body from diseases and cancer, but it is also involved in allergies, excessive reactions to common and often harmless substances in the environment.

immunologist
   The immunology specialist is an _____. In some cases, immunology is combined with the identification and treatment of allergies.

16. The **endocrine** glands secrete chemical messengers called hormones into the bloodstream. These hormones play an important role in regulating the body's metabolism. The prefix endo- means "inside." The suffix -crine, from the combining form crin/o, means "to secrete." Glands that secrete hormones into the bloodstream are endocrine glands.

endocrinologist
   The science of the endocrine glands and the hormones they produce is **endocrinology**. A specialist in endocrinology is an _____.

17. The combining form radi/o means radiation (sometimes radi/o is used to mean radius, a bone of the forearm, but usually it refers to radiation). **Radio+logy** is the use of various forms of radiation (e.g., x-rays) in the diagnosis and treatment of disease. The physician who specializes in radiology is a diagnostic imaging specialist, called a

radiologist
   _____.

18. **Onco+logy**, a rapidly changing specialty, involves the study of malignancy. The combining form onc/o means "tumor." Oncology is particularly concerned with malignant tumors and their treatment. **Malignant** means "tending to become worse, spread, and cause death." *Cancer* refers to any of a large group of diseases that are characterized by the presence of malignant cells.

oncologist
   A specialist who practices oncology is an _____
   A **radiation oncologist** has special training in the use of radiation to treat cancer.

19. The word *tumor* is used in different ways. It sometimes means a swelling or enlargement, but it often refers to a spontaneous new growth of tissue that forms an abnormal mass. This latter definition is also called a **neoplasm**. A **benign** tumor is not cancerous, so it does not spread to other parts of the body. Benign is the opposite of malignant (Fig. 2.9). Write the term you just

neoplasm
   learned that means a spontaneous new growth of tissue: _____.

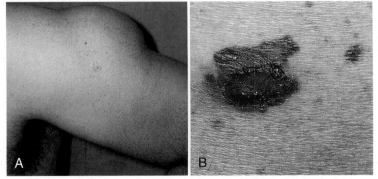

Fig. 2.9 Two Types of Tumors. **A,** A benign tumor, a lipoma, which consists of mature fat cells. **B,** Malignant melanoma, a type of skin cancer. Benign and malignant tumors have different characteristics; however, definitive diagnosis is possible by microscopic study of the cells of a suspicious tumor. **melan/o** = black; **-oma** = tumor

gastroenterology

20. **Gastro+entero+logy** is the study of diseases affecting the gastrointestinal tract, including the stomach and intestines. Write the name of this specialty that deals with the stomach and intestines: _____. A physician who specializes in gastric and intestinal disorders is a **gastroenterologist**.

geriatrician

21. Three combining forms—ger/a, ger/o, and geront/o—mean "old age" or "the aged." The scientific study of all aspects of the aging process and issues encountered by older persons is **gerontology**. The branch of medicine that deals with the problems of aging and the diseases of elderly persons is **geriatrics**. A physician who specializes in gerontology is a _____.

    The selection of the correct combining form may be confusing. Common usage determines which term is proper. Practice will help you remember.

BUILD IT!

EXERCISE 4

Write terms using these words parts.

1. ne/o + nat/o + -logy   _____
2. ot/o + laryng/o + -logy   _____
3. rheumat/o + -logist   _____
4. endo- + -crine   _____
5. onc/o + -logist   _____
6. gastr/o + enter/o + -logist _____

FIND IT!

EXERCISE 5

Draw a slash before the suffixes in the following list of new adjectives (descriptive terms). Then, find the meanings of the word parts within the definition. Think! Draw the slash, then perform the remainder of the activity as a mental exercise. This is one way to begin recognizing unfamiliar words. When you are working in your chosen profession, you may need to use a medical dictionary to know the full meaning of a term.

Term	Definition
1. **cardiac**	pertaining to the heart
2. **dermal**	pertaining to the skin
3. **dermatologic, dermatological**	pertaining to the skin or dermatology
4. **gastric**	pertaining to the stomach
5. **gynecologic, gynecological**	pertaining to the female reproductive tract or to gynecology
6. **neurologic, neurological**	pertaining to neurology or the nervous system
7. **obstetric, obstetrical**	pertaining to obstetrics
8. **ophthalmic, ophthalmologic, ophthalmological**	pertaining to the eye or ophthalmology
9. **otic**	pertaining to the ear
10. **pediatric**	pertaining to pediatrics or the health of children
11. **radiologic, radiological**	pertaining to radiation or radiology
12. **urologic, urological, urinary**	pertaining to urology, or sometimes, urine

or ideas. In some ways, it is similar to using a computer program because it tells you immediately if you are right. The primary difference is that here you write your answers in the blanks provided. It is a proven and easy way to learn medical terminology.

Pathology is the general study of the characteristics, causes, and effects of disease. *Cellular* pathology is the study of cellular changes in disease. *Clinical* pathology is the study of disease by the use of laboratory tests and methods. A medical **pathologist** usually specializes in either *clinical* or *surgical* pathology. A clinical pathologist is especially concerned with the use of laboratory methods in clinical diagnosis.

Tissues and organs that are removed in surgery are sent to the surgical pathology laboratory. The physician who studies those tissues and organs to determine the cause of disease is a surgical pathologist. Sometimes during a surgery, the surgical pathologist performs a frozen section method to determine how the operation should be modified or completed.

The terms **pathologic** and **pathological** mean "morbid" (diseased or unwholesome) or "pertaining to a condition that is caused by or that involves a disease process."

The term *surgery* is derived from a Greek word that means "handwork." Surgery includes several branches of medicine that treat disease, injuries, and deformities by manual or operative procedures. Surgery also refers to the work performed by a surgeon or the place where surgery is performed. Small surgical incisions through the skin and the use of scopes to access various body cavities provide a faster, less painful recovery with fewer visible scars.

A **neurosurgeon** specializes in surgery of the nervous system. Neurosurgery is surgery involving the brain, spinal cord, or peripheral nerves. General surgery deals with all types of surgical procedures. **Plastic surgery** is the surgical repair or reconstruction of the body; it may be essential to restore the structure or its function, or it may be an **elective procedure** (one that is performed by choice and is not essential, such as a face lift to remove wrinkles). There are many other surgical specialties, such as those dealing exclusively with the head and neck, hand, and urinary system.

The use of surgical robotics has gained increasing popularity (Fig. 2.10). Robotic surgery offers the advantages of minimally invasive surgery, decreased blood loss, faster recovery, less pain after surgery, and shorter hospital stays. In addition to robotics, the use of scopes enables access to various body cavities, also providing a faster, less painful recovery with fewer visible scars.

> **QUICK TIP**
> Programmed learning is great for learning at your own speed.
>
> **path/o** = disease

> **QUICK TIP**
> A surgical procedure may be called a surgery, or (in lay terms) an operation.
>
> **neur/o** = nerve

> **QUICK TIP**
> The first robotic surgery in the United States was performed in 1997.

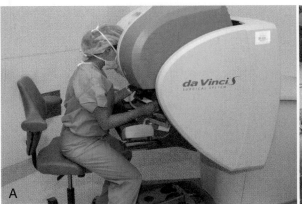
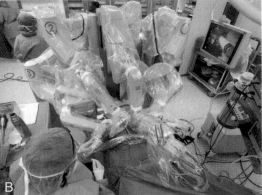

Fig. 2.10 Robotic Surgery. **A,** Surgeon seated at the surgical console. **B,** The surgical tower around the patient (view from the ceiling).

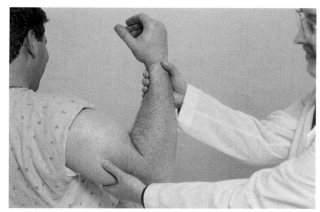

Fig. 2.11 Orthopedist Examining a Patient. Orthopedics is a branch of medicine that specializes in the prevention and correction of disorders of the muscular and skeletal systems of the body. **orth/o** = straight;   **ped/o** = child

orth/o = straight
ped/o = child

Ortho+ped+ics is a branch of surgery that deals with the preservation and restoration of the bones and associated structures. The specialist is called an **ortho+ped+ist**, or orthopedic surgeon (Fig. 2.11). The orthopedist originally straightened children's bones and corrected deformities. Today an orthopedist specializes in disorders of the bones and associated structures in people of all ages.

psych/o = mind

Psych+iatry is a medical specialty that deals with the causes, treatment, and prevention of mental, emotional, and behavioral disorders. A physician who specializes in psychiatry is a **psychiatrist**. Clinical psycho+logy is concerned with the diagnosis, treatment, and prevention of a wide range of personality and behavioral disorders. A person who is trained in this area is a clinical psychologist.

PSYCHIATRY IS DIFFERENT FROM *PSYCHOLOGY*

Clinical psychology is not a branch of medicine but a branch of psychology.

Physicians who specialize in the care of patients in intensive care are **intensivists**. The intensive care unit (ICU) is a place in the hospital that contains sophisticated monitoring devices and equipment for patients requiring close monitoring and care by specially trained personnel.

There are many other areas in which physicians specialize. Emergency medicine deals with very ill or injured patients who require immediate medical treatment. The emergency department is commonly called the "ER" (emergency room), but emergency department (ED) is the more accurate term. On arrival, patients are often prioritized according to their need for treatment. The method of sorting according to the patients' need for care is called **triage**.

Hospital+ists are physicians who specialize in the care of patients staying in the hospital. Hospitalists sometimes make rounds for physicians who are on vacation or choose to stay in their offices seeing patients.

An+esthesio+logy is the branch of medicine concerned with the administration of anesthetics and their effects. The physician who administers anesthetics during surgery is an **anesthesiologist**. The prefix *an-* means no, not, or without. Although the literal interpretation of anesthesiology is "the study of no feeling," you need to remember that it is the branch of medicine concerned with the administration of drugs that produce a loss of feeling.

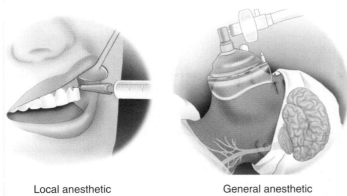

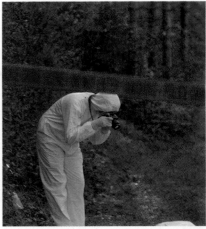

Local anesthetic   General anesthetic

Fig. 2.12 Local Versus General Anesthetic. Local anesthetics eliminate sensation in a defined area of the body. General anesthetics are inhaled or are given by intravenous injection and act on the brain, causing absence of sensation and consciousness.

an- = no, not, or without;   **esthesi/o** = feeling

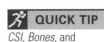

Fig. 2.13 Forensic Medicine. A forensic pathologist may examine, photograph, and collect specimens from a crime scene.

An **an+esthetist** is not a physician but is trained in administering anesthetics. An **anesthetic** is a drug or agent that is capable of producing an+esthes+ia, or loss of sensation or feeling. Anesthetic also means pertaining to anesthesia.

Anesthetics are classified as local or general according to their action. *Local* anesthetics affect a small area only, rather than the entire body, for brief surgical or dental procedures. *General* anesthetics act on the brain and cause loss of consciousness (Fig. 2.12). For another type of anesthesia, regional anesthesia, a local anesthetic is used to block a group of nerve fibers that detect sensations. For example, in epidural anesthesia, an anesthetic is injected into the epidural space surrounding the spinal cord to block pain in the legs or the abdomen during labor and childbirth.

Some people mistakenly associate anesthesia with normal sleep. A sleeping person can be awakened and normal awareness immediately restored, unlike someone who has been given a general anesthetic.

Preventive medicine is the branch of medicine involving the prevention of disease and also methods for increasing the abilities of the patient and community to resist disease and prolong life. A physician or scientist who studies the incidence, prevalence, spread, prevention, and control of disease in a community or a specific group of individuals is an **epidemiologist**. An epidemic attacks several people in a region at the same time. In a hospital, physicians who specialize in **epidemiology** may have the responsibility of directing infection control programs.

Some physicians specialize in sports medicine, which involves the prevention, diagnosis, and treatment of sports-related injuries. Physicians are often assisted by a **therapist**, a person with special skills who is trained in one or more areas of health care.

A specialist in **forensic medicine** deals with the legal aspects of health care (Fig. 2.13).

Aerospace medicine is concerned with the effects of living and working in an artificial environment beyond the Earth's atmosphere and the forces of gravity.

QUICK TIP

CSI, Bones, and similar TV series have familiarized people with forensic science.

Work the following reviews to test your understanding of the medical specialists.

MATCH IT!

EXERCISE 6

Match the medical specialists with the areas in which they specialize.

_____ 1. anesthesiologist
_____ 2. dermatologist
_____ 3. geriatrician
_____ 4. gynecologist
_____ 5. neonatologist
_____ 6. neurologist
_____ 7. oncologist
_____ 8. otolaryngologist
_____ 9. pathologist
_____ 10. pediatrician

A. children
B. disease in general
C. ear, nose, and throat
D. feeling or sensation
E. females
F. nervous system
G. newborns
H. older persons
I. skin
J. tumors

WRITE IT!

EXERCISE 7

Write the specialty associated with these conditions or situations.

1. heart attack _____
2. interpreting a radiograph _____
3. deficiency of the immune system _____
4. hormonal deficiency _____
5. nosebleed _____
6. miscarriage _____
7. irritable bowel disease _____
8. urinary infection _____
9. broken wrist _____
10. rheumatoid arthritis _____

Suffix
-pexy

Suffixes: Surgical Procedures

A list of suffixes pertaining to surgical procedures follows. Commit the meanings of these suffixes to memory. It is necessary to take some time now to memorize the suffixes and their meanings; this can be done in several ways. One way is to read each suffix, its meaning, and its *word association* (a familiar word associated with the suffix). Also, think of words you may know that can help you to remember the meaning. After you have studied the list for a few minutes and think you know it, use flashcards, or cover the column that contains the meanings and word associations and then check to make sure that you know each meaning.

All the suffixes in the following list form nouns when combined with other word parts.

SUFFIXES: SURGICAL PROCEDURES

Suffix	Meaning	Word Association
-centesis	surgical puncture to aspirate or remove fluid	**Amniocentesis** is puncture of the amnion for removing fluid for study or administering treatment to the fetus (Fig. 2.14).
-ectomy	excision (surgical removal or cutting out)	Appendectomy is **excision** of the appendix.
-lysis	process of loosening, freeing, or destroying	This suffix is also used in nonsurgical words to mean destruction or dissolving, as in **hemolysis**.
-pexy	surgical fixation (fastening in a fixed position)	**Mastopexy** is plastic surgery that fastens breasts in a fixed position to correct sagging.
-plasty	surgical repair	Plastic is derived from the same word root as -plasty. Plastic surgery repairs, restores, and reconstructs body structures. **Mammoplasty** is plastic surgery of the breast and is done for a variety of reasons.
-rrhaphy	suture (uniting a wound by stitches)	This suffix is not generally used in everyday language, but **angiorrhaphy** means **suture** of a blood vessel.
-scopy	visual examination with a lighted instrument (not always a surgical procedure)	**Microscopy** is visual examination of very small objects with a magnifying instrument (**microscope**) (Fig. 2.15). The suffix -scope means the instrument. Micro- means small.
-stomy	formation of an opening	A **tracheostomy** is a surgical procedure that forms a new opening into the trachea (windpipe).
-tome	an instrument used for cutting	A **microtome** is an instrument used for cutting thin sections of tissue for microscopic study.
-tomy	incision (cutting into tissue)	A **tracheotomy** is an **incision** of the trachea through the skin and muscles in the neck that overlie the **trachea** (windpipe).
-tripsy	surgical crushing	**Lithotripsy** is surgical crushing of a calculus (stone) (Fig. 2.16).

Use the electronic flashcards on the Evolve site or make your own set of flashcards using the above list. Study the word parts until you know their meanings.

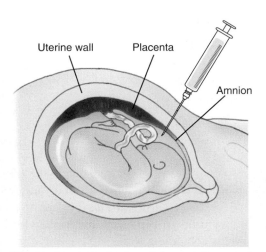

Fig. 2.14 Amniocentesis. Puncture of the amniotic sac is done to remove fluid for study of the fetal cells.
amni/o = amnion; **-centesis** = surgical puncture;
fet/o = fetus; **uter/o** = uterus

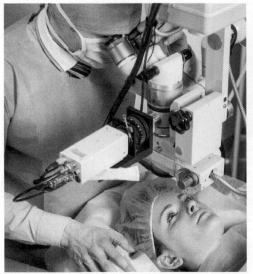

Fig. 2.15 Surgeon using a video microscope for eye surgery.
micro- = small; **-scope** = instrument for viewing

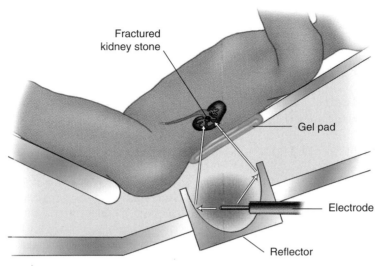

Fig. 2.16 Lithotripsy: Crushing of a Stone (Calculus). Extracorporeal shock wave lithotripsy, shown here, is used to crush certain urinary tract stones. Extracorporeal means outside the body. The reflector focuses a high-energy shock wave on the stone. The stone disintegrates into particles and is passed in the urine. Originally, lithotripsy referred only to the surgical technique of crushing the stone with an instrument.
lith/o = stone (calculus);   **-tripsy** = surgical crushing;   **extra-** = outside;   **corpor/o** = body

MATCH IT!   **EXERCISE 8**

Match the suffixes in the right column with their meanings in the left column.

_____ 1. instrument used for cutting	A. -centesis
_____ 2. instrument used for viewing	B. -ectomy
_____ 3. excision	C. -lysis
_____ 4. formation of an opening	D. -pexy
_____ 5. incision	E. -plasty
_____ 6. process of destroying	F. -rrhaphy
_____ 7. surgical crushing*	G. -scope
_____ 8. surgical fixation	H. -scopy
_____ 9. surgical puncture	I. -stomy
_____ 10. surgical repair	J. -tome
_____ 11. suture	K. -tomy
_____ 12. visual examination with an instrument	L. -tripsy

*Specifically means crushing and not "destruction by other means."

Combining
form
chir/o

Combining Forms for Selected Body Structures

You already know combining forms for several body structures used earlier to name the medical specialists. Additional combining forms are presented in the following list. This list is not intended to be complete. Many combining forms are presented in later chapters, which discuss major body systems. You should commit the following list to memory because subsequent chapters assume that you have learned these combining forms. Practice learning the material here in the same manner as you learned the list of suffixes pertaining to surgical procedures.

Read the term, its meaning, and its word association. When you think you know the material, use flashcards, or cover the two columns on the right and try to recall the meaning of each combining form. These combining forms will be used shortly to study medical terminology in more detail and to learn how to build words. Read on!

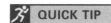

QUICK TIP

Chapters 3 to 5 assume that you learned the combining forms in this chapter. Later chapters build on these word parts.

COMBINING FORMS FOR SELECTED BODY STRUCTURE

Combining Form	Meaning	Word Association
aden/o	gland	**Adenoids** were so named because they resembled or were thought to be glands.
angi/o	vessel	An **angiogram** is an x-ray film of blood vessels filled with a contrast medium.
append/o, appendic/o	appendix	An **appendectomy** is excision of the appendix.
bi/o	life or living	**Biology** is the science of life and living things.
blephar/o	eyelid	**Blepharoptosis** is the drooping of the upper eyelid.
cerebr/o,* encephal/o	brain	**Cerebral** palsy is paralysis caused by a brain defect. **Encephalitis** is inflammation of the brain.
chir/o	hand	Writer's cramp is a type of **chirospasm**.
col/o	colon or large intestine	Coloscopy is visual examination of the colon, but the term **colonoscopy** is more commonly used.
cutane/o, derm/a, dermat/o	skin	**Cutaneous** means pertaining to the skin. A dermatologist is a specialist who treats diseases of the skin. Dermabrasion removes small scars, tattoos, or fine wrinkles from the skin.
faci/o	face	**Facial** pertains to the face.
hepat/o	liver	**Hepatitis** is an inflammatory condition of the liver.
mamm/o, mast/o	breast	**Mammography** is the use of x-rays to diagnose breast diseases. Mastectomy is surgical removal of the breast.
muscul/o, my/o	muscle	A person with well-developed muscles is **muscular**. **Myalgia** is muscle pain.
myel/o	bone marrow or spinal cord	**Myelopathy** has two meanings: any disease of the spinal cord, or any disease of the bone marrow.
oste/o	bone	**Osteoarthritis** is a common type of arthritis of older adults in which one or more joints undergo degenerative changes; it is named to include both bones and joints.
pulm/o, pulmon/o, pneum/o,† pneumon/o	lungs	**Pulmonary** means pertaining to the lungs. **Pneumatic** means pertaining to air or gas. **Pneumonia** is a lung condition.
tonsill/o	tonsil	**Tonsillitis** is inflammation of the tonsils.
trache/o	trachea (windpipe)	A tracheostomy is an operation that forms a new opening into the trachea.
vas/o	vessel; **ductus deferens**‡	**Vasectomy** is the removal of all or a segment of the vas deferens; it is a form of male sterilization.

Use the electronic flashcards on the Evolve site or make your own using the above list. Select the word parts just presented, and study them until you know their meanings.

cerebr/o sometimes means **cerebrum, the main portion of the brain.*
†pneum/o sometimes means "air" or "gas."
‡Also called the vas deferens, the excretory duct of the testicle.

CHOOSE IT!

EXERCISE 9

Circle the correct answer.

1. Which combining form means vessel? (aden/o, angi/o, chir/o, faci/o)
2. Which combining form means bone? (bi/o, blephar/o, myel/o, oste/o)
3. Which combining form means brain? (cutane/o, encephal/o, faci/o, vas/o)
4. Which combining form means breast? (cerebr/o, mast/o, pneumon/o, pulm/o)
5. Which combining form means skin? (derm/a, hepat/o, mamm/o, my/o)

FIND IT!

EXERCISE 10

Write the meanings of the suffixes in these new nouns. (Question 1 is done as an example.) A short definition is provided for each term.

Term/Meaning	Suffix
1. **colopexy** surgical fixation of the colon to the abdominal wall	-pexy, surgical fixation
2. **adenectomy** excision of a gland	
3. **colostomy** opening of some portion of the large intestine onto the abdominal surface	
4. **coloscopy** visual examination of the colon with a lighted instrument	
5. **hepatologist** a physician who specializes in liver diseases	
6. **mastectomy** removal of one or both breasts	
7. **mastopexy** surgical fixation of the breasts	
8. **neurectomy** partial or total excision of a nerve (partial or total is implied)	
9. **neurolysis** destruction of nerve tissue or loosening of adhesions surrounding a nerve	
10. **neuroplasty** surgical repair of a nerve or nerves	

---

col/o = colon
-stomy = formation of an opening
-pexy = surgical fixation

A colostomy is an opening of some portion of the large intestine onto the abdominal surface. This type of surgery is performed when solid waste (feces) cannot be eliminated through the normal opening because of some pathologic condition.

Colopexy is a surgical procedure in which the colon is sutured (surgically fixed, sewn, or otherwise attached) to the abdominal wall. The term *suture* has several meanings: the act of uniting a wound by stitches, the material used in closing a wound with stitches, or the stitch made to secure the edges of a wound. (If you study anatomy, you will learn that *suture* also refers to a type of joint in which the opposed surfaces are closely united, as in the skull.)

mast/o = breast
-ectomy = excision

Mastectomy may be performed when cancer of the breast is present. A breast biopsy is often done when a suspicious lump is found in the breast. A **biopsy** is excision of a small lump for microscopic examination, usually performed to establish a diagnosis (bi/o means life or living). The biopsy can be performed with a needle (needle biopsy) or by excision of the suspicious lump (**lumpectomy**).

mamm/o = breast
-plasty = surgical repair

Mammoplasty is plastic surgery of the breast and is done for a variety of reasons. Reduction mammoplasty is done to reduce the size of the breasts, whereas **augmentation mammoplasty** increases the size of the breasts (Fig. 2.17).

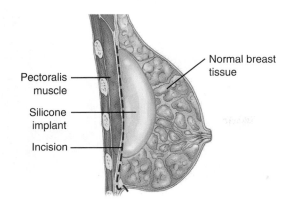

Pectoralis muscle

Normal breast tissue

Silicone implant

Incision

Fig. 2.17 Augmentation Mammoplasty. This surgical procedure to enlarge the breasts is achieved by inserting envelopes filled with silicone gel (shown here) or saline beneath normal breast tissue or beneath the muscle of the chest. The incision below the breast causes the least obvious scarring of several approaches that may be taken.

mamm/o = breast; **-plasty** = surgical repair

MATCH IT!
EXERCISE 11

Match the terms (1 to 6) with the correct specialists (A to L). Not all answers will be used.

_____ 1. amniocentesis
_____ 2. colonoscopy
_____ 3. eye infection
_____ 4. premature infant
_____ 5. skin biopsy
_____ 6. radiation of a neoplasm

A. cardiologist
B. dermatologist
C. endocrinologist
D. gastroenterologist
E. geriatrician
F. gynecologist

G. neonatologist
H. obstetrician
I. oncologist
J. ophthalmologist
K. otolaryngologist
L. pathologist

QUICK CASE STUDY | EXERCISE 12

Lily's gynecologist referred her to an obstetrician, who performed amniocentesis using a local anesthetic and ultrasound imaging. Define the following terms:

1. amniocentesis _____
2. anesthetic _____
3. gynecologist _____
4. obstetrician _____

PROGRAMMED LEARNING

Remember to cover the answers (left column) with folded paper or the bookmark. Write an answer in each blank, and then check your answer before proceeding to the next frame.

hepatic	1. Use -ic to write a word that means pertaining to the liver: _____.
my/o	2. Muscular means pertaining to muscle or describes someone with well-developed muscles. You also need to remember another combining form for muscle, which is _____.
myel/o	3. A combining form that means either bone marrow or the spinal cord is _____.
pneumectomy	4. Pulm/o, pulmon/o, and pneum/o mean lungs. Combine pneum/o and -ectomy to write a term that means excision of a lung:_____. See how easy it is to learn new words using the programmed method! You are already writing impressive medical terms.

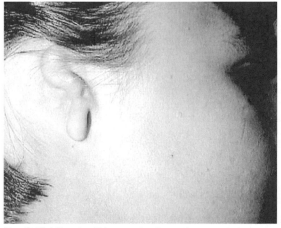

Fig. 2.18 Microtia. This example shows the unusual shape that resulted from underdevelopment of the external ear.
micro- = small; **ot/o** = ear

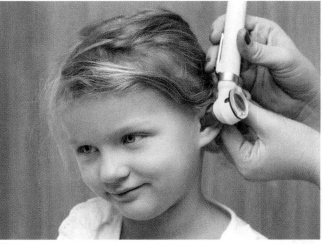

Fig. 2.19 Otoscopy. An otoscope is used to visually examine the eardrum.
ot/o = ear; **-scope** = instrument used for viewing; **-scopy** = visual examination

otoplasty	5. Surgical repair of the eye is **ophthalmoplasty**. Surgical repair of the ear is _____. (See Fig. 2.18 for an abnormality of the ear [**microtia**] that indicates a need for otoplasty.) Did you remember to check your answer immediately? Always be certain that you have spelled the word correctly.
	6. In addition to writing medical terms, you will learn how to divide words into their component parts and to analyze their meanings. Plus signs are used to show the component parts of a word, for example, oto+plasty. Observe that ot/o (ear) is joined to -plasty, the suffix you learned that means surgical repair. When analyzing difficult terms, look for familiar word parts. Divide **ophthalmoscopy** into its component parts:
ophthalmo+scopy	_____.
otoscopy	7. You learned that -scopy means visual examination. Ophthalmoscopy means examination of the eye. Visual examination of the ear is _____. These examinations are often called **otoscopic** and **ophthalmoscopic** examinations. (The person in Fig. 2.19 is undergoing otoscopy with an **otoscope**.) The instrument used in ophthalmoscopy is an **ophthalmoscope**.
skin	8. Cutane+ous means pertaining to the _____.
pertaining	9. In the previous frame, -ous is a suffix that means _____ to. (It can also mean "characterized by.")
skin	10. **Dermato+plasty** is surgical repair of the _____. This is skin grafting or transplantation of living skin to cover defects caused by injury, surgery, or disease.

dermatome	11. Use derm/a to write a term that means "an instrument used to incise the skin": _____.*
encephalotome	12. Use encephal/o to write a word that means an instrument for incising brain tissue: _____.
cerebrotomy	13. Two words that mean incision of the brain are **encephalotomy** and _____.
ophthalmoplasty	14. Surgical repair of the eye is _____.
angioplasty	15. Use angi/o to write a word that means surgical repair of vessels (blood vessels, in this case): _____.
angiorrhaphy	16. Use angio+plasty as a model to write a word that means suture of a vessel (especially a blood vessel): _____.
angiectomy	17. Use the last word you wrote as a model to form a word that means excision or cutting out of a blood vessel: _____.
appendectomy	18. Use append/o to write a word that means removal of the appendix: _____.
tonsillectomy	19. Write a word that means excision of the tonsils: _____.
puncture	20. The **amnion** is the thin transparent membrane that surrounds the fetus (unborn child). Amnio+centesis is surgical _____ of the amnion.

*Most anatomy books give a different meaning for *dermatome*. For terminology purposes, just be aware that *dermatome* has a second meaning.

WRITE IT! EXERCISE 13

Use -plasty to write terms for these meanings.
1. surgical repair of a vessel   _____
2. surgical repair of the breast   _____
3. surgical repair of the ear   _____
4. surgical repair of the eye   _____
5. surgical repair of the skin   _____

BUILD IT! EXERCISE 14

Combine the word parts to write terms.
1. excision of the appendix: append/o + -ectomy   _____
2. instrument for incising brain tissue: encephal/o + -tome   _____
3. instrument for viewing the eye: ophthalm/o + -scope   _____
4. pertaining to the ear: ot/o + -ic   _____
5. removal of the tonsils: tonsill/o + -ectomy   _____
6. surgical fixation of the colon: col/o + -pexy   _____
7. suture of a vessel: angi/o + -rrhaphy   _____
8. visual examination of the ear: ot/o + -scopy   _____

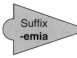

Suffixes: Symptoms and Diagnosis

Symptoms and *diagnosis* are frequently used terms, but they are sometimes used inaccurately. You will study both terms more in depth in Chapter 4. A *symptom* is a health change as perceived by the patient (example: "I don't feel well."), and *diagnosis* is the identification of a disease or condition by scientific evaluation. Several important suffixes pertain to symptoms and diagnosis.

Commit the following suffixes and their meanings to memory. Remember to read each suffix, its meaning, and the word association presented (most form nouns, but exceptions are noted.) Practice looking for the suffix in a term (Fig. 2.20). Be certain that you are familiar with this information before proceeding to Exercises 15 and 16.

SUFFIXES: SYMPTOMS OR DIAGNOSIS

Suffix	Meaning	Word Association
-algia, -dynia	pain	**Neuralgia** is pain along the course of a nerve. Both **otodynia** and **otalgia** mean pain in the ear.
-cele	**hernia** (protrusion of all or part of an organ through a wall of the cavity that contains it. See Fig. 5.19).	An **encephalocele** is a hernia of the brain through an opening in the skull.
-ectasia, -ectasis	**dilatation** (dilation, enlargement or stretching of a structure or part)	**Angiectasis** means dilation of a blood or lymph vessel. **Neurectasia** is stretching of a nerve.
-edema	swelling	**Edema** means the presence of abnormally large amounts of fluid in the tissues; the term is usually applied to an accumulation of excessive fluid in the subcutaneous tissues, resulting in swelling. **Lymphedema** is an abnormal accumulation of tissue fluid brought about by lymphatic vessel disruption (Fig. 2.21).
-emesis	vomiting	**Emesis** is a word that means vomiting.
-emia	condition of the blood	**Bacteremia** is the presence of bacteria in the blood.
-ia, -iasis	condition	**Hysteria** is a condition so named because long ago hysterical women were thought to suffer from a condition of the uterus (hyster/o). **Psoriasis** is a disease condition of the skin marked by itchy lesions (from the Greek word *psora*, meaning "itch"). (See Fig. 12.19.)

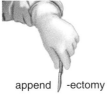

append | -ectomy

Fig. 2.20 Look for the Suffix. Then seeing a new term, look for a suffix ending and think of its meaning, then look for other parts you recognize, e.g., append/ectomy, angi/ectasis, hyper/emesis, cardio/megaly. osteo/malacia.

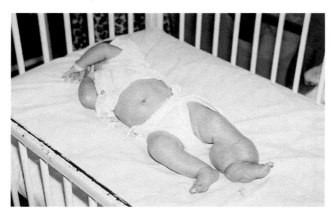

Fig. 2.21 Lymphedema. This particular type of lymphedema exists at birth and most often involves the legs. Another type, secondary lymphedema, may follow obstruction of lymphatic vessels. **lymph/o** = lymph, lymphatics;   **-edema** = swelling;   **lymphat/o** = lymphatics

SUFFIXES: SYMPTOMS OR DIAGNOSIS—cont'd

Suffix	Meaning	Word Association
-itis	inflammation	**Appendicitis** is **inflammation** of the appendix (see Fig. 9.10). **Otitis** is inflammation of the ear.
-lith	stone or calculus	Another name for a gallstone is **cholelith**.
-malacia	soft, softening	**Osteomalacia** is softening of the bones.
-mania	excessive preoccupation	In **kleptomania**, an excessive preoccupation leads to stealing on impulse.
-megaly	enlargement	You may be more familiar with mega-. Both mega- and megal- mean large, as in megalopolis, a large city, and megaton, a large explosive force.
-oid (forms adjectives and nouns)	resembling	**Mucoid** (an adjective) means similar to or resembling mucus. **Paranoid** (an adjective) means resembling **paranoia**, a psychotic disorder characterized by delusions of persecution.
-oma	tumor	**Carcinoma** is cancer (CA), or a cancerous tumor.
-osis	condition (often an abnormal condition; sometimes an increase)	**Neurosis** is a nervous condition (disorder) that is not caused by a demonstrable structural change.
-pathy	disease	The suffix -pathy is derived from the same source as many words that contain path/o; for example, **pathogenic** (an adjective) organisms can cause disease.
-penia	deficiency	**Calcipenia** means a deficiency of calcium.
-phobia	abnormal fear	**Phobia** means an obsessive, irrational fear of a specific object, activity, or a physical situation, such as fear of heights. "Hydrophobia" is an obsolete term for rabies.*
-ptosis	prolapse (sagging)	**Ptosis** means sagging. It also refers to drooping or sagging eyelids.
-rrhage, -rrhagia	excessive bleeding or hemorrhage	**Hemorrhage** is abnormal internal or external bleeding but can also be a verb. It often refers to the loss of a large amount of blood.
-rrhea	flow or discharge	A urethral or vaginal discharge is a primary feature of **gonorrhea**.
-rrhexis	rupture	**Cardiorrhexis** literally means "ruptured heart." One might think of a lover's broken heart, but cardiorrhexis is a pathologic condition in which the heart ruptures.
-spasm	twitching, cramp	**Spasm** means involuntary and sudden movement or convulsive muscular contraction. When contractions are strong and painful, they are often called "cramps."
-stasis	stopping, controlling	**Stasis** means slowing or stopping. It may be intentional (Fig. 2.22), or it may result from an abnormal state of health.

Use the electronic flashcards on the Evolve site or make your own set of flashcards using the above list. Select the word parts just presented and study them until you know their meanings.

*A viral disease transmitted to humans by the bite of an infected animal, rabies was given the name *hydrophobia* after it was observed that stricken animals avoided water, as though they had a fear of it. Actually, rabid animals avoid water because they cannot swallow as a result of the paralysis caused by the virus.

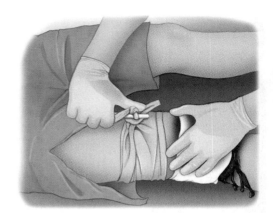

Fig. 2.22 Controlling Hemorrhage. Stasis of hemorrhaging is provided by compression (applying pressure) and a tourniquet (tight band). Tourniquets are used *only* when direct pressure applied to the wound or pressure points does not stop the bleeding.

MATCH IT!

EXERCISE 15

Match the suffixes in the right column with their meanings in the left column.

_____ 1. condition
_____ 2. controlling
_____ 3. dilatation
_____ 4. enlargement
_____ 5. excessive preoccupation
_____ 6. hernia
_____ 7. inflammation
_____ 8. pain
_____ 9. softening
_____ 10. vomiting

A. -algia
B. -cele
C. -ectasis
D. -emesis
E. -iasis
F. -itis
G. -malacia
H. -mania
I. -megaly
J. -stasis

CHOOSE IT!

EXERCISE 16

Circle the correct answer to complete each sentence.

1. The suffix -penia means (resembling, condition, deficiency, rupture).
2. The suffix -rrhexis means (resembling, rupture, preoccupation, cramp).
3. The suffix -oid means (flow, hemorrhage, resembling, condition).
4. The suffix -phobia means (abnormal fear, excessive preoccupation, deficiency, stopping).
5. The suffix -ptosis means (disease, fear, prolapse, decreased).
6. The suffix that means tumor is (-oid, -oma, -osis, -rrhagia).
7. The suffix meaning disease is (-pathy, -penia, -phobia, -ptosis).
8. The suffix that means flow or discharge is (-rrhage, -rrhea, -rrhexis, -penia).
9. Several of the suffixes that you learned are also words. One suffix that means cramp or twitching and that can also stand alone as a word is (ptosis, phobia, spasm, stasis).
10. Excessive bleeding is represented by the suffix (-rrhea, -rrhage, -rrhexis, -pathy).

PROGRAMMED LEARNING

Remember to cover the answers (left column) with folded paper or the bookmark. Write an answer in each blank, and then check your answer before proceeding to the next frame.

inflammation	1. In studying the suffixes pertaining to symptoms or diagnosis, you learned that -itis means _____. **Mastitis** is inflammation of the breast.
ophthalmitis	2. The combining form for eye is ophthalm/o. Write a word that means inflammation of the eye: _____.
appendicitis	3. Using the combining form appendic/o (meaning appendix), write a word that means inflammation of the appendix: _____. (See how easy it is to write medical terms using this method!)
pain	4. When analyzing the term neur+algia, we see that it is derived from neur/o (meaning nerve) and the suffix -algia. Neur+algia means _____ along a nerve.
pain	5. **Ophthalm+algia** is _____ of the eye.
hernia	6. The Suffixes: Symptoms or Diagnosis list on pages 36-37 contains a word meaning "protrusion of all or part of an organ through the wall of the cavity that normally contains it." This word is _____.
-cele	7. The suffix that means hernia is _____.
hernia (or herniation)	8. An encephalo+cele is _____ of the brain through an opening in the skull. (This is also called a cerebral hernia.)
hernia	9. Gastr/o means stomach. A **gastro+cele** is a _____ of the stomach.
vomiting	10. **Hyper+emesis** means excessive _____. Hyper- means excessive or above normal.
vomiting	11. **Hemat+emesis** is _____ of blood. Hemat/o means blood.
prolapse	12. The word *ptosis* means sag or prolapse. Blepharo+ptosis is _____ of the eyelid. Blephar/o means eyelid.
-rrhagia	13. The suffix -rrhage means excessive bleeding. Another suffix for forming words to indicate hemorrhage is _____.
bleeding	14. **Ophthalmo+rrhagia** is hemorrhage or excessive _____ from the eye.
discharge	15. Another suffix beginning with a double r is -rrhea. In the sexually transmitted disease gono+rrhea, -rrhea refers to the heavy _____ that is characteristic of the disease.
rupture	16. Cardi/o means heart. Cardio+rrhexis is _____ of the heart.
ophthalmorrhexis	17. Using ophthalm/o and the suffix for rupture, write a word that means rupture of the eyeball: _____. Translated literally, the word means rupture of the eye.

chirospasm	18. Chir/o means hand. The word that means cramping of the hand is _____. This is sometimes called "writer's cramp."
angiectasis	19. Using angi/o, write a word that means dilation of a blood or lymph vessel: _____.
softening	20. Osteo+malacia is a disease marked by increased _____ of the bone (oste/o means bone).
preoccupation	21. You have probably heard of the word *pyromaniac*. **Pyro+mania** is excessive _____ with fire. **Pyromaniacs** enjoy watching or setting fires (pyr/o means fire).
pyrophobia	22. Add another suffix to pyr/o to form a word that means abnormal fear of fire: _____.
enlargement	23. **Cardio+megaly** is _____ of the heart.
resembling	24. Muc/o means mucus. Muc+oid means _____ mucus.
tumor	25. Carcinoma is a synonym for cancer (Fig. 2.23). Carcin+oma is a cancerous growth or malignant _____.
skin	26. **Dermat+itis** is inflammation of the _____. It is evidenced by itching, redness, and various skin lesions (Fig. 2.24).
condition	27. The suffix -osis means condition, but it sometimes implies a disease or abnormal increase. **Dermat+osis** is a skin _____. (Specifically, a dermatosis is any skin condition in which inflammation is not necessarily a symptom.)
dermatitis	28. A skin condition involving inflammation is called _____.
disease	29. Another suffix you learned that means disease is -pathy. **Ophthalmo+pathy** refers to any _____ of the eye.
phlebostasis	30. Perhaps you are familiar with the word **phlebitis**, which means inflammation of a vein. Add another suffix to phleb/o to write a word that means "controlling the flow of blood in a vein by means of compression": _____.
deficiency	31. Calci+penia means a _____ of calcium in body tissues and fluids.
condition	32. Lith/o is a combining form that means stone or calculus. **Lith+iasis** is a _____ in which a stone or calculus is present.

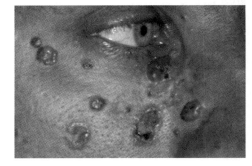

Fig. 2.23 Basal Cell Carcinoma. This is a common type of skin cancer.
carcin/o = cancer; **-oma** = tumor

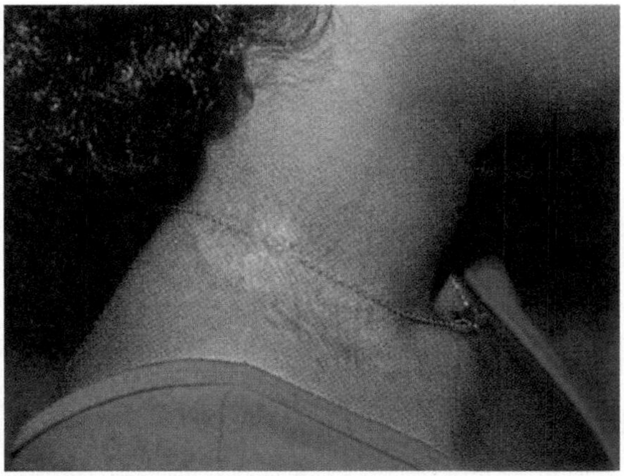

Fig. 2.24 Dermatitis. This example of allergic dermatitis is caused by the metal nickel and usually results from contact with jewelry, metal clasps, or coins. Other types of allergic dermatitis may be caused by contact with poison ivy, other metals, or chemicals, including latex, dyes, and perfumes.
dermat/o = skin; **-itis** = inflammation

WRITE IT! EXERCISE 17

Write terms for these meanings.

1. inflammation of a vein _____
2. inflammation of the appendix _____
3. inflammation of the ear _____
4. inflammation of the eye _____
5. inflammation of the skin _____

BUILD IT! EXERCISE 18

Combine the word parts to write terms.

1. cramping of the hand: chir/o + -spasm _____
2. dilation of a vessel: angi/o + -ectasis _____
3. excessive preoccupation with fire: pyr/o + -mania _____
4. hemorrhage from the eye: ophthalm/o + -rrhagia _____
5. herniation of the brain: encephal/o + -cele _____
6. herniation of the stomach: gastr/o + -cele _____
7. skin condition lacking inflammation: dermat/o + -osis _____
8. pain along a nerve: neur/o + -algia _____
9. painful eye: ophthalm/o + -algia _____
10. prolapse of the eyelid: blephar/o + -ptosis _____
11. rupture of the heart: cardi/o + -rrhexis _____
12. vomiting of blood: hemat/o + -emesis _____

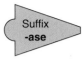

Suffix
-ase

Miscellaneous Suffixes

Commit the following list of suffixes and their meanings to memory. Some important suffixes have been omitted, but they will be presented with their associated combining forms in subsequent chapters.

MISCELLANEOUS SUFFIXES

Suffix	Meaning	Use in Sentence
-able, -ible	capable of, able to	(adjective) Preventable means "capable of being prevented." Illegible describes writing that is not capable of being read.
-ac, -al, -an, -ar, -ary, -eal, -ic, -ive, -tic	pertaining to	(adjective) Cardiac, **thermal, median, alveolar, salivary, peritoneal, lymphatic, invasive,** and **nephrotic** mean pertaining to the heart, heat, middle, alveoli, saliva, peritoneum, lymphatic system, invasion, and kidney, respectively.
-ase	enzyme	(noun) **Lactase** is an enzyme that breaks down lactose.
-eum, -ium	membrane	(noun) The **peritoneum** lines the abdominal cavity (see Fig. 5.14). The membrane that lines the heart is **endocardium**.
-ia, -ism	condition or theory	(noun) **Synergism** is a condition in which two agents, such as medications, produce a greater effect than the total effects of each agent alone.
-iac	one who suffers	(noun) A **hemophiliac** is one who suffers from (is afflicted by) **hemophilia**.
-opia	vision	(noun) **Diplopia** is double vision.
-ose	sugar	(noun) **Lactose** is a sugar found in milk.
-ous	pertaining to or characterized by	(adjective) **Cancerous** means pertaining to cancer.
-y	state or condition	(noun) **Atrophy** is a condition of wasting away of a cell, tissue, organ, or part.

Use the electronic flashcards on the Evolve site or make your own set of flashcards using the above list. Select the word parts just presented and study them until you know their meanings.

WRITE IT!

EXERCISE 19

Write the meaning of each underlined suffix. (Some meanings may have more than one word; e.g., the first answer is "capable of.")

1. coagul<u>able</u>   _____
2. derm<u>al</u>   _____
3. gluc<u>ose</u>   _____
4. lact<u>ase</u>   _____
5. neuro<u>logist</u>   _____
6. ot<u>ic</u>   _____
7. periton<u>eum</u>   _____
8. synerg<u>ism</u>   _____
9. oto<u>logist</u>   _____
10. tonsill<u>ar</u>   _____

PROGRAMMED LEARNING

Remember to cover the answers (left column) with folded paper or the bookmark. Write an answer in each blank, and then check your answer before proceeding to the next frame.

studies	1. You have learned that -ist means one who and that -logist means one who _____. The suffixes -ist and -logist are both used to form nouns. The suffix -logist is derived from log/o, meaning knowledge or study, and from -ist, but -logist is used so frequently that it is more convenient to learn the suffix form. The suffix -logist often refers to a specialist. In medicine, a specialist is a person who has advanced education and training in one area of practice, such as internal medicine, dermatology, or cardiology.
specialist	2. A patho+logist is a _____ in pathology, the medical specialty that studies the nature and cause of disease.
pertaining	3. Log/o is combined with -y so often that we learn -logy as a suffix form that means "the study of." Whether pathology is divided as patho+logy or patho+log+y, the meaning is the same. Patho+log+ic means _____ to pathology or disease. (Pathological is another term that means the same as pathologic, but pathologic is the preferred form.)
pertaining	4. A neurologist treats neural disorders. **Neur+al** means _____ to the nerves or nervous system.
pertaining	5. Many suffixes mean pertaining to, and you will have an opportunity to practice using them as you progress through the material. You learned earlier that mamm/o means breast. **Mamm+ary** is an adjective that means _____ to the breast.
enzyme	6. **Enzymat+ic** (occasionally enzym+ic) means pertaining to enzymes, substances that facilitate chemical reactions. The suffix that means enzyme is -ase. By its suffix, we know that lact+ase has something to do with an _____.
lactase	7. Lact/o means milk. Lact+ase is an enzyme that acts on a sugar called lactose that is present in milk. Enzymes are usually named by adding -ase to the combining form of the substance on which they act. Translated literally, lact+ose means milk sugar. The enzyme that acts on lactose is called _____.
fat	8. Adip/o and lip/o mean fat. Fats are also called **lipids** or **adipose** tissue, which should help you to remember the combining form. **Lip+ase** is an enzyme that breaks down _____.
amylase	9. Amyl/o means starch. Write the term that means an enzyme that breaks down starch: _____.
starch	10. The suffix for destruction is -lysis. **Amylo+lysis** is the destruction (digestion) of _____. In amylolysis, starch is broken down into sugar.
sugar	11. Glyc/o means sugar. **Glyco+lysis** is the breaking down of _____, which is accomplished by enzymes. These enzymes are named according to the specific sugar on which they act. Sucrase is an enzyme that acts on sucrose, common table sugar.
protease	12. Protein/o or prote/o means protein. Two words that mean "an enzyme that breaks down protein" are **proteinase** and _____. The breaking down or digestion of proteins is **proteo+lysis**. Proteins, as well as most substances we eat, must be broken down chemically before they can be absorbed by the body.

Miscellaneous Word Parts

If you do not recognize the meanings of the new word parts in the following list, commit them to memory before proceeding. Remember, **bold type** indicates that a term is included in the Quick & Easy List and is pronounced on the Evolve site.

MISCELLANEOUS WORD PARTS

Word Part	Meaning	Word Association
adip/o, lip/o	fat	Lipids are fats or fatlike substances. Adipose means fatty.
amyl/o	starch	Amylase is an enzyme that breaks down starch.
glyc/o	sugar	In **hypoglycemia**, the blood sugar level is too low.
hemat/o	blood	Hematemesis is the vomiting of blood.
lact/o	milk	Milk is secreted by a woman during **lactation**.
lith/o	stone	Lithology is the study of rocks.
micro-	small	A microscope is an instrument used to view small (microscopic) objects.
muc/o	mucus	Generally, **mucous** membranes secrete **mucus**.
prote/o, protein/o	protein	**Proteinuria** is an excess of proteins in urine.
pyr/o	fire	Pyromaniacs enjoy setting fires or seeing fires burn.

Use the electronic flashcards on the Evolve site or make your own set of flashcards using the above list. Select the word parts just presented and study them until you know their meanings.

MATCH IT! EXERCISE 20

Match the words in the left column with their corresponding combining forms in the right column.

_____ 1. blood
_____ 2. fat
_____ 3. fire
_____ 4. milk
_____ 5. mucus
_____ 6. protein
_____ 7. starch
_____ 8. stone
_____ 9. sugar

A. adip/o
B. amyl/o
C. glyc/o
D. hemat/o
E. lact/o
F. lith/o
G. muc/o
H. prote/o
I. pyr/o

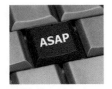

Abbreviations

Selected abbreviations are presented in Appendix I.

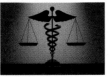

Pharmacology

The various ways a drug can be administered are called the routes of administration (most commonly by mouth or by injection). The generic name of a drug is used by any company (e.g., acetaminophen), whereas the trade name or brand name is the property of only one company (e.g., Tylenol). Drugs are generally grouped into classes based on their major effects or mechanisms of actions. If a drug acts on many sites away from where the drug is administered, the effect is said to be systemic. See http://evolve.else vier.com/Leonard/quick for pharmacologic terms.

Preparing for a Q&E Test

Study the Word Parts
Review all lists of word parts and their meanings for the chapter you are studying, using the flashcards you prepared or the flashcards on the Evolve site. Review the cards several times before the test.

Practice With the Self-Test
Work the Self-Test. The review helps you know if you have learned the material. After completing all sections of the review, check your answers with those in Appendix III. Find additional games and quizzes on the Evolve site at http://evolve.elsevier.com/Le onard/quick to help you review.

Review With Quick Connect
Use Quick Connect to assure that you understood the major concepts of Chapters 1 and 2; can divide terms into prefixes, suffixes, and combining forms; and can identify or conceptualize the meanings of terms by understanding the word parts.

Practice With the Q&E List of Terms
While looking at the terms listed at the end of each chapter, listen to the pronunciations on the Evolve site. Look closely at the spelling, and be sure that you know its meaning. If you can't recall its meaning, reread the frames that pertain to the term. (The index in the back of the book may help you locate the page on which the term appears.) Once you've mastered the chapter, you may want to use the audio files on Evolve to test your recognition and spelling of terms.

  Be Careful With These!

-*ist* (one who) versus -*iatry* (medical profession or treatment)
-*logy* (study of) versus -*logist* (one who studies; specialist)
ne/o (new) versus *neur/o* (nerve)

intern (one in postgraduate training) versus *internist* (a physician)

A Career as an Anesthesiology Assistant

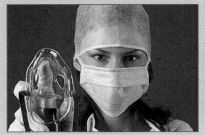

Terry Shapiro works with anesthesiologists to develop and implement anesthesia care plans. Terry loves the combination of vital work and patient interaction; she talks with patients before surgery, helps during surgery, and follows patients after surgery. She monitors patients' physiology and helps with the anesthetics. Terry knows her work is vital to successful surgery and that her role in the health care team is critical. For more information, visit the website of the American Academy of Anesthesiology Assistants: www.anesthetist.org.

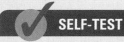

SELF-TEST

Work the following exercises to test your understanding of the material in Chapter 2. It is best to do all the exercises before checking your answers against the answers in Appendix III. Pay particular attention to spelling. If most of your answers are correct, you are ready to move on to Chapter 3.

A. FINDING!   Find the combining forms and suffixes and write their meanings (the first is done as an example).

1. amylolysis   *amyl/o (starch) + -lysis (destruction)*
2. appendicitis   _____
3. blepharoptosis   _____
4. dermatologist   _____
5. lipase   _____
6. mucoid   _____
7. neuroplasty   _____
8. ophthalmorrhagia _____
9. otic   _____
10. tonsillectomy   _____

B. WRITING!   Write the meanings of the underlined word parts in each of these terms.

1. <u>aden</u>oid   _____
2. <u>dermat</u>osis   _____
3. cardio<u>logy</u>   _____
4. <u>chiro</u>spasm   _____
5. colo<u>pexy</u>   _____
6. lact<u>ose</u>   _____
7. <u>mammo</u>plasty   _____
8. <u>neur</u>al   _____
9. <u>ophthalmo</u>scope _____
10. osteo<u>malacia</u> _____

C. MATCHING!   Match the medical specialists with the areas in which they specialize.

_____ 1. anesthesiologist   A. children
_____ 2. dermatologist   B. drugs that produce loss of feeling or sensation
_____ 3. endocrinologist   C. ear, nose, and throat
_____ 4. geriatrician   D. eyes
_____ 5. gynecologist   E. females
_____ 6. neurologist   F. hormones and the glands that secrete them
_____ 7. oncologist   G. mental, emotional, and behavioral disorders
_____ 8. ophthalmologist   H. nervous system
_____ 9. otolaryngologist   I. nose
_____ 10. pediatrician   J. older persons
_____ 11. psychiatrist   K. skin
_____ 12. rhinologist   L. tumors

D. IDENTIFYING!   *Label these illustrations using one of the following: anesthetic, anesthetist, cutaneous, dermatitis, mammoplasty, mastopexy, otoplasty, otoscopy.*

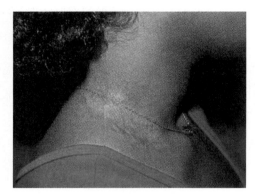

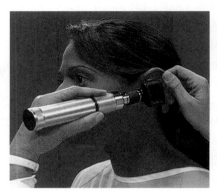

1. inflammation of the skin _____

2. visual examination of the ear _____

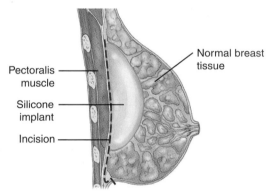

Pectoralis muscle
Normal breast tissue
Silicone implant
Incision

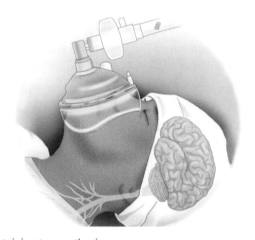

3. surgical repair of the breast _____

4. pertaining to anesthesia _____

E. WRITING!   *Write one word for each of the following meanings.*

1. enzyme that breaks down starch   _____
2. examination of the eye   _____
3. incision of the trachea   _____
4. inflammation of the appendix   _____
5. inflammation of the ear   _____
6. pertaining to a nerve   _____
7. removal of the tonsils   _____
8. skin specialist   _____
9. surgical crushing of a stone   _____
10. surgical removal of a breast   _____

F. CHOOSING!   *Circle the one correct answer (A, B, C, or D) for each question.*

1. Which term means the abnormal accumulation of fluid in the tissue and results in swelling?
   (A) dilatation   (B) edema   (C) emesis   (D) ptosis

2. Which of the following terms is a condition in which a calculus is present?
   (A) diplopia   (B) lithiasis   (C) neurotripsy   (D) pathology

3. Which branch of medicine specializes in the study of the nature and cause of disease?
   (A) cardiology   (B) dermatology   (C) pathology   (D) urology

4. Which of the following terms means pertaining to the ear?
   (A) dermatologic   (B) neural   (C) ophthalmic   (D) otic

5. Which of the following terms means an enzyme that breaks down starches?
   (A) adipose   (B) amylase   (C) lipase   (D) lipid

6. What does mastopexy mean?   (A) enlarged breasts   (B) inflammation of the breast   (C) surgical fixation of the breast   (D) surgical removal of a breast

7. Which of the following terms means excision of a small piece of living tissue for microscopic examination?
   (A) biopsy   (B) emesis   (C) ptosis   (D) stasis

8. Which term means pertaining to the skin?
   (A) blepharal   (B) cutaneous   (C) hernia   (D) suture

9. Which of the following terms means pain along the course of a nerve?
   (A) neuralgia   (B) neurocele   (C) neuroplasty   (D) neurosis

10. Which term means stretching of a structure?
    (A) dilatation   (B) ptosis   (C) prolapse   (D) spasm

11. A 65-year-old man has a history of heart problems. Which type of specialist should he see for care of his heart condition?   (A) cardiologist   (B) endocrinologist   (C) laryngologist   (D) orthopedist

12. Cynthia is pregnant. Which type of specialist should she see to care for her during her pregnancy, labor, and delivery?
    (A) gerontologist   (B) obstetrician   (C) orthopedist   (D) otologist

13. Which term means a person who is not a physician, but is trained in administering drugs that cause a loss of feeling?
    (A) anesthesiologist   (B) anesthesist   (C) anesthetics   (D) anesthetist

14. Which of the following physicians specializes in the diagnosis and treatment of newborns through the age of 28 days?
    (A) geriatrician   (B) gynecologist   (C) neonatologist   (D) urologist

15. John suffers from persistent digestive problems. To which specialist in disorders of the stomach and intestines is John referred?
    (A) gastroenterologist   (B) immunologist   (C) rheumatologist   (D) toxicologist

16. Sally injures her arm while ice skating. The emergency department physician orders an x-ray examination. Which type of physician is a specialist in interpreting x-ray images?
    (A) gynecologist   (B) ophthalmologist   (C) plastic surgeon   (D) radiologist

17. Sally's x-ray image reveals a fractured radius, one of the bones of her forearm. Dr. Bonelly, a bone specialist, puts a cast on Sally's arm. Which type of specialist is Dr. Bonelly?
    (A) dermatologist   (B) orthopedist   (C) otologist   (D) rhinologist

18. Which physician specializes in diagnosis of disease using clinical laboratory results?
    (A) clinical pathologist   (B) gastroenterologist   (C) internist   (D) surgical pathologist

G. HEALTH CARE REPORTING   *XI. Circle the correct answer in Questions 1 through 5 after reading the following chart note.*

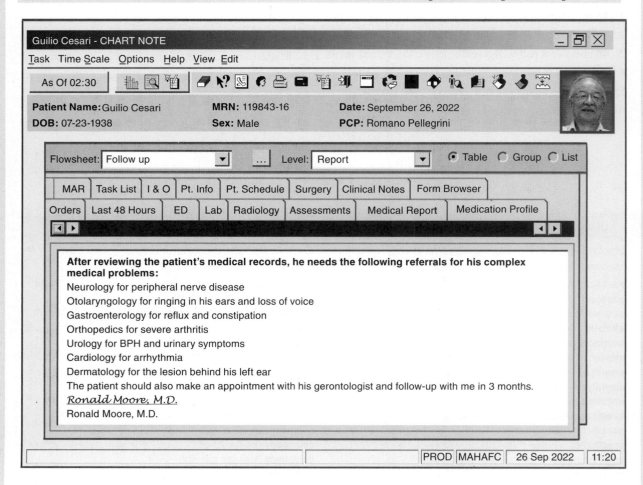

Guilio Cesari - CHART NOTE

Task Time Scale Options Help View Edit

As Of 02:30

Patient Name: Guilio Cesari   **MRN:** 119843-16   **Date:** September 26, 2022
DOB: 07-23-1938   **Sex:** Male   **PCP:** Romano Pellegrini

Flowsheet: Follow up   …   Level: Report   ● Table ○ Group ○ List

MAR | Task List | I & O | Pt. Info | Pt. Schedule | Surgery | Clinical Notes | Form Browser

Orders | Last 48 Hours | ED | Lab | Radiology | Assessments | Medical Report | Medication Profile

After reviewing the patient's medical records, he needs the following referrals for his complex medical problems:
Neurology for peripheral nerve disease
Otolaryngology for ringing in his ears and loss of voice
Gastroenterology for reflux and constipation
Orthopedics for severe arthritis
Urology for BPH and urinary symptoms
Cardiology for arrhythmia
Dermatology for the lesion behind his left ear
The patient should also make an appointment with his gerontologist and follow-up with me in 3 months.
Ronald Moore, M.D.
Ronald Moore, M.D.

PROD | MAHAFC | 26 Sep 2022 | 11:20

Circle the correct answer.

1. Which medical specialist deals with all aspects of aging and older persons? (cardiologist, gerontologist, obstetrician, urologist)
2. Dermatology is a medical specialty that primarily involves disorders of what type? (eye, gland, muscle, skin)
3. Orthopedics does NOT include preservation and restoration of the (bones, kidney function, structures associated with the bones)
4. Otolaryngology does NOT involve treating disorders of the (ears, lungs, nose, throat).
5. Gastroenterology is a specialty that does NOT include disorders of the (intestines, kidneys, stomach).

H. SPELLING AND PRONOUNCING!   *Circle all incorrectly spelled terms, and write their correct spelling. Then pronounce the terms.*

angiorrhaphy   chirospazm   incizion   mammoplasty   rheumatology

---

I. QUICK CHALLENGE!   *Find one incorrect term in each sentence and write it correctly.*

1. An endocrinologist specializes in pregnancy, labor, and delivery. _____

2. Skin grafting or transplantation of living skin to cover defects is known as dermatome. _____

3. Angiectomy is suture of a vessel, especially a blood vessel. _____

4. Involuntary or convulsive muscular contraction is stasis. _____

5. Sucrose is an enzyme that acts on common table sugar. _____

*Use Appendix III to check your answers.

 QUICK & EASY (Q&E) LIST

Use the Evolve website (http://evolve.elsevier.com/Leonard/quick) to review the terms presented in Chapter 2. Look closely at the spelling of each term as it is pronounced.

adenectomy *(ad-uh-**nek**-tuh-mē)*
adenoids *(**ad**-uh-noidz)*
adipose *(**ad**-i-pōs)*
alveolar *(al-**vē**-uh-lur)*
amniocentesis *(am-nē-ō-sen-**tē**-sis)*
amnion *(**am**-nē-on)*
amylase *(**am**-uh-lās)*
amylolysis *(am-uh-**lol**-uh-sis)*
anesthesiologist *(an-us-thē-zē-**ol**-uh-jist)*
anesthesiology *(an-us-thē-zē-**ol**-uh-jē)*
anesthetic *(an-us-**thet**-ik)*
anesthetist *(uh-**nes**-thuh-tist)*
angiectasis *(an-jē-**ek**-tuh-sis)*
angiectomy *(an-jē-**ek**-tuh-mē)*
angiogram *(**an**-jē-ō-gram)*
angioplasty *(**an**-jē-ō-plas-tē)*
angiorrhaphy *(an-jē-**or**-uh-fē)*
appendectomy *(ap-en-**dek**-tuh-mē)*
appendicitis *(uh-pen-di-**sī**-tis)*
atrophy *(**at**-ruh-fē)*
augmentation mammoplasty *(awg-men-**tā**-shun **mam**-ō-plas-tē)*
bacteremia *(bak-tur-**ē**-mē-uh)*
benign *(buh-**nīn**)*
biology *(bī-**ol**-uh-jē)*
biopsy *(**bī**-op-sē)*
blepharoptosis *(blef-uh-rop-**tō**-sis)*
calcipenia *(kal-si-**pē**-nē-uh)*
cancerous *(**kan**-sur-us)*
carcinoma *(kahr-si-**nō**-muh)*
cardiac *(**kahr**-dē-ak)*

cardiologist *(kahr-dē-**ol**-uh-jist)*
cardiology *(kahr-dē-**ol**-uh-jē)*
cardiomegaly *(kahr-dē-ō-**meg**-uh-lē)*
cardiorrhexis *(kahr-dē-ō-**rek**-sis)*
cerebral *(suh-**rē**-brul, **ser**-uh-brul)*
cerebrotomy *(ser-uh-**brot**-uh-mē)*
cerebrum *(**ser**-uh-brum, suh-**rē**-brum)*
chirospasm *(**kī**-rō-spaz-um)*
cholelith *(**kō**-luh-lith)*
colonoscopy *(kō-lun-**os**-kuh-pē)*
colopexy *(**kō**-lō-pek-sē)*
coloscopy *(kō-**los**-kō-pē)*
colostomy *(kuh-**los**-tuh-mē)*
cutaneous *(kū-**tā**-nē-us)*
dermal *(**dur**-mul)*
dermatitis *(dur-muh-**tī**-tis)*
dermatologic *(dur-muh-tō-**loj**-ik)*
dermatological *(dur-muh-tō-**loj**-i-kul)*
dermatologist *(dur-muh-**tol**-uh-jist)*
dermatology *(dur-muh-**tol**-uh-jē)*
dermatome *(**dur**-muh-tōm)*
dermatoplasty *(**dur**-muh-tō-plas-tē)*
dermatosis *(dur-muh-**tō**-sis)*
dilatation *(dil-uh-**tā**-shun)*
diplopia *(di-**plō**-pē-uh)*
ductus deferens *(**duk**-tus **def**-ur-enz)*
edema *(uh-**dē**-muh)*
elective procedure *(ē-**lek**-tiv prō-**sē**-jur)*
emesis *(**em**-uh-sis)*
encephalitis *(en-sef-uh-**lī**-tis)*
encephalocele *(en-**sef**-uh-lō-sēl)*

QUICK & EASY (Q&E) LIST—cont'd

encephalotome *(en-**sef**-uh-luh-tōm)*
encephalotomy *(en-sef-uh-**lot**-uh-mē)*
endocardium *(en-dō-**kahr**-dē-um)*
endocrine *(**en**-dō-krin, **en**-dō-krīn)*
endocrinologist *(en-dō-kri-**nol**-uh-jist)*
endocrinology *(en-dō-kri-**nol**-uh-jē)*
enzymatic *(en-zī-**mat**-ik)*
epidemiologist *(ep-i-dē-mē-**ol**-uh-jist)*
epidemiology *(ep-i-dē-mē-**ol**-uh-jē)*
excision *(ek-**sizh**-un)*
facial *(**fā**-shul)*
forensic medicine *(fuh-**ren**-zik **med**-i-sin)*
gastric *(**gas**-trik)*
gastrocele *(**gas**-trō-sēl)*
gastroenterologist *(gas-trō-en-tur-**ol**-uh-jist)*
gastroenterology *(gas-trō-en-tur-**ol**-uh-jē)*
geriatrician *(jer-ē-uh-**trish**-un)*
geriatrics *(jer-ē-**at**-riks)*
gerontology *(jer-on-**tol**-uh-jē)*
glycolysis *(glī-**kol**-uh-sis)*
gonorrhea *(gon-ō-**rē**-uh)*
gynecologic *(gī-nuh-kō-**loj**-ik)*
gynecological *(gī-nuh-kō-**loj**-i-kul)*
gynecologist *(gī-nuh-**kol**-uh-jist)*
gynecology *(gī-nuh-**kol**-uh-jē)*
hematemesis *(hē-muh-**tem**-uh-sis)*
hemolysis *(hē-**mol**-uh-sis)*
hemophilia *(hē-mō-**fil**-ē-uh)*
hemophiliac *(hē-mō-**fil**-ē-ak)*
hemorrhage *(**hem**-uh-raj)*
hepatitis *(hep-uh-t**ī**-tis)*
hepatologist *(hep-uh-**tol**-uh-jist)*
hernia *(**hur**-nē-uh)*
hospitalist *(**hos**-pi-tul-ist)*
hyperemesis *(hī-pur-**em**-uh-sis)*
hypoglycemia *(hī-pō-glī-**sē**-mē-uh)*
hysteria *(his-**ter**-ē-uh)*
immunologist *(im-ū-**nol**-uh-jist)*
immunology *(im-ū-**nol**-uh-jē)*
incision *(in-**sizh**-un)*
inflammation *(in-fluh-**mā**-shun)*
intensivist *(in-**ten**-si-vist)*
internist *(in-**tur**-nist)*
invasive *(in-**vā**-siv)*
kleptomania *(klep-tō-**mā**-nē-uh)*
lactase *(**lak**-tās)*
lactation *(lak-**tā**-shun)*
lactose *(**lak**-tōs)*
lipase *(**lip**-ās, **lī**-pās)*
lipids *(**lip**-idz)*

lithiasis *(li-**thī**-uh-sis)*
lithotripsy *(**lith**-ō-trip-sē)*
lumpectomy *(lum-**pek**-tuh-mē)*
lymphatic *(lim-**fat**-ik)*
lymphedema *(lim-fuh-**dē**-muh)*
malignant *(muh-**lig**-nunt)*
mammary *(**mam**-uh-rē)*
mammography *(muh-**mog**-ruh-fē)*
mammoplasty *(**mam**-ō-plas-tē)*
mastectomy *(mas-**tek**-tuh-mē)*
mastitis *(mas-t**ī**-tis)*
mastopexy *(**mas**-tō-pek-sē)*
median *(**mē**-dē-un)*
microscope *(**mī**-krō-skōp)*
microscopy *(mī-**kros**-kuh-pē)*
microtia *(mī-**krō**-shuh)*
microtome *(**mī**-krō-tōm)*
mucoid *(**mū**-koid)*
mucous *(**mū**-kus)*
mucus *(**mū**-kus)*
muscular *(**mus**-kū-lur)*
myalgia *(mī-**al**-juh)*
myelopathy *(mī-uh-**lop**-uh-thē)*
neonatologist *(nē-ō-nā-**tol**-uh-jist)*
neonatology *(nē-ō-nā-**tol**-uh-jē)*
neoplasm *(**nē**-ō-plaz-um)*
nephrotic *(nuh-**frot**-ik)*
neural *(**noor**-ul)*
neuralgia *(noo-**ral**-juh)*
neurectasia *(noor-uk-**tā**-zhuh)*
neurectomy *(noo-**rek**-tuh-mē)*
neurologic *(noor-uh-**loj**-ik)*
neurological *(noor-uh-**loj**-i-kul)*
neurologist *(noo-**rol**-uh-jist)*
neurology *(noo-**rol**-uh-jē)*
neurolysis *(noo-**rol**-i-sis)*
neuroplasty *(**noor**-ō-plas-tē)*
neurosis *(noo-**rō**-sis)*
neurosurgeon *(**noor**-ō-sur-jun)*
obstetric *(ob-**stet**-rik)*
obstetrical *(ob-**stet**-ri-kul)*
obstetrician *(ob-stuh-**tri**-shun)*
obstetrics *(ob-**stet**-riks)*
oncologist *(ong-**kol**-uh-jist)*
oncology *(ong-**kol**-uh-jē)*
ophthalmalgia *(of-thul-**mal**-juh)*
ophthalmic *(of-**thal**-mik)*
ophthalmitis *(of-thul-**mī**-tis)*
ophthalmologic *(of-thul-muh-**loj**-ik)*
ophthalmological *(of-thul-muh-**log**-i-kul)*

QUICK & EASY (Q&E) LIST—cont'd

ophthalmologist *(of-thul-**mol**-uh-jist)*
ophthalmology *(of-thul-**mol**-uh-jē)*
ophthalmopathy *(of-thul-**mop**-uh-thē)*
ophthalmoplasty *(of-**thal**-mō-plas-tē)*
ophthalmorrhagia *(of-thal-mō-**rā**-juh)*
ophthalmorrhexis *(of-thal-mō-**rek**-sis)*
ophthalmoscope *(of-**thal**-mō-skōp)*
ophthalmoscopic *(of-thal-muh-**skop**-ik)*
ophthalmoscopy *(of-thul-**mos**-kuh-pē)*
orthopedics *(or-thō-**pē**-diks)*
orthopedist *(or-thō-**pē**-dist)*
osteoarthritis *(os-tē-ō-ahr-**thrī**-tis)*
osteomalacia *(os-tē-ō-muh-**lā**-shuh)*
otalgia *(ō-**tal**-juh)*
otic *(ō-tik)*
otitis *(ō-**tī**-tis)*
otodynia *(ō-tō-**din**-ē-uh)*
otolaryngologist *(ō-tō-lar-ing-**gol**-uh-jist)*
otolaryngology *(ō-tō-lar-ing-**gol**-uh-jē)*
otologist *(ō-**tol**-uh-jist)*
otology *(ō-**tol**-uh-jē)*
otoplasty *(**ō**-tō-plas-tē)*
otoscope *(**ō**-tō-skōp)*
otoscopic *(ō-tō-**skop**-ik)*
otoscopy *(ō-**tos**-kuh-pē)*
paranoia *(par-uh-**noi**-ah)*
paranoid *(**par**-uh-noid)*
pathogenic *(path-ō-**jen**-ik)*
pathologic *(path-ō-**loj**-ik)*
pathological *(path-ō-**loj**-i-kul)*
pathologist *(puh-**thol**-uh-jist)*
pathology *(puh-**thol**-uh-jē)*
pediatrician *(pē-dē-uh-**tri**-shun)*
pediatric *(pē-dē-**at**-rik)*
pediatrics *(pē-dē-**at**-riks)*
peritoneal *(per-i-tō-**nē**-uhl)*
peritoneum *(per-i-tō-**nē**-um)*
phlebitis *(fluh-**bī**-tis)*
phlebostasis *(fluh-**bos**-tuh-sis)*
phobia *(**fō**-bē-uh)*
plastic surgery *(**plas**-tik **sur**-jur-ē)*
pneumatic *(noo-**mat**-ik)*

pneumonia *(noo-**mōn**-yuh)*
protease *(**prō**-tē-ās)*
proteinase *(**prō**-tēn-ās)*
proteinuria *(prō-tē-**nū**-rē-uh)*
proteolysis *(prō-tē-**ol**-i-sis)*
psoriasis *(suh-**rī**-uh-sis)*
psychiatrist *(sī-**kī**-uh-trist)*
psychiatry *(sī-**kī**-uh-trē)*
ptosis *(**tō**-sis)*
pulmonary *(**pool**-mō-nar-ē)*
pyromania *(pī-rō-**mā**-nē-uh)*
pyromaniac *(pī-rō-**mā**-nē-ak)*
pyrophobia *(pī-rō-**fō**-bē-uh)*
radiation oncologist *(rā-dē-**ā**-shun ong-**kol**-uh-jist)*
radiologic *(rā-dē-ō-**loj**-ik)*
radiological *(rā-dē-ō-**loj**-i-kul)*
radiologist *(rā-dē-**ol**-uh-jist)*
radiology *(rā-dē-**ol**-uh-jē)*
rheumatism *(r$\overline{oo}$-muh-tiz-um)*
rheumatologist *(r$\overline{oo}$-muh-**tol**-uh-jist)*
rheumatology *(r$\overline{oo}$-muh-**tol**-uh-jē)*
rhinologist *(rī-**nol**-uh-jist)*
rhinology *(rī-**nol**-uh-jē)*
salivary *(**sal**-i-var-ē)*
spasm *(**spaz**-um)*
stasis *(**stā**-sis)*
suture *(**s$\overline{oo}$**-chur)*
synergism *(**sin**-ur-jizm)*
therapist *(**ther**-uh-pist)*
thermal *(**thur**-mul)*
tonsillectomy *(ton-si-**lek**-tuh-mē)*
tonsillitis *(ton-si-**lī**-tis)*
trachea *(**trā**-kē-uh)*
tracheostomy *(trā-kē-**os**-tuh-mē)*
tracheotomy *(trā-kē-**ot**-uh-mē)*
triage *(trē-**ahzh**, **trē**-ahzh)*
urinary *(**ū**-ri-nar-ē)*
urologic *(ū-ruh-**loj**-ik)*
urological *(ū-ruh-**loj**-i-kul)*
urologist *(ū-**rol**-uh-jist)*
urology *(ū-**rol**-uh-jē)*
vasectomy *(vuh-**sek**-tuh-mē)*

Don't forget the games and other activities available at *http://evolve.elsevier.com/Leonard/quick*.

QUICK CONNECT

Review all lists of word parts and their meanings for Chapter 2, using the flashcards you prepared or the flashcards on the Evolve site.

Terms in bold typeface in *Quick & Easy Medical Terminology* are included in the Q&E List at the end of the chapter.

Suffixes added to other word parts form nouns, adjectives, and verbs (Examples: cardiology, cardiac, dilate)
When a combining form is joined with a suffix that begins with a vowel, the combining vowel is almost always dropped
   (Example: cardi/o + -ac = cardiac).

cardi/o + -logy = cardiology

ped/o + -iatrician = pediatrician

Most medical specialties end in -logy. Exceptions in Chapter 2 are geriatrics, obstetrics, orthopedics, pediatrics, psychiatry (with these names of specialists: geriatrician, obstetrician, orthopedist or orthopedic surgeon, pediatrician, psychiatrist).

Combining form for tumor is onc/o. Tumors can be benign (not cancerous) or malignant. (Oncology is particularly concerned with malignant tumors and their treatment.) Malignant means tending to become worse, spread, and can cause death. Tumor often refers to a spontaneous new growth of tissue that forms an abnormal mass (neoplasm).

Cancer: Any of a large group of diseases that are characterized by the presence of malignant cells. Distinguish between

- gerontology (scientific study of all aspects of aging) vs geriatrics (branch of medicine that deals with problems and diseases of elderly persons).
- clinical pathologist vs. surgical pathologist
- general surgery vs. plastic surgery vs. neurosurgery vs. orthopedic surgery vs. elective surgery
- psychiatry vs. psychology
- anesthesiologist vs. anesthetist vs. anesthetic (general vs. local)
- pulmonary vs. pneumatic vs. pneumonia
- ophthalmoscope vs. ophthalmoscopy; otoscope vs. otoscopy vs. otoscopic
- terms ending in -osis vs. terms ending in -itis.
- the suffixes -ose and -ase
- the suffixes -ia and -iac
- -tomy vs. -ectomy vs. -stomy vs. -tripsy
- -tome vs. -tomy
- -itis vs. -osis
- incision vs. excision

Recognize synonyms such as cutaneous and dermal; pathologic and pathological; protease and proteinase.

Remember the meanings of terms such as ductus deferens, edema, emesis, endocrine, hernia, lipids, mucus, ptosis, spasm, stasis, suture, and other boldface terms that are not easily broken down into their word parts.

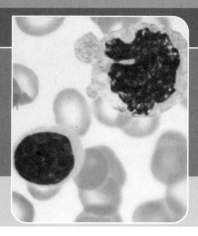

CHAPTER 3

Essential Prefixes and More

Prefixes are used to name many of the body's cells, including several types of blood cells. Various prefixes are joined with the suffix -cyte. Shown are red blood cells, erythrocytes, and white blood cells, leukocytes.

OBJECTIVES

After completing Chapter 3, you will be able to:

1. Write the meaning of Chapter 3 word parts or match word parts with their meanings.
2. Use prefixes for numbers, quantities, position, and direction to write medical terms.
3. Use combining forms for colors to write medical terms.
4. Identify and combine word parts correctly.
5. Write the correct term when presented with its definition or match terms with their definitions.
6. Build and analyze medical terms with Chapter 3 word parts.
7. Spell medical terms correctly.

Prefix
dys-

How Prefixes Are Used to Form Words

Prefixes are emphasized in this chapter, although you are already familiar with many of them. Several new combining forms and suffixes are also introduced.

Instead of only memorizing lists of prefixes, you will learn to combine them with other word parts. Learning new terms will help you remember the prefixes that are presented.

A *prefix* is placed before a word to modify its meaning. Most prefixes, including those ending with a vowel, can be added to the remainder of the word without change. Exceptions are noted. Prefixes are grouped here as follows: (1) prefixes used in numbers or quantities, (2) prefixes used in position or direction, and (3) miscellaneous prefixes.

 QUICK TIP

Written alone, **pre**fixes **pre**cede the hyphen.

Prefix
tri-

Prefixes: Numbers or Quantities

Many of the prefixes in the following table are used in everyday language. Common words are given to help you associate prefixes with their meanings. Commit their meanings to memory.

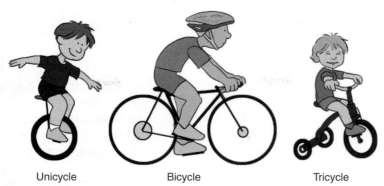

| Unicycle | Bicycle | Tricycle |

Fig. 3.1 Memory Jogger for the Prefixes uni-, bi-, and tri-. The terms *unicycle*, *bicycle*, and *tricycle* describe the number of wheels each cycle has.

PREFIXES: NUMBERS OR QUANTITIES

Prefix	Meaning	Word Association
Specific Numbers		
mono-, uni-	one	A *monorail* is a single rail that serves as a track for a wheeled vehicle. A *monocular* scope has one eyepiece. A *unicorn* has one horn, and a *unicycle* has one wheel.
bi-, di-	two	A *bicycle* has two wheels. *Carbon dioxide* contains two atoms of oxygen.
tri-	three	A *tricycle* has three wheels (Fig. 3.1).
quad-, quadri-, tetra-	four	*Quadruplets* are four offspring born at one birth. *Quadriplegia* is paralysis of all four extremities (arms and legs). A *tetrahedron* is a solid figure having four faces.
centi-	one hundred, one-hundredth	*Centigrade* is a measurement of temperature that is divided into 100 degrees, with 0° representing the freezing point and 100° representing the boiling point (Fig. 3.2). A *centimeter* is $\frac{1}{100}$ of a meter.
milli-	one-thousandth	A *millimeter* is $\frac{1}{1000}$ of a meter.

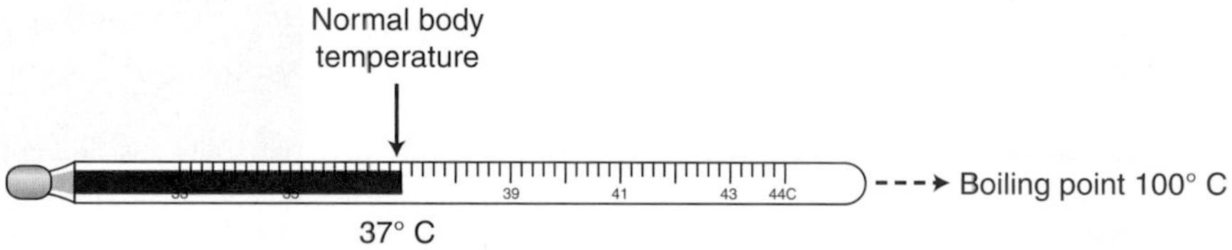

Normal body
temperature
↓

37° C   ---→ Boiling point 100° C

Fig. 3.2 Degrees Centigrade. Centigrade, or degrees Celsius, is so named because 0° is the freezing point and 100° is the boiling point of water at sea level using this temperature scale. The normal adult body temperature, as measured orally, is 37° Centigrade (37° C).

PREFIXES: NUMBERS OR QUANTITIES—cont'd

Prefix	Meaning	Word Association
Quantities		
diplo-	double	**Diplopia** means double vision (two images of a single object are seen).
hemi-, semi-	half, partly	Each of Earth's *hemispheres* is half of the Earth. A *semipermeable* membrane is one that allows the passage of some substances but prevents the passage of others (Fig. 3.3).
hyper-	excessive, more than normal	*Hyperactive* means excessively active. **Hyperglycemia** means an above-normal amount of sugar in the blood.
hypo-	under, less than normal	*Hypoplasia* means underdevelopment of an organ or tissue. **Hypoglycemia** is a condition characterized by a below-normal amount of sugar in the blood.
multi-, poly-	many	A *multitude* means many or several. *Multipurpose* means serving many purposes. *Polyunsaturated* fats have many unsaturated chemical bonds. *Polysaccharides* are complex carbohydrates generally composed of many molecules of simpler sugars.
nulli-	none	The word *null* means having no value, amounting to nothing, or equal to zero.
pan-	all	**Pandemic** means occurring throughout (i.e., affecting all) the population of a country, people, or the world.
primi-	first	*Primary* means standing first in rank or importance.
super-, ultra-	excessive	**Supervitaminosis** is a condition resulting from excessive ingestion (swallowing or taking by mouth) of vitamins. *Ultraviolet* (UV) describes light beyond the visible spectrum at its violet end. UV rays cause sunburn and skin tanning but are also used in the diagnosis and treatment of disease (Fig. 3.4).

Use the electronic flashcards on the Evolve site or make your own set of flashcards using the above list. Select the word parts just presented and study them until you know their meaning. Do this each time a set of word parts is presented.

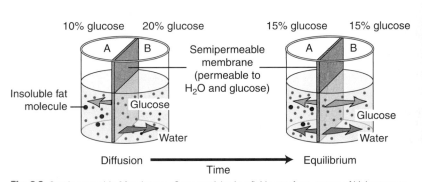

Fig. 3.3 Semipermeable Membrane. Some particles in a fluid move from an area of higher concentration to an area of lower concentration, but other particles cannot move across the membrane because of size, charge, or solubility. **semi-** = partly

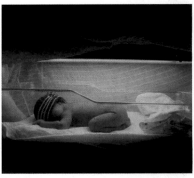

Fig. 3.4 Baby Receiving Ultraviolet Therapy. This treatment, sometimes called a bililight, is used to treat increased bilirubin in newborns. **ultra-** = beyond

MATCH IT!

EXERCISE 1

Match the prefixes in the left column with their meaning in the right column (a choice may be used more than once).

_____ 1. bi-	**A.** one
_____ 2. di-	**B.** two
_____ 3. centi-	**C.** three
_____ 4. milli-	**D.** four
_____ 5. mono-	**E.** one hundred or 1/100
_____ 6. quad-	**F.** 1/1000
_____ 7. tri-	
_____ 8. uni-	

*Use Appendix III, Answers, to check all your answers to the exercises in Chapter 3.

FIND IT!

EXERCISE 2

Find the prefix in each of these terms. Write each prefix and its meaning.

	Prefix	Meaning
1. diplopia	_____	_____
2. hyperglycemia	_____	_____
3. hemisphere	_____	_____
4. hypodermic	_____	_____
5. pandemic	_____	_____
6. polysaccharides	_____	_____
7. primary	_____	_____
8. quadriplegic	_____	_____
9. semipermeable	_____	_____
10. supervitaminosis	_____	_____
11. tetrahedron	_____	_____
12. ultraviolet	_____	_____

Prefixes: Position or Direction

Commit the meanings of the prefixes in the following table to memory. Familiar words are also listed to help you remember the prefixes.

Prefix
dia-

PREFIXES: POSITION OR DIRECTION

Prefix	Meaning	Word Association
ab-	away from	*Abduct* means to carry away by force or to draw away from a given position.
ad-	toward	In drug *addiction* (now called *chemical dependency*), one is "drawn toward" a habit-forming drug. In other words, one has a compulsive physiologic need for a certain drug.
ante-, pre-	before in time or in place	An *anteroom* is an outer room that is generally entered before a more important room.
		Prerenal pertains to the area in front of (literally, "before in place") the kidney.

PREFIXES: POSITION OR DIRECTION—cont'd

Prefix	Meaning	Word Association
circum-, peri-	around	The *perimeter* is the outer boundary or the line that is drawn around the outside of an area. The *circumference* is the line that is drawn around a circle.
contra-	against or opposed	**Contralateral** means affecting the opposite side.
dia-	through	The *diameter* passes through the center of a circle.
ecto-, ex-, exo-, extra-	outside, without, away from	To *export* is to carry or send away to another place. The skeletons of some animals, such as insects, are on the outer surface and are called *exoskeletons*. Extranuclear means outside a nucleus.
en-, end-, endo-	inside	*Enclose* means to close up inside something, hold in, or include. **Endotracheal** means within the trachea.
epi-	above, on	An *epitaph* is often inscribed on the tombstone or above the grave of the person buried there.
hypo-, infra-, sub-	beneath, under	**Hypodermic** means pertaining to the area below the skin. A **subcutaneous** injection places a small amount of medication below the skin layer into the subcutaneous tissue. Four types of hypodermic injections are shown in Fig. 3.5.
inter-	between	An *interval* is a space of time between events.
intra-	within	*Intracollegiate* activities are those within a college or engaged in by members of a college. See Fig. 3.5 for explanations of the terms **intramuscular**, **intradermal**, and **intravenous**.
ipsi-	same	**Ipsilateral** means pertaining to or affecting the same side of the body. (Compare with contralateral, Fig. 3.6).
meso-, mid-	middle	The **mesoderm** is the middle of three tissue layers that form during the development of an embryo.
para-	near, beside, or abnormal	Two *parallel* lines run beside each other.
per-	through or by	To *perspire* is to excrete fluid through the pores of the skin. *Permeable* means allowing certain substances to pass through.
post-	after, behind	To *postdate* is to assign a date to something after the date it actually occurred, such as when one postdates a check. **Postnasal** means behind the nose.
retro-	behind, backward	*Retroactive* means extending back to a prior time or condition. *Retrospection* means looking backward in time or surveying the past.
super-, supra-	above, beyond	**Superficial** means on or near the surface (Fig. 3.7). **Suprarenal** pertains to a location above each kidney.
sym-, syn-	joined, together	A **syndrome** is a set of symptoms that occur together and collectively characterize a particular disease or condition. In *symbiosis*, two organisms of different species beneficially coexist.
trans-	across	A **transdermal** drug is one that can be absorbed through (or across) unbroken skin, such as the nitroglycerin patch to relieve *angina pectoris*, chest pain caused by heart disease (Fig. 3.8).

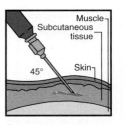 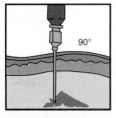 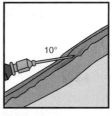 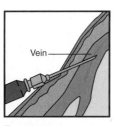

A subcutaneous   B intramuscular   C intradermal   D intravenous

Fig. 3.5 Using Prefixes in Naming Types of Injections. Note how the prefixes sub- and intra- are added to terms and used to describe the correct position of the needle. **A,** A subcutaneous injection places a small amount of medication (0.5 to 2 mL) below the skin layer into the subcutaneous tissue. The needle is inserted at a 45-degree angle. **B,** An intramuscular injection deposits medication into a muscular layer. As much as 3 to 5 mL may be administered in one injection; depending on the size of the patient, a needle 1 to 3 inches long is used. **C,** An intradermal injection places very small amounts into the outer layers of the skin with a short, fine-gauge needle. This type of injection is often used to test allergic reactions. **D,** An intravenous injection is used to administer medications directly into the bloodstream for immediate effect. A few milliliters of medication, or much larger amounts given over a long period, may be administered after venipuncture of the selected vein has been performed.
cutane/o, derm/a, = skin;   **muscul/o** = muscle;   **ven/o** = vein

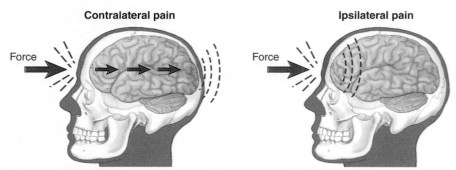

Fig. 3.6 Contralateral and Ipsilateral Are Opposites. If an injury to the forehead causes pain in the back of the skull, that's contralateral pain; however, if the same injury causes pain in the front of the skull, that's ipsilateral pain.

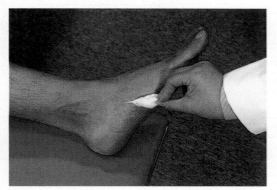

Fig. 3.7 Testing for Superficial Tactile Sensation. Superficial sensation is the perception of feelings in the superficial layers of the skin, responding in this case to the slight touch of a cotton ball.

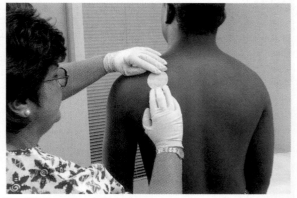

Fig. 3.8 Transdermal Drug Delivery. Application of a nitroglycerin patch. **trans-** = across;   **derm/a** = skin

WRITE IT!

EXERCISE 3

Write answers in the blank lines to complete the sentences. (Although an answer may require more than one word, it is represented by one blank line.)

1. The prefix ab- means _____, but ad- means _____.
2. Postnasal pertains to the region _____ the nose.
3. Two prefixes that have opposite meanings are endo- and ecto-, which mean _____ and _____, respectively.
4. Inter- means _____, and intra- means _____.
5. Suprarenal glands are located _____ each kidney.
6. An intravenous injection administers medication directly into or _____ the bloodstream.
7. Contra- means _____ or opposed.
8. Infra- means _____ or under.
9. Ipsilateral means pertaining to or affecting the _____ side.
10. Mid- means _____.
11. Para- means _____, beside, or abnormal.
12. Both intramuscular injections and intradermal injections deliver medication into (in other words, _____) the muscle and outer layers of the skin, respectively.
13. Abduction means drawing _____ from a given position.
14. Extranuclear means _____ the nucleus.
15. Endotracheal means _____ the trachea.

FIND IT!

EXERCISE 4

Find the prefix in each of these terms. Write each prefix and its meaning.

	Prefix	Meaning
1. circumference	_____	_____
2. diameter	_____	_____
3. exoskeleton	_____	_____
4. endotracheal	_____	_____
5. epitaph	_____	_____
6. hypodermic	_____	_____
7. mesoderm	_____	_____
8. perimeter	_____	_____
9. perspire	_____	_____
10. prerenal	_____	_____
11. retroactive	_____	_____
12. subcutaneous	_____	_____
13. supernormal	_____	_____
14. syndrome	_____	_____
15. transdermal	_____	_____

Miscellaneous Prefixes

The following list contains additional prefixes that you should commit to memory. Their meanings should be easy to remember because many of them are used in every-day language.

Note that some prefixes have more than one meaning and may pertain to two classifications, such as position and time. Two examples are ante- and post-, which you also saw in the prefixes related to position.

MISCELLANEOUS PREFIXES

Prefix	Meaning	Word Association
Related to Description		
anti-, contra-	against	An *antiperspirant* acts against perspiration. A **contraceptive** acts against or prevents conception (the beginning of pregnancy). **Contralateral** means affecting the opposite side (see Fig. 3.6). (The *i* in anti- is sometimes dropped before a vowel.)
brady-	slow	**Bradycardia** means a decreased pulse rate, but its literal translation is "a slow heart condition" (Fig. 3.9).
dys-	bad, difficult, disordered	Reading is very difficult when one has **dyslexia**. This disorder is thought to be an inability to organize written symbols.
eu-	good, normal	**Euthanasia** is "mercy killing," thought by some to be a good, painless death when a person has a terminal, intolerably painful condition.
mal-	bad, abnormal	*Maladjusted* means poorly or badly adjusted.
pro-	favoring, supporting	To *prolong* is to make something longer; in other words, to support making it longer.
tachy-	fast	**Tachycardia** means an increased pulse rate, but its literal translation is "a fast heart condition" (see Fig. 3.9).

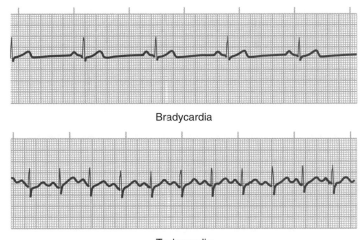

Bradycardia

Tachycardia

Fig. 3.9 Bradycardia and Tachycardia Are Opposites. A graphic record of the heartbeats (an electrocardiogram) shows many abnormalities, including abnormal slowness (bradycardia) and an increased rate (tachycardia). Each record represents slightly more than 6 seconds of heart activity.
brady- = slow;   **tachy-** = fast

MISCELLANEOUS PREFIXES—cont'd

Prefix	Meaning	Word Association
Related to Time		
ante-, pre-, pro-	before	**Antepartum** means before childbirth. *Premarital* means existing or occurring before marriage. *Proactive* involves taking action before an anticipated event or occurrence.
post-	after or behind	**Postpartum** means after childbirth.
Related to Size		
macro-, mega-, megalo-	large or great	**Macroscopic** structures are large enough to be seen by the naked eye. A **megadose** is a dose that greatly exceeds the usual prescribed amount. **Megalomania** is an abnormal mental state characterized by delusions of greatness.
micro-	small	A **microscope** is used to view very small objects.
Related to Negation		
a-, an-	no, not, without	*Rule:* Use a- before a consonant. Use an- before a vowel and often the letter h. **Asymptomatic** means without symptoms. *Anesthesia* means without feeling.
in-	not or inside (in)	*Inconsistent* means not consistent. *Inhale* means "to breathe in."
non-	not	A **noncancerous** tumor is not malignant.

MATCH IT! EXERCISE 5

Match the prefixes in the left columns with their meanings in the right column (a choice may be used more than once).

_____ 1. dys-
_____ 2. tachy-
_____ 3. brady-
_____ 4. anti-
_____ 5. in-
_____ 6. mal-
_____ 7. a-

_____ 8. contra-
_____ 9. eu-
_____ 10. an-
_____ 11. pro-
_____ 12. ante-
_____ 13. post-
_____ 14. macro-

A. after
B. against
C. bad
D. before
E. fast
F. favoring, supporting
G. good, normal
H. large
I. not
J. slow

MATCH IT! EXERCISE 6

Match the clues in the left column with prefixes in the right column.

_____ 1. opposite of post-
_____ 2. opposite of micro-

A. megalo-
B. non-
C. pre-

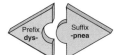

Recognizing Prefixes in Terms

You are now ready to recognize prefixes in terms. Several words in the following exercises contain prefixes that you have learned.

Write the prefix and its meaning for these new terms (Question 1 is done as an example).

Term/Meaning	Prefix	Meaning
1. **bradyphasia** slowness of speech	brady-	slow
2. **tachyphasia** fast speech		
3. **hypothyroidism** decreased activity of the thyroid gland		
4. **hyperthyroidism** increased activity of the thyroid gland		
5. **incontinence** not having **continence***		
6. **malabsorption** poor absorption		
7. **antacid** acts against acidity, especially an agent acting against acidity in the digestive tract		
8. **incompatible** not capable of uniting; not compatible		
9. **dysphonia** weak voice		
10. **contraindication** any condition that renders some particular form of treatment improper		
11. **anticonvulsive** agent that suppresses convulsions		
12. **para-appendicitis** inflammation of tissue adjacent to or near the appendix		
13. **parathyroids** small glands that lie near the thyroid gland, sometimes embedded within the gland		
14. **hyposecretion** less-than-normal secretion		
15. **hypersecretion** greater-than-normal secretion		
16. **euthyroid** pertaining to a normal (or normally functioning) thyroid gland		
17. **hypoparathyroidism** insufficient secretion of parathyroid glands		
18. **hyperparathyroidism** excessive activity of parathyroid glands		

FIND IT! EXERCISE 7

***Continence** is the ability to resist or control the urge to defecate or urinate.

Complete the sentences by writing in the blank a word or words that correspond to the underlined prefix.

1. **Unilateral** means _____ side of the body only, but **bilateral** means both (literally two) sides of the body.

2. **Primigravida** refers to a woman who is pregnant for the _____ time.

3. Translated literally, **hemiplegia** means paralysis of _____ of the body. In this case, it means one side of the body.

4. A **tripara** is a woman who has had _____ pregnancies that resulted in viable offspring. This can be viewed as births of live offspring but does not reflect the result of multiple births.

5. **Bifocal** means having _____ focal distances. In eyeglasses, the upper part of the lens is generally used for distant vision and the lower section for near vision.

6. A **nullipara** is a woman who has borne _____ children.

7. **Semiconscious** is being _____ aware of one's surroundings.

8. **Multicellular** means composed of _____ cells. **Unicellular** means made up of a single cell, such as bacteria (singular, bacterium).

9. **Polydipsia** literally means _____ thirsts. It actually means excessive thirst.

10. **Quadriplegia** is paralysis of all _____ extremities.

11. **Mononuclear** describes a cell that has how many nuclei? _____

12. The term **hypocalcemia** indicates something about the amount of calcium in the blood. It means that the amount of calcium is _____.

13. Translated literally, **macrocephaly** means _____ head. It actually means excessive size of the head.

14. **Hyperlipemia** means having an _____ amount of fat in the blood.

15. Multiple sclerosis is a chronic, progressive disease of the central nervous system characterized by destruction of the myelin sheaths of neurons (nerve cells). The damaged myelin sheaths deteriorate to scleroses (scler/o means hard), hardened scars, or plaques. The disorder is called multiple **sclerosis** because of the _____ scleroses formed on the neurons.

16. **Microorganisms** are _____ living organisms, usually microscopic, such as bacteria, rickettsiae, viruses, molds, yeasts, and protozoa (Fig. 3.10).

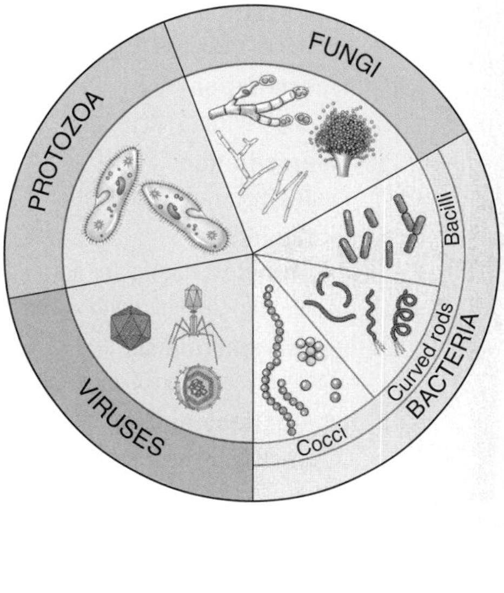

WRITE IT!

EXERCISE 8

Fig. 3.10 Types of Microorganisms. Organisms that have characteristics of both viruses and bacteria, such as Rickettsia, are not included here. (Organisms are not drawn to scale.)

Using Prefixes to Write Terms

Learn new terms by writing answers in the blank spaces in the next exercise. After you complete it, you will study additional combining forms in three groups: (1) combining forms that pertain to colors, (2) combining forms that have the same root as several common suffixes, and (3) miscellaneous combining forms.

WRITE IT! **EXERCISE 9**

Write a word in each blank space to complete the terms in this exercise.

1. Small flaps on certain valves of the heart are called cusps. If two flaps are present, the valve is called a **bicuspid** valve. If _____ flaps are present, the valve is called a **tricuspid** valve.

2. **Abduction** moves a bone or limb away from the midline of the body (Fig. 3.11); the muscle responsible is an **abductor**. **Adduction** moves a bone or limb toward the middle of the body (Fig. 3.11); thus an **adductor** is a muscle that draws a body part _____ the axis or midline of the body.

3. **Dermal** refers to the skin. Write a word that refers to a procedure that is performed through (literally, across) the skin: _____.

4. **Dysphasia** is _____ or impairment in speech.

5. Use a prefix with -kinesia to write a word that means an abnormal condition characterized by slowness of all voluntary movement: _____.

6. **Aerobic** means living only in the presence of oxygen; living without _____ is **anaerobic**.

7. Esthesia means feeling or sensation; partial or complete loss of sensation is _____.

8. **Febrile** refers to a fever; _____ fever is **afebrile**.

9. Hydrous means containing water; without or lacking _____ is **anhydrous**.

10. **Symptomatic** means of the nature of a symptom or concerning a symptom; "_____ symptoms" defines asymptomatic.

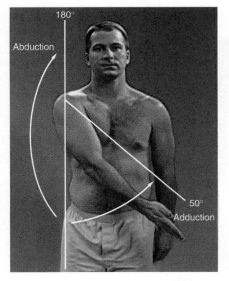

Fig. 3.11 Comparison of Abduction and Adduction. Abduction moves a bone or limb away from the midline of the body. Adduction moves a bone or limb toward the midline of the body.
ab- = away from;   **ad-** = toward

Combining
form
cyan/o

Combining Forms for Colors

Commit the combining forms for colors and their meanings in the following list to memory. Again, word association (familiar words derived from the same root) is included to facilitate learning the word parts.

COMBINING FORMS FOR COLORS

Combining Form	Meaning	Word Association
alb/o, albin/o, leuk/o (leuc/o)	white	An **albino** is an individual with congenital absence of pigment in the skin, hair, and eyes. The skin and hair appear white because of lack of pigment (Fig. 3.12). The Latin term *alba* means white. **Leukemia** is a malignant disease of the blood-forming organs characterized by a marked increase in the number of **leukocytes** (white blood cells), including immature leukocytes.
chlor/o	green	Chlorophyll is the green pigment contained in chloroplasts in the leaves of plants and is the reason that plants are green.
cyan/o	blue	Deficiency of oxygen in the blood can cause a condition called **cyanosis**, a slightly bluish, slatelike skin discoloration (Fig. 3.13).
erythr/o	red	**Erythrocytes** are red blood cells.
melan/o	black	A **melancholy** person is sad. In ancient times, people thought the bodies of melancholy persons produced a black bile that caused sadness. A melanoma is a malignant skin cancer (see Fig. 2.7, *B*).
xanth/o	yellow	Xanthophyll is a yellow pigment in plants. A condition called **jaundice** is often associated with a yellow appearance in the patient; however, it is derived from French and does not use xanth/o as a combining form. Jaundice is characterized by a yellowish discoloration of the skin (Fig. 3.14), mucous membranes, and white outer part of the eyeballs.

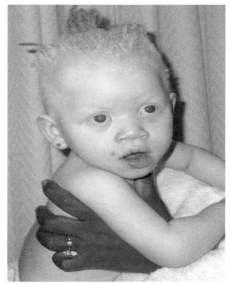

Fig. 3.12 Partial Albinism. The white hair and pale skin are characteristic of this condition; however, note the melanin pigment in the eyes. **albin/o** = white; **melan/o** = black

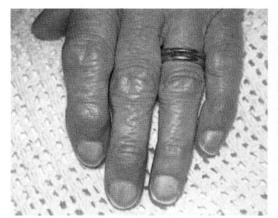

Fig. 3.13 Cyanosis. This bluish discoloration of the skin is caused by a deficiency of oxygen in the blood. Cyanosis is generally not as obvious as it is in this patient. **cyan/o** = blue

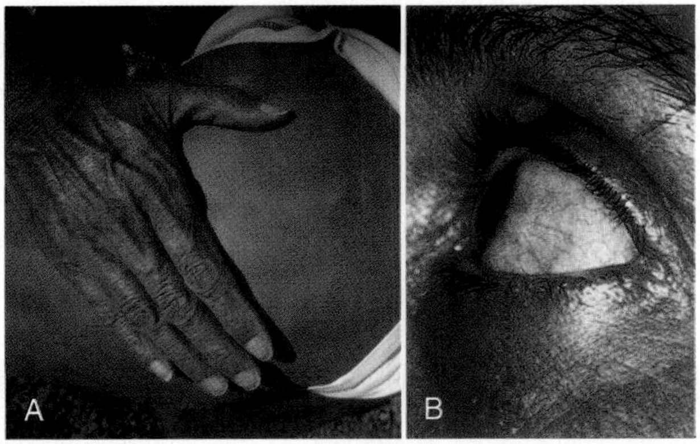

Fig. 3.14 Jaundice. **A,** Note the contrast between the examiner's hand and the yellow discoloration of the skin of a patient with a chronic liver disorder. **B,** The sclera (the white outer part of the eyeball) has become yellow.

WRITE IT!   EXERCISE 10

Write the meaning of each underlined word part in the blank spaces.

1. **erythrocytosis** _____ ; _____
2. **xanth osis** _____ ; _____
3. **melan oma** _____ ; _____
4. **leuko derma** _____ ; _____
5. **chlor opia** _____ ; _____
6. **albin ism** _____ ; _____
7. **cyano tic** _____ ; _____

WRITE IT!   EXERCISE 11

Write a word in each blank to complete the descriptions of these new terms.

1. **Antifebrile** means acting _____ fever or the drug that does so.
2. **Acyanotic** means _____ a blue skin discoloration.
3. **Melanocytes** are body cells capable of producing melanin, a _____ or dark brown pigment that naturally occurs in the hair and skin, for example.
4. A **multipara** is a _____ who has been pregnant more than once (literal translation, many).
5. **Hyperopia**, means farsightedness, the inability of the eye to focus on nearby objects. The literal translation of hyperopia is _____ vision.
6. Chlorophyll is the _____ pigment in plants.
7. Xanthophyll is the _____ pigment in plants.
8. Leukocytes are _____ blood cells.
9. Deficiency of oxygen in the blood can result in a slightly bluish appearance of the skin called _____ .
10. A term for red blood cells is _____ .
11. A malignant disease characterized by an increase in white blood cells is _____ .
12. A condition that is often associated with a yellow appearance of the skin is _____ .

Combining
form
gram/o

Combining Forms and Related Suffixes

Several combining forms have related suffixes that are frequently used in writing medical terms. Commit the following list to memory. All these suffixes are used to form nouns, with the exception of those ending in -ic and -tic. (The suffixes -genic, -lytic, -phagic, and -trophic are used to form adjectives, words that modify or describe nouns. The suffix -ic can also be used to form words with several of the combining forms presented.)

SELECT COMBINING FORMS AND RELATED SUFFIXES

Combining Form	Suffixes	Meaning
cyt/o	-cyte	cell
gen/o		beginning, origin (sometimes genes)
	-genic	produced by or in
	-genesis	producing or forming
gram/o		to record
	-gram	a record
	-graph	instrument for recording
	-graphy	process of recording
kinesi/o	-kinesia, -kinesis	movement, motion
leps/o	-lepsy	seizure
lys/o		destruction, dissolving
	-lysin	that which destroys
	-lysis	process of destroying
	-lytic*	capable of or producing destruction
malac/o		soft, softening
	-malacia	abnormal softening
megal/o		large, enlarged
	-megaly	enlargement
metr/o		measure, uterine tissue
	-meter	instrument used to measure
	-metry	process of measuring
path/o	-pathy	disease
phag/o		eat, ingest
	-phagia, -phagic, -phagy	eating, swallowing
phas/o	-phasia	speech
pleg/o	-plegia	paralysis
schis/o, schiz/o, schist/o	-schisis	split, cleft
scler/o		hard
	-sclerosis	hardening
scop/o		to examine, to view
	-scope	instrument used for viewing
	-scopy	process of examining visually
troph/o	-trophic, -trophy	nutrition

*Careful! Note the change in *s* to *t* in the spelling of -*lytic*.

WRITE IT!

EXERCISE 12

Write a word in each blank to complete these sentences. Several new word parts are introduced in this exercise.

1. An **electro+cardio+gram** (electr/o, electricity; cardi/o, heart) is a record (tracing) of the electrical impulses of the heart. **Electrocardiography** is the _____ of recording the electrical impulses of the heart, and an **electrocardiograph** is the _____ used (Fig. 3.15). The abbreviation for electrocardiogram is ECG (also EKG, from the German term).

2. A micro+scope is an instrument for viewing small objects that must be magnified so they can be studied. **Microscopy** is the _____ of viewing things with a microscope.

3. **Hemo+lysis** (hem/o, blood; lysis, destruction) is the destruction of red blood cells that results in the liberation of **hemoglobin**, a red pigment in the cells. The term for a substance that causes hemolysis is _____. **Hemolyze** is a verb that means to destroy red blood cells and cause them to release hemoglobin. **Hemolytic** substances cause hemolysis and are known as **hemolysins**.

4. Cephal/o means head. **Cephalo+metry** is measurement of the dimensions of the head (see Fig. 4.5). A device or instrument for measuring the head is a _____.

5. A **carcino+gen** is a substance or agent that produces cancer. The production or origin of cancer is called _____. A **carcinogenic** substance causes _____.

6. **Ophthalmo+pathy** is any _____ of the eye.

7. **Dys+trophic** muscle deteriorates because of defective nutrition or metabolism. A **dystrophy** is any disorder caused by defective metabolism or _____.

8. Ingestion is the act of eating (oral taking of substances into the body). Ingest means to _____.

9. Tele+kinesis is the concept of controlling _____ of an object by the powers of the mind.

10. An erythrocyte is a red (blood) _____.

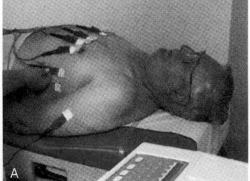

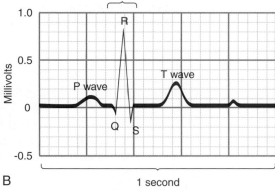

Fig. 3.15 Electrocardiography. **A,** Patient undergoing electrocardiography, the technique that produces graphic records of the electrical activity of the heart muscle. The instrument, an electrocardiograph, is shown. The electrical impulses given off by the heart are picked up by electrodes (sensors) and conducted into the electrocardiograph through wires. **B,** An enlarged section of the tracing called an *electrocardiogram*, or ECG. It represents the heart's electrical impulses, which are picked up and conducted to the electrocardiograph by electrodes or leads connected to the body. The pattern of the graphic recording indicates the heart's rhythm and other actions. The normal ECG is composed of the labeled parts shown in the drawing. Each labeled segment represents a different part of the heartbeat.

electr/o = electric;   **cardi/o** = heart;   **-graphy** = process of recording;   **-graph** = recording instrument;   **-gram** = a record

Write the meaning of the underlined word part in these new terms. A brief definition is provided for each term.

Term	Meaning of Word Part	Meaning of Term
1. <u>kinesio</u>therapy	_____	treatment through movement
2. osteo<u>malacia</u>	_____	softening of bone
3. dys<u>phagia</u>	_____	difficulty swallowing
4. cardio<u>megaly</u>	_____	enlarged heart
5. arterio<u>sclerosis</u>	_____	hardening of the arteries
6. <u>phago</u>cyte	_____	cell that ingests
7. a<u>phasia</u>	_____	inability to speak
8. quadri<u>plegia</u>	_____	paralysis of all four limbs
9. <u>schizo</u>phrenia	_____	psychosis with distortions of reality
10. dys<u>kinesia</u>	_____	difficulty in executing movement
11. <u>megalo</u>cyte	_____	large cell
12. rachi<u>schisis</u>	_____	split spine (spina bifida)

Combining
form
blast/o

Miscellaneous Combining Forms

Commit the following combining forms to memory.

MISCELLANEOUS COMBINING FORMS

Combining Form	Meaning	Word Association
aer/o	air	*Aeroplane* is the British spelling of airplane.
blast/o	embryonic form	The names of early (**embryonic**) forms have -blast endings. For example, embryonic bone cells are **osteoblasts**.
cancer/o, carcin/o	cancer	A **carcinoma** is a cancerous tumor.
cephal/o	head	**Cephalic** means pertaining to the head.
cry/o	cold	**Cryotherapy** uses cold temperatures to treat certain conditions.
crypt/o	hidden	A *cryptic* remark has a hidden meaning. A cryptogram is a message written in code, so it has a hidden meaning.
dips/o	thirst	*Polydipsia* means excessive thirst.
electr/o	electricity	Electr/o will be easy to remember because the combining form is contained in its meaning, electricity.
fibr/o	fiber	**Fibrous** means containing, consisting of, or resembling fiber.
hist/o	tissue	**Histocompatibility** is a measure of the compatibility of tissue of a donor and recipient.
myc/o	fungus	**Mycology** is a branch of botany that deals with fungi (plural of fungus).
narc/o	stupor	**Narcotics** are so named because they produce insensibility or stupor.
necr/o	dead	**Necrosis** is localized tissue death in response to disease or injury (see Fig. 12.17).
optic/o, opt/o	vision	**Optical** pertains to vision. An **optometrist** tests the eyes to measure visual acuity and prescribes corrective lenses, if necessary.
phon/o	voice	We hear someone's voice when we speak with that person by *phone*.
phot/o	light	Photography produces images on a film by the action of radiant energy, especially light.
py/o	pus	**Pyogenic** means "pus producing."

MISCELLANEOUS COMBINING FORMS—cont'd

Combining Form	Meaning	Word Association
therm/o	heat	*Thermal* clothing is designed to prevent loss of body heat.
top/o	position, place	*Topography* is often concerned with the making of maps or charts to show relative positions and elevations of a particular place or region.
trache/o	trachea (windpipe)	*Endotracheal* means within or through the trachea.

PROGRAMMED LEARNING

Remember to cover the answers (left column) with folded paper or the bookmark. Write an answer in each blank, and then check your answer before proceeding to the next frame.

large (enlarged)	1. A megalo+cyte is a large cell. (This term usually refers to an extremely large red blood cell.) You have learned that megalo- means _____.
red	2. You learned earlier that erythr/o means red. Translated literally, an erythro+cyte is a _____ cell. (This is an abbreviated way of saying red blood cell, a blood cell that carries oxygen.)
leukocyte	3. With erythro+cyte as a model, use leuk/o to write a word that means white cell (or white blood cell): _____.
cytoscopy	4. Combine cyt/o and the suffix that means process of visually examining to form a new word that means examination of cells: _____. (Congratulations if you answered this correctly. You can see that you really are learning medical terms. You might even have written a word that you've never seen before!)
cytology	5. Write a word that means the study of cells: _____.
black	6. A melan+oma, one type of skin cancer, is a malignant pigmented mole or tumor (see Fig. 2.6, *B*). Translated literally, a **melanoma** is a _____ tumor. Carcin+oma is a synonym for cancer. The combining form carcin/o means cancer, and -oma means tumor.
cancer	7. Carcino+gens are agents that cause _____.
psychogenesis	8. Change psycho+genic to a word that means the origin and development of the mind, or the formation of mental traits: _____.
formation	9. **Litho+genesis** is the _____ of stones, or calculi. A **calculus** is an abnormal concretion that forms within the body, such as a kidney stone (see Fig. 10.12).
dissolving (or destruction)	10. **Litho+lysis** means _____ of stones. Drinking large amounts of water can sometimes dissolve small stones in the bladder. A common surgical procedure crushes small stones using an instrument called a **lithotrite** or using ultrasonic energy from a source outside the body.
stones	11. **Lith+iasis** is a condition marked by the formation of _____.

sugar	12. **Glyco+lysis** is the breaking down of sugar by an enzyme in the body. In Chapter 2 you learned that glyc/o means _____. Most sugars that we consume are converted to **glyco+gen** and stored for future conversion into glucose, which is used for performing work. Sugars and starches (carbohydrates) are important in providing the body with energy. Glucose is the most important carbohydrate in metabolism because cells use glucose for energy.
fat (fatty)	13. **Lipids** are fats that are used by our bodies to store energy on a long-term basis. Fats also act as insulation against cold. You learned previously that lip/o means fat. A **lip+oma** is a benign tumor composed of _____ tissue (see Fig. 2.7, *A*).
destruction	14. Remembering that -lysis means dissolving or destruction, **electro+lysis** is _____ using an electric current. Electrolysis is sometimes used to remove unwanted hair.
electroencephalo-graphy	15. An **electro+encephalo+gram** (EEG) is a record produced by the electrical impulses of the brain. The process of recording the electrical impulses of the brain is _____ (Fig. 3.16).
electroencephalo-graph	16. Now write the name of the instrument used in electroencephalography: _____.
cephalometer	17. The combining form, encephal/o, is derived from en- (meaning inside) and cephal/o (meaning head). Cephalo+metry is measurement of the head. Change the suffix to write a word that means an instrument used to measure the head: _____.
light	18. Photo+graphy is the process of making images on sensitized material (film) by exposure to light or other radiant energy. What we call a photograph is actually a "photogram," but the picture is commonly called a photograph. Translated literally, **photo+phobia** is abnormal fear of _____. It means unusual sensitivity of the eyes to light. A person with measles may experience photophobia.
fear	19. **Necro+phobia** is abnormal _____ of death or dead bodies.

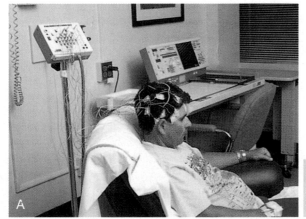
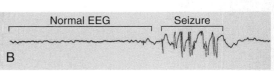

Fig. 3.16 Electroencephalography. **A,** In this technique that produces a graphic record of the electrical activity of the brain, electrodes are attached to various areas of the patient's head, and the patient generally remains quiet with the eyes closed during the procedure. In certain cases, prescribed activities may be requested. **B,** An electroencephalogram (EEG) showing a normal pattern, followed by seizure activity.

electr/o = electricity;   **encephal/o** = brain;   **-gram** = record;   **-graph** = process of recording

dead	20. Translated literally, necr+osis means a _____ condition. Necrosis is the death of areas of tissue or bone surrounded by healthy tissue.
fire	21. **Pyro+phobia** is abnormal fear of fire. You learned in Chapter 2 that pyr/o means _____.
fire	22. **Pyro+mania** is abnormal preoccupation with _____. A **pyromaniac** derives pleasure from seeing or setting fires.
fever	23. A **pyro+gen** is any substance that produces fever. In this new term, the meaning is implied. In an infection, pyrogenic bacteria produce or cause _____ in their *host*, the individual who is harboring the bacteria. **Pyrogenic** means producing fever. (Note: Be sure to distinguish between *pyogenic* and *pyrogenic*.)
producing	24. Using pyro+genic as a model, pyo+genic means _____ pus.
pus	25. **Pyo+derma** is any acute, inflammatory disease of the skin in which _____ is produced.
study	26. **Histo+logy** is the _____ of the structure, function, and composition of tissues.
histologist	27. Write a word that means one who specializes in histology: _____.
tissue	28. **Histo+logic** means pertaining to _____.
tissue	29. Histologic compatibility refers to _____ that is suitable for transplantation to another individual.
stupor	30. A narco+tic is a drug that produces insensibility or _____.
stupor	31. **Narco+lepsy** is a chronic ailment that consists of recurrent attacks of drowsiness and _____, or sleep.
seizure	32. You probably have heard of **epi+lepsy**, a brain disorder characterized by sudden, brief attacks of altered consciousness, motor activity, or sensory phenomena. Convulsive seizures are the most common form of these attacks, and this is the basis for the term epilepsy. The suffix -lepsy means _____.
thirst	33. **Poly+dips+ia** is a condition characterized by excessive _____. Translated literally, polydipsia means many thirsts.
place	34. The term *ectopic* results when ecto- is joined with top/o and -ic (note the omission of the syllable *to*). In an **ectopic** pregnancy, the embryo is implanted outside the uterus. In other words, the embryo is implanted outside the usual _____.
vision	35. An **optic+ian** specializes in the translation, filling, and adapting of prescriptions, products, and accessories for _____.
heat	36. **Hyper+therm+ia** is a serious condition in which the body temperature is greatly elevated because of retention of body _____.
hidden	37. **Crypt+orchid+ism** is a developmental defect in which the testicles remain in the abdominal cavity. Because the testes cannot be seen, they might be considered _____; thus the name cryptorchidism.
fiber	38. **Fibr+in** is the essential portion of a blood clot. By its name, we know that fibrin has the characteristic of a _____.

Write the combining forms and their meanings for these new terms. A short definition is provided for each term.

Term/Meaning	Combining Form(s)	Meaning of Combining Form(s)
1. **aerosol** suspension of fine particles in a gas or in the air	_____	_____
2. **aphonia** absence or loss of voice	_____	_____
3. **carcinogenesis** origin of cancer	_____	_____
4. **cryosurgery** destruction of tissue by extremely cold temperatures	_____	_____
5. **electrosurgery** surgery performed with high-frequency electric current	_____	_____
6. **erythroblast** embryonic form of red blood cell	_____	_____
7. **lithotripsy** surgical crushing of a stone	_____	_____
8. **mycodermatitis** skin inflammation caused by fungus	_____	_____
9. **necrotic** pertaining to the death of tissue	_____	_____
10. **psychogenic** originating in the mind	_____	_____
11. **pyogenesis** formation of pus	_____	_____
12. **sclerotic** hard; affected with sclerosis	_____	_____

! Be Careful With These!

in- (not) versus *in-* (inside)
infra- (under) versus *intra-* (within)
pro- (before) versus *pro-* (favoring, supporting)
py/o (pus) versus *pyr/o* (fire)

Similar Endings

-gram versus *-graph* versus *-graphy*
-meter versus *-metry*
-scope versus *-scopy*

Opposites

ab- (away from) versus *ad-* (toward)
ante-, pre- (before) versus *post-* (after)
en-, end-, endo- (inside) versus *ecto-, exo-, extra-* (outside)
hyper- (more than normal) versus *hypo-* (less than normal)
macro- (large) versus *micro-* (small)
nulli- (none) versus *pan-* (all)
super-, supra- (above) versus *hypo-, infra-, sub-* (below)

Reminder:
- Review the word parts and their meanings
- Work the Self-Test and check your answers
- Practice with the Q&E List, being sure you know the meaning and can spell and pronounce each term correctly
- Prepare for the test with QUICK CONNECT

A Career as a Histology Technician

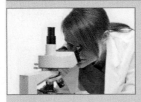

As a histology technician, Terre Cumberland prepares thin slices of tissue collected as biopsies for examination by a pathologist. Terre enjoys her work, knowing that how she prepares the samples gives crucial information to the physicians treating the patient. She plans to continue her education to become a histotechnologist, in which she will identify tissue structures and their staining characteristics and will have some supervisory responsibilities. The American Society for Clinical Pathology explains that a histotechnologist's expertise would qualify Terre to manage even unexpected situations in the laboratory, such as technical or instrument problems. For more information, visit the following website: http://www.ascp.org/content/careers/learn-about-careers.

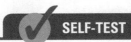 **SELF-TEST**

Work the following exercises to test your understanding of the material in Chapter 3. It is best to do all the exercises before checking your answers against the answers in Appendix III. Pay particular attention to spelling. If most of your answers are correct, you are ready to move on to Chapter 4.

A. MATCHING!   *Match the word parts in the left column with the meanings in the right column.*

_____ 1. blast/o	**A.** after
_____ 2. cry/o	**B.** bad or abnormal
_____ 3. crypt/o	**C.** before
_____ 4. kinesi/o	**D.** cold
_____ 5. lys/o	**E.** destruction
_____ 6. macro-	**F.** embryonic form
_____ 7. mal-	**G.** fast
_____ 8. post-	**H.** hidden
_____ 9. pro-	**I.** large
_____ 10. tachy-	**J.** movement

B. MATCHING!   *Match the terms in the left column with the colors suggested by the combining form.*

_____ 1. albinism	**A.** black
_____ 2. chloroplast	**B.** blue
_____ 3. cyanosis	**C.** green
_____ 4. erythrocyte	**D.** red
_____ 5. melancholy	**E.** white
_____ 6. xanthophyll	**F.** yellow

C. IDENTIFYING!

Label these illustrations using one of the following: albino, contralateral, cyanotic, electrocardiography, electroencephalography, ipsilateral, mononuclear, polydipsia.

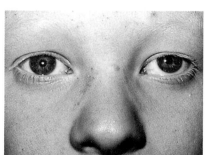

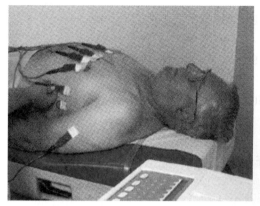

1. Person who has albinism _____

2. Process related to an ECG _____

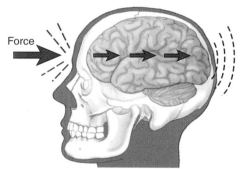

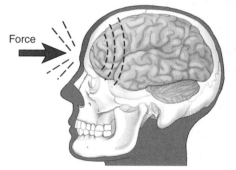

3. Affecting the opposite side _____

4. Affecting the same side _____

D. CHOOSING!

Circle the one correct answer (A, B, C, or D) for each question.

1. Which term means a white blood cell?
   (A) chlorocyte **(B)** erythrocyte **(C)** leukocyte **(D)** melanocyte

2. Which of the following means recording the electrical impulses of the brain?
   (A) electroencephalogram **(B)** electroencephalograph **(C)** electroencephalography **(D)** electroencephology

3. Which term means a substance that causes cancer?
   (A) cancerous **(B)** carcinogen **(C)** carcinogenic **(D)** carcinogenesis

4. Which term means an inflammation of the skin caused by a fungus?
   (A) cutaneous **(B)** dermatology **(C)** dermatosis **(D)** mycodermatitis

5. Which term means destruction of red blood cells resulting in the liberation of hemoglobin?
   (A) hemolysin **(B)** hemolysis **(C)** hemolytic **(D)** hemostasis

6. Which term means able to live without oxygen?
   (A) aerobic   (B) aerosol   (C) anaerobic   (D) a-aerobic

7. What does bradycardia mean?
   (A) decreased blood pressure   (B) decreased pulse rate   (C) increased blood pressure   (D) increased pulse rate

8. What is the term for any condition that renders some particular line of treatment improper?
   (A) antipathology   (B) contraindication   (C) continence   (D) incontinence

9. Which of the following specifically means a cell that can ingest and destroy particulate substances?
   (A) erythrocyte   (B) leukocyte   (C) melanocyte   (D) phagocyte

10. Which term means a fever-producing agent?
    (A) pyoderma   (B) pyogen   (C) pyrogen   (D) pyrophobia

E. HEALTH CARE REPORTING!   *Read the following Office Note. Then circle the correct answers to the questions that follow the note.*

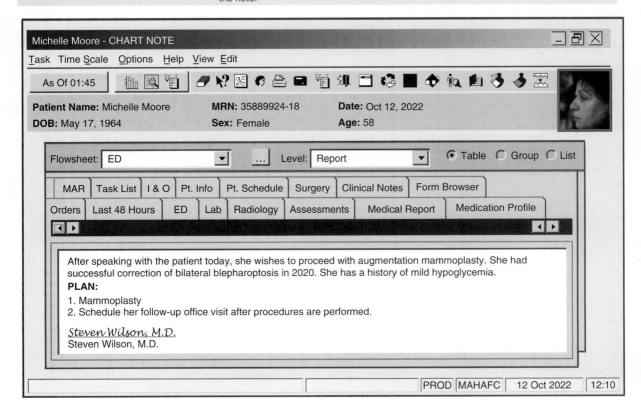

1. The organ(s) involved in mammoplasty is the (breast(s), ear, lips, nose).
2. The term "bilateral" refers to both (cells, colors, ears, sides).
3. The suffix in blepharoptosis means (cancerous, drooping, split, surgical fixation).
4. Blepharoptosis relates to which body part? (breast, ear, eyelid, head)
5. Hypoglycemia describes which of the following? (blood sugar, pulse, skin, vision)

F. WRITING!   *Write one-word terms for these meanings.*

1. difficult or weak voice   _____
2. malignant pigmented tumor   _____
3. increased amount of lipids in the blood   _____
4. composed of many cells   _____
5. excessive thirst   _____
6. increased pulse rate   _____
7. inside the trachea   _____
8. measurement of the head   _____
9. paralysis of one side of the body   _____
10. slowness of all body movement   _____

G. SPELLING AND PRONOUNCING!   *Circle all incorrectly spelled terms, and write their correct spelling. Pronounce all five terms.*

intramuscular   distrofy   opthalmopathy   pioderma   sindrome

H. QUICK CHALLENGE!   *Read the history from a health report and define the underlined terms.*

HISTORY: Stroke in Jan. 2013 with resulting <u>hemiplegia</u>, <u>dysphasia</u> and <u>dysphagia</u>; <u>narcolepsy</u> diagnosed in 2000; malignant <u>melanoma</u> diagnosed in Jan. 2015.

1. hemiplegia   _____
2. dysphasia   _____
3. dysphagia   _____
4. narcolepsy   _____
5. melanoma   _____

*Use Appendix III to check your answers.

QUICK & EASY (Q&E) LIST

Use the Evolve website (http://evolve.elsevier.com/Leonard/quick) to review the terms presented in Chapter 3. Look closely at the spelling of each term as it is pronounced.

abduction *(ab-**duk**-shun)*
abductor *(ab-**duk**-tor)*
acyanotic *(ā-sī-uh-**not**-ik)*
adduction *(uh-**duk**-shun)*
adductor *(uh-**duk**-tur)*
aerobic *(ār-ō-bik)*
aerosol *(**ār**-ō-sol)*

afebrile *(ā-**feb**-ril)*
albinism *(**al**-bi-niz-um)*
albino *(al-**bī**-nō)*
anaerobic *(an-uh-**rō**-bik)*
anhydrous *(an-**hī**-drus)*
antacid *(ant-**as**-id)*
antepartum *(an-tē-**pahr**-tum)*

QUICK & EASY (Q&E) LIST—cont'd

anticonvulsive (an-tē-kun-**vul**-siv)
antifebrile (an-tē-**feb**-ril)
aphasia (uh-**fā**-zhuh)
aphonia (ā-**fō**-nē-uh)
arteriosclerosis (ahr-tēr-ē-ō-skluh-**rō**-sis)
asymptomatic (ā-simp-tō-**mat**-ik)
bicuspid (bī-**kus**-pid)
bifocal (bī-**fō**-kul)
bilateral (bī-**lat**-ur-ul)
bradycardia (brad-ē-**kahr**-dē-uh)
bradyphasia (brad-i-**fā**-zhuh)
calculus (**kal**-kū-lus)
carcinogen (kahr-**sin**-uh-jen)
carcinogenesis (kahr-si-nō-**jen**-uh-sis)
carcinogenic (kahr-sin-ō-**jen**-ik)
carcinoma (kahr-si-**nō**-muh)
cardiomegaly (kahr-dē-ō-**meg**-uh-lē)
cephalic (suh-**fal**-ik)
cephalometer (sef-uh-**lom**-uh-tur)
cephalometry (sef-uh-**lom**-uh-trē)
chloropia (klor-**ōp**-ē-uh)
continence (**kon**-ti-nuns)
contraceptive (kon-truh-**sep**-tiv)
contraindication (kon-truh-in-di-**kā**-shun)
contralateral (kon-truh-**lat**-ur-ul)
cryosurgery (krī-ō-**sur**-jur-ē)
cryotherapy (krī-ō-**ther**-uh-pē)
cryptorchidism (krip-**tor**-ki-diz-um)
cyanosis (sī-uh-**nō**-sis)
cyanotic (sī-uh-**not**-ik)
cytology (sī-**tol**-uh-jē)
cytoscopy (sī-**tos**-kuh-pē)
dermal (**dur**-mul)
diplopia (di-**plō**-pē-uh)
dyskinesia (dis-ki-**nē**-zhuh)
dyslexia (dis-**lek**-sē-uh)
dysphagia (dis-**fā**-jē-uh)
dysphasia (dis-**fā**-zhuh)
dysphonia (dis-**fō**-nē-uh)
dystrophic (dis-**trō**-fik)
dystrophy (**dis**-truh-fē)
ectopic (ek-**top**-ik)
electrocardiogram (ē-lek-trō-**kahr**-dē-ō-gram)
electrocardiograph (ē-lek-trō-**kahr**-dē-ō-graf)
electrocardiography (ē-lek-trō-kahr-dē-**og**-ruh-fē)
electroencephalogram (ē-lek-trō-en-**sef**-uh-lō-gram)
electroencephalograph (ē-lek-trō-en-**sef**-uh-lō-graf)

electroencephalography (ē-lek-trō-en-sef-uh-**log**-ruh-fē)
electrolysis (ē-lek-**trol**-uh-sis)
electrosurgery (ē-lek-trō-**sur**-jur-ē)
embryonic (em-brē-**on**-ik)
endotracheal (en-dō-**trā**-kē-ul)
epilepsy (**ep**-i-lep-sē)
erythroblast (uh-**rith**-rō-blast)
erythrocyte (uh-**rith**-rō-sīt)
erythrocytosis (uh-rith-rō-sī-**tō**-sis)
euthanasia (ū-thuh-**nā**-zhuh)
euthyroid (ū-**thī**-roid)
febrile (**feb**-ril)
fibrin (**fī**-brin)
fibrous (**fī**-brus)
glycogen (**glī**-kō-jun)
glycolysis (glī-**kol**-uh-sis)
hemiplegia (hem-ē-**plē**-juh)
hemoglobin (**hē**-mō-glō-bin)
hemolysin (hē-**mol**-uh-sin)
hemolysis (hē-**mol**-uh-sis)
hemolytic (hē-mō-**lit**-ik)
hemolyze (**hē**-mō-līz)
histocompatibility (his-tō-kum-pat-i-**bil**-i-tē)
histologic (his-tō-**log**-ik)
histologist (his-**tol**-uh-jist)
histology (his-**tol**-uh-jē)
hyperglycemia (hī-pur-glī-**sē**-mē-uh)
hyperlipemia (hī-pur-lī-**pē**-mē-uh)
hyperopia (hī-pur-**ōp**-ē-uh)
hyperparathyroidism (hī-pur-par-uh-**thī**-roid-iz-um)
hypersecretion (hī-pur-sē-**krē**-shun)
hyperthermia (hī-pur-**thur**-mē-uh)
hyperthyroidism (hī-pur-**thī**-roid-iz-um)
hypocalcemia (hī-pō-kal-**sē**-mē-uh)
hypodermic (hī-pō-**dur**-mik)
hypoglycemia (hī-pō-glī-**sē**-mē-uh)
hypoparathyroidism (hī-pō-par-uh-**thī**-roid-iz-um)
hyposecretion (hī-pō-suh-**krē**-shun)
hypothyroidism (hī-pō-**thī**-roid-iz-um)
incompatible (in-kum-**pat**-i-bul)
incontinence (in-**kon**-ti-nuns)
intradermal (in-truh-**dur**-mul)
intramuscular (in-truh-**mus**-kū-lur)
intravenous (in-truh-**vē**-nus)
ipsilateral (ip-si-**lat**-ur-ul)
jaundice (**jawn**-dis)
kinesiotherapy (ki-nē-sē-ō-**ther**-uh-pē)

QUICK & EASY (Q&E) LIST—cont'd

leukemia *(lōō-**kē**-mē-uh)*
leukocyte *(**lōō**-kō-sīt)*
leukoderma *(lōō-kō-**dur**-muh)*
lipid *(**lip**-id)*
lipoma *(lip-**ō**-muh)*
lithiasis *(li-**thī**-uh-sĭs)*
lithogenesis *(lith-ō-**jen**-uh-sis)*
litholysis *(li-**thol**-i-sis)*
lithotripsy *(**lith**-ō-trip-sē)*
lithotrite *(**lith**-ō-trīt)*
macrocephaly *(mak-rō-**sef**-uh-lē)*
macroscopic *(mak-rō-**skop**-ik)*
malabsorption *(mal-ub-**sorp**-shun)*
megadose *(**meg**-uh-dōs)*
megalocyte *(**meg**-uh-lō-sīt)*
megalomania *(meg-uh-lō-**mā**-nē-uh)*
melancholy *(**mel**-un-kol-ē)*
melanocyte *(**mel**-uh-nō-sīt)*
melanoma *(mel-uh-**nō**-muh)*
mesoderm *(**mez**-ō-durm)*
microorganism *(mī-krō-**or**-gan-iz-um)*
microscope *(**mī**-krō-skōp)*
microscopy *(mī-**kros**-kuh-pē)*
mononuclear *(mon-ō-**nōō**-klē-ur)*
multicellular *(mul-tē-**sel**-ū-lur)*
multipara *(mul-**tip**-uh-ruh)*
mycodermatitis *(mī-kō-der-muh-t ī-tis)*
mycology *(mī-**kol**-uh-jē)*
narcolepsy *(**nahr**-kō-lep-sē)*
narcotic *(nahr-**kot**-ik)*
necrophobia *(nek-rō-**fō**-bē-uh)*
necrosis *(nuh-**krō**-sis)*
necrotic *(nuh-**krot**-ik)*
noncancerous *(non-**kan**-sur-us)*
nullipara *(nuh-**lip**-uh-ruh)*
ophthalmopathy *(of-thul-**mop**-uh-thē)*
optical *(**op**-ti-kul)*
optician *(op-**tish**-un)*
optometrist *(op-**tom**-uh-trist)*
osteoblast *(**os**-tē-ō-blast)*

osteomalacia *(os-tē-ō-muh-**lā**-shuh)*
pandemic *(pan-**dem**-ik)*
para-appendicitis *(par-uh-uh-pen-di-**sī**-tis)*
parathyroids *(par-uh-**thī**-roidz)*
phagocyte *(**fā**-gō-sīt)*
photophobia *(fō-tō-**fō**-bē-uh)*
polydipsia *(pol-ē-**dip**-sē-uh)*
postnasal *(pōst-**nā**-zul)*
postpartum *(pōst-**pahr**-tum)*
prerenal *(prē-**rē**-nul)*
primigravida *(prī-mi-**grav**-i-duh)*
psychogenesis *(sī-kō-**jen**-uh-sis)*
psychogenic *(sī-kō-**jen**-ik)*
pyoderma *(pī-ō-**dur**-muh)*
pyogenesis *(pī-ō-**jen**-uh-sis)*
pyogenic *(pī-ō-**jen**-ik)*
pyrogen *(**pī**-rō-jun)*
pyrogenic *(pī-rō-**jen**-ik)*
pyromania *(pī-rō-**mā**-nē-uh)*
pyromaniac *(pī-rō-**mā**-nē-ak)*
pyrophobia *(pī-rō-**fō**-bē-uh)*
quadriplegia *(kwod-ri-**plē**-juh)*
rachischisis *(rā-**kis**-ki-sis)*
schizophrenia *(skit-sō-**fren**-ē-uh)*
sclerosis *(skluh-**rō**-sis)*
sclerotic *(skluh-**rot**-ik)*
semiconscious *(sem-ē-**kon**-shus)*
subcutaneous *(sub-kū-**tā**-nē-us)*
superficial *(sōō-pur-**fish**-ul)*
supervitaminosis *(sōō-pur-vī-tuh-min-**ō**-sis)*
suprarenal *(sōō-pruh-**rē**-nul)*
symptomatic *(simp-tō-**mat**-ik)*
syndrome *(**sin**-drōm)*
tachycardia *(tak-i-**kahr**-dē-uh)*
tachyphasia *(tak-ē-**fā**-zhuh)*
transdermal *(trans-**dur**-mul)*
tricuspid *(trī-**kus**-pid)*
tripara *(**trip**-uh-ruh)*
unicellular *(ū-ni-**sel**-ū-lur)*
unilateral *(ū-ni-**lat**-ur-ul)*
xanthosis *(zan-**thō**-sis)*

Don't forget the games and other activities available at http://evolve.elsevier.com/Leonard/quick.

QUICK CONNECT

Review all lists of word parts and their meanings for Chapter 3 using the flashcards you prepared or the flashcards on the Evolve site.

A prefix is placed before a word to modify its meaning. Most prefixes, including those ending with a vowel, can be added to the remainder of the word without change.

Prefixes for numbers or quantities:

½ = hemi-, semi-

1 = mono-, uni-

2 = bi-, di-

3 = tri-

4 = quad-, quadri-, tetra-

100 (or one-hundredth) = centi-

1,000 = milli-

double = diplo-

hypo- (under or below) vs. hyper- (excessive, more than normal)

many = multi-, poly-

none = nulli-

all = pan-

first = primi-

excessive = super-, ultra-

Remember these opposites for position or direction:

ab- vs. ad-

ante-, pre- vs. post-

en-, end-, endo-, intra- vs. ecto-, ex-, exo-, extra-

sub- vs. super-, supra-

More opposites:

ante-, pre-, post- vs. anti-, contra- vs. pro-

brady- vs. tachy-

dys-, mal- vs. eu-

macro- vs. micro-

Prefixes related to negation: a-, an- (no, not, or without) vs. in- (not or inside) vs. non- (not)

Remember the meanings of these combining forms for colors: alb/o, albin/o, leuk/o vs. chlor/o vs. cyan/o, vs. erythr/o vs. melan/o, vs. xanth/o

Be sure to remember the meanings of these combining forms and their associated suffixes: cyt/o, gen/o, gram/o, kinesi/o, leps/o, lys/o, malac/o, metr/o, path/o, phag/o, phas/o, pleg/o, schist/o (schiz/o or schist/o), scler/o, scop/o, trop/o

Distinguish these similar looking terms:

adduction and adductor
asymptomatic and symptomatic
carcinogen, carcinogenesis, and carcinogenic
cephalic, cephalometer, and cephalometry
cryosurgery vs. electrosurgery
dystrophic and dystrophy
electrocardiogram, electrocardiograph, and electrocardiography
electroencephalogram, electroencephalograph, and electroencephalography
fiber and fibrin
hemolyze, hemolysis, hemolysin, hemolytic
histologic and histology
ingest and ingestion
lipid and lipoma
lithiasis, lithogenesis, litholysis, lithotripsy
microscope and microscopy
narcolepsy and narcotic
pyoderma and pyogenesis
pyromania, pyromaniac, and pyrophobia
pyrogen and pyrogenic
sclerosis and sclerotic
superficial, supervitaminosis, and suprarenal
tachycardia and tachyphasia

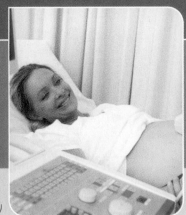

CHAPTER 4

Diagnostic Procedures and Therapeutic Interventions

(Ultrasound has many diagnostic applications, including fetal monitoring.)

CONTENTS

Signs and Symptoms in Diagnosis
Basic Examination Procedures
Common Diagnostic Tests and Procedures
Diagnostic Radiology

Radiation and Other Therapeutic Interventions
 SELF-TEST
QUICK & EASY (Q&E) LIST
QUICK CONNECT

OBJECTIVES

After completing Chapter 4, you will be able to:

1. Identify the difference between signs and symptoms.
2. List the vital signs and the four basic examination procedures.
3. Match diagnostic terms with their meanings.
4. Match therapeutic interventions with their meanings.
5. Write the meanings of Chapter 4 word parts, or match word parts with their meanings.
6. Build and analyze medical terms with Chapter 4 word parts.
7. Spell medical terms correctly.

When the body is in a healthy state, it functions normally, and the physical and chemical characteristics of the body substances are generally within a certain acceptable range, known as the *normal range.* The abbreviation WNL, meaning "within normal limits," is sometimes used to describe the results of a laboratory or other diagnostic test (e.g., range of motion). Pathologic means pertaining to a condition that is caused by or involves a disease process. When a pathologic condition exists, changes take place within the body and may cause an alteration in the physical and chemical characteristics of body substances, as evidenced by abnormal laboratory values or results.

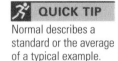
QUICK TIP
Normal describes a standard or the average of a typical example.

HEALTH CARE CONNECTION

The International Classification of Diseases (ICD) is used to code and classify diagnoses and mortality data from death certificates. Many countries use ICD, which was published in 1993 by the World Health Organization (WHO). Over the years, the system has been changed to allow its use not only in mortality (death) statistics, but also in reporting disease.

Medical professionals use Current Procedural Terminology (CPT) codes, which are numbers assigned to every service provided to the patient, including medical, surgical, and diagnostic services. The codes (i.e., 90658 indicates an influenza shot) are used on insurance forms by insurers to determine the amount of reimbursement and are maintained by the American Medical Association (AMA). Medical coders and physicians are familiar with both the ICD and CPT codes.

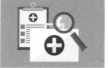

Signs and Symptoms in Diagnosis

An examiner looks for signs of change from what is expected in the normal range. A **symptom** is a change that is perceived by the patient, which may or may not be confirmed by the examiner, e.g., a headache. Another symptom, itching, may be accompanied by a rash, which is a sign that can be noted by an examiner. At times, the examiner may note a change from what is expected but has not been noted by the patient.

WORD ORIGIN

Physicians see, feel, hear, and smell signs (*signa* [L.], marks).

WORD ORIGIN

acute (*acutus* [L.], sharp); think of acute appendicitis.
chronic (*chronos* [G.], time); think of chronic alcoholism.

QUICK TIP

Blood, urine, sweat, and tears are examples of body fluids.

SIGNS VERSUS SYMPTOMS

Signs are objective, or definitive, evidence of an illness or disordered function that are perceived by an examiner, such as fever, a rash, or evidence established by radiologic or laboratory testing.
Symptoms (Sx) are subjective evidence as perceived by the patient, such as pain.

Diagnosis (Dx) is the identification of a disease or condition by a scientific evaluation of physical signs, symptoms, history, tests, and procedures. **Prognosis** means the predicted outcome of a disease.

A disease is often described as acute or chronic. **Acute** means having a short and relatively severe course. The opposite of acute is **chronic**, meaning that the disease exists over a long time.

Diagnostic terms are used to describe the signs and symptoms of disease and the tests used to establish a diagnosis. The tests include clinical studies (e.g., measuring blood pressure), laboratory tests (e.g., determination of blood gases), and **radio+logic** studies, which relate to the use of radiation (e.g., chest x-ray image). Laboratory (lab) tests, ranging from simple to sophisticated studies, identify and quantify substances to evaluate organ functions or establish a diagnosis. Various body fluids are collected and sent to the laboratory for testing, most often blood and urine. In addition, fluids are collected from various body cavities or wounds. A small sample or part taken from the body to represent the nature of the whole is called a **specimen**.

WRITE IT!*

EXERCISE 1

Write terms for these meanings.

1. descriptive of a disease with a short, relatively severe course _____
2. descriptive of a disease that exists over a long period _____
3. identification of a disease or condition by scientific evaluation _____
4. predicted outcome of a disease _____

*Use Appendix III, Answers, to check your answers to all the exercises throughout Chapter 4.

MATCH IT!

EXERCISE 2

Choose A or B from the right column to classify the items in the left column as a sign or a symptom.

_____ 1. blood pressure reading   A. sign
_____ 2. definitive evidence of a disease   B. symptom
_____ 3. subjective evidence perceived by a patient
_____ 4. itching
_____ 5. rash

Basic Examination Procedures

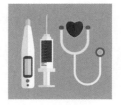

Basic examinations are performed to assess the patient's condition. Vital signs are measured and recorded for most patients. Vital signs are the measurements of pulse rate, respiration rate, and body temperature.

The **pulse** (sometimes abbreviated P) is the rhythmic expansion of an artery that occurs as the heart beats; it may be felt with a finger or measured electronically (Fig. 4.1). The pulse results from the expansion and contraction of an artery as blood is forced from the heart. The pulse rate is the count of the heartbeats per minute. A normal pulse rate in a resting state is 60 to 100 beats per minute.

Respiration (R) refers either to the exchange of oxygen and carbon dioxide within the body or to breathing. The respiration (or respiratory) rate is the number of breaths per minute. The rise and fall of the patient's chest is observed while counting the number of breaths and noting the ease with which breathing is accomplished.

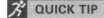

> **QUICK TIP**
> Normal respiration rate is 12 to 20 breaths/min for teenagers and adults.

Body temperature can be measured through several routes, including the mouth, the rectum, the armpit, and the external opening of the ear canal. T is the abbreviation for temperature. Thermo+meters are instruments used to measure temperature. Originally, a thermometer consisted of a sealed glass tube, marked in degrees Celsius or Fahrenheit, and contained a liquid such as mercury. The liquid rises or falls as it expands or contracts according to changes in temperature. Electronic measurement of body temperature has reduced the time required for accurate readings. Some devices for electronic temperature measurement have a probe that is covered by a disposable sheath and placed under the tongue with the mouth tightly closed, in the rectum, or under the arm with the arm held close to the body (Fig. 4.2). The **tympanic thermometer** has a specially designed probe tip that is placed at the external opening of the ear canal. The temporal artery scanner and the forehead thermometer are especially useful for taking temperatures of young children and babies.

> **therm/o** = heat (also used to write terms about temperature)
> **-meter** = instrument used to measure

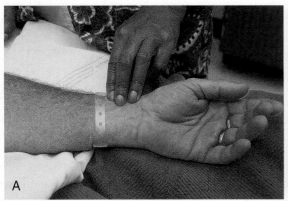
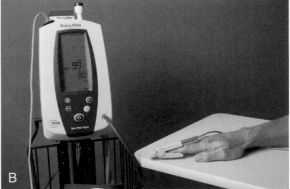

Fig. 4.1 Assessment of the Radial Pulse. **A,** The pulse is an intermittent throbbing sensation felt when the fingers are pressed against an artery, such as the radial artery. Radi/o sometimes means radiant energy, but in this case it is used to mean *radius*, a bone of the forearm, for which the artery is named. **B,** Pulse can also be monitored electronically using a special clip-like device on the fingertip or earlobe. The oximeter shown indicates a blood oxygen level of 99 and a pulse rate of 90.

radi/o = radius or radiant energy

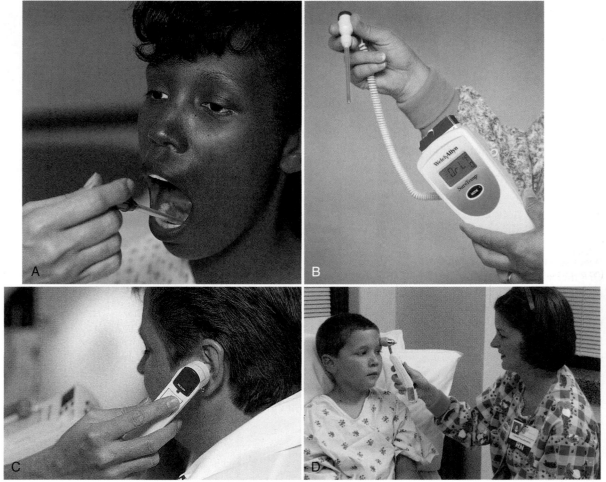

Fig. 4.2 Devices for Temperature Measurement. **A,** The original oral thermometer, which sometimes is used in homes, contains a liquid that expands or contracts according to changes in temperature. **B,** A thermometer for measuring temperature orally, rectally, or under the arm. **C,** A tympanic membrane thermometer, which uses a probe placed in the ear. **D,** A temporal artery thermometer works well for babies and small children.
or/o = mouth;   **rect/o** = rectum;   **therm/o** = heat

VITAL SIGNS

Vital signs actually include only the measurements of pulse rate, respiration rate, and body temperature. However, they can vary and sometimes include other measurements. Although not strictly a vital sign, blood pressure is customarily included. For more information about vital signs, visit https://www.nlm.nih.gov/medlineplus/ency/article/002341.htm

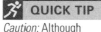 **QUICK TIP**

Caution: Although sometimes included, blood pressure is not strictly a vital sign.

Blood pressure (BP) is the pressure exerted by the circulating volume of blood on the walls of the arteries and veins and on the chambers of the heart. Indirect measurement of blood pressure is made with a stethoscope and a blood pressure cuff. The readings generally consist of two numbers expressed as a fraction, with the first number representing the maximum pressure on the artery and the second number representing the amount of pressure that still exists when the heart is relaxed (in other words, not contracting). The standard unit of measurement is millimeters of mercury (mm Hg). For example, a healthy adult has a blood pressure of approximately 120/80 mm Hg.

The higher reading is the **systolic pressure**, and the lower reading is the **diastolic pressure** (Fig. 4.3). The pressure in both arms is sometimes taken to check for differences in the two readings.

WORD ORIGIN

systole (G.), contraction

QUICK CASE STUDY | EXERCISE 3

Louis feels weak and uses a home blood pressure apparatus. His blood pressure is shown in Fig. 4.3F. Write either "systolic" or "diastolic" to complete the sentences.

1. The value 147 in Fig. 4.3F represents the _____ pressure.
2. The value 77 in Fig. 4.3F represents the _____ pressure.

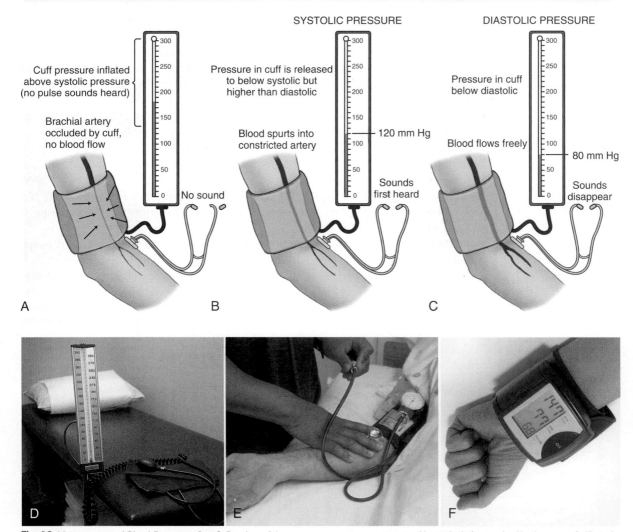

Fig. 4.3 Measurement of Blood Pressure. **A** to **C,** Drawings of the mercury manometer apparatus, an older method of measuring blood pressure, facilitate the understanding of blood pressure readings. **A,** No sounds are heard because the pressure in the cuff is higher than the systolic pressure. **B,** The first sound heard (a systolic pressure of 120 mm Hg) is noted. **C,** The last sound heard (80 mm Hg) represents the diastolic pressure. This example represents a normal blood pressure reading of 120/80 mm Hg (the height of mercury in a graduated column on the blood pressure apparatus). **D** to **F,** Three types of instruments for indirect measurement of blood pressure: mercury, aneroid, and automatic digital. **D,** This type of apparatus has been used in healthcare for more than a century. **E,** Aneroid types have an easy-to-read dial, and wall-mounted models are recommended because mechanical jarring may result in less accurate readings. **F,** An automatic digital instrument that a person can use at home.

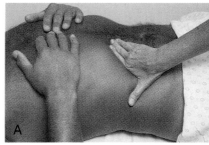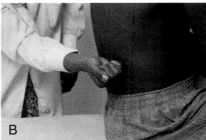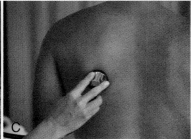

Fig. 4.4 Three Aspects of the Physical Examination. **A,** Palpation. **B,** Percussion. **C,** Auscultation with a stethoscope aids in assessment of the internal organs.

A person's history is a record of past events and factors that may have a bearing on one's present condition. The history of present illness is obtained by the medical professional from the patient regarding the onset, duration, and character of the present illness.

The history and physical examination, an investigation to determine the state of health, become part of a patient's medical record. The following four techniques are useful in the physical examination:

- **Inspection**. The examiner uses the eyes and ears to observe and listen to the patient. Inspection could reveal superficial abnormalities, such as a rash.
- **Palpation**. The examiner feels the texture, size, consistency, and location of certain body parts with the hands (Fig. 4.4, *A*). Palpation sometimes reveals deep abnormalities, such as an enlarged liver.
- **Percussion**. The examiner taps the body with the fingertips or fist to evaluate the size, borders, and consistency of internal organs and to determine the amount of fluid in a body cavity (Fig. 4.4, *B*).
- **Auscultation**. The examiner listens for sounds within the body to evaluate the heart, blood vessels, lungs, intestines, or other organs, or to detect the fetal heart sound. Auscultation is performed most frequently with a stethoscope (Fig. 4.4, *C*). A **stethoscope** is an instrument consisting of two earpieces connected by flexible tubing; the diaphragm is placed against the patient's skin to hear sounds within the body.

steth/o = chest
-scope = instrument
used for viewing

WRITE IT!
EXERCISE 4

Write an answer in each blank to complete these sentences.

1. The rhythmic expansion of an artery that occurs as the heart beats is called the

   _____.

2. Counting the number of breaths per minute measures the _____ rate.

3. An electronic instrument that measures body temperature by placing the probe at the opening of the external ear is called a tympanic _____.

4. Blood pressure is represented as a fraction, with the higher reading representing the _____ pressure.

5. Application of the fingers with light pressure to the surface of the body during physical examination is called _____.

6. Tapping the body with the fingertips or fist during physical examination is _____.

7. Listening for sounds within the body using a stethoscope is called _____.

Common Diagnostic Tests and Procedures

The diagnostic process helps determine a patient's health status. You have already studied several tests and procedures that aid in this process. Laboratory analyses of blood, urine, and stool specimens, along with diagnostic radiology (presented in the next section), assist the physician in establishing a diagnosis. Work the following exercises to review the word parts and terms from previous chapters.

MATCH IT!
EXERCISE 5

Match the following suffixes with their meanings.

_____ 1.   -gram
_____ 2.   -graph
_____ 3.   -graphy
_____ 4.   -meter
_____ 5.   -metry
_____ 6.   -scope
_____ 7.   -scopy

A. a record
B. instrument for recording
C. instrument used in a visual examination
D. instrument used to measure
E. process of measuring
F. process of recording
G. visual examination with a lighted instrument

WRITE IT!
EXERCISE 6

Write terms for these diagnostic instruments and procedures, which you studied in Chapter 3.

1. instrument used to record the electrical impulses of the heart   _____
2. recording the electrical impulses of the heart (see Fig. 3.15)   _____
3. the record produced in electrocardiography   _____
4. measurement of the dimensions of the head (Fig. 4.5)   _____
5. instrument used to examine the eye   _____
6. examination of the eye with an ophthalmoscope (Fig. 4.6)   _____
7. instrument for viewing microscopic objects   _____
8. visual examination of the ear (see Fig. 2.17)   _____

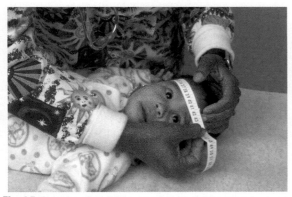

Fig. 4.5 Cephalometry. Appropriate placement of the measuring tape to obtain the head circumference of an infant.
cephal/o = head; **-metry** = measurement

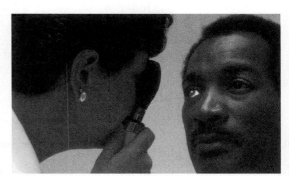

Fig. 4.6 Ophthalmoscopy. Proper technique for visually examining the interior of the eye with an ophthalmoscope.
ophthalm/o = eye; **-scopy** = visual examination

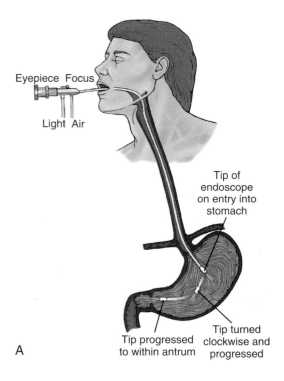

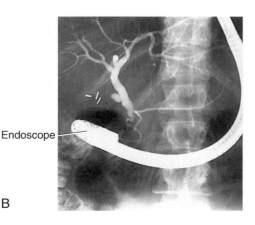

Fig. 4.7 Example of a Flexible Endoscope. **A,** This endoscope is being used to examine the interior of the stomach through the esophagus. Depending on the structure to be examined, the physician chooses either a flexible or a rigid endoscope. Most of the interior stomach can be examined, including the antrum, located in the lower part of the stomach. **B,** A radiographic view of the placement of the endoscope.

endo- = inside
-scope = instrument for viewing

An **endo+scope** is an illuminated instrument for the visualization of the interior of a body cavity or organ (Fig. 4.7). Although the endoscope is generally introduced through a natural opening (e.g., mouth, rectum), it may also be inserted through an incision, such as into the chest cavity through an incision in the chest wall. The visual inspection of the body by means of an endoscope is **endoscopy**. **Endo+scop+ic** means pertaining to endoscopy or performed using an endoscope.

A **catheter** is a hollow flexible tube that can be inserted into a cavity of the body to withdraw or instill fluids, perform tests, or visualize a vessel or cavity. The introduction of a catheter is **catheterization** and to introduce a catheter is to **catheterize** (Fig. 4.8). The Latin term **cannula** is also used to mean a hollow, flexible tube that is inserted into vessels or cavities.

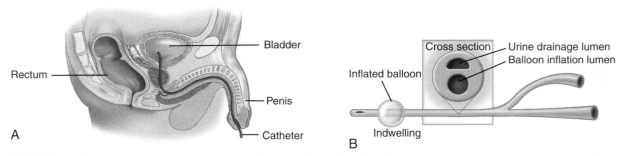

Fig. 4.8 Urinary Catheter. **A,** The most common route of catheterization is insertion of the catheter through the external opening of the urethra and into the bladder. This procedure is done to drain or remove fluid from the bladder or to introduce fluids for various tests or treatments. **B,** A Foley catheter has a balloon tip that is filled with a sterile liquid after it has been placed in the bladder. This is a type of indwelling catheter and is used when continuous draining is desired. Lumen means a tubular space or channel within a structure.

WRITE IT! EXERCISE 7

Write terms for these meanings.

1. visual inspection of the body using an endoscope _____
2. the process of inserting a catheter into the body _____
3. to introduce a catheter into the body _____
4. a hollow flexible tube; catheter _____

Diagnostic Radiology

Radiology is the branch of medicine concerned with x-rays, radioactive substances, and the diagnosis and treatment of disease by using any of the various sources of radiant energy. Several of these procedures are noninvasive, whereas an **invasive procedure** requires entry of a body cavity (e.g., cardiac catheterization) or interruption of normal body function (e.g., surgical incision).

Diagnostic radiology is used to establish or confirm a diagnosis. Digital radiography uses a computer to store and manipulate radiographic data. For example, in **computed radiography**, the image data are converted to electronic signals, digitized, and immediately displayed on a monitor or recorded on film.

Learn the word parts pertaining to radiology and their meanings.

radi/o = radiant energy
-graphy = process of recording

WORD PARTS: RADIOLOGY

Combining Form	Meaning
ech/o, son/o	sound
electr/o	electricity
fluor/o	emitting or reflecting light
radi/o*	radiant energy
tom/o	to cut
Prefix	
ultra-	excessive

Use the electronic flashcards on the Evolve site or make your own set of flashcards using the above list. Select the word parts just presented, and study them until you know their meaning.

*Sometimes means *radius*, a bone of the forearm.

FIND IT! EXERCISE 8

Find the combining forms used in these terms, and write the combining form and its meaning.

	Combining Form	Meaning
1. **echogram**	_____	_____
2. **fluoroscope**	_____	_____
3. **radiography**	_____	_____
4. **tomogram**	_____	_____
5. **ultrasonography**	_____	_____

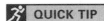
Radio+graphy was the predominant means of diagnostic imaging for many years, with x-rays providing image data (film) of internal structures. An x-ray image is a **radio+graph**; however, the suffix -graph refers to an instrument used for recording. The radiograph is made by projecting x-rays through organs or structures of the body onto a digital image receptor. X-rays that pass through the patient expose the digital image receptor to create the image. X-radiation passes through different substances in the body to varying degrees. Where penetration is greater, the image is black or darker; where the x-rays are absorbed by the subject, the image is white or light gray. Thus, air appears black, fat appears dark gray, muscle tissue appears light gray, and bone appears very light or white. Very dense substances, such as lead or steel, appear white because they absorb the rays and prevent them from reaching the image receptor (Fig. 4.9).

Substances that do not permit the passage of x-rays are described as **radiopaque**. **Radiolucent** describes substances that readily permit the passage of x-rays.

Additional diagnostic imaging modalities include the following:
- Computed tomography (CT)
- Magnetic resonance imaging (MRI)
- Sono+graphy, also called **echo+graphy**, ultra+sono+graphy, and **ultra+sound**
- Contrast imaging
- Nuclear imaging (placing radioactive materials into body organs for the purpose of imaging)

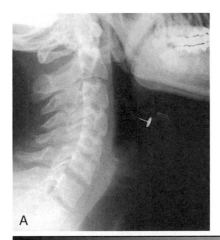

Fig. 4.9 Penetration of X-radiation by Various Substances in an X-ray Image. **A,** Radiograph of an aspirated thumbtack. The lodged tack appears white because it absorbs most of the x-rays and prevents them from reaching the image receptor. Note also the different appearances of air, soft tissue, bone, and teeth. **B,** Schematic representation of how substances appear on an x-ray image, depending on the amount of x-radiation the substance absorbs.

Computed tomography uses ionizing radiation to produce a detailed image of a cross section of tissue, similar to what one would see if the body or body part were actually cut into sections. The procedure, however, is painless and noninvasive. Fig. 4.10 shows a CT (or CAT) scanner and a **tomogram**, the record produced.

Magnetic resonance imaging creates images of internal structures based on the magnetic properties of chemical elements within the body and uses a powerful magnetic field and radio wave pulses rather than ionizing radiation such as x-rays. MRI produces superior soft tissue resolution for distinguishing adjacent structures (Fig. 4.11). Patients must remain motionless for a time and may experience anxiety because of being somewhat enclosed inside the scanner. Open MRI scanners have eliminated much of the anxiety and can accommodate larger patients.

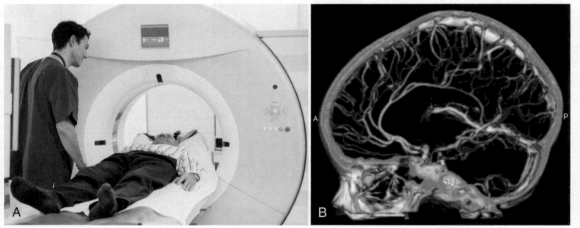

Fig. 4.10 Computed Tomography (CT) of the Brain. **A,** Positioning of a patient for CT. **B,** CT image of the blood vessels of the brain after injection of a contrast dye.
tom/o = to cut;   **-graphy** = process of recording

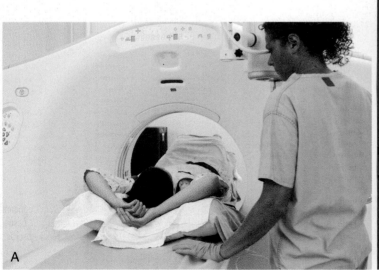
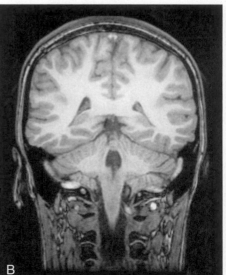

Fig. 4.11 Magnetic Resonance Imaging (MRI). **A,** MRI scanner. **B,** MR image of the head.

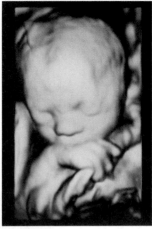

ultra- = beyond
son/o = sound
-graphy = process of
recording

Fig. 4.12 Three-Dimensional Sonogram of a Fetus. This three-dimensional ultrasound image shows a normal fetal face in late pregnancy. Sonograms provide important information to the obstetrician and pictures for the parents as the fetus develops.

ultra- = beyond
son/o = sound
-gram = process of
recording

Also called **ultrasonography**, *ultrasound imaging*, and other names, **sonography** is the process of imaging deep structures of the body by sending and receiving high-frequency sound waves that are reflected back as echoes from internal tissues and structures. Conventional sonography provides two-dimensional images, but the more recent scanners are capable of showing a three-dimensional perspective. The record produced is called a **sonogram** or an **echogram**. Sonography is very safe and does not use ionizing radiation. It has many medical applications, including imaging of the fetus (Fig. 4.12).

Contrast imaging is the use of radiopaque materials to make internal organs visible on x-ray images. A contrast medium may be swallowed, introduced into a body cavity, or injected into a vessel, resulting in greater visibility of internal organs or cavities outlined by the contrast material (Fig. 4.13).

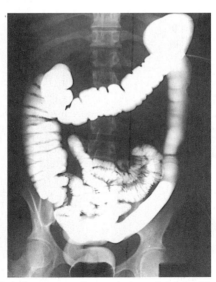

Fig. 4.13 Contrast Imaging. In this example of a barium enema, radiopaque barium sulfate is used to make the large intestine clearly visible.

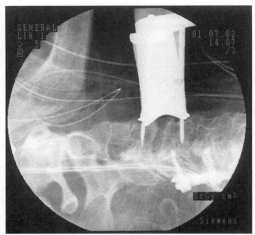

Fig. 4.14 Fluoroscopy. The image produced by the fluoroscope is magnified and brightened electronically, then projected on a monitor screen.

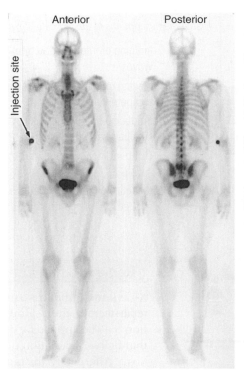

Fig. 4.15 Nuclear Medicine. Administration of a radiopharmaceutical allows its accumulation in a specific organ or structure, providing information about function and, to some degree, structure.
radi/o = radiant energy;   **pharmaceut/i** = drugs or medicine;
-al = pertaining to

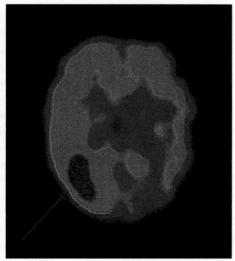

Fig. 4.16 PET Scan. Image of the brain of a 6-month-old male with seizures. Arrow demonstrates focal area.

Fluoroscopy is the visual examination of an internal organ using a **fluoroscope** (Fig. 4.14). This technique offers continuous x-ray imaging of the motion of internal structures and immediate serial images, such as during surgery. Radiography provides a record of the image at a particular point in time.

fluor/o = emitting or reflecting light
-scopy = visual examination

Nuclear medicine scans involve administering radio+pharmaceuticals to a patient orally, into the vein, or by having the patient breathe the material in vapor form. **Pharmaceuticals** are medicinal drugs, and radiopharmaceuticals are those that are radioactive. Computerized scanners called *gamma cameras* detect the radioactivity emitted by the patient and map its location to form an image of the organ or system (Fig. 4.15).

Positron emission tomography (PET), a type of nuclear medicine scan, combines computed tomography and radioactive substances to produce enhanced images of selected body structures, especially the heart, blood vessels, and the brain (Fig. 4.16). The radioactive materials used in PET are very short-lived, so the patient is exposed to extremely small amounts of radiation.

Match the descriptions in the left column with the imaging modalities in the right column.

_____ 1. Imaging of internal structures by measuring and recording sound waves

_____ 2. Placing radioactive materials into body organs and using computerized scanners

_____ 3. Producing detailed images of cross sections of tissue as though cuts had been made

_____ 4. Using radiopaque materials to make internal organs or vessels visible

_____ 5. Visualizing internal structures based on the magnetic properties of chemical elements

A. computed tomography
B. contrast imaging
C. magnetic resonance imaging
D. nuclear medicine
E. sonography

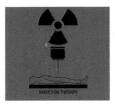

radi/o = radiant energy
-therapy = treatment

Radiation and Other Therapeutic Interventions

X-rays and radioactive materials are helpful in diagnosing disease and are also used in **radio+therapy**, the treatment of tumors using radiation to destroy cancer cells. The radiation may be applied by directing a beam of radiation toward the tumor with a machine that delivers radiation doses many times higher in intensity than those used for diagnosis. Alternately, the radiation may be introduced through the bloodstream or may be surgically implanted. **Radiation oncology** is a type of radiation therapy (Fig. 4.17).

Radiotherapy can produce undesirable side effects because of incidental destruction of normal body tissues. Most of the side effects disappear with time and include nausea and vomiting, hair loss, ulceration or dryness of mucous membranes, and suppression of bone marrow activity.

Therapeutic means "pertaining to therapy." Learn the word parts for treatment and their meanings.

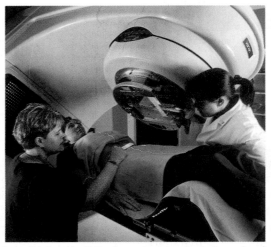

Fig. 4.17 Radiation Oncology. This type of radiation therapy treats neoplastic disease by using powerful x-rays or gamma rays to prevent the malignant cells from increasing in number.

WORD PARTS: TREATMENT

Combining Form	Meaning
algesi/o	sensitivity to pain
chem/o	chemical
pharmac/o, pharmaceut/i	drugs or medicine
plast/o	repair
therapeut/o	treatment
tox/o	poison
Suffix	
-therapy	treatment

FIND IT!
EXERCISE 10

Find the combining forms used in these terms, and write the combining form and its meaning.

	Combining Form	Meaning
1. **algesia**	_____	_____
2. **chemotherapy**	_____	_____
3. **pharmaceutical**	_____	_____
4. **therapeutic**	_____	_____
5. **toxic**	_____	_____

PROGRAMMED LEARNING

Remember to cover the answers (left column) with folded paper or the bookmark. Write an answer in each blank, and then check your answer before proceeding to the next frame.

treat	1. Therapeutic radiology uses radiation to _____ cancer. Radiation therapy, also called *radiation oncology*, is the treatment of cancer using ionizing radiation, such as x-rays.
cells	2. In addition to radiation, several approaches are used to treat cancer, including surgery to remove the cancer and **chemo+therapy**, treatment of disease by chemical agents. The combining form chem/o means chemical. **Cyto+tox+ic** agents are used in cancer treatment to kill cancer _____.
new	3. A neoplasm is a _____ growth of tissue (a tumor) that is either benign or malignant. **Anti+neo+plast+ics** are medications that are used to treat neoplasms. Malignant tumors are called *carcinomas*. Many malignant tumors are curable if detected and treated at an early stage. Invasive carcinoma is a malignant tumor that infiltrates and destroys surrounding tissues and may continue spreading. **Remission**, whether spontaneous or the result of therapy, is the disappearance of the characteristics of a malignant tissue.

4. **Pharmaco**+**therapy** is the treatment of diseases with drugs or medicine. Write an adjective that means "pertaining to treatment" by combining therapeut/o + -ic: _____. A second meaning of this term is curative.

therapeutic

   Radiopharmaceuticals are used to treat certain cancers or tissue hyperfunction and also to assess internal functions.

5. An **an**+**alges**+**ic** is a drug that relieves pain. The term results from combining an- + algesi/o + -ic. Notice that one *i* is omitted to facilitate pronunciation. The combining form algesi/o means sensitivity to _____.

pain

   An analgesic such as aspirin is a type of pharmaceutical. The term *pharmaceutical* refers to pharmacy or drugs, but it also means a medicinal drug. Some drugs require a physician's prescription and others, such as aspirin, are over-the-counter (OTC) drugs; in other words, not requiring a prescription.

6 **Narcotic** means pertaining to a substance that produces insensibility or _____. The term also means a narcotic drug. Narcotic analgesics alter perception of pain, induce a feeling of euphoria, and may induce sleep. Repeated use of narcotics may result in physical and psychologic dependence. In large amounts, as in an overdose (OD), narcotics can depress respiration.

stupor

7. **Anti**+**microbials** are drugs that destroy or inhibit growth of microbes (microorganisms). **Anti**+**bio**+**tics** are antimicrobial agents that are derived from cultures of a microorganism or produced semisynthetically and used to treat infections. Literal translation of antimicrobials indicates that they are used _____ microbes.

against

8. Both heat and cold are used to treat disease, especially to relieve pain and speed healing. Treating with heat is **thermo**+**therapy**, which can be helpful in relaxing muscles and promoting blood circulation. It may be administered as dry heat (e.g., heat lamps, electrical pads) or moist heat (e.g., warm compresses, warm water soaks). Write the term that means treatment of disease with heat: _____.

thermotherapy

   Photo/therapy is treatment of disorders with light, such as the use of bilirubin lights for jaundice of newborns.

9. Use thermotherapy as a model to write a term that means treatment using cold temperatures: _____. Cold compresses, such as an ice pack, are used to reduce pain and swelling, especially after surgery. You learned in Chapter 3 that destruction of tissue by use of a subfreezing temperature is cryosurgery.

cryotherapy

BUILD IT! **EXERCISE 11**

Combine the words parts to write terms.

1. an- + algesi/o + -ic   _____
2. anti- + ne/o + plast/o + -ic   _____
3. chem/o + -therapy   _____
4. cry/o + -therapy   _____
5. cyt/o + tox/o + -ic   _____
6. pharmac/o + -therapy   _____
7. radi/o + -therapy   _____
8. therm/o + -therapy   _____

QUICK CASE STUDY | EXERCISE 12

Andrea Parker, a 66-year-old female, is a smoker and has a history of chronic bronchitis. She is coughing and short of breath. T 100.8; P 98; BP 160/94; R 28. ECG: Normal. Chest x-ray shows an unidentified opacity in the superior segment of the left lower lobe. CT scan of the chest with contrast: Multiple nodules throughout the left lung, as well as a well-defined nodular opacity (12 × 13 × 9 mm) in the superior segment of the left lower lobe. Dx: Upper respiratory tract infection; unidentified nodules in the left lung. Treatment Plan: Antibiotics for the respiratory tract infection; biopsy of the large pulmonary nodule, left lower lobe.

1. Abbreviations for blood pressure, pulse, and temperature are _____, _____, and _____, respectively.
2. Which radiologic abbreviation represents a test that uses contrast agents? _____
3. What is the meaning of Dx? _____
4. Is a chest x-ray invasive? _____

Be Careful with These!

catheter (instrument) versus *catheterize* (verb) versus *catheterization* (the process)
diagnosis (disease ID) versus *prognosis* (predicted outcome)
palpation (part of physical exam) versus *palpitation* (heart flutter)
radiograph (same as radiogram, x-ray record) produced in *radiography*
sonogram or *echogram* (the record produced in *sonography*, the process)
tomogram (the tomographic record) versus *tomography* (the process)

Opposites

acute versus *chronic*
diastolic pressure versus *systolic* pressure
radiopaque versus *radiolucent*
signs (objective) versus *symptoms* (subjective)

A Career as a Radiologic Technologist

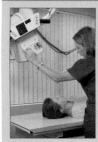

Radiologic technologists (RTs) play a vital role in diagnosis. They perform diagnostic imaging examinations, creating the images that radiologists evaluate. RTs work with many types of imaging, including plain x-ray examinations, magnetic resonance imaging, computed tomography, mammography, sonography, fluoroscopy, and bone density exams. RTs can also be trained to administer radiation therapy treatments. Meet Jeanne Jones, an RT who works at a community hospital. She is positioning a patient for an x-ray examination of the head. Jeanne loves her work because she knows that both radiologists and patients count on her to provide the best diagnostic images possible. To learn more, visit this website: www.asrt.org.

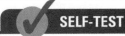

SELF-TEST

Work the following exercises to test your understanding of the material in Chapter 4. It is best to do all the exercises before checking your answers against the answers in Appendix III. Pay particular attention to spelling. If most of your answers are correct, you are ready to move on to Chapter 5.

A. MATCHING!   *Choose A or B from the right column to classify the descriptions as a sign or a symptom.*

_____ 1. The patient says he has a sore throat.

_____ 2. The patient has a fever.

_____ 3. The patient's blood pressure is elevated.

_____ 4. The patient has an abnormal laboratory result.

_____ 5. The patient says she has a headache.

A. sign

B. symptom

Match the terms in the left column with their descriptions in the right column.

_____ 6. auscultation

_____ 7. inspection

_____ 8. palpation

_____ 9. percussion

A. feeling internal body parts with the hands on the external surface

B. tapping the patient's body with the fingertips or fist

C. using a stethoscope to listen for sounds within the body

D. using the eyes to observe the patient

B. WRITING!   *List the three vital signs. (Remember: Blood pressure is not strictly a vital sign.)*

1. _____

2. _____

3. _____

C. CHOOSING!   *Circle the one correct answer (A, B, C, or D) for each question.*

1. Which term means "the probable outcome of a disease"?
   (A) diagnosis   **(B)** prognosis   **(C)** sign   **(D)** symptom

2. Which diagnostic procedure produces a detailed image of a cross section of tissue, similar to what one would see if the organ were actually cut into sections?
   (A) computed tomography   **(B)** contrast imaging   **(C)** electrocardiography   **(D)** nuclear medicine imaging

3. What is the term for the rhythmic expansion of an artery as the heart beats?
   (A) blood pressure   **(B)** pulse   **(C)** respiration   **(D)** systolic pressure

4. Which diagnostic procedure creates images based on the magnetic properties of chemical elements in the body?
   (A) computed tomography   **(B)** magnetic resonance imaging   **(C)** nuclear scanning   **(D)** positron emission tomography

5. Which of the following is the same as radiation therapy?
   (A) diagnostic radiology   **(B)** fluoroscopy   **(C)** positron tomography   **(D)** radiation oncology

D. IDENTIFYING THE ILLUSTRATION *Label these illustrations using one of the following: auscultation, cephalometry, echography, inspection, ophthalmoscopy, palpation, percussion, sonography, tympanic thermometer.*

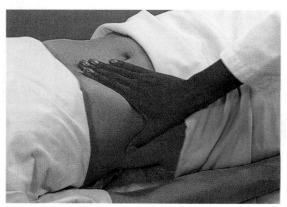

1. Feeling the texture, size, consistency, and location of body parts with the hands

_____

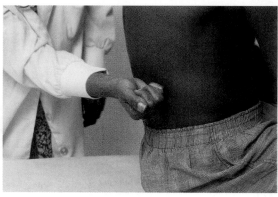

2. Tapping the body with the fingertips or fists to evaluate internal organs _____

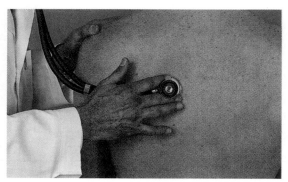

3. Listening for sounds within the body, often using a stethoscope _____

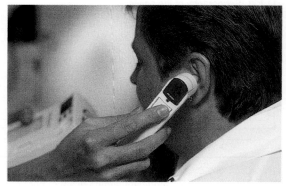

4. Instrument for measuring temperature

_____

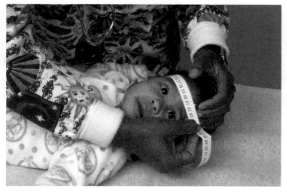

5. Measurement of the head _____

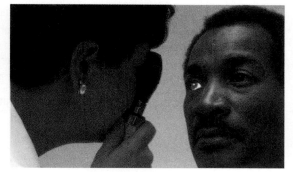

6. Visual examination of the eye _____

E. HEALTH CARE REPORTING!

Read the following Office Note. Then circle the correct answer to the questions that follow the report.

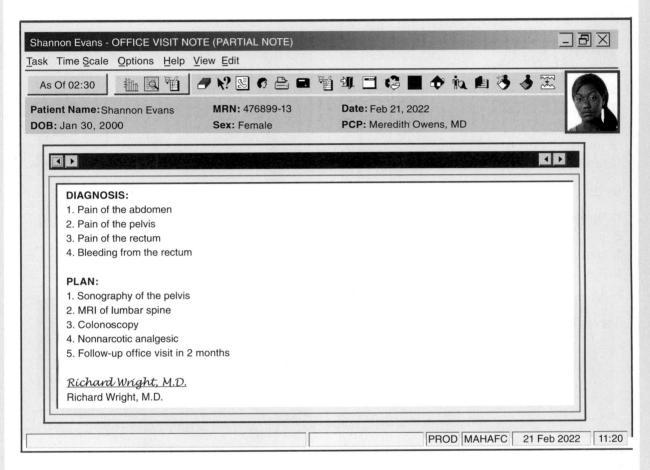

Shannon Evans - OFFICE VISIT NOTE (PARTIAL NOTE)

Task Time Scale Options Help View Edit

As Of 02:30

Patient Name: Shannon Evans   **MRN:** 476899-13   **Date:** Feb 21, 2022
DOB: Jan 30, 2000   **Sex:** Female   **PCP:** Meredith Owens, MD

DIAGNOSIS:
1. Pain of the abdomen
2. Pain of the pelvis
3. Pain of the rectum
4. Bleeding from the rectum

PLAN:
1. Sonography of the pelvis
2. MRI of lumbar spine
3. Colonoscopy
4. Nonnarcotic analgesic
5. Follow-up office visit in 2 months

Richard Wright, M.D.
Richard Wright, M.D.

PROD MAHAFC   21 Feb 2022   11:20

1. The patient is having a medical imaging exam of her pelvis that uses (radio waves, radioactive materials, sound waves, x-rays).
2. The patient was prescribed medication to treat (cancer, inflammation, fever, pain).
3. The "M" in the abbreviation "MRI" stands for (magnetic, medical, motion, muscular).
4. An alternate term for sonography is (fluoroscopy, radiography, tomography, ultrasound imaging).

F. SPELLING AND PRONOUNCING!

Circle all incorrectly spelled terms, and write their correct spelling. Then pronounce the terms.

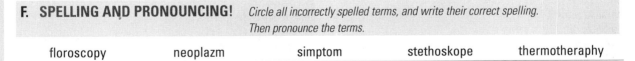

| floroscopy | neoplazm | simptom | stethoskope | thermotheraphy |

G. WRITING!   *Write a term for each definition.*

1. drug that produces insensibility or stupor   _____
2. drug that relieves pain   _____
3. objective evidence of an illness   _____
4. pertaining to therapy   _____
5. treatment of disease by chemical agents   _____
6. having severe symptoms and lasting a short time   _____
7. permitting the passage of x-rays   _____
8. not allowing passage of x-rays   _____
9. showing little change or slow progression   _____
10. small sample, intended to represent the nature of the whole   _____

H. QUICK CHALLENGE!   *Find an incorrect term in each sentence and write it correctly.*

1. Narcoleptic analgesics alter perception of pain and may induce sleep.   _____
2. Tomography means the treatment of malignant tumors using radiation.   _____
3. Invasive describes substances that readily permit the passage of x-rays.   _____
4. Direct palpation involves striking the fingers directly on the body surface.   _____
5. A term that is sometimes used in place of a catheter is a prognosis.   _____

*Use Appendix III to check your answers.

QUICK & EASY (Q&E) LIST

Use the Evolve website (http://evolve.elsevier.com/Leonard/quick) to review the terms presented in Chapter 4. Look closely at the spelling of each term as it is pronounced.

acute *(uh-**kūt**)*
algesia *(al-jē-zē-uh)*
analgesic *(an-ul-**jē**-zik)*
antibiotic *(an-tē-bī-**ot**-ik)*
antimicrobial *(an-tē-mī-**krō**-bē-ul)*
antineoplastics *(an-tē-nē-ō-**plas**-tiks)*
auscultation *(aws-kul-**tā**-shun)*
blood pressure *(blud **presh**-ur)*
cannula *(**kan**-ū-luh)*
catheter *(**kath**-uh-tur)*
catheterization *(kath-uh-tur-i-**zā**-shun)*
catheterize *(**kath**-uh-ter-īz)*
chemotherapy *(kē-mō-**ther**-uh-pē)*
chronic *(**kron**-ik)*
computed radiography *(kom-**pū**-tid rā-dē-**og**-ruh-fē)*
computed tomography *(kom-**pū**-tid tō-**mog**-ruh-fē)*
cryotherapy *(krī-ō-**ther**-uh-pē)*

cytotoxic *(sī-tō-**tok**-sik)*
diagnosis *(dī-ug-**nō**-sis)*
diastolic pressure *(dī-uh-**stol**-ik **presh**-ur)*
echogram *(**ek**-ō-gram)*
echography *(uh-**kog**-ruh-fē)*
endoscope *(**en**-dō-skōp)*
endoscopic *(en-dō-**skop**-ik)*
endoscopy *(en-**dos**-kuh-pē)*
fluoroscope *(**floor**-ō-skōp)*
fluoroscopy *(floo-**ros**-kuh-pē)*
inspection *(in-**spek**-shun)*
invasive procedure *(in-**vā**-siv prō-**sē**-jur)*
magnetic resonance imaging *(mag-**net**-ik **rez**-ō-nuns **im**-uh-jing)*
narcotic *(nahr-**kot**-ik)*
neoplasm *(**nē**-ō-plaz-um)*
palpation *(pal-**pā**-shun)*

QUICK & EASY (Q&E) LIST—cont'd

percussion (pur-**kuh**-shun)
pharmaceutical (fahr-muh-**soo**-ti-kul)
pharmacotherapy (fahr-muh-kō-**ther**-uh-pē)
phototherapy (fō-tō-**ther**-uh-pē)
positron emission tomography (**poz**-i-tron ē-**mish**-un tō-**mog**-ruh-fē)
prognosis (prog-**nō**-sis)
pulse (puls)
radiation oncology (rā-dē-**ā**-shun ong-**kol**-uh-jē)
radiograph (**rā**-dē-ō-graf)
radiography (rā-dē-**og**-ruh-fē)
radiologic (rā-dē-ō-**loj**-ik)
radiolucent (rā-dē-ō-**loo**-sunt)
radiopaque (rā-dē-ō-**pāk**)
radiopharmaceuticals (rā-dē-ō-fahr-muh-**soo**-ti-kulz)
radiotherapy (rā-dē-ō-**ther**-uh-pē)

remission (rē-**mish**-un)
respiration (res-pi-**rā**-shun)
sign (sīn)
sonogram (**son**-ō-gram)
sonography (suh-**nog**-ruh-fē)
specimen (**spes**-i-mun)
stethoscope (**steth**-ō-skōp)
symptom (**simp**-tum)
systolic pressure (sis-**tol**-ik **presh**-ur)
therapeutic (ther-uh-**pū**-tik)
thermotherapy (thur-mō-**ther**-uh-pē)
tomogram (**tō**-mō-gram)
toxic (**tok**-sik)
tympanic thermometer (tim-**pan**-ik thur-**mom**-uh-tur)
ultrasonography (ul-truh-suh-**nog**-ruh-fē)
ultrasound (**ul**-truh-sound)

Don't forget the games and other activities available at http://evolve.elsevier.com/Leonard/quick.

QUICK CONNECT

Review all lists of word parts and their meanings for Chapter 4, using the flashcards you prepared or the flashcards on the Evolve site.

The normal range of a healthy body is when the physical and chemical characteristics are within acceptable limits. Results of a diagnostic test are sometimes reported as "within normal limits" (WNL). Pathologic conditions are caused by or involve a disease process. The International Classification of Diseases (ICD) code is used to classify diagnoses and procedures. Procedure codes (CPT codes) are standard terminology and coding for medical services and procedures.

Distinguish the meanings and examples of signs vs. symptoms. Signs are *objective* evidence of illness or disordered function; symptoms are *subjective* evidence as perceived by the patient.

Diagnosis vs. prognosis: The identification of a disease or condition (diagnosis) vs. the probable outcome of a disease (prognosis).

Acute describes a disease (having a short and relatively severe course) vs. chronic (existing over a long time). Diagnostic clinical studies include measuring vital signs, radiology studies and laboratory tests. A specimen is a small sample or part of a whole that is collected to represent the nature of the whole.

Know the meanings of the vital signs: pulse, respiration, and body temperature. (Blood pressure is not strictly a vital sign, but is often included in other measurements.)

Measuring body temperature: Temperature can be measured orally, rectally, under the arm, via a probe placed in the ear, or using a touch-free digital forehead thermometer.

Blood pressure is the pressure exerted by the circulating volume of blood on the walls of the arteries and veins and on the chambers of the heart. Systolic pressure (higher reading that represents maximum pressure on the artery) vs. systolic pressure (pressure that exists when the heart is relaxed).

Four techniques useful in the physical exam: Distinguish inspection, palpation, percussion and auscultation (frequently performed using a stethoscope).

Common nonradiologic diagnostic techniques: cephalometry, ophthalmoscopy, electrocardiography, cephalometry, ophthalmoscopy, otoscopy, microscopy, endoscopy, catheterization.

Distinguish between diagnostic radiology terms presented in this chapter, including: radiography, computed tomography, echography (sonography, ultrasound, ultrasonography), magnetic resonance imaging, and nuclear imaging. Using radiopaque materials, contrast imaging makes many internal organs visible that would not be visible in standard radiology (related terms: radiopaque vs. radiolucent). Fluoroscopy is visual examination of an internal organ using a fluoroscope. PET scans combine computed tomography and radioactive substances to produce enhanced images.

Distinguish types of therapeutic interventions: radiation oncology, chemotherapy, antineoplastics, radiopharmaceuticals, analgesics, narcotics, antimicrobials, antibiotics, thermotherapy, cryotherapy, and phototherapy.

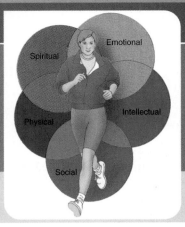

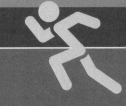

CHAPTER 5

The Body as a Whole

Holistic health views the individual as an integrated system rather than one or more separate parts.

OBJECTIVES

After completing Chapter 5, you will be able to:

1. Recognize the relationship of cells, tissues, and organs, and list the major body systems.
2. List four types of tissue, and recognize five general terms for abnormal tissue development.
3. Recognize the directional terms and planes of the body, match them with their descriptions, and write their combining forms.
4. Identify the body cavities, the body regions, and the four abdominal quadrants.
5. Recognize and write the terms for diagnostic procedures and disorders presented in Chapter 5.
6. Recognize the meanings of Chapter 5 word parts and use them to build and analyze medical terms.
7. Write terms pertaining to body fluids and their disorders, as well as associated terms.
8. Write terms about body defenses, immunity, and bioterrorism when given their definitions, or match them with their meanings.
9. Spell medical terms correctly.

Organization of the Body

All parts of the human body, from atoms to visible structures, work together as a functioning whole. Starting with the simplest and proceeding to the most complex, the eight levels of organization in the body are represented in Fig. 5.1.

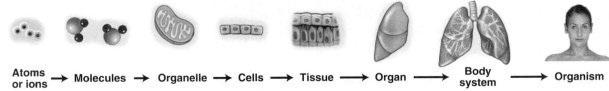

Atoms or ions → **Molecules** → **Organelle** → **Cells** → **Tissue** → **Organ** → **Body system** → **Organism**

Fig. 5.1 Organizational Scheme of the Body. The formation of the human organism progresses from different levels of complexity. All its parts, from tiny atoms to visible structures, work together to make a functioning whole.

WRITE IT!*
EXERCISE 1

Which is simpler? Decide which of the two choices is simpler, then write the name of the simpler organizational level of the body in the blank. (Question 1 is done as an example.)

1. cell versus organ   <u>cell</u>
2. organ versus tissue   _____
3. organ versus body system   _____
4. body system versus organism   _____
5. organelle versus tissue   _____

*Use Appendix III, Answers, to check all your answers to the exercises in Chapter 5.

THE CELL IS THE FUNDAMENTAL UNIT OF LIFE

A fertilized human egg resulted from penetration of an egg by a sperm, each contributing 23 unpaired chromosomes, thus resulting in a total of 46 chromosomes (23 pairs). Every human begins life as a single cell, a fertilized egg (Fig. 5.2). Rapid chemical changes in the membrane of the fertilized egg prevent the penetration of additional sperm. This single cell divides into two cells, then four, eight, and so on, until maturity. Humans in the early stages of development until the end of the eighth week are referred to as embryos (Fig. 5.2, *C*). During development, cells become specialized. Cells that have the ability to divide without limit and give rise to specialized cells are called **stem cells**. They are abundant in a fetus and in the cord blood of a newborn. Stem cells are used in bone marrow transplants and can be used in research for organ or tissue regeneration.

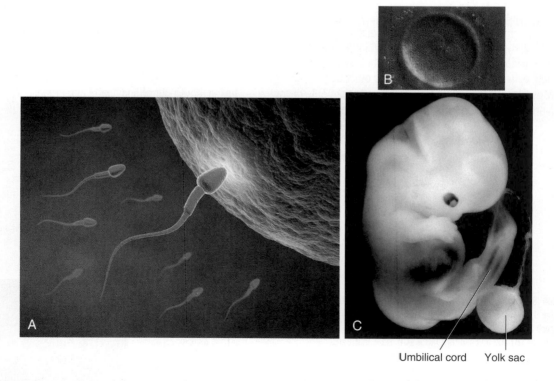

Umbilical cord   Yolk sac

Fig. 5.2 Life begins as a single cell. **A,** Drawing showing only one of several sperm penetrates the egg. **B,** This fertilized human egg shows the joining of the male and female nuclei, which determines the gender and the characteristics of the individual who will develop. **C,** Human embryo.

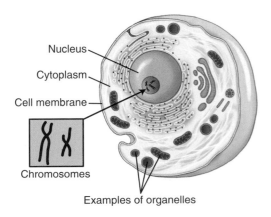

Nucleus

Cytoplasm

Cell membrane

Chromosomes

Examples of organelles

Fig. 5.3 Basic Cell Structure (Diagrammatic Representation). Chromosomes are threadlike structures in the nucleus of a cell that function in the transmission of genetic information. Each chromosome consists of a double strand of deoxyribonucleic acid (DNA).

somat/o = body

Nerve cells, muscle cells, and blood cells are examples of different types of somatic, or body, cells. In humans, each **somatic cell** has 23 pairs of chromosomes (Fig. 5.3). Somat+ic cells account for all the body's cells except the reproductive cells—the sperm and eggs (ova). Groups of cells that perform the same basic activity are called *tissues*. Somatic cells are surrounded by a cell membrane and have a nucleus that contains genetic information, cytoplasm (the liquid portion outside the nucleus), and organelles (cytoplasmic inclusions).

THE FOUR MAIN TYPES OF TISSUE (FIG. 5.4)

A. Epithelial tissue forms the covering of both internal and external surfaces (skin and lining of cavities). Cells are joined by small amounts of cementing substances.
B. Connective tissue supports and binds other body tissue and parts (bone and fat cells, for example).
C. Muscular tissue is composed of fibers that are able to contract, causing movement of body parts and organs.
D. Nervous tissue conducts impulses that connect the brain and spinal cord with other parts of the body.

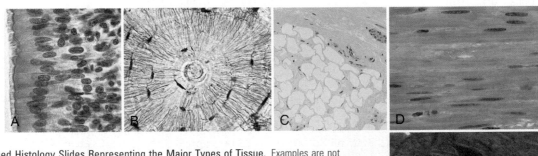

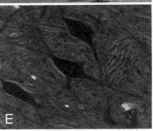

Fig. 5.4 Stained Histology Slides Representing the Major Types of Tissue. Examples are not shown at the same magnification. **A,** Epithelial cells of the type shown are made up of several layers of cells, such as those found on the outer layers of the skin. **B** and **C,** Two types of connective tissue are shown (bone **[B]** and adipose [fat] tissue **[C]**). Note that the center of the compact bone has a canal, which carries blood vessels throughout the bone. Adipose tissue is composed of large fat cells. **D,** Muscle tissue showing more than a dozen long, slender central nuclei within narrow cells that lie parallel to each other. **E,** Note the large nerve cells with numerous cytoplasmic extensions.

MATCH IT!
EXERCISE 2

Match the types of tissue and their functions.

_____ 1. connective
_____ 2. epithelial
_____ 3. muscular
_____ 4. nervous

A. conducting impulses
B. contracting
C. covering
D. supporting and protecting

Two or more tissue types that work together to perform one or more functions and form a more complex structure make up *organs.* The skin, stomach, and ear are examples of organs.

A *body system* consists of several organs that work together to accomplish a set of functions. Body systems are covered in Chapters 6 through 15 of this book. Some systems are combined in the same chapter; for example, the skeletal and muscular systems are presented in Chapter 6. Table 5.1 lists major body systems and functions.

The most complex level in the organizational scheme is the organism, the human body. **Homeo**+**stasis** refers to the constant internal environment that is naturally maintained by the body.

home/o = sameness
-stasis = controlling

TABLE 5.1   MAJOR BODY SYSTEMS

Body System (Chapter)	Major Functions
Muscular system (6)	Makes movement possible
Skeletal system (6)	Provides protection, form, and shape for the body; stores minerals and forms some blood cells
Cardiovascular system (7)	Delivers oxygen, nutrients, and vital substances throughout the body; transports cellular waste products to the lungs and kidneys for excretion
Lymphatic system (7)	Helps maintain the internal fluid environment; produces some types of blood cells; regulates immunity
Respiratory system (8)	Brings oxygen into the body and removes carbon dioxide and some water waste
Digestive system (9)	Provides the body with water, nutrients, and minerals; removes solid wastes
Urinary system (10)	Filters blood to remove wastes of cellular metabolism; maintains the electrolyte and fluid balance
Reproductive system (11)	Facilitates procreation (producing offspring)
Integumentary system (12)	Provides external covering for protection; regulates body temperature and water content
Nervous system (13, 14)	Coordinates the reception of stimuli; transmits messages to stimulate movement
Endocrine system (15)	Secretes hormones and helps regulate body activities

With the exception of nerve cells, body cells are constantly being replaced. Various cells have different life spans, and in addition, cells can become damaged (e.g., physical damage, insufficient oxygen, or exposure to toxins or bacteria). Pathologists use terms to describe abnormal changes in tissue or organ formation. Learn the word parts in the following table.

QUICK TIP

Think of homeostasis as equilibrium.

WORD PARTS: ABNORMAL DEVELOPMENT OF TISSUE

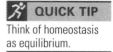

Prefix	Meaning	Suffix	Meaning
ana-	upward, excessive or again	-plasia	development or formation of tissue

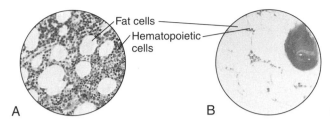

Fat cells
Hematopoietic cells

Fig. 5.5 Biopsy smears help compare normal and hypoplastic (pertaining to incomplete development) bone marrow tissue. **A,** Stained normal bone marrow tissue shows many precursors of blood cells. **B,** Stained hypoplastic bone marrow tissue has few cells, and many of those may be abnormal in appearance. **hypo-** = below normal;   **-plasia** = development

A   B

a- = without
-plasia = formation or development
dys- = bad
hypo- = below normal
hyper- = above normal

> **⚐ QUICK TIP**
>
> Be aware that hyperplasia and hypertrophy are sometimes used interchangeably.

Terms used to describe abnormal changes in tissue or organ formation usually contain the suffix -plasia.
- **a+plasia**: The lack of development of an organ or tissue
- **dys+plasia**: Any abnormal development of tissues, recognized by cells that differ in size, shape, and appearance
- **hypo+plasia**: Underdevelopment of an organ or a tissue; less severe than aplasia
- **hyper+plasia**: An abnormal increase in the number of normal cells in tissue (Fig. 5.5)
- **hyper+trophy**: An increase in the size of an organ caused by an increase in the size of existing cells rather than the number of cells (as in hyperplasia). Fig. 5.6 shows a comparison of the two terms.

Hypertrophy of skeletal muscles is brought about by exercise and is typically seen in body builders; however, hypertrophy of the heart is a common pathologic finding in cardiac disease as an adaptation to increased workload.

HEALTH CARE CONNECTION

Gradual atrophy (decrease in size) of our brain occurs as we age. Unless brain-destroying drugs are used, most of us will have more brain cells than we'll ever use. For example, many older people's brains function into their early one hundreds. It was originally believed that the primary cells of the nervous system (neurons) were not replaced if they were damaged; however, research shows that a limited production of new neurons may occur after cerebral injury.

Unlike other terms ending in -plasia, **anaplasia** is characteristic of malignant tumors. Ana+plasia (in this case, meaning upward, or an earlier stage of development)

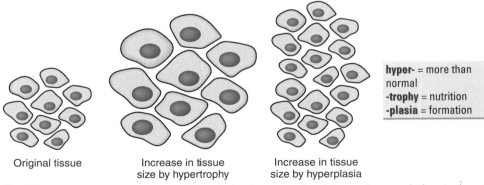

Original tissue   Increase in tissue size by hypertrophy   Increase in tissue size by hyperplasia

hyper- = more than normal
-trophy = nutrition
-plasia = formation

Fig. 5.6 Comparison of Hypertrophy and Hyperplasia. A representation of tissue enlargement by hypertrophy and hyperplasia.

refers to a change in the structure and orientation of cells, characterized by a loss of differentiation and reversal to a more primitive form. The microscopic appearance of cells from a malignant tumor shows new features that are not characteristic of their tissue of origin.

MATCH IT! EXERCISE 3	*Match the description with the correct condition.*

1. _____ increase in size of an organ due to an increase in the number of normal cells
2. _____ increase in the size of an organ caused by an increase in the size of the cells
3. _____ lack of development
4. _____ underdevelopment

A. aplasia
B. hyperplasia
C. hypertrophy
D. hypoplasia

Reference Planes

Anatomists use directional terms and planes to describe the position and direction of various body structures or parts. Locations and positions are described relative to the body in the **anatomic position**; that is, the position a person is in while standing erect with the arms at the sides and the palms forward (Fig. 5.7).

Unless otherwise stated, descriptions of location and position assume that the body is in the anatomic position.

Commit to memory the directional terms, their combining forms, and their meanings as presented in the following table.

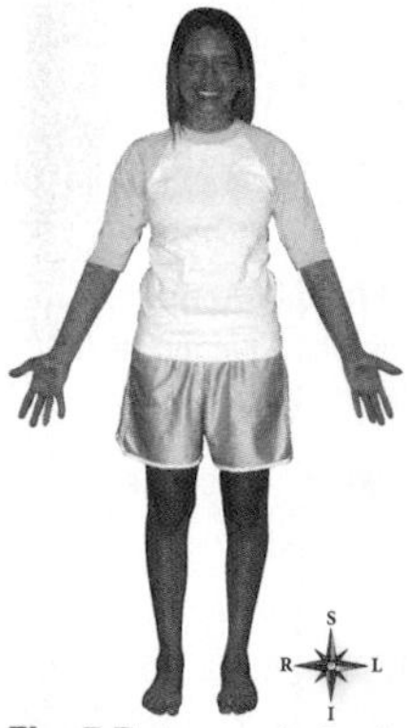

Fig. 5.7 Anatomic Position. Standing erect with the face directed to the front, the upper limbs at the sides, and the palms turned forward.

DIRECTIONAL TERMS

Combining Form	Term	Meaning
anter/o	**anterior**	nearer to or toward the front; ventral
poster/o	**posterior**	nearer to or toward the back; dorsal; situated behind
ventr/o	**ventral**	belly side; same as anterior surface in humans
dors/o	**dorsal**	directed toward or situated on the back side; same as posterior surface in humans
medi/o	**medial, median**	middle or nearer the middle; the prefix mid- also means middle
later/o	**lateral**	toward the side; denoting a position farther from the midline of the body or from a structure
super/o	**superior**	uppermost or above
infer/o	**inferior**	lowermost or below
proxim/o	**proximal**	nearer the origin or point of attachment
dist/o	**distal**	far or distant from the origin or point of attachment
cephal/o	**cephalad**	toward the head
caud/o	**caudad**	toward the tail or in an inferior direction in humans
intern/o	**internal**	inside, within (L., *internus*)
extern/o	**external**	outside (L., *externus*)

Use the electronic flashcards on the Evolve site or make your own set of flashcards using the above list. Select the word parts just presented, and study them until you know their meaning. Do this each time a set of word parts is presented.

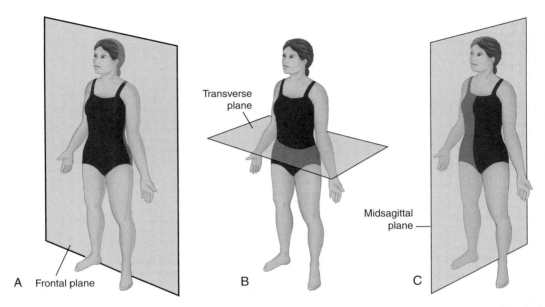

Fig. 5.8 Reference Planes of the Body. **A,** Frontal plane. **B,** Transverse plane. **C,** Midsagittal plane. The midsagittal plane is a special sagittal plane that is located in the center to create two equal portions.

trans- = across

Terms such as *plane* and *aspect* are used to describe the orientation of the body. Three reference planes (imaginary flat surfaces) are as follows (Fig. 5.8):

- **frontal** (coronal) **plane**: Divides the body into front and back portions.
- **transverse plane**: Divides the body into upper and lower portions
- **sagittal plane**: Divides the body into right and left sides. A **midsagittal plane** divides the body into two equal halves.

Six important aspects are shown in Fig. 5.9 and are used to describe locations:

- anterior (front)
- posterior (behind)
- lateral (side)

- medial (middle)
- superior (uppermost)
- inferior (lowermost)

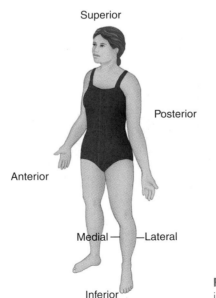

anter/o = front
poster/o = behind
later/o = side
medi/o = middle
super/o = uppermost
infer/o = lowermost

Fig. 5.9 Aspects of the Body. Note the terms with opposite meanings: *inferior* vs. *superior, anterior* vs. *posterior, medial* vs. *lateral.*

WRITE IT!
EXERCISE 4

Write the meanings of the combining forms, and then provide the corresponding anatomic term. (Question 1 is done as an example.)

Combining Form	Meaning	Anatomic Term
1. anter/o	*front*	*anterior*
2. caud/o		
3. cephal/o		
4. dist/o		
5. dors/o		
6. infer/o		
7. later/o		
8. medi/o		
9. poster/o		
10. proxim/o		
11. super/o		
12. ventr/o		

FIND IT!
EXERCISE 5

Write the combining forms and their meanings for these new terms. (Question 1 is done as an example.) A short definition is provided for each term.

Term/Meaning	Combining Forms	
1. **anteromedian** located in front and toward the middle	*anter/o, front*	*medi/o, middle*
2. **posteroexternal** situated on the outer side of a posterior aspect		
3. **posteromedian** situated in the middle of the back		
4. **dorsolateral** pertaining to the back and the side		
5. **posterolateral** pertaining to a position behind and to the side		
6. **anterolateral** pertaining to the front and one side		
7. **mediolateral** pertaining to the middle and one side		
8. **anterosuperior** indicates a position in front and above		
9. **posterosuperior** indicates a position behind and above		
10. **inferomedian** situated in the middle of the underside		

WRITE IT! **EXERCISE 6**

Using terms from the list of directional terms, write terms that mean the opposite of these terms.

1. anterior _____
2. inferior _____
3. proximal _____
4. ventral (in humans) _____

PROGRAMMED LEARNING

Remember to cover the answers (left column) with folded paper or the bookmark. Write an answer in each blank, and then check your answer before proceeding to the next frame.

anterior	1. The body is facing forward in the anatomic position. Anterior means toward the front; therefore the anatomic position refers to the _____ aspect, or front of the body. Antero+superior means in front of and at a higher level.
back	2. **Postero+internal** means situated toward the _____ and the inner side.
front	3. In radiology, directional terms are used to specify the direction of the x-ray beam from its source to its exit surface before striking the image receptor. In an **antero+posterior** projection, the x-ray beam strikes the anterior aspect of the body first. In other words, the beam passes from the _____ of the body to the back.
back	4. **Postero+anterior** means from the posterior to the anterior surface; in other words, from _____ to front. (Fig. 5.10 shows three radiographic positions.)

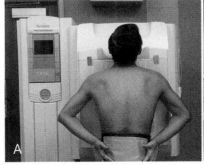
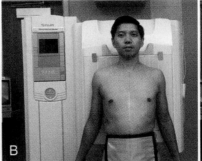
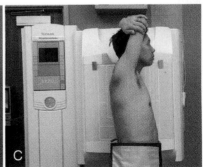

Posteroanterior projection   Anteroposterior projection   Left lateral projection

Fig. 5.10 Patient Positioning for a Chest X-Ray. **A,** In a posteroanterior (PA) projection, the anterior aspect of the chest is closest to the image receptor. **B,** In an anteroposterior (AP) projection, the posterior aspect of the chest is closest to the image receptor. **C,** In a left lateral chest projection, the left side of the patient is placed against the image receptor.

poster/o = posterior
anter/o = anterior (front)
later/o = side

back	5. Dorsal also means directed toward or situated on the back side. **Dorso+ventral** pertains to the _____ and belly surfaces. Dorsoventral sometimes means passing from the back to the belly surface. For example, the path of a bullet resulting from a shot in the back could be described as dorsoventral.
ventral	6. The term for belly side is _____.
anterior	7. In humans, the ventral surface is the same as the _____ aspect of the body.
posterior	8. Similarly, the dorsal surface in humans is the same as the _____ aspect of the body.
median	9. Two terms that mean middle are medial and _____.
tail	10. Caudad means toward the tail. **Caud+al** means pertaining to the _____ or to a tail-like structure. Sometimes caudal is also used to mean inferior in position.
near	11. Proximal describes the position of structures that are nearer their origin or point of attachment. The combining form proxim/o is used in words that refer to proximal, or _____.
nearer	12. The proximal end of the thigh bone joins with the hip bone. This means that the proximal end of the thigh bone is _____ the hip bone than is the other end of the thigh bone.
distal	13. Distal is the opposite of proximal. Distal means far or distant. It also means away from the origin or point of attachment. The lower end of the thigh bone is _____ to the hip bone.
distant	14. Distal is derived from the same word root as distant, which should help you to remember the term. The combining form tel/e also means distant. A **tele+cardio+gram**, for example, is a tracing of the electrical impulses of the heart recorded by a machine _____ from the patient.
telecardiogram	15. Telecardiograms can be sent by telephone. With a _____, the cardiologist and the patient may be in different cities.
up	16. Physicians rely on additional positions for examination or surgery. **Prone** and **supine** are terms used to describe the position of a person who is lying on the belly (with the face down or to either side) and lying on the back, respectively (Fig. 5.11). If a person is supine, is the face turned up or downward? _____

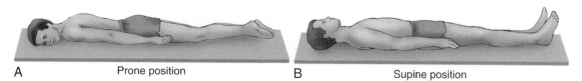

A   Prone position   B   Supine position

Fig. 5.11 Comparison of Prone and Supine Positions. **A,** Prone: lying face downward. **B,** Supine: lying on the back.

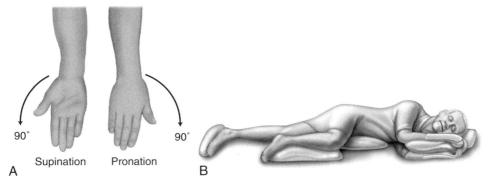

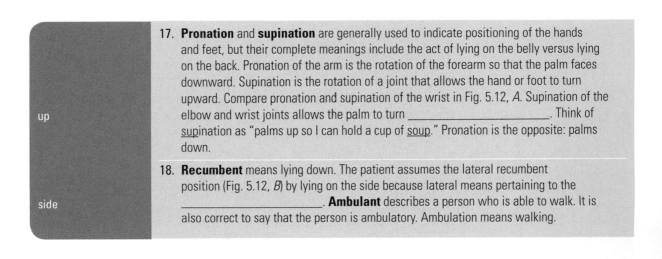

Lateral (recumbent) position

Fig. 5.12 Supination, Pronation, and the Lateral Recumbent Position. **A,** Supination and pronation: turning the palm of the hand upward (supination) or downward (pronation). **B,** The lateral recumbent position (also called the *Sims position*) is sometimes used in surgery. The patient lies on the left side with the right knee and thigh flexed (bent) and the upper limb parallel along the back.

17. **Pronation** and **supination** are generally used to indicate positioning of the hands and feet, but their complete meanings include the act of lying on the belly versus lying on the back. Pronation of the arm is the rotation of the forearm so that the palm faces downward. Supination is the rotation of a joint that allows the hand or foot to turn upward. Compare pronation and supination of the wrist in Fig. 5.12, *A.* Supination of the elbow and wrist joints allows the palm to turn _____. Think of supination as "palms up so I can hold a cup of <u>soup</u>." Pronation is the opposite: palms down.

up

18. **Recumbent** means lying down. The patient assumes the lateral recumbent position (Fig. 5.12, *B*) by lying on the side because lateral means pertaining to the _____. **Ambulant** describes a person who is able to walk. It is also correct to say that the person is ambulatory. Ambulation means walking.

side

MATCH IT! **EXERCISE 7**

Match the terms with the descriptions.

_____ 1. ambulant
_____ 2. distal
_____ 3. prone
_____ 4. proximal
_____ 5. recumbent
_____ 6. supine

A. away from the origin or point of attachment
B. describes a person who is lying face down
C. describes a person who is able to walk
D. describes a person who is lying on the back
E. lying down
F. nearer the origin or point of attachment

Body Cavities

The body has two major cavities, which are spaces within the body that contain internal organs. The two principal body cavities are the *dorsal cavity*, located near the posterior part of the body, and the *ventral cavity*, located near the anterior part (Fig. 5.13).

The dorsal cavity is divided into the **cranial** and **spinal** cavities. The cranial cavity contains the brain, and the spinal cavity contains the spinal cord and the beginnings of the spinal nerves. The other principal body cavity is the ventral cavity. Large organs contained in the ventral cavity are called **viscera**. The ventral cavity is subdivided into the **thoracic** cavity and the **abdominopelvic** (abdominal and pelvic) cavity. The muscular **diaphragm** divides the thoracic and abdominopelvic cavities. The diaphragm is a dome-shaped partition that functions in respiration (see Fig. 8.1).

thorac/o = chest

The abdominopelvic cavity can be thought of as a single cavity or as two cavities, the abdominal and pelvic cavities, although no wall separates them. A membrane called the **periton+eum** lines the abdominopelvic cavity and enfolds the internal organs (Fig. 5.14). As do all serous membranes, the peritoneum secretes a lubricating fluid that allows the organs to glide against one another or against the cavity wall. A sticking

periton/o = peritoneum **-eum** = membrane

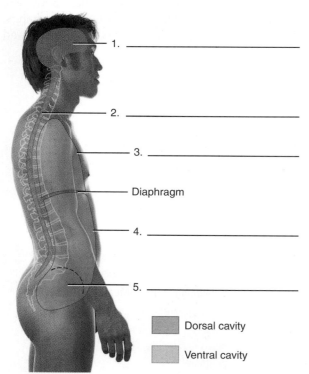

1. _____
2. _____
3. _____
— Diaphragm
4. _____
5. _____

☐ Dorsal cavity
☐ Ventral cavity

Fig. 5.13 The Dorsal and Ventral Cavities. Label the numbered structures as you read. The dorsal cavity is divided into the cranial cavity *(1)* and spinal cavity *(2)*. The ventral cavity is divided into the thoracic cavity *(3)* and the abdominopelvic cavity, which is subdivided into the abdominal cavity *(4)* and the pelvic cavity *(5)*.

dors/o = back;   **ventr/o** = belly;   **crani/o** = skull;   **spin/o** = spine;   **thorac/o** = chest;   **abdomin/o** = abdomen;   **pelv/i** = pelvis

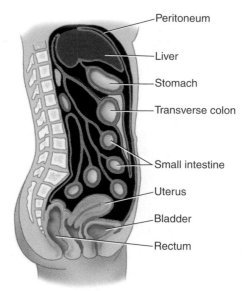

— Peritoneum
— Liver
— Stomach
— Transverse colon
— Small intestine
— Uterus
— Bladder
— Rectum

Fig. 5.14 The Peritoneum *(tan shading)* in a Median Sagittal Section of a Female. The free surface of the peritoneum is smooth and lubricated by a fluid that permits the viscera to glide easily against the abdominal wall and against one another.

together of two structures that are normally separated is called an **adhesion**. Abdominal adhesions are usually caused by inflammation or trauma (injury) and are treated surgically if they cause intestinal obstruction or excessive discomfort (see Fig. 11.18).

MATCH IT!
EXERCISE 8

Choose A or B from the right column to identify the body cavities in the left column as a dorsal or a ventral cavity.

_____ 1. abdominopelvic cavity   **A.** dorsal cavity
_____ 2. cranial cavity   **B.** ventral cavity
_____ 3. spinal cavity
_____ 4. thoracic cavity

Body Regions

The major regions of the body are the following:
- Head   • Torso
- Neck   • Extremities

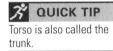

QUICK TIP

Torso is also called the trunk.

The head contains the brain and special sense organs, such as the mouth, the nose, the eyes, and the ears. Our senses include sight, hearing, smell, taste, touch, and pressure. The neck connects the head with the **torso**, which includes the chest, abdomen, and pelvis. The extremities are the four limbs (arms and legs). The arms, wrists, hands, and fingers make up the upper extremities. The thighs, knees, legs, ankles, feet, and toes make up the lower extremities.

WRITE IT!
EXERCISE 9

List the four major regions of the body.

_____
_____
_____
_____

Commit the combining forms in the following table to memory.

COMBINING FORMS FOR SELECT BODY REGIONS OR STRUCTURES

Combining Form	Meaning	Combining Form	Meaning
abdomin/o	abdomen	omphal/o, umbilic/o	umbilicus (navel)
acr/o	extremities (arms and legs)	onych/o	nail
blephar/o	eyelid	pelv/i	pelvis
cyst/o	cyst, bladder, or sac	periton/o	peritoneum
dactyl/o	digit (toes, fingers, or both)	som/a, somat/o	body
lapar/o	abdominal wall	thorac/o	chest (thorax)

Use the electronic flashcards on the Evolve site, or make your own set of flashcards using the Combining Forms list. Select the word parts just presented, and study them until you know their meaning.

WRITE IT!
EXERCISE 10

Write combining forms for these meanings.

1. abdominal wall _____
2. body _____
3. digit _____
4. extremities _____

5. eyelid _____
6. nail _____
7. chest _____
8. umbilicus _____

Acral means pertaining to the extremities of the body (arms and legs). **Acro+dermat+itis** is dermatitis of the extremities. In **acro+cyan+osis**, cyanosis of the extremities, the arms and legs appear bluish (Fig. 5.15). Abnormal coldness of the extremities is **acrohypothermy**. **Acromegaly** is a disorder in which there is abnormal enlargement of the body extremities, including the nose, jaws, fingers, and toes, caused by hypersecretion of growth hormone after maturity (see Fig. 15.8).

acr/o = extremities
hypo- = below normal
therm/o = temperature
-y = condition
-megaly = enlarged

The chest is also called the **thorax**. The chest and pelvis are the upper part and lower part of the torso, respectively. The **abdomen** is the portion of the body trunk that is located between the chest and the pelvis. The division of the abdomen into quadrants is the convenient method of using imaginary lines to divide the abdomen into regions. **Abdominal quadrants** are often used to describe the location of pain or body structures. The four abdominal quadrants are the right upper quadrant (RUQ), left upper quadrant (LUQ), right lower quadrant (RLQ), and left lower quadrant (LLQ) (Fig. 5.16).

Thoracic means pertaining to the chest. Thoracic surgery is another way of saying "chest surgery." Surgical puncture of the chest wall for aspiration of fluids could be called **thoracocentesis**, but **thoracentesis** is the more common term.

thorac/o = thorax or chest

The **pelvis** is the lower portion of the body trunk. The word *pelvis* can refer to any basinlike structure, so you will also see it in other terms (e.g., the *renal pelvis*, a funnel-shaped structure in the kidney). **Pelvic** means pertaining to a pelvis, usually the bony pelvis, as is the case here. In cephalopelvic disproportion, the head of the fetus is too large for the pelvis of the mother. In such cases, vaginal delivery is difficult or impossible. **Cephalo+pelvic** refers to the head of the fetus and the maternal pelvis.

cephal/o = head
pelv/i = pelvis

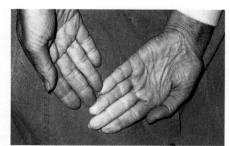

Fig. 5.15 Acrocyanosis. This blueness of the extremities is often accompanied by pain and is usually brought on by cold or emotional stimuli. **acr/o** = extremities; **cyan/o** = blue; **-osis** = condition

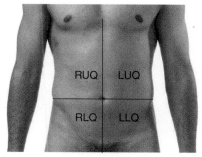

Fig. 5.16 Abdominal Quadrants. The four quadrants in this anatomic division of the abdomen are determined by drawing a vertical and horizontal line through the umbilicus. RUQ, LUQ, RLQ, and LLQ are abbreviations for right upper quadrant, left upper quadrant, right lower quadrant, and left lower quadrant, respectively. **abdomin/o** = abdomen; **quad-** = four

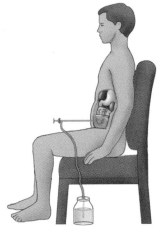

Fig. 5.17 Abdominal Paracentesis. In this surgical puncturing of the abdomen, fluid is withdrawn for diagnosis or to remove excess fluid.
abdomin/o = abdomen; **para-** = beside;
-centesis = surgical puncture

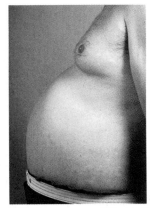

Fig. 5.18 Ascites. This abnormal accumulation of a fluid in the peritoneal cavity is treated with dietary therapy and drugs. Abdominal paracentesis may be performed to relieve the pressure of the accumulated fluid.
periton/o = peritoneum; **-al, -eal** = pertaining to;
abdomin/o = abdomen

abdomin/o = abdomen
-centesis = surgical puncture

periton/o = peritoneum
-itis = inflammation

omphal/o = umbilicus
-cele = hernia

Abdominothoracic is an adjective that pertains to the abdomen and the thorax. **Abdomino+centesis**, usually called abdominal **paracentesis**, is a surgical procedure that is performed to remove excess fluids from the abdominal cavity or to inject a therapeutic agent (Fig. 5.17).

Abnormal accumulation of fluid in the peritoneal cavity is called **ascites** (Fig. 5.18). **Periton+itis** can result if infectious microorganisms gain access by way of surgical incisions or by the rupture or perforation of viscera or associated structures (as in rupture of the appendix). Microorganisms can also spread to the peritoneum from the bloodstream or lymphatic vessels. *Omphalos* is Greek for the **umbilicus**, or navel. Many new terms can be formed using omphal/o with various suffixes that you have already learned. Congenital herniation of the navel is an **omphalo+cele**. A *hernia* is protrusion of an organ through an abnormal opening in the wall of the cavity that surrounds it. Types of abdominal hernias include umbilical, **femoral**, incisional, and **inguinal** (Fig. 5.19).

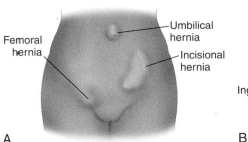

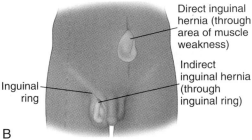

femor/o = femur (thigh bone)
inguin/o = groin

A

B

Fig. 5.19 Common Types of Abdominal Hernias. **A,** *Umbilical* hernias result from a weakness in the abdominal wall around the umbilicus. An *incisional* hernia is herniation through an inadequately healed surgical incision. In a *femoral* hernia, a loop of intestine descends through the femoral canal into the groin (femoral means pertaining to the thigh). **B,** *Inguinal* hernias are of two types. A *direct* hernia occurs through an area of weakness in the abdominal wall. In an *indirect* hernia, a loop of intestine descends through the inguinal canal, an opening in the abdominal wall for passage of the spermatic cord in males, and a ligament of the uterus in females.

Many additional terms can be written using the combining forms you've learned.

Write the combining form and suffix and their meanings for these new terms. (Question 1 is done as an example.)
A short definition is provided for each term.

Term/Meaning	Combining Form	Meaning
1. **acral** pertaining to the extremities (arms and legs)	*acr/o, extremities*	*-al, pertaining to*
2. **blepharal** pertaining to the eyelid		
3. **blepharoplasty** surgical repair of one or both eyelids		
4. **blepharoplegia** paralysis of one or both eyelids		
5. **blepharospasm** twitching of the eyelid		
6. **blepharotomy** incision of the eyelid		
7. **cephalgia, cephalodynia** pain in the head; headache		
8. **cephalometry** measurement of the dimensions of the head		
9. **laparotomy** incision into the abdominal wall		
10. **laparoscopy** examination of the interior of the abdominal wall		
11. **laparoscope** an instrument that is inserted into the peritoneal cavity to inspect it		
12. **omphalic, umbilical** pertaining to the umbilicus		
13. **omphalitis** inflammation of the umbilicus		
14. **omphalorrhagia** umbilical hemorrhage		
15. **omphalorrhexis** rupture of the umbilicus		

FIND IT!   **EXERCISE 11**

QUICK CASE STUDY | EXERCISE 12

Write a term from the report to complete each sentence.

Emily's physician ordered chest x-rays. In the first image, she was positioned with her chest nearest the image receptor. In the second image, she was standing with her left side against the image receptor. Choose from the following directional terms to describe the projections: anteroposterior, posteroanterior, left lateral, right lateral

1. Which term is correct for the first position? _____
2. Which term is correct for the second position? _____

Write terms for these descriptions.

1. cyanosis of the extremities _____
2. examination of the interior of the abdomen _____
3. inflammation of the peritoneum _____
4. measurement of the head _____
5. pertaining to the abdomen and the chest _____
6. pertaining to the arms and legs _____
7. plastic surgery of the eyelid _____
8. rupture of the umbilicus _____
9. shortened term for thoracocentesis _____
10. surgical incision of the chest wall _____
11. pertaining to the head of the fetus and maternal pelvis _____
12. abnormal accumulation of fluid in the peritoneal cavity _____
13. herniation of the umbilicus _____
14. abnormal coldness of the extremities _____

WORD ORIGIN

palma (L.), hand;
also the tree
planta (L.), sole
of the foot

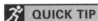 **QUICK TIP**

Think of planting your
foot to remember that
plantar pertains to the
sole.

---

onych/o = nails
phag/o = eat
-ist = one who

Remember that when a person is in the anatomic position, the palms (anterior surface of the hands) are facing forward. **Palmar** means pertaining to the palm. **Plantar** means the sole, or undersurface, of the foot. Compare palmar and plantar (Fig. 5.20).

A finger or toe is a digit. The combining form dactyl/o is often used in words that pertain to the fingers and toes. **Dactylo+graphy** is the study of fingerprints. **Dactylospasm** means cramping of a finger or toe. Inflammation of the bones of the fingers and toes is **dactylitis**.

Chiro+pody means pertaining to the hands and feet. It is also the art or profession of a **chiropodist**, a specialist who treats corns, bunions, and other afflictions of the hands and feet. Cramping of the hand, such as writer's cramp, is **chirospasm**. Plastic surgery of the hand is **chiroplasty**.

The combining form onych/o refers to the nails. An **onycho+phag+ist** habitually bites the nails. **Onychopathy** is any disease of the nails, and **onycho+myc+osis** means a disease of the nails caused by a fungus. Surgical removal of the nail is **onychectomy**, which also means declawing of an animal.

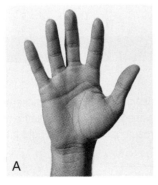
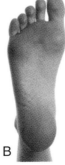

Fig. 5.20 Palmar vs. Plantar. **A,** Palmar pertains to the inside surface of the hands. **B,** Plantar pertains to the sole of the foot.

Write the combining forms and suffixes and their meanings for these new terms. A short definition is provided for each term.

Term/Meaning	Combining Form	Suffix
1. **blepharedema**		
swelling of the eyelid, as from blepharitis and crying		
2. **blepharitis** (Fig. 5.21)		
inflammation of the eyelid		
3. **blepharoptosis** (Fig. 5.22)		
prolapse (drooping) of the upper eyelid		
4. **onychomalacia**		
softening of the nails		
5. **thoracodynia**		
pain in the thorax, as distinguished from chest pain caused by angina pectoris, a heart condition		
6. **thoracostomy** (Fig. 5.23)		
providing an opening into the chest wall for drainage		
7. **thoracotomy**		
surgical incision of the chest wall		
8. **thoracoplasty**		
chest wall surgery in which portions of the ribs are removed to collapse areas of the lung		
9. **thoracoscopy**		
diagnostic examination of the chest cavity		

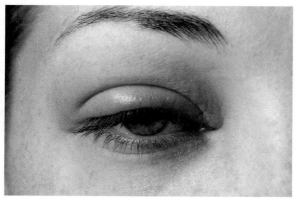

Fig. 5.21 Blepharitis. Note the swollen and inflamed upper eyelid.
blephar/o = eyelid;   **-itis** = inflammation

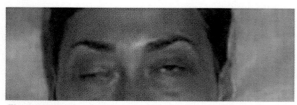

Fig. 5.22 Blepharoptosis. Note the drooping of the right upper eyelid.
blephar/o = eyelid;   **-ptosis** = drooping.

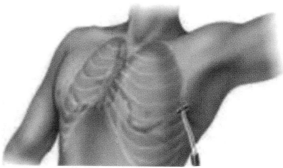

Fig. 5.23 Thoracostomy. An incision is made into the chest wall to insert a drainage tube after an injury or surgery.
thorac/o = chest;   **-stomy** = formation of an opening.

Body Fluids

Fluids constitute more than 60% of an adult's weight under normal conditions (Fig. 5.24). These fluids are vital in the transport of nutrients to all cells and removal of wastes from the body. Fluid balance is maintained through intake and output of water.

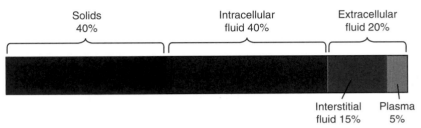

Fig. 5.24 Body Weight and Fluid Compartments. Fluid makes up 60% of the adult's body weight, and most of this is intracellular fluid. Two types of extracellular fluid are interstitial fluid and plasma. Plasma is the fluid part of the blood.

Water leaves the body by way of urine, feces, sweat, tears, and other fluid discharges (e.g., pus, sputum, mucus). Blood and lymph, two of the body's main fluids, are circulated through two separate but interconnected networks.

Water is the most important component of body fluids. These fluids are not distributed evenly throughout the body, and they move back and forth between compartments that are separated by cell membranes. Body fluids are found either within the cells (**intra**+**cellular**) or outside the cells (**extra**+**cellular**). Approximately one-fourth of the extracellular fluid is plasma, the fluid part of the blood. Another type of extracellular fluid, called **interstitial** fluid, fills the spaces between most of the cells of the body. Accumulation of fluid in the interstitial compartment results in a condition called **edema** (see Fig. 2.18). Several word parts that relate to body fluids are presented next. Commit the word parts to memory.

intra- = within
extra- = outside
inter- = between

SELECT WORD PARTS THAT PERTAIN TO BODY FLUIDS

Combining Form/Word Part	Meaning
crin/o, -crine	secrete
dacry/o, lacrim/o	tear, tearing, crying
-emia	condition of the blood
hem/o, hemat/o	blood
hidr/o	sweat or perspiration
hydr/o	water
lymph/o	lymph (sometimes refers to the lymphatics)
muc/o	mucus
-poiesis	production
-poietin	substance that causes production
py/o	pus
sial/o	saliva (sometimes refers to salivary glands)
ur/o	urine (sometimes refers to the urinary tract)

MATCH IT!

EXERCISE 15

Match the word parts with their meanings.

_____ 1. crin/o
_____ 2. dacry/o
_____ 3. hidr/o
_____ 4. hydr/o
_____ 5. -poiesis
_____ 6. -poietin
_____ 7. py/o
_____ 8. sial/o

A. perspiration
B. production
C. pus
D. saliva
E. secrete
F. substance that causes production
G. tear
H. water

PROGRAMMED LEARNING

Remember to cover the answers (left column) with folded paper or the bookmark. Write an answer in each blank, and then check your answer before proceeding to the next frame.

crying tears	1. The combining forms dacry/o and lacrim/o mean tear, as in crying. The **lacrimal** gland produces fluid that keeps the eye moist. Tears are lacrimal fluid. If more lacrimal fluid is produced than can be removed, the person is _____ or "tearing."
	2. **Lacrimation** refers to crying, or the discharge of _____.
inflammation	3. Ophthalmitis may lead to excessive lacrimation. **Ophthalm+itis** refers to _____ of the eye.
stone	4. **Calculi** (stones or concretions) sometimes form in the lacrimal passages. A **dacryo+lith** is a lacrimal _____ or calculus. Dacryoliths are also called "tear stones."
stones	5. **Dacryo+lith+iasis** is the presence of lacrimal _____.
dacryocyst	6. The **dacryo+cyst** is the tear sac. The dacryocyst collects lacrimal fluid. Another name for the tear sac is _____.
inflammation	7. **Dacryo+cyst+itis** is _____ of the tear sac.
dacryolith	8. Write the word that means tear stone: _____.
sialolith	9. Stones can also occur in a salivary gland or duct. The combining form sial/o is used to form words that pertain to a **salivary** gland or to the fluid of these glands, called **saliva**. Use dacryo+lith as a model to write a word that means a salivary calculus: _____.
salivary	10. **Sialo+graphy** is x-ray imaging of the ducts of the _____ glands. Sialography sometimes demonstrates the presence of calculi in the salivary ducts.
inside	11. In addition to salivary glands, the body contains many other types of glands. On the basis of the presence or absence of ducts, glands are classified as exocrine or endocrine glands. You previously learned that endo- means _____. The prefix exo- in this case means outside.

12. The combining form crin/o and the suffix -crine mean secrete. **Exo+crine** glands have ducts that carry their secretions to an epithelial surface, sometimes to the outside (e.g., sweat glands secrete perspiration onto the skin surface). Salivary glands also have ducts. Are salivary glands exocrine or endocrine glands? _____

exocrine

13. Sweat glands are also called **sudoriferous** glands, because the Latin word *sudor* means sweat. The combining form for sweat that you will use, however, is hidr/o. **Hidr+osis** means the formation and excretion of _____. A second meaning of hidrosis is excessive sweating, but **diaphoresis** is the term that is usually used to mean excessive sweating.

sweat

14. Remembering that aden/o means gland, **hidr+aden+itis** is inflammation of a _____ gland. (Notice that when hidr/o is joined with aden/o, the *o* is dropped from hidr/o to make it easier to pronounce.)

sweat

15. Now write a word that means tumor of a sweat gland: _____.

hidradenoma

16. **Endo+crine** glands are ductless and secrete their hormones into the bloodstream. There are many ductless glands, including the sex glands, the thyroid, and the adrenal glands. Ductless glands are classified as _____ glands.

endocrine

17. The combining form hydr/o means water. Do not confuse hydr/o and hidr/o. Remembering that a water hydrant is spelled with a *y* might help. **Hydro+therapy** refers to treatment using _____.

water

18. The combining form ur/o means urine. Translated literally, **an+uria** means without _____. Production of less than 100 mL of urine in 24 hours constitutes anuria.

urine

19. Using poly- and -uria, write a word that means excessive urination: _____

polyuria

20. **Hemat+uria** is _____ in the urine.

blood

21. **Lymph** is another type of body fluid. It is a transparent fluid found in **lymphatic** vessels. The lymphatic system (also called the lymphatics) collects tissue fluids from all parts of the body and returns the fluids to the blood circulation. Lymph/o usually refers to the lymphatics but sometimes refers to its fluid, _____.

lymph

22. The combining form muc/o means **mucus**. **Mucoid** means resembling _____.

mucus

23. **Mucous** means pertaining to mucus. Notice the slight difference in the spelling of mucous and mucus. Mucous also means secreting, producing, containing, or covered with mucus. The adjective that means pertaining to mucus is _____.

mucous

24. Membranes that line passages and cavities that communicate with the air (example: the mouth) are called mucous membranes. A mucous membrane is also called a **mucosa**. Mucous membranes usually contain mucus-secreting cells. Passages and cavities that communicate with the air are lined with _____ membranes.

mucous

25. **Muco+lytic** agents, including those used to treat certain diseases (e.g., bronchial asthma), break up or destroy _____.

mucus

py/o = pus
-genic = produced by

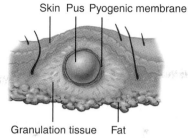

Skin Pus Pyogenic membrane

Granulation tissue   Fat

Fig. 5.25 Abscess. The pus is contained within a thin, pyogenic membrane surrounded by harder granulation tissue, the tissue's response to the infection.

pus	26. Pus is a type of body fluid that is the liquid product of inflammation. The combining form py/o means pus. **Py+uria** is _____ in the urine.
pus	27. **Pyo+genic** microorganisms are those that produce _____. A localized collection of pus in a cavity surrounded by healthy tissue is called an **abscess** (Fig. 5.25). **Purulent** means producing or containing pus.
brain	28. Another type of fluid, **cerebrospinal fluid**, flows through and protects the brain and spinal cord. Dividing cerebrospinal into its component parts, cerebr/o means _____ and spinal means pertaining to the spine.
head	29. **Hydrocephalus** is a condition characterized by an abnormal accumulation of cerebrospinal fluid (CSF). The combining forms hydr/o and cephal/o mean water and _____, respectively.
nervous	30. When hydrocephalus occurs in an infant, the head enlarges at an abnormal rate because the soft bones of the skull push apart (Fig. 5.26). If hydrocephalus occurs later in life, the bones of the skull forming the skull have fused, so symptoms are primarily neurologic. Neuro+logic means pertaining to the _____ system.

hydr/o = water
cephal/o = head

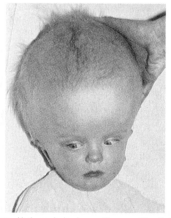

Fig. 5.26 Four-Month-Old Child With Hydrocephalus. Hydrocephalus is usually caused by obstruction of the flow of cerebrospinal fluid. If hydrocephalus occurs in an infant, the soft bones of the skull push apart as the head increases in size.

Blood

Blood circulates through the heart and blood vessels, carrying oxygen, nutrients, vitamins, antibodies, and other needed substances. It carries away carbon dioxide and other wastes.

Study the following word parts.

SELECT WORD PARTS PERTAINING TO BLOOD			
Combining Form	**Meaning**	**Suffix**	**Meaning**
coagul/o	coagulation	-cyte	cell
cyt/o	cell	-osis	generally, "increased" or "abnormal" when describing cellular components
erythr/o	red		
hem/a, hemat/o	blood	-penia	deficiency
immun/o	immune	-poiesis	production
leuk/o	white		
thromb/o	clot (thrombus)		

WRITE IT!
EXERCISE 16

Write the combining form for these meanings.

1. cell _____
2. clot _____
3. coagulation _____

4. red _____
5. white _____

MATCH IT!
EXERCISE 17

Match the meanings with the word parts.

_____ 1. blood   A. -cyte
_____ 2. cell   B. hemat/o
_____ 3. deficiency   C. -osis
_____ 4. increased or abnormal   D. -penia
_____ 5. production   E. -poiesis

Approximately half of the blood is composed of formed elements (cells or cell fragments), and the remainder is a straw-colored fluid, **plasma** (Fig. 5.27). The cells are packed at the bottom of the tube when treated blood is spun in a **centrifuge**.

erythr/o = red
-**cyte** = cell
leuk/o = white
thromb/o = clot

THE THREE FORMED ELEMENTS FOUND IN BLOOD
• Erythrocytes (red blood cells)
• Leukocytes (white blood cells)
• Blood platelets (also called thrombocytes)

Hemato+logy is the study of blood and the blood-forming tissues. The blood-forming tissues are bone marrow and lymphoid tissue (spleen, tonsils, and lymph nodes). Hemat/o means blood, but in the word *hematology*, the definition includes the blood-forming tissues.

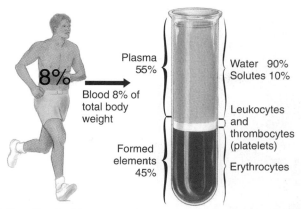

Fig. 5.27 Composition of the Blood. The cells and cell fragments are heavier than the liquid matrix, the plasma. When treated blood is spun in a centrifuge, the heavier elements (erythrocytes, leukocytes, and blood platelets) are packed into the bottom of the tube.

WRITE IT! EXERCISE 18

Write terms for the formed elements of the blood.

1. blood platelets _____
2. red blood cells _____
3. white blood cells _____

Hemolysis is the destruction of red blood cells with the liberation of hemoglobin.

Hemodialysis is the process of diffusing blood through a semipermeable membrane to remove toxic materials from the bodies of persons with impaired kidney function.

A **hematoma** is a localized collection of blood, usually clotted, in an organ, tissue, or space, resulting from a break in the wall of a blood vessel. The word hematoma is derived from the former meaning of tumor, a swelling, so named because there is a raised area whenever a hematoma occurs. Hematomas can occur almost anywhere in the body and are usually not serious. Bruises are familiar forms of hematomas. Hematomas that occur inside the skull, however, are dangerous (Fig. 5.28).

hem/o = blood
-lysis = destruction

hemat/o = blood
-oma = tumor

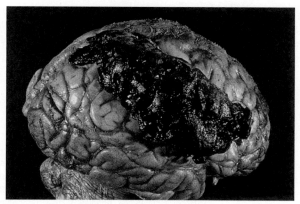

Fig. 5.28 Cerebral Hematoma. Note the large hematoma in this postmortem photograph of the brain.
cerebr/o = brain; **hemat/o** = blood

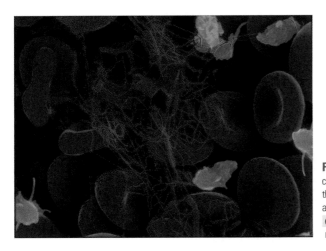

Fig. 5.29 Blood Coagulation. This scanning electron micrograph has been colored to emphasize the different structures. Red blood cells *(red)* are entangled with the fibrin *(yellow).* Note the thin center and the thick edges that give red blood cells a concave appearance. The platelets *(blue),* which initiate clotting, are also visible. **coagul/o** = coagulation; **micro-** = small; **-graph** = instrument for recording; **fibr/o** = fiber or fibrous

Blood **coagulation** (blood clotting), the transforming of blood from a liquid to a solid, occurs when blood is removed from the body (Fig. 5.29). **Fibrin** forms in the clot, entangling trapped cells. A substance that delays or prevents blood from clotting is an **anticoagulant**. Blood can be treated with an anticoagulant as soon as it is removed from the body, which prevents coagulation. In a blood transfusion, blood from the donor is transferred into a blood vessel of the recipient. Some blood transfusions require the use of whole blood, whereas in other types of transfusions only part of the blood is needed. The white cells, red cells, plasma, and blood platelets are blood fractions that can be used in a transfusion. A transfusion reaction is any adverse effect that occurs after a transfusion that is attributed to the transfusion.

CAUTION

Don't confuse *coagulation* (a chemical reaction, clotting) with *agglutination* (an antigen-antibody reaction). Read on to learn more about antigens and antibodies.

BLOOD TRANSFUSION REACTION

ABO and Rh factors on the surface of red blood cells are genetically determined and may cause a transfusion reaction in another person who is lacking these factors. In the laboratory, one's blood type is determined by mixing blood with commercially prepared sera (plural of serum) and observing for agglutination, aggregates or small clumps of erythrocytes that may be visible macroscopically (Fig. 5.30). There are also several other factors that can cause a transfusion reaction, and the adverse effect ranges from acute reactions, which are life threatening, to relatively benign allergic reactions.

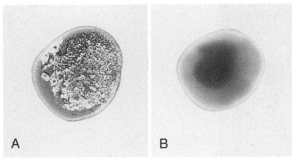

A   Agglutination

B   No agglutination

Fig. 5.30 Observing Macroscopic Agglutination in the Laboratory. **A,** This test, performed on a glass slide using blood and commercially prepared serum, results in visible small clumps (agglutination). **B,** Absence of macroscopic agglutination. Although there is no visible clumping, microscopic examination is required to verify that agglutination has not occurred.

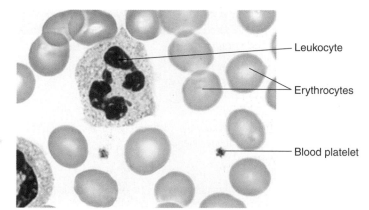

Fig. 5.31 Stained Blood. There are normally many more erythrocytes (red blood cells) than leukocytes (white blood cells). Only one leukocyte is shown here, although there are many types, each containing a nucleus. Platelets (tiny cell fragments) are also shown.

erythr/o = red;   **-cyte** = cell;   **leuk/o** = white

Some patients tend to form clots within blood vessels. **Thrombosis**, formation of internal blood clots, is a serious condition that can cause death. Special anticoagulant therapy is indicated for such persons to prevent internal clot formation.

> **thromb/o** = clot
> **-osis** = condition

Blood can be stained so that erythrocytes, leukocytes, and platelets can easily be recognized. Circulating erythrocytes in normal blood do not contain a nucleus, unlike leukocytes. There are several types of leukocytes, and all still have a nucleus in circulating blood (Fig. 5.31).

A red blood cell (RBC) count, often called a red cell count, is enumeration of the number of erythrocytes. A white blood cell (WBC) count, often shortened to white cell count, is the enumeration of the leukocytes. A differential WBC count is an examination and enumeration of the distribution of the various types of leukocytes in a stained blood smear. This laboratory test provides information related to infections and various diseases. All three of these tests are included in a complete blood count (CBC).

Blood **platelets** are small structures in the blood that are important for blood clotting. Blood platelets are also called **thrombo+cytes**, but they are not really cells, only cell fragments. A reduction in the number of blood platelets is called **thrombocytopenia** or **thrombopenia**. This results in a prolonged clotting time.

> **thromb/o** = blood clot
> **-cyte** = cell
> **-penia** = deficiency

Erythrocytes contain **hemoglobin** (hem/o, blood + globin, a type of protein). Hemoglobin is a red, iron-containing pigment that transports oxygen to the tissues and waste carbon dioxide to the lungs, where it is exchanged for fresh oxygen. **An+emia** is a condition in which the number of red blood cells or the concentration of hemoglobin (or both) is decreased. **Pallor** (paleness) and tachycardia are some typical signs of mild anemia, whereas more serious problems, such as difficult breathing, shortness of breath (SOB), headache, fainting, and even congestive heart failure, can occur in severe anemia. **Sickle cell anemia**, one of a group of disorders known as sickle cell disease, is an inherited red blood cell disorder in which the red blood cells do not have sufficient hemoglobin to transport oxygen throughout the body.

> **QUICK TIP**
> Anemia is a broad classification of disease. Compare with erythropenia, a decrease in erythrocytes.

> **an-** = without
> **-emia** = blood

The major function of **leukocytes** is body defense, helping to combat infection. Many leukocytes are highly **phago+cytic**. **Phagocytes** are cells that can ingest and destroy particulate substances such as bacteria, protozoa, cells, and cell debris. **Leukopenia**, or **leukocytopenia**, is an abnormal decrease in the total number of white blood cells. **Leukocytosis** is an abnormal increase in the total number of white blood cells. Leukocytosis can be transitory, but it is often associated with a bacterial infection.

> **phag/o** = eat
> **cyt/o** = cell
> **leuk/o** = white
> **-penia** = deficiency

TABLE 5.2	CHANGES IN NUMBERS OF FORMED ELEMENTS OF BLOOD	
Cell (Function)	**Common Name**	**Condition/Deficiency**
erythrocyte (transports oxygen)	red blood cell (RBC)	**erythrocytosis** (erythr/o, red + cyt/o, cell + -osis, condition) **erythrocytopenia**, **erythropenia** (erythr/o, red + cyt/o, cell + -penia, deficiency)
leukocyte (body defense)	white blood cell (WBC)	**leukocytosis** (leuk/o, white + cyt/o, cell + -osis, condition) **leukopenia**, **leukocytopenia** (leuk/o, white + cyt/o, cell + -penia, deficiency)
thrombocyte (blood clotting)	platelet (blood platelet)	**thrombocytosis** (thromb/o, clot + cyt/o, cell + -osis, condition) **thrombopenia**, **thrombocytopenia** (thromb/o, clot + cyt/o, cell + -penia, deficiency)

-emia = blood

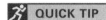 **QUICK TIP**

Leukemia is a disease. Leukocytosis is descriptive of the leukocytes only.

Leukemia is a progressive, malignant disease of the blood-forming organs. It is characterized by a marked increase in the number of leukocytes and by the presence of immature forms of leukocytes in the blood and bone marrow. Leukemias are classified according to the type of leukocyte in greatest number and according to the severity of the disease (acute or chronic).

Table 5.2 summarizes terms associated with changes in the numbers of different blood cells.

hemat/o = blood
-poiesis = production

HEMATOPOIESIS IS THE FORMATION AND DEVELOPMENT OF BLOOD CELLS

Hematopoiesis generally takes place in the bone marrow, but some types of white blood cells are produced in lymphoid tissue. **Erythro+poietin** (-poietin, substance that causes production), a hormone produced mainly in the kidneys and released into the bloodstream, causes the production of red blood cells. By studying their word parts, you obtain only a partial insight into the meanings of **erythropoiesis** and erythropoietin. Various proteins are produced by the body to stimulate the production of the different types of white blood cells.

Perhaps you are familiar with the pheresis department in a hospital and wonder how its name came about. It can't be broken down because it is derived from Greek *aphairesis,* removal. The term refers to a procedure in which blood is temporarily withdrawn, a fraction is retained, and the remainder is returned to the donor.

MATCH IT!
EXERCISE 19

Match the descriptions with the cell types in the right column (a choice may be used more than once).

_____ 1. red blood cell

_____ 2. white blood cell

_____ 3. cell that is often decreased in anemia

_____ 4. major cell type that is increased in leukemia

_____ 5. has an important function in blood clotting

A. blood platelet

B. erythrocyte

C. leukocyte

WRITE IT!

EXERCISE 20

Write a term in each blank to complete these sentences.

1. The fluid portion of blood is called _____.
2. A term for a localized collection of blood in an organ, tissue, or space is _____.
3. Destruction of erythrocytes with the liberation of hemoglobin is _____.
4. The process of diffusing blood through a semipermeable membrane to remove toxic materials is called _____.
5. Another term for clotting of blood when it is removed from the body is _____.
6. A substance that prevents blood from clotting when it is removed from the body is called a(n) _____.
7. The term for formation of internal blood clots is _____.
8. A shortened term for thrombocytopenia is _____.
9. The condition in which erythrocytes, hemoglobin, or both are decreased is _____.
10. Cells that can digest and destroy particulate matter are called _____.
11. The formation and development of blood cells is _____.
12. An abnormal increase in the number of white blood cells is _____.
13. A shorter term that means the same as leukocytopenia is _____.
14. A term that has the opposite meaning of erythrocytopenia is _____.

Body Defenses and Immunity

Susceptibility is being vulnerable to a disease or disorder. **Resistance** is the body's natural ability to counteract microorganisms or toxins. Our immune system usually protects us from pathogenic organisms. Unlike most body systems, the immune system is not contained within a single set of organs, but depends on several body systems.

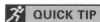 **QUICK TIP**

Barriers against microbes may be mechanical, fluid, or chemical (stomach acids).

THE BODY'S FIRST LINE OF DEFENSE IS *NONSPECIFIC RESISTANCE* (DIRECTED AGAINST ALL PATHOGENS)

Several body systems or structures help prevent foreign substances from entering the body:
- Intact skin: no cuts or open sores.
- Tearing apparatus of the eyes: fluids contain destructive enzymes; wash out microorganisms.
- Urinary system: urine's composition and outflow aid in ridding the body of microorganisms.
- Mucous membranes: mucus traps foreign particles.
- Digestive system: acids and enzymes produced by the stomach destroy many invaders that are swallowed.
- Respiratory system: moist respiratory membranes and hairs in the nose trap some organisms that are breathed; coughing and sneezing help expel foreign matter.
- Lymphatic system: lymphatic structures trap pathogens and produce cells that are vital to immunity.

This initial defense mechanism also includes **inflammation** (a protective response of body tissue that increases circulation to an area after irritation or injury), **phagocytosis** (ingestion and destruction of microorganisms), and production of interferon and complement. **Interferon** is a cell-produced protein that protects the cells from viral infection. **Complement** is a protein that not only promotes inflammation and phagocytosis, but also causes bacterial cells to rupture.

While the body's first line of defense is occurring, another type of defense (specific) is also taking place.

THE SECOND TYPE OF DEFENSE, *SELECTIVE OR SPECIFIC RESISTANCE* (DIRECTED AGAINST PARTICULAR PATHOGENS), IS CALLED IMMUNITY

The body's ability to counteract the effects of infectious organisms is **immunity**. This immune reaction, known as the antigen-antibody reaction, attacks foreign substances and destroys them. An **antigen** is any substance (e.g., bacterium, virus, toxin) that the body regards as foreign. An **antibody** is a disease-fighting protein produced by the immune system in response to the presence of a specific antigen. The body produces many types of antibodies, and each type of antibody destroys or neutralizes a specific type of antigen that caused its production. Two types of lymphocytes, T lymphocytes (also called T cells) and B lymphocytes (B cells), are involved in specific resistance.

🏃 QUICK TIP

Lymphocytes of specific resistance

B cells   T cells

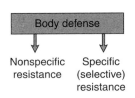

Body defense

Nonspecific resistance   Specific (selective) resistance

MATCH IT!
EXERCISE 21

Choose A or B from the right column to classify the characteristics as examples of specific or nonspecific resistance.

_____ 1. Antigen-antibody reaction destroys microorganisms.
_____ 2. Digestive acids destroy many swallowed microorganisms.
_____ 3. Sneezing expels foreign matter.
_____ 4. The immune reaction attacks foreign substances.
_____ 5. Urine aids in eliminating microorganisms.

A. specific resistance
B. nonspecific resistance

Antibodies are generally acquired by having a disease or by receiving a vaccination. **Immunization** is the process by which resistance to an infectious disease is induced or augmented. Active immunity occurs when the individual's own body produces an immune response to a harmful antigen. Passive immunity results when the immune agents develop in another person or animal and then are transferred to an individual who was not previously immune. This second type of immunity is "borrowed" immunity that provides immediate protection but is effective for only a short time.

Natural   Artificial

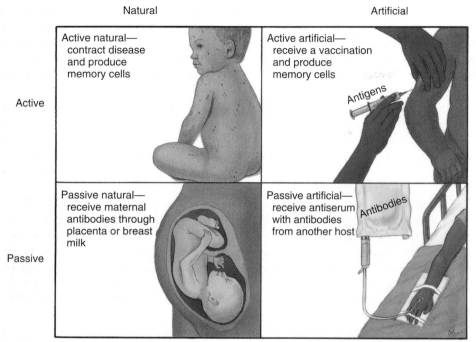

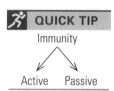

Fig. 5.32 Four Types of Specific Immunity. Active natural immunity and passive natural immunity, as the names imply, occur through the normal activities of either an individual contracting a disease or a fetus being exposed to maternal antibodies. Both active artificial and passive artificial immunities require deliberate actions of receiving vaccinations or antibodies.

In both active and passive immunity, the recognition of specific antigens is called *specific immunity*. The terms *natural* and *artificial* refer to how the immunity is obtained (Fig. 5.32).

QUICK TIP

Immunity

Active   Passive

MATCH IT!
EXERCISE 22

Choose A or B to classify the events as active or passive immunity.

_____ 1. having a disease

_____ 2. receiving a vaccination

_____ 3. receiving antibodies from a host

_____ 4. receiving antibodies through the placenta

A. active immunity

B. passive immunity

A **vaccination** is the administration of antigenic material (inactivated or killed microbes or their products) to induce immunity. Vaccinations are available to immunize against many diseases, including typhoid, diphtheria, polio, measles, and mumps. Depending on its type, a vaccine is administered orally or by injection or is sprayed into the nostrils.

An **immuno+compromised** person is one whose immune response has been weakened by a disease or an **immunosuppressive** agent. Radiation and certain drugs are **immunosuppressants**.

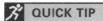 **QUICK TIP**

AIDS has a long
debilitating course,
generally resulting
in AIDS-wasting
syndrome.

Immunodeficiency diseases are caused by a defect in the immune system and are characterized by a susceptibility to infections and chronic diseases. Acquired immunodeficiency syndrome (AIDS) is a viral disease involving a defect in immunity that is manifested by various *opportunistic infections*. These infections are caused by normally nonpathogenic organisms in a host with decreased resistance. There is no known cure for AIDS, and the prognosis is poor. AIDS is caused by either of two types of the human immunodeficiency virus, HIV-1 or HIV-2. AIDS is transmitted by sexual intercourse or exposure to contaminated body fluid of an infected person. It was originally found in homosexual men and intravenous (IV) drug users but now occurs increasingly among heterosexual men and women and babies born of HIV-infected mothers.

HEALTH CARE CONNECTION

David Vetter, "the boy in the bubble," was born with a rare immunodeficiency disease. He spent his 12 years of life inside a sterile isolator, with a layer of plastic shielding him from microorganisms. He died 2 weeks after being removed from the "bubble." Read David's story, which was presented on https://www.cbsnews.com/pictures/bubble-boy-40-years-later-look-back-at-heartbreaking-case/.

Occasionally, the interaction of our defense mechanisms with an antigen results in injury. This excessive reaction to an antigen is called **hypersensitivity**. **Allergies** are conditions in which the body reacts with an exaggerated immune response to common, harmless substances, most of which are found in the environment.

WORD ORIGIN

ana-, excessive;
phylaxis (G.), a guarding

ANAPHYLAXIS/ANAPHYLACTIC REACTIONS ARE LIFE-THREATENING

Anaphylactic reactions are exaggerated hypersensitivity reactions to a previously encountered antigen (-phylaxis, protection). With a wide range in the severity of symptoms, **anaphylaxis** may include generalized itching, difficult breathing, airway obstruction, and shock. Insect stings and penicillin are two common causes of *anaphylactic shock*, a severe and sometimes fatal systemic hypersensitivity reaction.

The body's defense mechanisms, particularly the phagocytes, are important in impeding the spread of cancer and other diseases. You learned that **benign** means "favorable for recovery" and "not having a tendency to spread." **Malignant** means tending to grow worse, to spread, and possibly become life-threatening. Cancer cells are malignant, exhibiting the properties of invasion and **metastasis** (spreading from one part of the body to another part). Cancer cells **metastasize** (spread to sites away from where they originate) by several means, including the bloodstream, lymphatic system, and direct extension to neighboring tissue (Fig. 5.33).

A neoplasm that is at the original site where it first arose is called a **primary tumor** (example, lung cancer that has originated in the lung). That cancer can metastasize and spread to other tissues (**metastatic cancer**). An example of metastatic cancer is advanced lung cancer that has spread to nearby organs, such as the liver. The immune system acts against cancer cells to block or impede their spread and invasion of sites distant from their source.

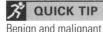 **QUICK TIP**

Benign and malignant
are opposites.

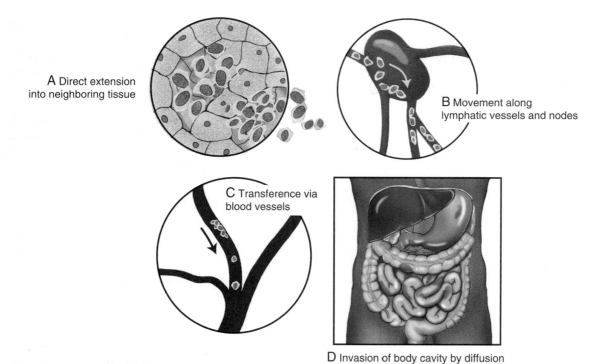

A Direct extension into neighboring tissue

B Movement along lymphatic vessels and nodes

C Transference via blood vessels

D Invasion of body cavity by diffusion

Fig. 5.33 Modes of Metastasis of Cancer. **A,** Extension into neighboring tissue. **B,** Invasion of the lymphatic system. **C,** Cancer cells are picked up and spread to other parts by the blood. **D,** Invasion of a body cavity.

WRITE IT!   EXERCISE 23

Write words in the blanks to complete these sentences.

1. A foreign substance that induces production of antibodies is called a(n) _____.
2. Lack of resistance is being _____ to a disease.
3. Phagocytosis of pathogens is part of the body's _____ defense mechanism.
4. Antibody-mediated immunity is part of the body's _____ defense mechanism.
5. _____ immunity occurs when an individual's body produces an immune response to a harmful antigen.
6. AIDS is an abbreviation for acquired _____ syndrome.

Pathogens

A **pathogen** is a microorganism that is capable of causing or producing a disease. You learned earlier that pathogenic means capable of causing or producing disease.

PATHOGENS ARE ANY DISEASE-PRODUCING AGENT OR MICROORGANISM

Our immune system is not always able to prevent *infection*, the invasion of the body by pathogenic microorganisms that cause disease.

The Centers for Disease Control and Prevention (CDC) is a U.S. government agency that provides services for the investigation, identification, prevention, and control of disease.

Types of pathogenic microorganisms include viruses, bacteria, fungi, and protozoa.

- A **virus** is a minute microorganism that replicates only within a cell of a living plant or animal, because viruses have no independent metabolic activity. Pathogenic viruses are responsible for human diseases such as influenza, hepatitis, and fever blisters.
- Microbiologists classify **bacteria** according to their shape. Most bacteria are easy to study and grow in the laboratory. A special staining technique (called Gram staining) serves as a primary means of identifying and classifying bacteria into three major types: **cocci**, **bacilli**, or **spirilla** (Fig. 5.34). Certain types of pathogenic bacteria cause sexually transmitted infections (STIs). Learn more about gonorrhea and syphilis and other types of sexually transmitted diseases (STDs) in Chapter 11.
- **Fungi** are microorganisms that feed by absorbing organic molecules from their surroundings. They may be parasitic and may invade living organic substances. Yeasts and molds are included in this group.
- **Protozoa** are the simplest organisms of the animal kingdom. Like fungi, only a few species of protozoa are pathogenic.

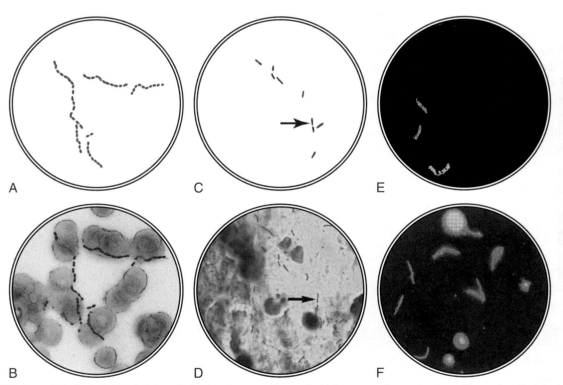

Fig. 5.34 Bacteria in Body Fluids. **A,** Schematic drawing of gram-positive cocci, which appear as tiny purple spheres. The cocci are in chains in this example. **B,** Gram-positive cocci in a Gram stain of a direct smear. Note the small size of the bacteria (which stain purple) compared with the much larger cells. **C,** Schematic of gram-negative bacilli, which appear as tiny pinkish rods. **D,** Gram-negative bacilli *(arrow)* in the presence of numerous leukocytes in a Gram stain of a direct smear. **E,** Schematic of spirochetes, which appear as long, tightly coiled spirals. **F,** Spirochetes in a preparation from material collected from a chancre, a skin lesion that occurs in syphilis.

VIRUSES ARE MUCH SMALLER THAN BACTERIA, FUNGI, AND PROTOZOA

Because of their small size, visualization of viruses generally requires the use of an electron microscope, which uses a beam of electrons rather than visible light. The magnified image is about 1000 times greater than that produced by an optic (light) microscope. Coronavirus diesease 2019 (COVID-19) is a highly contagious respiratory illness, caused by a coronavirus first discovered in 2019 (Fig. 5.35)

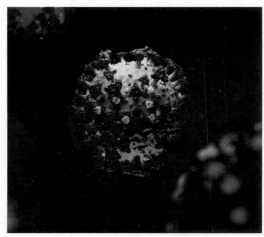

Fig. 5.35 COVID-19 virus, seen using an electron microscope. The virus was so named by the World Health Organization.

A microbiologist uses a light microscope to view most bacteria, fungi, or protozoa. Typical laboratory microscopes provide low-power and high-power magnifications of ×100 and ×400, meaning 100 times and 400 times the actual sizes of the objects viewed. Each microscopically viewed area is called a field of vision. As an estimation of quantity, microscopy laboratory reports often cite the number of organisms per high-power field (HPF), not just in reporting bacteria, but also in other areas such as the study of urine or in hematology. Sometimes the number of organisms or cells per low-power field (LPF) is reported.

WRITE IT! EXERCISE 24

List four general types of microorganisms.

1. _____
2. _____
3. _____
4. _____

Bioterrorism

Weapons of mass destruction (WMD) have been a concern for many years but have come to the forefront as acts of terrorism have increased. Health care providers must be trained to recognize and deal with these emergencies. The Federal Emergency Management Agency (FEMA) and the Centers for Disease Control and Prevention (CDC) use the following categories to define weapons of mass destruction:

- Biological
- Nuclear/Radiological
- Chemical
- Explosive
- Combined Hazards

bi/o = life

Bio+terrorism is the use of pathogenic biological agents to cause terror in a population. High-priority agents include microorganisms that pose a risk to national security largely for the following reasons:

1. They can be easily disseminated (distributed over a general area) or transmitted from person to person.
2. They cause high mortality rates and a major public health impact.
3. They can cause public panic and social disruption.
4. They require special action for public health preparedness.

WRITE IT!

EXERCISE 25

Write words in the blanks to complete these sentences.

1. WMD is an abbreviation for _____ of mass destruction.
2. CDC is an abbreviation for Centers for _____ Control and Prevention.
3. The use of pathogenic biological agents to cause terror in a population is called _____.
4. A term that means scattered or distributed over a general area is _____.

ⓘ Be Careful With These!

Opposites

anter/o versus *poster/o,* and *ventr/o* versus *dors/o*
proxim/o versus *dist/o* or *tel/e,* and *medial* versus *lateral*
prone versus *supine* (*pronation* versus *supination*)

Know the Difference!

anaplasia, aplasia, dysplasia, hypoplasia, hyperplasia, and *hypertrophy*
dacry/o (tears) versus *dactyl/o* (digits)
hemolysis and *hemodialysis*
hidr/o (sweat) versus *hydr/o* (water)
leukemia and *leukocytosis*
nonspecific resistance and *immunity*

A Career as a Phlebotomist

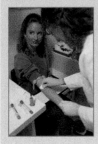

Meet Amy Thompson, a phlebotomy technician, or phlebotomist. Amy loves her job because she works with people, helping them by collecting blood samples to obtain valuable information for their physicians. As a member of the medical team in a large hospital, Amy is often the patient's only contact with the medical laboratory. Phlebotomists practice quality patient contact, safety, and professional behavior. Amy is cognizant of her essential role in the medical process and how she can help make diagnostic testing easier for patients. For more information on this career, visit this website: www.aspt.org or www.nationalphlebotomy.org.

Work the following exercises to test your understanding of the material in Chapter 5. It is best to do all the exercises before checking your answers against the answers in Appendix III. Pay particular attention to spelling. If most of your answers are correct, you are ready to move on to Chapter 6.

A. LABELING!   *Use the following terms to label planes #1 through #3 (frontal, sagittal, transverse) and aspects #4 through #6 (inferior, lateral, superior) in the illustration.*

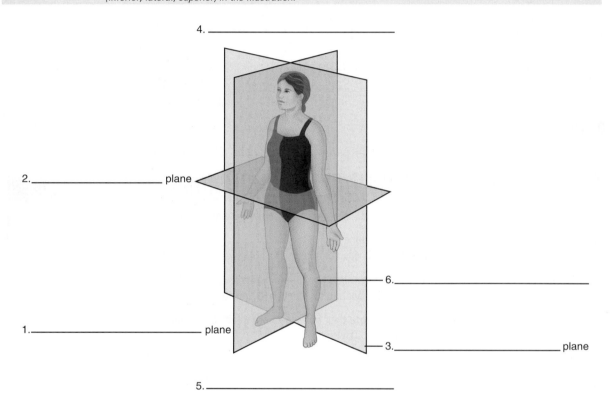

4. _____

2. _____ plane

6. _____

1. _____ plane

3. _____ plane

5. _____

B. MATCHING!   *Match the directional aspects of the body with the meanings in the right column.*

_____ 1. anterior	A. above
_____ 2. caudad	B. below
_____ 3. cephalad	C. far
_____ 4. distal	D. middle
_____ 5. dorsal	E. nearer the origin
_____ 6. inferior	F. toward the back
_____ 7. lateral	G. toward the front
_____ 8. medial	H. toward the head
_____ 9. proximal	I. toward the side
_____ 10. superior	J. toward the tail

C. IDENTIFYING!
Label these illustrations using one of the following: edema, hemolysis, hidrosis, hyperplasia, hypertrophy, hypoplasia.

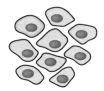

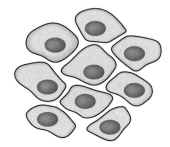

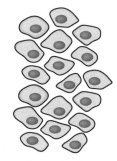

Original tissue

1. Increase tissue size by

_____

2. Increase tissue size by

_____

D. CHOOSING!   *Circle the one correct answer (A, B, C, or D) for each question.*

1. Which term means the opposite of distal?   (A) proximal   (B) inferior   (C) superior   (D) ventral

2. What membrane lines the abdominopelvic cavity and enfolds the internal organs?
   (A) lymph   (B) pericardium   (C) peritoneum   (D) visceral

3. Which term means inflammation of the navel?   (A) dactylitis   (B) dermatitis   (C) omphalitis   (D) sialitis

4. Which term means the presence of lacrimal stones?
   (A) allergic rhinitis   (B) dacryocystitis   (C) dacryolithiasis   (D) sialitis

5. Which term means a sticking together of two structures that are normally separated?
   (A) abdominocentesis   (B) adhesion   (C) laparogastrotomy   (D) mucosa

6. Which glands are ductless and therefore secrete their hormones into the bloodstream?
   (A) endocrine   (B) exocrine   (C) salivary   (D) sudoriferous

7. Which term means formation and excretion of sweat?   (A) adrenal   (B) ascites   (C) hidradenoma   (D) hidrosis

8. Which term means belly side?   (A) lateral   (B) posterior   (C) superior   (D) ventral

9. What is the term for the fluid part of the blood?   (A) intracellular   (B) lymph   (C) plasma   (D) thrombosis

10. Which term means pertaining to an immune response that has been weakened by disease or by an agent that suppresses the immune system?
    (A) immunocompromised   (B) malignancy   (C) resistance   (D) susceptibility

E. WRITING!   *List the four main types of tissue.*

1. _____   3. _____
2. _____   4. _____

F. SPELLING AND PRONOUNCING!   *Circle all incorrectly spelled terms, and write the correct spelling. Pronounce all 5 terms after correcting their spelling.*

anafalaxis   fibren   hypertrofy   immunosupressant   supination

G. WRITING!   *Write one word for each of these meanings.*

1. substance that induces an immune response _____
2. substance that prevents coagulation   _____
3. formation and development of blood cells   _____
4. in front and to one side   _____
5. lack of development of an organ or tissue   _____
6. pertaining to the abdomen and thorax   _____
7. presence of a thrombus   _____
8. use of pathogenic agents to cause terror   _____
9. white blood cells   _____
10. within a cell   _____

H. QUICK CHALLENGE!   *Find an incorrect term in each sentence and write the correct term.*

1. Homeostasis is a form of treatment that utilizes water.   _____
2. The noun *metastasize* means spreading from one part of the body to another part.   _____
3. Infection is a protective response of body tissue that increases circulation to an area.   _____
4. An omphalocele is a cavity containing pus, formed as a result of suppuration.   _____
5. Active artificial immunity is acquired by contracting disease and producing memory cells.   _____

*Use Appendix III to check your answers.

QUICK & EASY (Q&E) LIST

Use the Evolve website (http://evolve.elsevier.com/Leonard/quick) to review the terms presented in Chapter 5. Look closely at the spelling of each term as it is pronounced.

abdomen (***ab***-duh-mun)
abdominal quadrant (ab-***dom***-i-nul ***kwod***-runt)
abdominocentesis (ab-dom-i-nō-sen-***tē***-sis)
abdominopelvic (ab-dom-i-nō-***pel***-vik)
abdominothoracic (ab-dom-i-nō-thuh-***ras***-ik)
abscess (***ab***-ses)
acral (***ak***-rul)
acrocyanosis (ak-rō-sī-uh-***nō***-sis)
acrodermatitis (ak-rō-dur-muh-***tī***-tis)
acrohypothermy (ak-rō-***hī***-pō-thur-mē)
acromegaly (ak-rō-***meg***-uh-lē)
adhesion (ad-***hē***-zhun)
allergy (***al***-ur-jē)

ambulant (***am***-bū-lunt)
anaphylaxis (an-uh-fuh-***lak***-sis)
anaplasia (an-uh-***plā***-zhuh)
anatomic position (an-uh-***tom***-ik puh-***zish***-un)
anemia (uh-***nē***-mē-uh)
anterior (an-***tēr***-ē-ur)
anterolateral (an-tur-ō-***lat***-ur-ul)
anteromedian (an-tur-ō-***mē***-dē-un)
anteroposterior (an-tur-ō-pos-***tēr***-ē-ur)
anterosuperior (an-tur-ō-s$\overline{oo}$-***pēr***-ē-ur)
antibody (***an***-ti-bod-ē)
anticoagulant (an-tē-kō-***ag***-ū-lunt)
antigen (***an***-ti-jun)

QUICK & EASY (Q&E) LIST—cont'd

anuria *(an-ū-rē-uh)*
aplasia *(uh-**plā**-zhuh)*
ascites *(uh-**sī**-tēz)*
bacilli *(buh-**sil**-ī)*
bacteria *(bak-**tēr**-ē-uh)*
benign *(buh-**nīn**)*
blepharal *(**blef**-uh-rul)*
blepharedema *(blef-uh-ri-**dē**-muh)*
blepharitis *(blef-uh-**rī**-tis)*
blepharoplasty *(**blef**-uh-rō-plas-tē)*
blepharoplegia *(blef-uh-rō-**plē**-juh)*
blepharoptosis *(blef-uh-rop-**tō**-sis)*
blepharospasm *(**blef**-uh-rō-spaz-um)*
blepharotomy *(blef-uh-**rot**-uh-mē)*
calculi *(**kal**-kū-lī)*
caudad *(**kaw**-dad)*
caudal *(**kaw**-dul)*
centrifuge *(**sen**-tri-fūj)*
cephalad *(**sef**-uh-lad)*
cephalgia *(suh-**fal**-juh)*
cephalodynia *(sef-uh-lō-**din**-ē-uh)*
cephalometry *(sef-uh-**lom**-uh-trē)*
cephalopelvic *(sef-uh-lō-**pel**-vik)*
cerebrospinal fluid *(ser-uh-brō-**spī**-nul **floo**-id)*
chiroplasty *(**kī**-rō-plas-tē)*
chiropodist *(kī-**rop**-uh-dist)*
chiropody *(kī-**rop**-uh-dē)*
chirospasm *(**kī**-rō-spaz-um)*
coagulation *(kō-ag-ū-**lā**-shun)*
cocci *(**kok**-sī)*
complement *(**kom**-pluh-munt)*
cranial *(**krā**-nē-ul)*
dacryocyst *(**dak**-rē-ō-sist)*
dacryocystitis *(dak-rē-ō-sis-**tī**-tis)*
dacryolith *(**dak**-rē-ō-lith)*
dacryolithiasis *(dak-rē-ō-li-**thī**-uh-sis)*
dactylitis *(dak-tuh-**lī**-tis)*
dactylography *(dak-tuh-**log**-ruh-fē)*
dactylospasm *(**dak**-tuh-lō-spaz-um)*
diaphoresis *(dī-uh-fuh-**rē**-sis)*
diaphragm *(**dī**-uh-fram)*
distal *(**dis**-tul)*
dorsal *(**dor**-sul)*
dorsolateral *(dor-sō-**lat**-ur-ul)*
dorsoventral *(dor-sō-**ven**-trul)*
dysplasia *(dis-**plā**-zhuh)*
edema *(uh-**dē**-muh)*
endocrine *(**en**-dō-krin, **en**-dō-krīn)*
erythrocyte *(uh-**rith**-rō-sīt)*
erythrocytopenia *(uh-rith-rō-sī-tō-**pē**-nē-uh)*
erythrocytosis *(uh-rith-rō-sī-**tō**-sis)*

erythropenia *(uh-rith-rō-**pē**-nē-uh)*
erythropoiesis *(uh-rith-rō-poi-**ē**-sis)*
erythropoietin *(uh-rith-rō-**poi**-uh-tin)*
exocrine *(**ek**-sō-krin)*
external *(ek-**stur**-nul)*
extracellular *(eks-truh-**sel**-ū-lur)*
femoral *(**fem**-uh-rul)*
fibrin *(**fī**-brin)*
frontal plane *(**frun**-tul plān)*
fungi *(**fun**-jī)*
hematology *(hē-muh-**tol**-uh-jē)*
hematoma *(hē-muh-**tō**-muh)*
hematopoiesis *(hē-muh-tō-poi-**ē**-sis)*
hematuria *(hē-muh-**tū**-rē-uh)*
hemodialysis *(hē-mō-dī-**al**-uh-sis)*
hemoglobin *(**hē**-mō-glō-bin)*
hemolysis *(hē-**mol**-uh-sis)*
hidradenitis *(hī-drad-uh-**nī**-tis)*
hidradenoma *(hī-drad-uh-**nō**-muh)*
hidrosis *(hī-**drō**-sis)*
homeostasis *(hō-mē-ō-**stā**-sis)*
hydrocephalus *(hī-drō-**sef**-uh-lus)*
hydrotherapy *(hī-drō-**ther**-uh-pē)*
hyperplasia *(hī-pur-**plā**-zhuh)*
hypersensitivity *(hī-pur-sen-si-**tiv**-i-tē)*
hypertrophy *(hī-**pur**-truh-fē)*
hypoplasia *(hī-pō-**plā**-zhuh)*
immunity *(i-**mū**-ni-tē)*
immunization *(im-ū-ni-**zā**-shun)*
immunocompromised *(im-ū-nō-**kom**-pruh-mīzd)*
immunodeficiency *(im-ū-nō-duh-**fish**-un-sē)*
immunosuppressant *(im-ū-nō-suh-**pres**-unt)*
immunosuppressive *(im-ū-nō-suh-**pres**-iv)*
inferior *(in-**fēr**-ē-ur)*
inferomedian *(in-fur-ō-**mē**-dē-un)*
inflammation *(in-fluh-**mā**-shun)*
inguinal *(**ing**-gwi-nul)*
interferon *(in-tur-**fēr**-on)*
internal *(in-**tur**-nul)*
interstitial *(in-tur-**stish**-ul)*
intracellular *(in-truh-**sel**-ū-lur)*
lacrimal *(**lak**-ri-mul)*
lacrimation *(lak-ri-**mā**-shun)*
laparoscope *(**lap**-uh-rō-skōp)*
laparoscopy *(lap-uh-**ros**-kuh-pē)*
laparotomy *(lap-uh-**rot**-uh-mē)*
lateral *(**lat**-ur-ul)*
leukemia *(loo-**kē**-mē-uh)*
leukocyte *(**loo**-kō-sīt)*
leukocytopenia *(loo-kō-sī-tō-**pē**-nē-uh)*
leukocytosis *(loo-kō-sī-**tō**-sis)*

QUICK & EASY (Q&E) LIST—cont'd

leukopenia *(l o͞o -kō-__pē__-nē-uh)*
lymph *(limf)*
lymphatic *(lim-__fat__-ik)*
malignant *(muh-__lig__-nunt)*
medial *(__mē__-dē-ul)*
median *(__mē__-dē-un)*
mediolateral *(mē-dē-ō-__lat__-ur-ul)*
metastasis *(muh-__tas__-tuh-sis)*
metastasize *(muh-__tas__-tuh-sīz)*
metastatic cancer *(met-uh-__sta__-tik-__kan__-sur)*
midsagittal plane *(mid-__saj__-i-tul plān)*
mucoid *(__mū__-koid)*
mucolytic *(mū-kō-__lit__-ik)*
mucosa *(mū-__kō__-suh)*
mucous *(__mū__-kus)*
mucus *(__mū__-kus)*
omphalic *(om-__fal__-ik)*
omphalitis *(om-fuh-__lī__-tis)*
omphalocele *(__om__-fuh-lō-sēl)*
omphalorrhagia *(om-fuh-lō-__rā__-juh)*
omphalorrhexis *(om-fuh-lō-__rek__-sis)*
onychectomy *(on-i-__kek__-tuh-mē)*
onychomalacia *(on-i-kō-muh-__lā__-shuh)*
onychomycosis *(on-i-kō-mī-__kō__-sis)*
onychopathy *(on-i-__kop__-uh-thē)*
onychophagist *(on-i-__kof__-uh-jist)*
ophthalmitis *(of-thul-__mī__-tis)*
pallor *(__pal__-ur)*
palmar *(__pahl__-mur)*
paracentesis *(par-uh-sen-__tē__-sis)*
pathogen *(__path__-ō-jun)*
pelvic *(__pel__-vik)*
pelvis *(__pel__-vis)*
peritoneum *(per-i-tō-__nē__-um)*
peritonitis *(per-i-tō-__nī__-tis)*
phagocyte *(__fā__-gō-sīt)*
phagocytic *(fā-gō-__sit__-ik)*
phagocytosis *(fā-gō-sī-__tō__-sis)*
plantar *(__plan__-tur)*
plasma *(__plaz__-muh)*
platelets *(__plāt__-luts)*
polyuria *(pol-ē-__ū__-rē-uh)*
posterior *(pos-__tēr__-ē-ur)*
posteroanterior *(pos-tur-ō-an-__tēr__-ē-ur)*
posteroexternal *(pos-tur-ō-ek-__stur__-nul)*
posterointernal *(pos-tur-ō-in-__tur__-nul)*
posterolateral *(pos-tur-ō-__lat__-ur-ul)*
posteromedian *(pos-tur-ō-__mē__-dē-un)*
posterosuperior *(pos-tur-ō- s o͞o -__pēr__-ē-ur)*

primary tumor *(__prī__-mar-ē t o͞o -mur)*
pronation *(prō-__nā__-shun)*
prone *(prōn)*
protozoa *(prō-tō-__zō__-uh)*
proximal *(__prok__-si-mul)*
purulent *(__pū__-roo-lunt)*
pyogenic *(pī-ō-__jen__-ik)*
pyuria *(pī-__ū__-rē-uh)*
recumbent *(rē-__kum__-bunt)*
resistance *(rē-__zis__-tuns)*
sagittal plane *(__saj__-i-tul plān)*
saliva *(suh-__lī__-vuh)*
salivary *(__sal__-i-var-ē)*
sialography *(sī-uh-__log__-ruh-fē)*
sialolith *(sī-__al__-ō-lith)*
sickle cell anemia *(__sik__-ul sel uh- __nē__-me- uh)*
somatic cell *(sō-__mat__-ik sel)*
spinal *(__spī__-nul)*
spirilla *(spī-__ril__-uh)*
stem cells *(stem selz)*
sudoriferous *(s o͞o -dō-__rif__-ur-us)*
superior *(s o͞o -__pēr__-ē-ur)*
supination *(s o͞o -pi-__nā__-shun)*
supine *(s o͞o -pīn, s o͞o -__pīn__)*
susceptibility *(suh-sep-ti-__bil__-i-tē)*
telecardiogram *(tel-uh-__kahr__-dē-ō-gram)*
thoracentesis *(thor-uh-sen-__tē__-sis)*
thoracic *(thuh-__ras__-ik)*
thoracocentesis *(thor-uh-kō-sen-__tē__-sis)*
thoracodynia *(thor-uh-kō-__din__-ē-uh)*
thoracoplasty *(__thor__-uh-kō-plas-tē)*
thoracoscopy *(thor-uh-__kos__-kuh-pē)*
thoracostomy *(thor-uh-__kos__-tuh-mē)*
thoracotomy *(thor-uh-__kot__-uh-mē)*
thorax *(__thor__-aks)*
thrombocyte *(__throm__-bō-sīt)*
thrombocytopenia *(throm-bō-sī-tō-__pē__-nē-uh)*
thrombocytosis *(throm-bō-sī-__tō__-sis)*
thrombopenia *(throm-bō-__pē__-nē-uh)*
thrombosis *(throm-__bō__-sis)*
torso *(__tor__-sō)*
transverse plane *(trans-__vurs__ plān)*
umbilical *(um-__bil__-i-kul)*
umbilicus *(um-__bil__-i-kus)*
vaccination *(vak-si-__nā__-shun)*
ventral *(__ven__-trul)*
virus *(__vī__-rus)*
viscera *(__vis__-ur-uh)*

Don't forget the games and other activities available at http://evolve.elsevier.com/Leonard/quick.

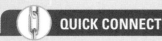
QUICK CONNECT

Review all lists of word parts and their meanings for Chapter 4, using the flashcards you prepared of the flashcards on the Evolve site.

Understand the levels of organization of the body, recognize their relationship, and sequence them from simpler to more complex: atoms, molecules, organelles, cells, tissue, organ, body system, organism. Recognize which of these (the cell) is the fundamental unit of life. Understand the significance of stem cells (divide without limit and give rise to specialized cells).

Understand the significance of reproductive cells (sperm or ovum with 23 unpaired chromosomes) vs. somatic cells (23 pairs of chromosomes). Recognize that somatic cells that perform the same basic activity are called tissues. Major structures in somatic cells are a cell membrane, nucleus (including chromosomes), cytoplasm, organelles.

Know the functions and differences in the four main types of tissue:

- epithelial tissue: forms the covering of both internal and external surfaces
- connective tissue: supports and binds other body tissue and parts
- muscular tissue: fibers that contract, causing movement of body parts and organs
- nervous tissue: conducts impulses that connect the brain and spinal cord with other body parts

Recognize the major body systems and their main functions:

- muscular: body movement
- skeletal: protection, form, and body shape; stores minerals and forms some blood cells
- cardiovascular: delivers oxygen, nutrients, and vital substances throughout the body; transports waste products to the lungs and kidneys
- lymphatic: helps maintain the internal fluid environment, produces some blood cells, regulates immunity
- respiratory: brings oxygen to the body and removes carbon dioxide and some water waste
- digestive: provides water, nutrients, and minerals; maintains the electrolyte and fluid balance
- urinary: filters blood, maintains electrolyte and fluid balance
- reproductive: facilitates procreation
- integumentary: provides external covering; regulates body temperatures and water content
- nervous system: coordinates reception of stimuli, transmits messages to stimulate movement
- endocrine: secretes hormones and helps regulate body activities

Differentiate these terms used to describe changes in tissue or organ formation: aplasia vs. dysplasia vs. hypoplasia vs. hypertrophy (Know that a similar looking term, anaplasia, is a change in cells that is characteristic of malignant tumors.)

BODY PLANES: FRONTAL VS. TRANSVERSE VS. SAGITTAL

Body Directional terms and aspects:

Know the meanings of these directional terms: anterior, posterior, ventral, dorsal, medial/median, lateral, superior, inferior, proximal, distal, cephalad, caudad, internal, external.

Six body aspects: anterior vs. posterior vs. lateral vs. medial vs. superior vs. interior. Understand the meanings of terms when body aspects are combined with directional terms.

Differentiate these terms: pronation, supination, recumbent, ambulant

Major body cavities: dorsal (cranial and spinal cavities), ventral contains the viscera (subdivided by the diaphragm into thoracic and abdominal cavities)

Body regions: head, neck, torso, extremities

Recognize words using acr/o (which means extremities).

Abdomen: The portion of the body trunk located between the chest and pelvis. Know the names and meanings of the four abdominal quadrants. Know the meanings of the types of abdominal hernias.

Differentiate these terms: palmar vs. plantar; thoracotomy vs. thoracostomy.

Write terms pertaining to body fluids and three formed elements of blood. Recognize terms related to changes in the numbers of erythrocytes, leukocytes, and thrombocytes.

Recognize the meanings of terms related to the body defenses and immunity, including the ways in which cancer cells metastasize.

Name and describe four types of pathogenic microorganisms.

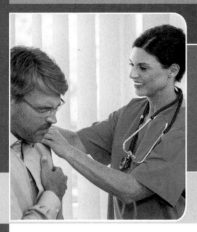

CHAPTER **6**

Musculoskeletal System

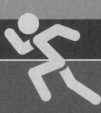

Orthopedics, a branch of surgery, specializes in the prevention and correction of musculoskeletal disorders.

OBJECTIVES

After completing Chapter 6, you will be able to:

1. Recognize or write the functions of the musculoskeletal system.
2. Recognize or write the meanings of Chapter 6 word parts and use them to build and analyze medical terms.
3. Write terms for selected structures of the musculoskeletal system or match terms with their descriptions.

4. Write the names of the diagnostic terms and pathologies related to the musculoskeletal system when given their descriptions, or match terms with their meanings.
5. Match surgical and therapeutic interventions for the musculoskeletal system, or write the names of the interventions when given their descriptions.
6. Spell terms for the musculoskeletal system correctly.

 Function First

The musculoskeletal system provides protection, support, and movement for the body. Bones store mineral salts and are important in **hematopoiesis**, the normal production of blood cells in the bone marrow. Muscles move an organ or part of the body by contracting and relaxing. Because of the close association of the body's skeleton and muscles, the two systems are often referred to as one, the musculoskeletal system. Muscles are also closely related to the nervous system because nerve impulses stimulate the muscles to contract.

hemat/o = blood
-poiesis = production

muscul/o = muscle

In addition to support and movement, the bones function in the formation of blood cells, storage of fat in the bone marrow, and storage and release of minerals, especially calcium.

EXERCISE 1

Write words associated with functions of the musculoskeletal system; the first letter is provided. (Question 1 is done as an example.)

1. *protection*
2. *s*_____
3. *m*_____
4. *f*_____of blood cells
5. bone marrow storage of *f*_____
6. storage and release of *m*_____

*Use Appendix III, Answers, to check your answers to all the exercises in Chapter 6.

Structures of the Musculoskeletal System

Musculoskeletal means pertaining to the muscles and the skeleton. The musculoskeletal system includes all of the muscles, bones, joints and related structures. Bones, as well as muscles, function in the movement of body parts, protected by a cushion of fat (Fig. 6.1). The muscular system includes all types of muscle, including the ones you're most familiar with. The skeletal system consists of the bones and cartilage of the body, which collectively provide the supporting framework for the muscles and organs in addition to places for the attachment of tendons, ligaments, and muscles.

Orthopedics is the branch of medicine involved in prevention and correction of deformities or diseases of the musculoskeletal system, especially those of the bones, muscles, joints, ligaments, and tendons. Ortho+ped+ics was so named because the **orthopedist** originally aligned children's bones and corrected deformities. Today, however, an orthopedist treats musculoskeletal disorders in people of all ages.

> **orth/o** = straight
> **ped/o** = child
> **-ic** = pertaining to

Bone marrow is the soft tissue that fills the cavities of the bone (Fig. 6.2). Red marrow functions in the formation of erythrocytes, leukocytes, and platelets.

Calcium in bone is radiopaque; thus, bones block x-rays from reaching the image receptor. Bones are represented by light areas on radiographic images (See Fig. 4.9).

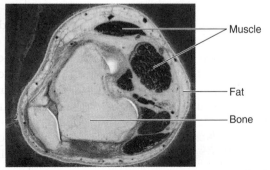

Fig. 6.1 Digitized Photograph of the Arm in Transverse Section. Bone, muscle, and fat are identified.

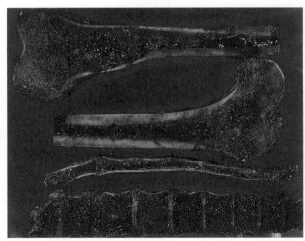

Fig. 6.2 The Interior Appearance of Bones, Split to Reveal Marrow. Note the red coloration of these bones, due to hemoglobin of red blood cells within the marrow. Note the width of the bones (from top to bottom), which are a lower leg bone, thigh bone, rib, and spinal bones.

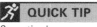

Major Bones of the Body

The adult human skeleton usually consists of 206 named bones (Fig. 6.3). The skull, spinal column, breastbone, and ribs are a major division of the skeleton; together these bones form the vertical axis of the body (shaded blue in Fig. 6.3). Write the name of the bones on Fig. 6.3 as you read the legend.

The following table lists the combining forms for the major bones, as well as their common names (when appropriate). Commit this information to memory.

MAJOR BONES OF THE BODY

Bone	Combining Form	Common Name
Bones That Form the Vertical Axis of the Body (Axial Skeleton)		
cranium	crani/o	skull
costa	cost/o	rib
sternum	stern/o	breastbone
spine	rachi/o, spin/o	backbone
vertebrae, in general	spondyl/o, vertebr/o	spinal bones
cervical vertebrae	cervic/o	⎫
thoracic vertebrae	thorac/o	⎪
lumbar vertebrae	lumb/o	⎬ spinal bones
sacrum (sacral vertebrae)	sacr/o	⎪
coccyx (coccygeal vertebrae)	coccyg/o	⎭ tail bone
Bones of the Appendicular Skeleton		
clavicle	clavicul/o	collarbone
scapula	scapul/o	shoulder blade
Bones of the Upper Extremities		
humerus	humer/o	upper arm bone
radius	radi/o	⎫ bones of the forearm
ulna	uln/o	⎭
carpals	carp/o	wrist bones
metacarpals	metacarp/o	bones of the hand
phalanges	phalang/o	bones of the fingers
Bones of the Pelvis	pelv/i	
ilium	ili/o	⎫
ischium	ischi/o	⎬ pelvic bones
pubis	pub/o	⎭
Bones of the Lower Extremities		
femur	femor/o	thigh bone
patella	patell/o	kneecap
fibula	fibul/o	⎫ bones of the lower leg
tibia	tibi/o	⎭
tarsals	tars/o	hindfoot bones, especially the ankle
calcaneus	calcane/o	heel bone
metatarsals	metatars/o	bones of the feet
phalanges	phalang/o	bones of the toes

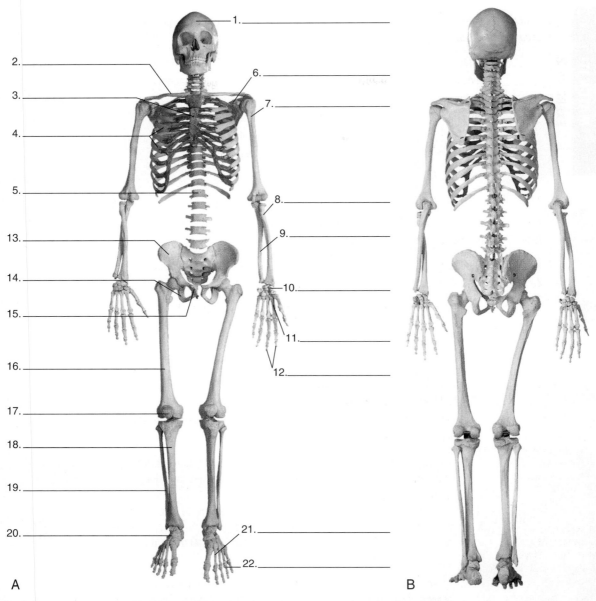

Fig. 6.3 **The Human Skeleton, With Major Bones Identified.** **A,** Anterior view. Label the bones as you read. The cranium *(1)* protects the brain and forms the framework of the face. The clavicle *(2)* is attached to the upper end of the sternum *(3)*. Also associated with the sternum are the ribs *(4)*, which support the chest wall and protect the lungs and heart. The vertebrae protect the spinal cord. A vertebra *(5)* is part of the vertebral or spinal column. The scapula *(6)* is a large triangular bone that joins the upper end of the longest bone of the arm, the humerus *(7)*. The bones of the forearm are the radius *(8)* and the ulna *(9)*. The wrist is composed of eight carpal bones, or carpals *(10)*. The bones of the palm are the metacarpals *(11)*, and the bones of the fingers are the phalanges *(12)*. The bones of the pelvis are the ilium *(13)*, the ischium *(14)*, and the pubis *(15)*. The femur *(16)* is the upper leg bone. The kneecap, or patella *(17)*, overlaps the bottom end of the femur and protects the knee joint, where the femur and tibia *(18)* meet. The smaller bone of the lower leg is the fibula *(19)*. The ankle is composed of seven tarsal bones, or tarsals *(20)*. The bones located between the ankle and toes are the metatarsals *(21)*. As with the bones of the fingers, bones of the toes are called phalanges *(22)*. **B,** Posterior view of the skeleton.

MATCH IT!
EXERCISE 2

Match the names of bones in the left columns with their common names in the right columns (a choice may be used more than once).

_____1. carpals   _____ 7. patella   A. ankle bones   G. shoulder blade
_____2. clavicle   _____ 8. phalanges   B. bones of the fingers or toes   H. skull
_____3. cranium   _____ 9. pubis   C. breastbone   I. thigh bone
_____4. femur   _____10. scapula   D. collarbone   J. wrist bones
_____5. ilium   _____11. sternum   E. pelvic bone
_____6. ischium   _____12. tarsals   F. kneecap

WRITE IT!
EXERCISE 3

Envision a person in the anatomic position. Write the names of the following bones in order (superior to inferior): femur, clavicle, fibula, humerus, tarsus, ulna

1. _____   4. _____
2. _____   5. _____
3. _____   6. _____

PROGRAMMED LEARNING

Remember to cover the answers (left column) with folded paper or the bookmark. Write an answer in each blank, and then check your answer before proceeding to the next frame.

bone	1. The axial skeleton forms the vertical axis of the body: skull, vertebrae, ribs, and sternum. The appendicular skeleton consists of the bones of the shoulders, upper extremities, hips, and lower extremities. The rigid nature of bone gives it the ability to provide shape and support for the body. However, bone also contains living cells and is richly supplied with blood vessels and nerves. The combining form oste/o means bone. **Oste+oid** means resembling _____.
calcium	2. The combining form calc/i means calcium. **Calcification** is the process by which organic tissue becomes hardened by deposits of calcium. Calcification normally occurs in bones and teeth; however, it is abnormal in soft tissue (e.g., deposition of calcium in the walls of arteries leads to arteriosclerosis). **De+calcification** is loss of _____ from bone or teeth. (The prefix de- means down, from, or reversing.) Osteomalacia is a consequence of decalcification without replacement of the lost calcium (See p. 170).
marrow	3. Bone marrow is the soft organic material that fills the central cavity of a bone. The combining form for bone marrow is myel/o, which also refers to the spinal cord. It is sometimes difficult to know which meaning is intended. When you see myel/o, you will need to decide if it means spinal cord or bone _____.

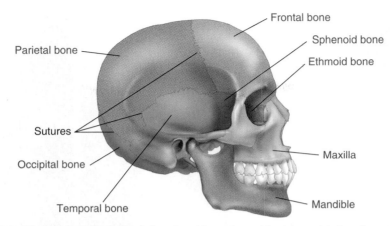

Fig. 6.4 The Skull, the Bony Structure of the Head. The skull consists of the cranium and the skeleton of the face. Sutures are immovable fibrous joints between many of the cranial bones. Blue labels are used for the cranial bones (parietal, occipital, temporal, frontal sphenoid, and ethmoid), whereas orange labels are used for the facial bones (only the maxilla and mandible are labeled).

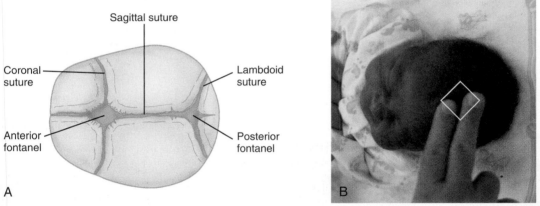

Fig. 6.5 Fontanels in an Infant. A, The anterior and posterior fontanels are located between soft cranial bones. Ossification of the sutures begins after completion of brain growth, about 6 years of age, and is finished by adulthood, at which time, the sutures have become immovable joints. **B,** Demonstration of the anterior fontanel of an infant.

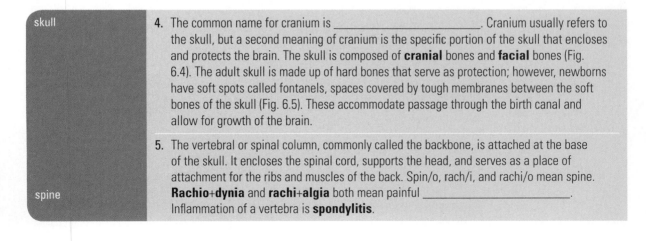

skull

4. The common name for cranium is _____. Cranium usually refers to the skull, but a second meaning of cranium is the specific portion of the skull that encloses and protects the brain. The skull is composed of **cranial** bones and **facial** bones (Fig. 6.4). The adult skull is made up of hard bones that serve as protection; however, newborns have soft spots called fontanels, spaces covered by tough membranes between the soft bones of the skull (Fig. 6.5). These accommodate passage through the birth canal and allow for growth of the brain.

5. The vertebral or spinal column, commonly called the backbone, is attached at the base of the skull. It encloses the spinal cord, supports the head, and serves as a place of attachment for the ribs and muscles of the back. Spin/o, rach/i, and rachi/o mean spine. **Rachio+dynia** and **rachi+algia** both mean painful _____. Inflammation of a vertebra is **spondylitis**.

spine

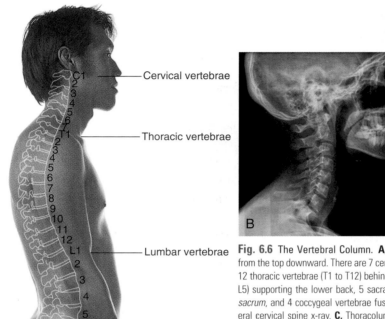

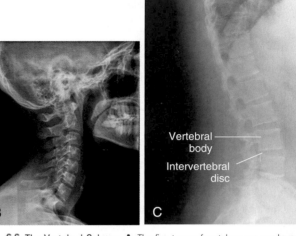

Fig. 6.6 The Vertebral Column. A, The five types of vertebrae are numbered from the top downward. There are 7 cervical vertebrae (C1 to C7) in the neck region, 12 thoracic vertebrae (T1 to T12) behind the chest cavity, 5 lumbar vertebrae (L1 to L5) supporting the lower back, 5 sacral vertebrae fused into one bone called the *sacrum*, and 4 coccygeal vertebrae fused into one bone called the *coccyx*. **B,** Lateral cervical spine x-ray. **C,** Thoracolumbar spine x-ray image with vertebral body and intervertebral disc labeled. **vertebr/o** = vertebra; **cervic/o** = neck; **thorac/o** = thorax (chest); **lumb/o** = lumbar; **sacr/o** = sacrum; **coccyg/o** = coccyx

Labels on figure A: Cervical vertebrae; Thoracic vertebrae; Lumbar vertebrae; Sacrum; Coccyx

Labels on figure C: Vertebral body; Intervertebral disc

	6. The vertebral column is composed of 33 vertebrae. The vertebrae are named and numbered from the top downward (Fig. 6.6A). The spinal cord is part of the central nervous system. It is a cylindrical structure located in the spinal canal, extending from the lower part of the brain to the upper part of the lumbar region. Spinal fluid or **cerebro+spin+al** (cerebr/o, brain + spin/o, spine) fluid is the clear, colorless liquid that circulates throughout the brain and _____ canal, the cavity within the vertebral column.
spinal	
between	7. **Inter+vertebral** means between two adjoining vertebrae. Cushions of cartilage _____ adjoining vertebrae are called intervertebral disks. These layers of cartilage absorb shock.
neck	8. The combining form cervic/o means either neck or the cervix of the uterus. In the naming of cervic+al vertebrae, cervical refers to the _____. Fig. 6.6A shows the seven cervical vertebrae, C1 through C7. Pads of cartilage, intervertebral disks, lie between the vertebrae (Fig. 6.6C)
thoracic	9. The combining form thorac/o means the thorax (or chest). As with other vertebrae, the thorac+ic vertebrae are so named because of their location. They are numbered T1 through T12. The thoracic vertebrae are part of the posterior (back) wall of the _____ cavity.
lower	10. The combining form lumb/o means the lower back. You may have heard the word **lumbago**, which is a general term for a dull, aching pain in the lower back. The lumb+ar vertebrae are located in the _____ back, numbered L1 through L5.

lumbar	11. The **thoraco+lumbar** region (Fig. 6.6 B) refers to the inferior thoracic vertebrae and the superior _____ vertebrae as a group.
sacral	12. The combining form sacr/o refers to the sacrum, the triangular bone below the lumbar vertebrae. Five **sacr+al** vertebrae are present at birth, but in the adult, they are fused to form one bone. The sacrum results from fusion of five _____ bones.
coccygeal	13. The coccyx is also the result of the natural fusion of vertebrae. The combining form coccyg/o means coccyx, or tail bone. This is located at the base of the spinal column and represents four fused **coccyg+eal** bones (-eal means pertaining to). The coccyx is the result of fusion of four _____ bones.
sternal	14. The **thorax** is the upper part of the trunk or cage of bone and cartilage containing the principal organs of respiration and circulation and covering part of the abdominal organs. It is formed ventrally by the sternum and costal cartilages and dorsally by the thoracic vertebrae and dorsal parts of the ribs (Fig. 6.7). Locate the elongated flattened sternum. Use the suffix -al (pertaining to) to write a word that means pertaining to the breastbone: _____.
ribs	15. The **thoracic cage** is the bony framework that surrounds the organs and soft tissues of the chest. It consists of the sternum, the ribs, and the vertebrae. **Cost+al** refers to the costae, or _____. There are 12 pairs of ribs, each one joined to a vertebra posteriorly (at the back). The first seven pairs, called "true ribs," attach directly to the sternum. The other five pairs, referred to as "false ribs," do not attach directly to the sternum (Fig. 6.8).
ribs	16. **Inter+costal** means between the _____. Intercostal muscles lie between the ribs and draw ribs together to increase the chest volume when breathing.

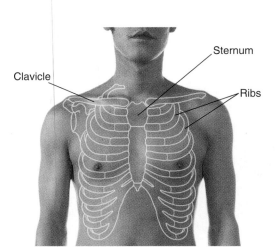

Fig. 6.7 The Thorax. The bones of the front part of the thorax are shown. The breastbone and ribs are part of the axial skeleton.

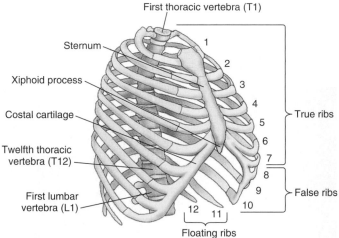

Fig. 6.8 The Thoracic Cage. The ribs exist in pairs, 12 on each side of the chest, and are numbered from 1 to 12, beginning with the top rib. The last two pairs of false ribs, the "floating ribs," are attached only on the posterior. **thorac/o** = chest; **-oid** = resembling; **cost/o** = rib; **lumb/o** = lumbar

below (under)	17. **Sub+costal** means _____ a rib or the ribs.
below	18. **Sub+sternal** indicates a location or position _____ the sternum.
sternum	19. **Sterno+costal** pertains to the _____ and the ribs.
vertebra	20. **Vertebro+costal** pertains to a rib and a _____.
rib	21. **Costo+vertebral** also means pertaining to a _____ and a vertebra. (Not all words can be reversed, as in vertebrocostal and costovertebral, but you will learn to recognize terms in which this can be done.)
	22. **Sterno+clavicular** is an adjective that pertains to the clavicle and the
sternum	_____.
clavicle	23. The clavicles attach to the sternum and either the right or left scapula. **Clavicul+ar** is an adjective that pertains to the _____. **Scapul+ar** refers to the scapula. The upper arm bones attach to the scapulae.
sternal	24. Sternal punctures are sometimes made with a needle to obtain a sample of bone marrow, the soft material that fills the central cavities of bones. Bone marrow samplings can be examined for abnormal cells. Puncture of the sternum with a needle is called a _____ puncture.
pelvis	25. The lower vertebrae make up part of the pelvis, the basin-like structure formed by the sacrum, the coccyx, and the pelvic girdle (pelvic bones). The combining form pelv/i means pelvis. **Pelv+ic** means pertaining to the _____.
pubis	26. Two hip bones help form the pelvis. Each hip bone consists of three separate bones (ilium, ischium, pubis) in the newborn, but eventually the three bones fuse to form one bone. By covering the right or left half of either Fig. 6.9, *A* or *B*, you are observing a hip bone. Locate the ilium, the ischium, and the _____, which fuse to make up the hip bone.

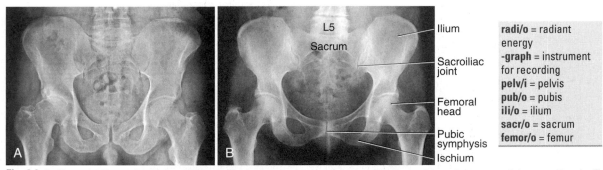

Fig. 6.9 Radiographs Comparing Male and Female Pelvis, Anterior Views. **A,** Male pelvis. Bones of the male are generally larger and heavier. The pelvic outlet, the space surrounded by the lower pelvic bones, is heart shaped. **B,** Female pelvis. The pelvic outlet is larger and more oval than that of the male. The size and shape of the female pelvis varies and is important in childbirth. L5 is the fifth lumbar vertebra. The pubic symphysis is the joint where the two pubic bones are joined.

ischium	27. **Ili+ac** refers to the ilium, and **ischi+al** means pertaining to the _____.
pubis	28. **Pub+ic** means pertaining to the _____.
ilium	29. **Ilio+pubic** refers to the _____ and the pubis.
ischiopubic	30. Use iliopubic as a model to write a word that means pertaining to the ischium and the pubis: _____.
ischiococcygeal	31. Use ischiopubic as a model to write a new term that means pertaining to the ischium and the coccyx: _____.
	32. The shoulder (Fig. 6.10) is the junction of the clavicle, scapula, and humerus (where the arm attaches to the trunk of the body).

🏃 **QUICK TIP**

The clavicles and scapulae are part of the appendicular skeleton.

	33. Technically, the arm is the portion of the upper limb of the body between the shoulder and the elbow. The bone of the upper arm is the humerus. Bones of the forearm are the ulna and the radius. The upper extremity is composed of the arm, forearm, and hand. Practice using the word parts you have learned for the bones of the arm and hand. **Humero+scapular** refers to the _____ and the scapula.
humerus	
ulna	34. **Humero+ulnar** refers to both the humerus and the _____.
ulnar	35. From the previous frame, you should now recognize the adjective that means pertaining to the ulna. It is _____.
humerus	36. **Humer+al** means pertaining to the _____.
radial	37. Use humeral as a model to write an adjective that means pertaining to the radius: _____.
carpectomy	38. The wrist, also known as the **carpus**, consists of eight small bones called the carpals (Fig. 6.11). Write a word that means excision of one or more bones of the wrist: _____.

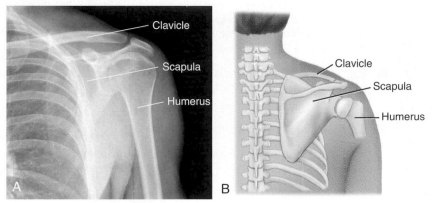

A, Anteroposterior radiograph. — Clavicle, Scapula, Humerus

B, Drawing — Clavicle, Scapula, Humerus

Fig. 6.10 Right Shoulder. **A,** Anteroposterior radiograph. **B,** Drawing of right shoulder, posterior view, shows the thin, flat, triangular scapula joining with the clavicle and humerus.

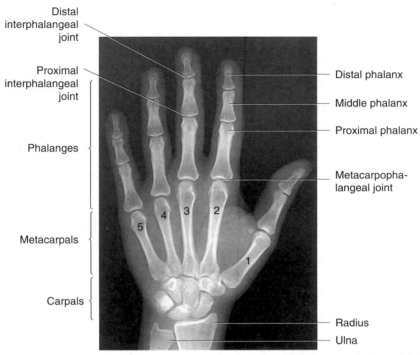

Fig. 6.11 Radiograph of the Human Hand. Bones of the forearm, the ulna and the radius, are identified, as are the bones of the hand. Eight small carpal bones make up the wrist (not all are visible). The palm contains five metacarpal bones, numbered 1 to 5. There are three phalanges in each finger except the thumb, which has two. **carp/o** = carpus (wrist bones);   **meta-** = change or next in a series;   **phalang/o** = phalanges; **dist/o** = far or distant from the origin or point of attachment;   **inter-** = between;   **proxim/o** = nearer the origin or point of attachment

carpal	39. **Carpal tunnel syndrome** is a complex of symptoms resulting from pressure on the median nerve in the carpal tunnel of the wrist. It causes pain, burning, or tingling in the fingers or hand. This complex of symptoms is called _____ tunnel syndrome.
next	40. The metacarpals are located between the carpals and the phalanges. The prefix meta- means change or next in a series. Meta+carpals lie _____ to the carpals.
fingers	41. The distal (far) ends of the metacarpals join with the fingers. **Carpo+phalang+eal** refers to the wrist and bones of the _____. There are two phalanges (singular, **phalanx**) in the thumb and three phalanges in each of the other four fingers. **Phalangitis** is inflammation of the bones of the fingers or toes.
leg	42. Each of the lower extremities is composed of the bones of the thigh, leg, patella (kneecap), and foot (Fig. 6.12). The femur is the longest and heaviest bone in the body. Femur is the name of the bone of the upper _____.
femur	43. **Ischio+femoral** pertains to the ischium and the _____.
femoral	44. From the previous frame, you should recognize the adjective that means pertaining to the femur. The word is _____. (This term also means the thigh.)
kneecap	45. **Patello+femoral** refers to the patella, or _____, and the femur.

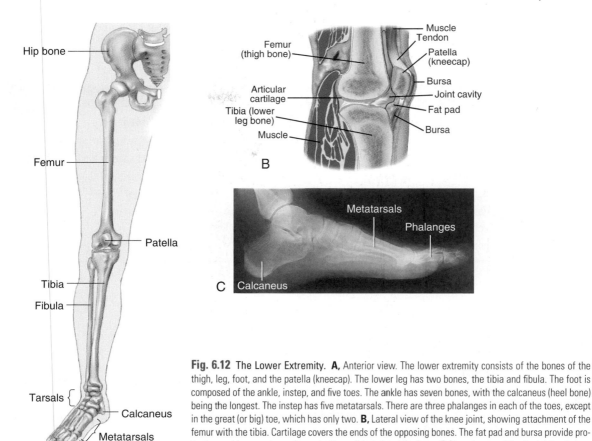

Fig. 6.12 The Lower Extremity. **A,** Anterior view. The lower extremity consists of the bones of the thigh, leg, foot, and the patella (kneecap). The lower leg has two bones, the tibia and fibula. The foot is composed of the ankle, instep, and five toes. The ankle has seven bones, with the calcaneus (heel bone) being the longest. The instep has five metatarsals. There are three phalanges in each of the toes, except in the great (or big) toe, which has only two. **B,** Lateral view of the knee joint, showing attachment of the femur with the tibia. Cartilage covers the ends of the opposing bones. The fat pad and bursa provide protective cushions, and muscles make it possible to bend the knee. **C,** X-ray image of the foot, lateral view. **articul/o** = joint;   **meta-** = change or next in a series;   **tars/o** = tarsus (ankle bones)

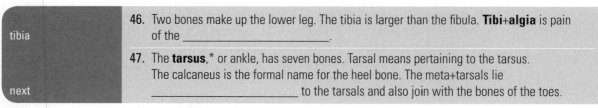

tibia	**46.** Two bones make up the lower leg. The tibia is larger than the fibula. **Tibi+algia** is pain of the _____.
next	**47.** The **tarsus,*** or ankle, has seven bones. Tarsal means pertaining to the tarsus. The calcaneus is the formal name for the heel bone. The meta+tarsals lie _____ to the tarsals and also join with the bones of the toes.

*Tarsus also means a curved plate of dense tissue that forms the supporting structure of the eyelid.

WRITE IT!
EXERCISE 4

Write adjectives that describe these structures. (Question 1 is done as an example.)

1. wrist   *carpal*
2. skull   _____
3. femur   _____
4. humerus   _____
5. vertebra   _____
6. lower back   _____

7. pelvis   _____
8. spine   _____
9. rib   _____
10. chest   _____
11. radius   _____
12. ulna   _____

Some additional word parts are presented in the following table. Be sure that you recognize their meanings.

ADDITIONAL WORD PARTS AND THEIR MEANINGS

Word Parts	Meaning	Word Parts	Meaning
ankyl/o	stiff	de-	down, from, or reversing
arthr/o	articulation, joint	meta-	change or next in a series
-asthenia	weakness	-sarcoma	malignant tumor of connective tissue
burs/o	bursa		
calc/i	calcium	ten/o, tend/o, tendin/o	tendon
cellul/o	little cell or compartment		
chondr/o	cartilage		

MATCH IT!

EXERCISE 5

Match the word parts in the left column with their meanings in the right column.

_____ 1. ankyl/o
_____ 2. arthr/o
_____ 3. -asthenia
_____ 4. chondr/o
_____ 5. de-
_____ 6. meta-

A. cartilage
B. change or next in a series
C. down, from, or reversing
D. joint
E. stiff
F. weakness

Cartilage

Cartilage is a specialized type of dense connective tissue that is elastic but strong and that can withstand considerable pressure or tension. Cartilage forms the major portion of the embryonic skeleton, but generally it is replaced by bone as the embryo matures. Cartilage does remain after birth, however, and is found chiefly in the joints (forming a covering of bone surfaces at the places where they meet), the thorax, and various rigid tubes, such as the larynx, trachea, nose, and ear. **Chondral** means pertaining to cartilage.

FIND IT!

EXERCISE 6

Write the combining form(s) and meanings for these new terms. A short definition is provided for each term.

Term	Combining Form(s) + Meaning	Meaning
1. **subchondral**	_____	beneath the cartilage
2. **vertebrochondral**	_____ _____	pertaining to a vertebra and its adjacent cartilage
3. **costochondral** (also **chondrocostal**)	_____ _____	pertaining to a rib and its cartilage

Muscles and Associated Structures

Muscle is composed of cells or fibers that contract and allow movement of an organ or part of the body. There are three main types of muscle tissue: cardiac (heart) muscle; smooth (**visceral** or **involuntary**) muscle found in the internal organs; and skeletal muscle, which is under conscious or voluntary control (Fig. 6.13). The muscular system, however, usually refers only to skeletal muscle.

The term **fascia** is used for the fibrous membrane that covers, supports, and separates muscles. **Tendons** are bands of strong fibrous tissue that attach the muscles to the bones. The combining forms ten/o and tend/o mean tendon.

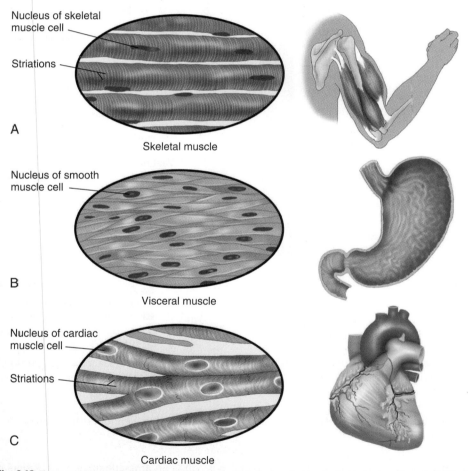

Nucleus of skeletal muscle cell

Striations

A

Skeletal muscle

Nucleus of smooth muscle cell

B

Visceral muscle

Nucleus of cardiac muscle cell

Striations

C

Cardiac muscle

Fig. 6.13 Types of Muscle. **A,** Voluntary, or skeletal, muscle is the type that is attached to bone and is controlled by the conscious part of the brain to produce movement. Under the microscope, voluntary muscle shows *striations*, alternate light and dark bands similar to those in the drawing. **B,** Visceral muscle is located in the walls of hollow internal structures, is involuntary, and lacks striations. It is also called smooth muscle. **C,** Cardiac muscle is involuntary but striated.

skelet/o = skeleton
micro- = small
-scope = instrument used for viewing
viscer/o = viscera (internal organs enclosed within a body cavity)
in- = not
cardi/o = heart

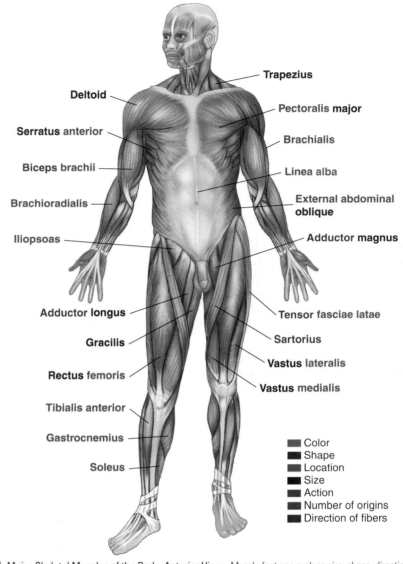

pector/o = chest
bi- = two
brachi/o = arm
radi/o = radius
abdomin/o = abdomen
ili/o = ilium
femor/o = femur
tibi/o = tibia

Trapezius
Deltoid
Pectoralis **major**
Serratus anterior
Brachialis
Biceps brachii
Linea alba
Brachioradialis
External abdominal oblique
Iliopsoas
Adductor **magnus**
Adductor **longus**
Tensor fasciae latae
Gracilis
Sartorius
Rectus femoris
Vastus lateralis
Vastus medialis
Tibialis anterior
Gastrocnemius
Soleus

Color
Shape
Location
Size
Action
Number of origins
Direction of fibers

Fig. 6.14 Major Skeletal Muscles of the Body, Anterior View. Muscle features such as size, shape, direction of fibers, location, number of attachments, origin, and action are often used in naming muscles. This is demonstrated by the use of color coding for the names. The meanings of the major word parts are identified.

More than 600 skeletal muscles control movement of the skeletal bones (Fig. 6.14).

Articulations and Associated Structures

The place of union between two or more bones is called an **articulation**, or joint. **Articular** means pertaining to a joint, and **nonarticular** means not related to or involving the joints. Cartilage or other tissue covers the articular surfaces of bones. Joints that have cavities between articulating bones are called **synovial** joints (joints covered with cartilage surrounded by a synovial membrane, **synovium**). The synovial membrane secretes synovial fluid (resembles egg white), which lubricates the joint and makes it freely movable. The elbow, knee, ankle, shoulder, and hip joints are examples of synovial joints.

WORD ORIGIN

synovia: syn (G.), together or with *ovum* (L.), egg

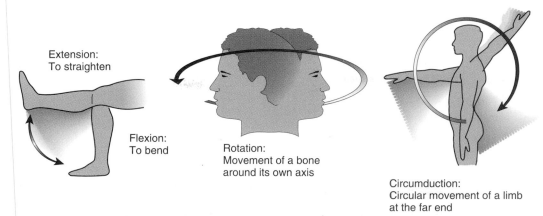

Extension:
To straighten

Flexion:
To bend

Rotation:
Movement of a bone
around its own axis

Circumduction:
Circular movement of a limb
at the far end

Fig. 6.15 Four Common Types of Joint Motion.

Movement tends to create friction between a bone and adjacent structures. **Bursae** are sacs of fluid located in areas of friction, especially in the joints (see Fig. 6.12, *B*). Four common types of joint motion are extension, flexion, rotation, and circumduction. Looking at Fig. 6.15, you can see that **extension** straightens a limb and the opposite movement, **flexion**, bends a limb. **Rotation** is the movement of a bone around its own axis, and a circular movement of a limb at the far end is **circumduction**. Remember that abduction and adduction mean movement of a limb away from or toward the midline or axis of the body, respectively. Refresh your memory of these terms by reviewing Fig. 3.11. The muscles responsible are **abductors** and **adductors**.

Range of motion (ROM) is the maximum amount of movement that a healthy joint is capable of, and it is measured in degrees of a circle (Fig. 6.16). ROM exercises are used to increase muscle strength and joint mobility and also to detect joint weakness or injury, such as rotator cuff tear (Fig. 6.17).

Ligaments are strong bands of fibrous connective tissue that connect bones or cartilage and serve to support and strengthen joints. Ligamentous means related to or resembling a ligament.

> 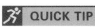 **QUICK TIP**
> Bursae is the plural of bursa.

> 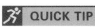 **QUICK TIP**
> Adhesives bring things together for bonding; adductors bring parts of the body toward its midline.

> 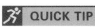 **QUICK TIP**
> The rotator cuff in the shoulder provides mobility and strength.

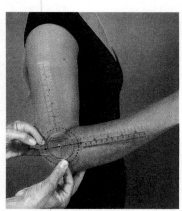

Fig. 6.16 Range of motion (ROM) and its measurement.

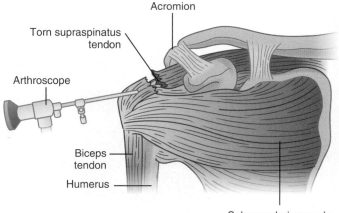

Acromion

Torn supraspinatus tendon

Arthroscope

Biceps tendon

Humerus

Subscapularis muscle
(located behind
the rib cage)

Fig. 6.17 A Torn Rotator Cuff. The acromion, the extension of the scapula, forms a joint with the clavicle. Manifestations of a tear in the rotator cuff include shoulder weakness and pain, as well as decreased ROM.

WRITE IT!   **EXERCISE 7**

Using combining forms and other word parts you have learned, write words in the blanks to complete the sentences. This exercise teaches you several new terms and is not a review.

1. **Fascial** means pertaining to _____.
2. **Myo+lysis** means _____ of muscle.
3. **Myo+pathy** means any _____ of muscle.
4. **Musculo+fascial** refers to or consists of _____ and fascia.
5. **My+algia** is muscle _____.

🚑 Diseases, Disorders, and Diagnostic Terms

Although injury is a primary cause of problems of the musculoskeletal system, the bones, muscles, and associated tissues are subject to various pathologies, including infections, malignancies, metabolic disturbances, congenital defects, and diseases of connective tissue, such as bone, cartilage, ligaments, and tendons, which bind and support other structures. The cause of some disorders is not known, such as chronic fatigue syndrome, characterized by disabling fatigue, or **fibro+my+algia**, characterized by widespread non+articular pain of the torso, extremities, and face. In **myo+fibro+sis**, tissue is replaced by fibrous tissue, and **myasthenia gravis** is characterized by fatigue and muscle weakness resulting from a defect in the conduction of nerve impulses.

non- = not
articul/o = joint
-ar = pertaining to

Stress and Trauma Injuries

A **dislocation** is the displacement of a bone from a joint (Fig. 6.18). **Fracture** (fx) is the breaking of a bone, usually from sudden injury. Bones may break spontaneously, as in osteomalacia or osteomyelitis. In a simple fracture, the bone is broken but does not puncture the skin surface. In a compound fracture, the broken bone is visible through an opening in the skin. Compare simple and compound fractures (Fig. 6.19).

A **sprain** is injury to a joint that causes pain and disability, with the severity depending on the degree of injury to ligaments or tendons. A **strain** is excessive use of a part of the body to the extent that it is injured or trauma to a muscle caused by violent contraction or excessive forcible stretch. A **myo+cele** is a condition in which muscle protrudes through

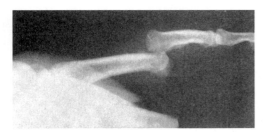

Fig. 6.18 Radiograph Demonstrating a Dislocation of the Finger. Dislocations, often the result of trauma, can occur in any synovial joint but are more common in the shoulder, hip, knee, and fingers. **radi/o** = radiant energy; **-graph** = recording instrument

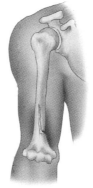 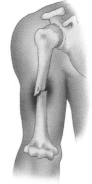 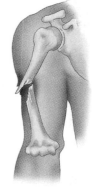

Incomplete, simple (closed)   Complete, simple (closed)   Compound (open)

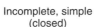

Fig. 6.19 Classification and Description of the Severity of Fractures. Fractures are classified as complete or incomplete and are described as open (compound) or closed.

its fascial covering. This is also called a fascial hernia. **Tendin+itis** means inflammation of a tendon (sometimes spelled **tendonitis**, not using the combining form).

> **tendin/o** = tendon
> **-itis** = inflammation

The vertebral column is composed of several bones and is, in effect, a strong, flexible rod that moves anteriorly (forward), posteriorly (backward), and laterally (from side to side). If the disks between the vertebrae become diseased, they sometimes rupture, resulting in a **herniated disk**, which can press on the spinal cord or on a spinal nerve, causing pain (Fig. 6.20). Although commonly called a "slipped disk," herniated disk is a more appropriate name.

In injuries of the spine, the greatest danger is that the spinal cord may be injured by the movement of a fractured vertebra. Cord injury can cause paralysis below the point of injury. **Para+plegia** is paralysis of the lower portion of the body and of both legs from a severe cord injury in the lumbar region. (Disease of the spinal cord can also cause paralysis.) **Quadri+plegia** or **tetra+plegia** is paralysis of the arms and legs. (In this term, quadri- refers to all four extremities, both arms and both legs.) Compare these terms (see Fig. 13.13).

> **para-** = beside
> **quadri-, tetra-** = four
> **-plegia** = paralysis

Paresis is motor weakness or partial paralysis. **Para+paresis** means partial paralysis of the lower limbs, and **quadriparesis** or **tetraparesis** affects all four extremities.

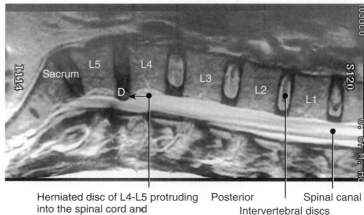

Anterior

L5 L4 L3 L2 L1
Sacrum
D
Posterior Spinal canal

Fig. 6.20 A Lumbar MRI Scan of a Herniated Disk. The superior vertebrae are located to the right in the scan.

Herniated disc of L4-L5 protruding into the spinal cord and compressing the nerve roots

Intervertebral discs

Combine the word parts to write terms for these descriptions.

1. replacement of normal tissue by fibrous tissue (my/o + fibr/o + -osis) _____
2. muscular weakness (my/o + -asthenia) _____
3. paralysis in the lower limbs and trunk (para- + -plegia) _____
4. paralysis of arms and legs (quadri- + -plegia) _____
5. fascial hernia (my/o + -cele) _____

Match the terms in the left column with their meanings in the right column.

_____ 1. compound fracture   A. bone broken, but does not protrude through skin
_____ 2. dislocation   B. bone broken, and protrudes through opening in skin
_____ 3. simple fracture   C. muscle injury caused by excessive use of body part
_____ 4. strain   D. displacement of a bone from a joint

cellul/o = little cell
-itis = inflammation
my/o = muscle

Infections

Cellulitis is an acute, spreading inflammation of the deep subcutaneous tissues (Fig. 6.21). If the muscle is also involved, it is called **myocellulitis**.

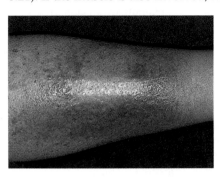

Fig. 6.21 Cellulitis. Note the acute, diffuse (spreading) infection of the skin and subcutaneous tissue. **cellul/o** = small cell;   **-itis** = inflammation; **sub-** = under; **cutane/o** = skin

oste/o = bone
chondr/o = cartilage

Osteitis is inflammation of a bone and may be caused by infection, degeneration, or trauma. Osteomyelitis, as mentioned earlier, is an infection of the bone and bone marrow and is caused by infectious microorganisms. **Osteochondritis** is inflammation of bone and cartilage and tends to attack the bone-forming (ossification) centers of the skeleton.

Myel+itis means inflammation of either the spinal cord or the bone marrow. **Myelo+fibr+osis** is replacement of bone marrow by fibrous tissue. **Osteo+myelitis** means inflammation of bone and the bone marrow.

Remembering that encephal/o means brain, **myelo+encephal+itis** means inflammation of the brain and spinal cord. Congratulations if you knew which meaning was intended by myel/o! Its meaning is not always immediately apparent, but you will be able to determine which meaning is intended by the context in which the terms appear.

Tumors and Malignancies

There are many types of benign tumors of the musculoskeletal system. The cause of bone tumors is largely unknown, unless cancer originates in other tissues and spreads to the bone.

Malignant bone tumors may be *primary* (originating in the bone) or *secondary* (originating in other tissue and metastasizing to the bone).

chondr/o = cartilage
-sarcoma = malignant tumor

Sarcomas are cancers that arise from connective tissue, such as muscle or bone, and in general, terms using the word part -sarcoma name or describe malignant tumors (but there are rare misnomers). A **chondro+sarcoma** is composed of masses of cartilage. A **fibro+sarcoma** is a malignant tumor containing much fibrous tissue. **Leukemias** are chronic or acute diseases of the blood-forming tissues characterized by unrestrained growth of leukocytes and their precursors.

Bone marrow is important in blood production and is involved in some types of leukemia. Leukemias are classified according to the predominant cell type and the severity of the disease (acute or chronic). Bone marrow studies are used to diagnose leukemia, identify tumors or other disorders of the bone marrow, and determine the extent of myelosuppression, or inhibition of the bone marrow. The posterior iliac crest is generally the preferred site for bone marrow aspiration (Fig. 6.22, *A*). In adults, the anterior iliac crest or the sternum may also be used. Smears of the bone marrow aspirate are stained and examined for numbers and types of cells (Fig. 6.22, *B*).

myel/o = bone marrow
-oma = tumor

Multiple myeloma is a disease characterized by the presence of many tumor masses in the bone and bone marrow. It is usually progressive and generally fatal.

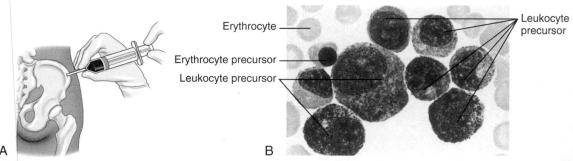

Fig. 6.22 Bone Marrow Aspiration. **A,** Aspiration of bone marrow from the posterior iliac crest. **B,** Stained bone marrow. Numerous erythrocytes and leukocytes are normally present in bone marrow, and many are precursors (earlier forms) of cells that are seen in circulating blood.
poster/o = behind; **ili/o** = ilium

Metabolic Disturbances

Metabolism is the sum of all the chemical processes that result in growth. Metabolic disorders result in a loss of homeostasis in the body (e.g., anything that upsets the delicate balance between bone destruction and bone formation).

Osteo+porosis is a metabolic disease in which reduced bone mass leads to subsequent fractures, most often affecting postmenopausal women, sedentary individuals, and patients receiving long-term steroid therapy. Osteoporosis may cause pain, especially in the lower back, and loss of height; spinal deformities are common. Fig. 6.23 shows the effect of the disease on height and shape of the spine with advancing years. Dowager's hump is an abnormal curvature of the spine from front to back often seen in osteoporosis (caused by multiple fractures of the thoracic vertebrae).

oste/o = bone
thorac/o = thorax (chest)

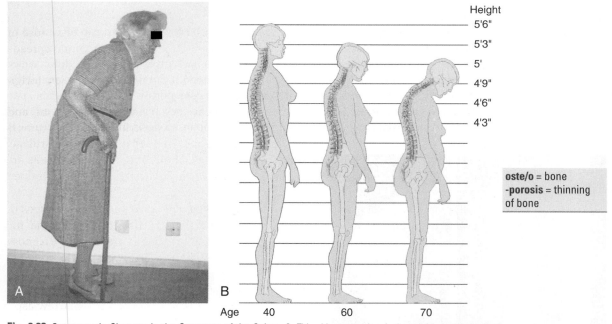

oste/o = bone
-porosis = thinning of bone

Fig. 6.23 Osteoporotic Changes in the Curvature of the Spine. **A,** This older woman's spinal condition is the result of osteoporotic and degenerative changes. **B,** The spine appears normal at age 40 years and shows osteoporotic changes at ages 60 and 70. These changes bring about a loss of as much as 6 to 9 inches in height and the so-called dowager's hump in the upper thoracic vertebrae.

Osteitis deformans (Paget disease) is a skeletal disease of elderly persons characterized by chronic bone inflammation. This results in the thickening and softening of bones and in the bowing of the long bones.

Osteo+malacia is a reversible skeletal disorder characterized by a defect in the mineralization of bone. The most common cause of osteomalacia is a deficiency of vitamin D, which is necessary for proper absorption of calcium. A specific term for softening of the vertebrae is **spondylo+malacia**.

BUILD IT!

EXERCISE 10

Combine the word parts to write terms for these descriptions.

1. acute inflammation of deep subcutaneous tissues (cellul/o + -itis) _____
2. infection of bone and bone marrow (oste/o + myel/o + -itis) _____
3. inflammation of bone and cartilage (oste/o + chondr/o + -itis) _____
4. malignant tumor composed of cartilage (chondr/o + -sarcoma) _____
5. malignant tumor containing fibrous tissue (fibr/o + -sarcoma) _____
6. disease characterized by unrestrained WBC growth (leuk/o + -emia) _____
7. abnormal loss of bone density and bone deterioration (oste/o + -porosis) _____
8. abnormal mineralization and softening of bone (oste/o + -malacia) _____

Congenital Defects

The skeletal system is affected by several developmental defects, including malformations of the spine. Some spinal malformations are congenital, and others can result from postural or nutritional defects or injury. **Spina bifida** is a congenital abnormality characterized by defective closure of the bones of the spine. It can be so extensive that it allows herniation of the spinal cord (see Fig. 13.14), or it might be evident only on radiologic examination, such as a CT or MRI scan.

Scoliosis is lateral curvature of the spine. It may be congenital but can be caused by other conditions, such as hip disease.

Exaggerated curvature of the spine from front to back gives rise to a condition called **kyphosis**, commonly known as humpback or hunchback. It can result from congenital disorders or from certain diseases, but it is also seen in osteoporosis affecting the spine, particularly in postmenopausal women with calcium deficiency. It is thought that ingestion of sufficient calcium can help prevent this problem. Compare scoliosis and kyphosis (Fig. 6.24).

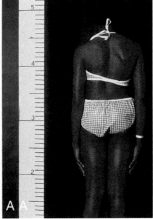
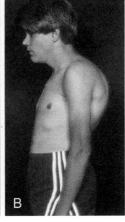

Fig. 6.24 Scoliosis and Kyphosis. **A,** Lateral curvature of the spine, scoliosis, is a common abnormality in childhood, especially in girls. **B,** Severe kyphosis of the thoracic spine. **later/o** = lateral or side;   **thorac/o** = chest

Muscular dystrophy is a group of inherited diseases characterized by weakness, atrophy (wasting) of muscle without involvement of the nervous system, and progressive disability and loss of strength.

Cranio+**cele** is a hernial protrusion of the brain through a defect in the skull. The feet and hands are also subject to congenital defects, such as the presence of extra fingers or toes, or webbing between adjacent digits. Flatfoot, also known as **tarso**+**ptosis**, is a relatively common inherited condition characterized by the flattening out of the arch of the foot.

dys- = bad **-trophy** = nutrition
crani/o = skull **-cele** = herniation

tars/o = ankle **-ptosis** = prolapsed

Arthritis and Connective Tissue Diseases

Connective tissue diseases affect tissue that supports and binds other body parts. The affected tissues include muscle, cartilage, tendons, vessels, and ligaments. **Arthr**+**itis** is any inflammatory condition of the joints characterized by pain, heat, swelling, redness, and limitation of movement.

Osteo+**arthritis**, also called degenerative joint disease (DJD), is a form of arthritis in which one or many joints undergo degenerative changes, particularly loss of articular cartilage. It is a chronic disease involving the bones and joints, especially joints that bear weight, which can also cause loss of spinal flexibility. Osteoarthritis is the most common type of arthritis and is often classified as a connective tissue disease. Connective tissue diseases are a group of acquired disorders that have immunologic and inflammatory changes in small blood vessels and connective tissue.

oste/o = bone **arthr/o** = joint **-itis** = inflammation

Rheumatoid arthritis (RA) is the second most common connective tissue disease. It is a chronic, systemic (pertaining to the whole body) disease that often results in joint deformities, particularly of the hands and feet (Fig. 6.25). (**Rheumatism** is a general term for acute and chronic conditions characterized by inflammation, soreness, and stiffness of muscles and by pain in joints and associated structures.)

There are many other types of arthritis, including **spondylarthritis** (inflammation of a vertebra), which can be thought of as arthritis of the spine. (For easier pronunciation, the *o* is dropped from spondyl/o when it is joined with arthritis.) **Rheumatoid spondylitis** causes inflammation of cartilage between the vertebrae and can eventually cause neighboring vertebrae to fuse. **Ankyl**+**osis** is an abnormal condition in which a joint is immobile and stiff. Sometimes the whole spine becomes stiffened, a condition called "poker spine" or ankylosing spondylitis. **Polyarthritis** is inflammation of more than one

spondyl/o = vertebra **arthr/o** = joint **-itis** = inflammation **poly-** = many
ankyl/o = stiff **burs/o** = bursa

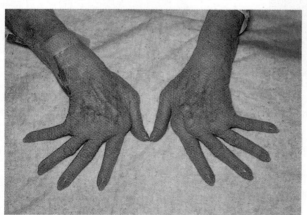

Fig. 6.25 Hand Deformity Characteristic of Chronic Rheumatoid Arthritis. Rheumatoid arthritis causes marked deformity of the joints in the hand, causing deviation of the fingers.
rheumat/o = rheumatism;   **arthr/o** = joint;   **-itis** = inflammation

hyper- = excessive
uric = uric acid
-emia = blood

joint. Both **arthralgia** and **arthrodynia** mean painful joint. **Burs+itis** is inflammation of a bursa, but does not necessarily include joint inflammation.

Lupus erythematosus (LE) is an autoimmune disease that involves connective tissue. The disease is named for the characteristic butterfly rash that appears across the bridge of the nose in some patients (see Fig. 12.13).

Gout is a painful metabolic disease that is a form of acute arthritis. It is characterized by inflammation of the joints, especially of those in the foot or knee. It is hereditary and results from **hyper+uric+emia** and from deposits of urates in and around joints.

The knee, a synovial joint, is subject to many injuries, including dislocation, sprain, and fracture. The most common injury is the tearing of the cartilage, which can often be repaired during arthroscopy.

Arthro+scopy is direct visualization of the interior of a joint using a special fiberoptic endoscope called an **arthro+scope**. It requires only a few small incisions (Fig. 6.26). Bits of diseased or damaged cartilage can be removed during this procedure. Incision of a joint is **arthrotomy**. **Arthropathy** refers to any disease of a joint.

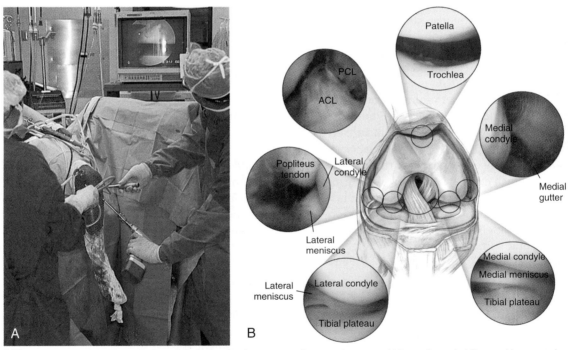

Fig. 6.26 Arthroscopy of the Knee. A, A specially designed endoscope, as well as an arthroscope, which contains optical fibers and lenses, are inserted. The physician sees the interior of the joint on a television monitor and may take material for biopsy or remove loose cartilage that interferes with movement. **B,** Six points of the knee that can be seen. **arthr/o** = joint; **-scopy** = visual examination; **endo-** = inside; **-scope** = instrument used for viewing

BUILD IT!
EXERCISE 11

Combine these word parts to write terms for the descriptions.

1. spinal arthritis (spondyl/o + arthr/o + -itis) _____
2. inflammation of more than one joint (poly- + arthr/o + -itis) _____
3. stiff joint (ankyl/o + -osis) _____
4. inflammation of a bursa (burs/o + -itis) _____
5. direct visualization of the interior of a joint (arthr/o + -scopy) _____

WRITE IT!

EXERCISE 12

Write the correct term in the blanks to complete each sentence.

1. A congenital abnormality characterized by defective closure of the spine is spina _____.
2. Lateral curvature of the spine is _____.
3. A group of inherited diseases characterized by weakness, wasting of muscle, and progressive disability is muscular _____.
4. An inflammatory condition of the joints characterized by pain and limitation of movement is _____.
5. Degenerative joint disease is also called _____.
6. A chronic, systemic type of arthritis is called _____ arthritis.
7. Painful joint is called either arthralgia or _____.
8. An autoimmune disease that involves connective tissue is lupus _____.
9. A painful inherited form of acute arthritis that involves urate deposits in the joints is _____.
10. A term for excessive uric acid in the blood is _____.

QUICK CASE STUDY | EXERCISE 13

Write the meaning of terms 1 through 4.

Prem Kamala, 70 years of age, fell while painting. He was diagnosed with scoliosis and osteoarthritis in 2020. Radiologic findings show a simple, complete fracture of the left fibula. He is able to move his left ankle and toes, suffers widespread arthralgia, and underwent right knee arthroscopy in 2013.

1. simple, complete fracture _____
2. fibula _____
3. arthralgia _____
4. arthroscopy _____
5. osteoarthritis _____
6. scoliosis _____

Surgical and Therapeutic Interventions

Orthopedic surgeons restore fractures to their normal positions by **reduction**, pulling the broken fragments into alignment. Management usually involves immobilization with a splint, bandage, cast, or traction. A cast immobilizes a broken bone until it heals. Traction is the use of a pulling force to a part of the body to produce alignment and rest while decreasing muscle spasm and correcting or preventing deformity.

A fracture is usually restored to its normal position by manipulation without surgery. This is called closed reduction. If a fracture must be exposed by surgery before the broken ends can be aligned, it is an open reduction. The fracture shown in Fig. 6.27, *A*, was corrected by surgery that included internal fixation to stabilize the alignment. Internal fixation uses pins, rods, plates, screws, or other materials to immobilize the fracture. After healing, the fixation devices may be removed or left in place. External fixation is used in both open and closed reductions. This method uses metal pins attached to a compression device outside the skin surface (Fig. 6.27, *B*).

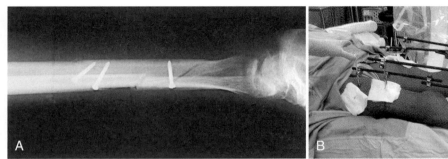

Fig. 6.27 Internal and External Fixation of Fractures. **A,** Lateral view of a lower leg break after reduction and internal fixation using screws. **B,** External fixation of a fracture using pins that are attached to a compression device. The pins are removed when the fracture is healed.

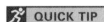

> **QUICK TIP**
> There is an abnormal loss of bone density in osteoporosis.

After a bone is broken, the body begins the healing process to repair the injury. Electrical bone stimulation, bone grafting, and ultrasound treatment may be used when healing is slow or does not occur.

Persons with osteoporosis are predisposed to fractures. Calcium therapy, vitamin D, and **anti-osteoporotics** are used to treat osteoporosis. Estrogen therapy, begun soon after the start of menopause, may help in the prevention and treatment of osteoporosis. Vertebral fractures can sometimes be repaired by **vertebro+plasty**. In this procedure, a cementlike substance is injected into the body of a fractured vertebra to stabilize and strengthen it and immediately remove pain.

Numerous surgeries are performed to straighten the toes, remove bunions (abnormal enlargement of the joint at the base of the great toe), and correct various deformities of the feet. A **bunion+ectomy** is excision of a bunion. Surgical repair to straighten the alignment of the toes is usually done at the same time.

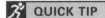

> **QUICK TIP**
> One *e* is often dropped. Ostectomy versus osteectomy.

Excision of a bone (or a portion of it) is **oste+ectomy**; this is usually written **ostectomy**. Excision of a rib is **cost+ectomy**. **Cranio+tomy** is incision into the skull; **crani+ectomy** is excision of a segment of the skull (Fig. 6.28). Plastic surgery to repair the skull is **cranio+plasty**.

Tendons may become damaged when a person sustains a deep wound and may require surgical repair or **tendo+plasty**. **Myo+plasty** is surgical repair of muscle. **Teno+myo+plasty** is surgical repair of tendon and muscle.

Muscle relaxants are prescribed to relieve muscle spasms, such as the spasms that accompany a herniated disk. If bed rest and other treatments do not alleviate

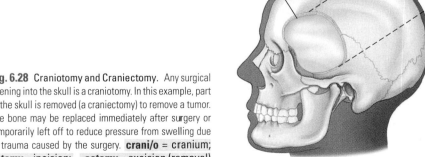

Fig. 6.28 Craniotomy and Craniectomy. Any surgical opening into the skull is a craniotomy. In this example, part of the skull is removed (a craniectomy) to remove a tumor. The bone may be replaced immediately after surgery or temporarily left off to reduce pressure from swelling due to trauma caused by the surgery. **crani/o** = cranium; **-tomy** = incision; **-ectomy** = excision (removal)

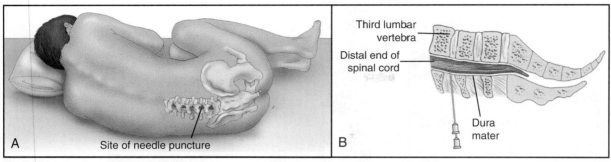

Fig. 6.29 Lumbar Puncture. The needle is inserted into the space between the third and fourth lumbar vertebrae. A specimen of cerebrospinal fluid may be collected for examination. A lumbar puncture is also necessary for injection of a spinal anesthetic.
cerebr/o = brain;   **spin/o** = spine;   **esthesi/o** = feeling

the problem, a **laminectomy** may be indicated. This is surgical removal of the bony posterior arch of a vertebra to permit surgical access to the disk so that the herniated material can be removed. Complete excision of an intervertebral disk is a **disk+ectomy**.

Spinal anesthesia is loss of feeling produced by an anesthetic injected into the spinal canal. Spinal puncture (also called spinal tap or lumbar puncture [Fig. 6.29]) is puncture of the spinal cavity with a needle, either to extract the spinal fluid for diagnostic purposes or to introduce agents into the spinal canal for anesthesia or radiographic studies, termed a **myelogram**.

Many drugs are available to treat different forms of arthritis and other connective tissue diseases. **Antiinflammatories** are generally used to reduce inflammation and pain, especially drugs classified as nonsteroidal antiinflammatory drugs (NSAIDs). Two examples are aspirin and ibuprofen. Physical therapy is an important part of arthritis treatment as well as restoring function after injury or surgery.

Cyclooxygenase-2 (COX-2) inhibitors are also frequently used to reduce the inflammation of arthritis and are less likely than aspirin or ibuprofen to cause stomach distress and ulcers. **Antiarthritics** are various forms of therapy that relieve the symptoms of arthritis. Disease-modifying antirheumatic drugs (DMARDs) may change the course of inflammatory conditions such as rheumatoid arthritis, slowing progression of the disease. They tend to be slower acting than NSAIDs and may be prescribed with antiinflammatories.

Torn cartilage or loose bodies in a joint space can be removed during arthroscopy. Excision of cartilage is **chondr+ectomy**. Excessive fluid can accumulate in a synovial joint after injury and must be extracted with a needle; this procedure is called **arthro+centesis**.

-centesis = surgical puncture

When other measures are inadequate to provide pain control for degenerative joint disease, surgery may be indicated, often total joint replacement. Replacement of hips, knees, elbows, wrists, shoulders, and finger or toe joints is common. Total knee replacement (Fig. 6.30) is the surgical insertion of a hinged device to relieve pain and restore motion to a knee that is severely affected by arthritis or injury. Any surgical reconstruction or replacement of a joint is called **arthro+plasty**.

Cancer treatment often induces **myelosuppression**. If the patient's bone marrow is destroyed with radiation and chemotherapy, bone marrow transplants (BMTs) are used to stimulate the production of normal blood.

myel/o = bone marrow
suppress = to inhibit

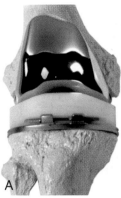 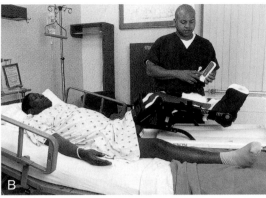

Fig. 6.30 Knee Replacement. A, With the patient under anesthesia, the diseased surfaces of the knee are removed and a hinged prosthesis, such as the one shown, is inserted into the medullary cavities of the femur and tibia. **B,** After surgery, progressive exercise sometimes includes a continuous passive motion machine.

MATCH IT!
EXERCISE 14

Match the surgical terms in the left column with their meanings in the right column.

_____ 1. closed reduction
_____ 2. internal fixation
_____ 3. open reduction
_____ 4. ostectomy

A. excision of a bone
B. surgically exposing and aligning a broken bone
C. pulling a broken bone into alignment without surgery
D. surgery using pins or other materials to immobilize a broken bone

WRITE IT!
EXERCISE 15

Write terms for these meanings.

1. excision of a disk   _____
2. inhibiting bone marrow activity   _____
3. medications that reduce inflammation   _____
4. surgical puncture of a synovial joint   _____
5. surgical repair of muscle   _____

WRITE IT!
EXERCISE 16

Write the correct term for #1 through #3.

2. _____
(bone removed)

1. _____
(bone incised)

Be Careful With These!

ankyl/o (stiff) does not mean ankle! *tars/o* means ankle. *coccyg/o* means *coccyx.*
metatars/o (bones of the foot) versus *metacarp/o* (bones of the hand)
paresis (incomplete paralysis) versus *paralysis.*
Note spelling of combining form for femur is *femor/o.*
Remember that *radi/o* can mean a bone of the forearm, not just radiation.

A Career as an Athletic Trainer

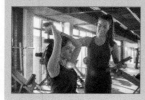 Tanya Palmer has been a certified athletic trainer for 10 years and never plans to stop personal training. She is passionate about helping others achieve their goals. Her educational preparation took 4 years, but Tanya knew it would be worth the effort. She has her own business working at an exercise facility, training individuals of all abilities and fitness levels. She also works for three high school athletic teams. For more information, visit this website: www.nata.org.

 SELF-TEST

Work the following exercises to test your understanding of the material in Chapter 6. It is best to do all the exercises before checking your answers against the answers in Appendix III. Pay particular attention to spelling. Study Chapters 6 through 15 in the order selected by your instructor.

A. MATCHING!   *Match the names of bones in the two left columns with their common names in the two right columns (a choice may be used more than once).*

_____ 1. carpals   _____ 10. phalanges   A. ankle bones   H. kneecap
_____ 2. clavicle   _____ 11. pubis   B. bone of the forearm   I. shoulder blade
_____ 3. cranium   _____ 12. radius   C. bone of the lower leg   J. skull
_____ 4. femur   _____ 13. scapula   D. bones of the fingers or toes   K. spinal bone
_____ 5. fibula   _____ 14. sternum   E. breastbone   L. thigh bone
_____ 6. humerus   _____ 15. tarsals   F. collarbone   M. upper arm bone
_____ 7. ilium   _____ 16. ulna   G. pelvic bone   N. wrist bones
_____ 8. ischium   _____ 17. vertebra
_____ 9. patella

B. SPELLING AND PRONOUNCING!   *Circle the terms that are incorrectly spelled, and write the correct spelling. Then pronounce the terms.*

ankilosis   coccyk   femural   flexsion   laminektomy

C. MATCHING!   *Match the connective tissues with their descriptions (each choice is used once).*

_____ 1. bone
_____ 2. bursa
_____ 3. cartilage
_____ 4. joint
_____ 5. ligament
_____ 6. synovial membrane
_____ 7. tendon

A. connects bones or cartilages
B. fluid-filled sac that helps reduce friction
C. fluid-secreting tissue lining the joint
D. place of union between two or more bones
E. provides protection and support for a joint
F. strong, fibrous tissue that attaches muscles to bones
G. the most rigid connective tissue

D. IDENTIFYING!   *Label the types of vertebrae as cervical, coccygeal, lumbar, sacral, or thoracic.*

1. _____ vertebrae
2. _____ vertebrae
3. _____ vertebrae
4. _____ vertebrae
5. _____ vertebrae

E. IDENTIFYING!   *Label the figures with the types of fractures (A, B, or C): **A**, Complete, simple; **B**, complete compound; **C**, incomplete, simple.*

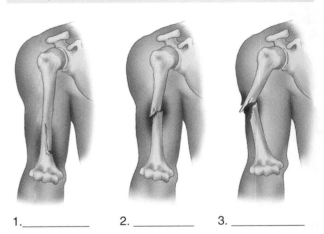

1._____   2. _____   3. _____

F. CHOOSING!   *Circle the one correct answer (A, B, C, or D) for each question.*

1. What does rachialgia mean?
   (A) fused spine   **(B)** painful spine   **(C)** the opposite of rachiodynia   **(D)** the same as spondylitis

2. What is the meaning of myocele?
   (A) fascial hernia   **(B)** fibrous muscle   **(C)** hardened muscle   **(D)** painful muscle

3. Which term means inflammation of the vertebrae?   (A) carpitis   (B) phalangitis   (C) spondylitis   (D) tarsitis

4. Which term means between the ribs?   (A) costovertebral   (B) intercostal   (C) intracostal   (D) subcostal

5. Which term means excision of a portion of the skull?
   (A) angiectomy   (B) coccygectomy   (C) craniectomy   (D) craniotomy

6. Which term indicates a broken bone that is visible through an opening in the skin?
   (A) closed fracture   (B) complete fracture   (C) compound fracture   (D) simple fracture

7. What is the meaning of articulation?
   (A) bone   (B) cartilage   (C) fascia   (D) joint

8. Which term means rupture of an intervertebral disk?
   (A) chondrosarcoma   (B) herniated disk   (C) spondylomalacia   (D) vertebrochondritis

9. What does osteoid mean?
   (A) growth of bone   (B) inflammation of bone   (C) resembling bone   (D) softening of bone

10. Which term refers to the bones located between the toes and the bones of the ankle?
    (A) carpals   (B) metacarpals   (C) metatarsals   (D) tarsals

G. WRITING!   *Write answers in the blanks to complete the sentences.*

1. In examining a male patient, Dr. Johnson asks him to straighten his leg. This joint motion is called
   _____.

2. A 60-year-old man undergoes a procedure in which the physician examines his right knee with an arthroscope. The name of the procedure is _____.

3. Seventy-year-old Esther has osteoporosis and has fractured a vertebra. Dr. Bonelly injects a cement-like substance into the vertebra to stabilize and strengthen it, in a procedure called _____.

4. Fourteen-year-old Mary has lateral curvature of the spine. This condition is called _____.

5. The orthopedist diagnoses an adult woman with carpal tunnel syndrome. This complex of symptoms results from pressure on the median nerve in the carpal tunnel of the _____.

H. WRITING!   *Write a one-word term for each of these meanings.*

1. destruction of muscle _____.
2. inflammation of the bone and cartilage _____.
3. inhibition of the bone marrow _____.
4. medications used to reduce inflammation _____.
5. medications used to treat osteoporosis _____.
6. pertaining to the collarbone _____.
7. pertaining to the neck _____.
8. pertaining to the upper arm bone _____.
9. prolapse of the ankle _____.
10. restoring a fracture to its normal position _____.

I. READING HEALTH CARE REPORTS   *Read the health report; then select one-word answers to complete the sentences.*

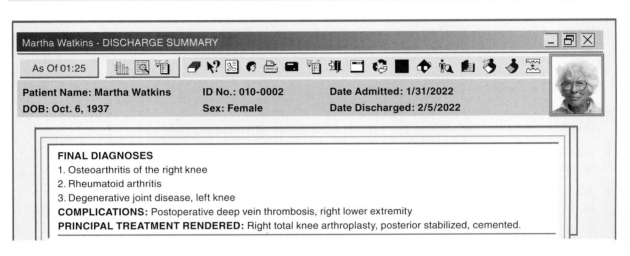

Martha Watkins - DISCHARGE SUMMARY

| As Of 01:25 | |

Patient Name: Martha Watkins   **ID No.: 010-0002**   **Date Admitted: 1/31/2022**
DOB: Oct. 6, 1937   **Sex: Female**   **Date Discharged: 2/5/2022**

FINAL DIAGNOSES
1. Osteoarthritis of the right knee
2. Rheumatoid arthritis
3. Degenerative joint disease, left knee
COMPLICATIONS: Postoperative deep vein thrombosis, right lower extremity
PRINCIPAL TREATMENT RENDERED: Right total knee arthroplasty, posterior stabilized, cemented.

1. A type of arthritis that often results in joint deformities is _____ arthritis.
2. An operation to restore the integrity and function of a joint is _____.
3. Another term for degenerative arthritis is _____.
4. The right leg and foot is the right _____.

J.   *Read the following ED visit note and select the correct answers on the following page.*

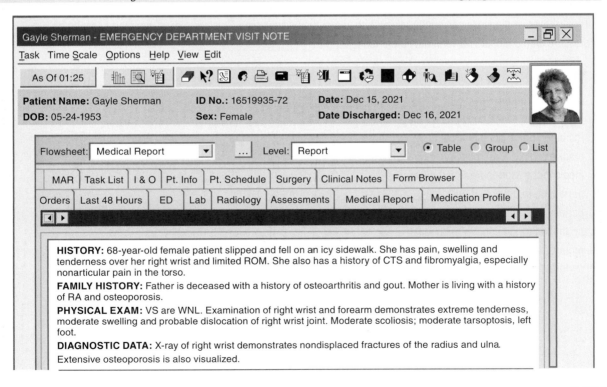

Gayle Sherman - EMERGENCY DEPARTMENT VISIT NOTE

Task   Time Scale   Options   Help   View   Edit

| As Of 01:25 | |

Patient Name: Gayle Sherman   **ID No.:** 16519935-72   **Date:** Dec 15, 2021
DOB: 05-24-1953   **Sex:** Female   **Date Discharged:** Dec 16, 2021

Flowsheet: Medical Report   ▼   ...   Level: Report   ▼   ⦿ Table   ○ Group   ○ List

| MAR | Task List | I & O | Pt. Info | Pt. Schedule | Surgery | Clinical Notes | Form Browser |

| Orders | Last 48 Hours | ED | Lab | Radiology | Assessments | Medical Report | Medication Profile |

HISTORY: 68-year-old female patient slipped and fell on an icy sidewalk. She has pain, swelling and tenderness over her right wrist and limited ROM. She also has a history of CTS and fibromyalgia, especially nonarticular pain in the torso.
FAMILY HISTORY: Father is deceased with a history of osteoarthritis and gout. Mother is living with a history of RA and osteoporosis.
PHYSICAL EXAM: VS are WNL. Examination of right wrist and forearm demonstrates extreme tenderness, moderate swelling and probable dislocation of right wrist joint. Moderate scoliosis; moderate tarsoptosis, left foot.
DIAGNOSTIC DATA: X-ray of right wrist demonstrates nondisplaced fractures of the radius and ulna. Extensive osteoporosis is also visualized.

1. A hereditary form of arthritis resulting in hyperuricemia is (gout, kyphosis, scoliosis, tarsoptosis).
2. Osteoarthritis refers to inflammation of a bone and a/an (intervertebral disk, ligament, joint, tendon).
3. Mrs. Sherman's history indicates widespread nonarticular pain in the torso. Nonarticular means not related to the (extremities, joints, muscles, torso).
4. There is a reduction in the amount of (bone, calcaneal, medullary, muscle) mass with increased porosity in osteoporosis.
5. Carpal tunnel syndrome refers to a disorder involving the (pelvis, skull, spine, wrist).

K. QUICK CHALLENGE!   *Find an incorrect term in each sentence and write the correct term.*

1. Adductors cause movement of a limb away from the axis of the body. _____
2. A circular movement of a limb at the far end is extension. _____
3. Hypouricemia is an excess or increased amount of uric acid in the blood. _____
4. A kyphosis is a malignant tumor containing much fibrous tissue. _____
5. Anti-osteoporotics are various forms of therapy that relieve arthritic symptoms. _____

*Use Appendix III to check your answers.

◆)) QUICK & EASY (Q&E) LIST

Use the Evolve website (http://evolve.elsevier.com/Leonard/quick) to review the terms presented in Chapter 6. Look closely at the spelling of each term as it is pronounced.

abductors *(ab-**duk**-torz)*
adductors *(uh-**duk**-turz)*
ankylosis *(ang-kuh-**lō**-sis)*
antiarthritics *(an-tē-ahr-**thrit**-iks)*
antiinflammatories *(an-tē-in-**flam**-uh-tor-ēz)*
anti-osteoporotics *(an-tē-os-tē-ō-puh-**rot**-iks)*
arthralgia *(ahr-**thral**-juh)*
arthritis *(ahr-**thrī**-tis)*
arthrocentesis *(ahr-thrō-sen-**tē**-sis)*
arthrodynia *(ahr-thrō-**din**-ē-uh)*
arthropathy *(ahr-**throp**-uh-thē)*
arthroplasty *(**ahr**-thrō-plas-tē)*
arthroscope *(**ahr**-thrō-skōp)*
arthroscopy *(ahr-**thros**-kuh-pē)*
arthrotomy *(ahr-**throt**-uh-mē)*
articulation *(ahr-tik-ū-**lā**-shun)*
articular *(ahr-**tik**-ū-lur)*
bone marrow *(bōn **mar**-ō)*
bunionectomy *(bun-yun-**ek**-tuh-mē)*
bursa *(**bur**-suh)*
bursitis *(bur-**sī**-tis)*

calcaneus *(kal-**kā**-nē-us)*
calcification *(kal-si-fi-**kā**-shun)*
carpal *(**kahr**-pul)*
carpal tunnel syndrome *(**kahr**-pul **tun**-ul **sin**-drōm)*
carpectomy *(kahr-**pek**-tuh-mē)*
carpophalangeal *(kahr-pō-fuh-**lan**-jē-ul)*
carpus *(**kahr**-pus)*
cartilage *(**kahr**-ti-luj)*
cellulitis *(sel-ū-**lī**-tis)*
cerebrospinal *(ser-uh-brō-**spī**-nul)*
cervical *(**sur**-vi-kul)*
chondral *(**kon**-drul)*
chondrectomy *(kon-**drek**-tuh-mē)*
chondrocostal *(kon-drō-**kos**-tul)*
chondrosarcoma *(kon-drō-sahr-**kō**-muh)*
circumduction *(sur-kum-**duk**-shun)*
clavicle *(**klav**-i-kul)*
clavicular *(kluh-**vik**-ū-lur)*
coccygeal *(kok-**sij**-ē-ul)*
coccyx *(**kok**-siks)*
costa *(**kos**-tuh)*

QUICK & EASY (Q&E) LIST—cont'd

costal (**kos**-tul)
costectomy (kos-**tek**-tuh-mē)
costochondral (kos-tō-**kon**-drul)
costovertebral (kos-tō-**vur**-tuh-brul)
cranial (**krā**-nē-ul)
craniectomy (krā-nē-**ek**-tuh-mē)
craniocele (**krā**-nē-ō-sēl)
cranioplasty (**krā**-nē-ō-plas-tē)
craniotomy (krā-nē-**ot**-uh-mē)
cranium (**krā**-nē-um)
decalcification (dē-kal-si-fi-**kā**-shun)
diskectomy (dis-**kek**-tuh-mē)
dislocation (dis-lō-**kā**-shun)
extension (ek-**sten**-shun)
facial (**fā**-shul)
fascia (**fash**-ē-uh)
fascial (**fash**-ē-ul)
femoral (**fem**-uh-rul)
femur (**fē**-mur)
fibromyalgia (fī-brō-mī-**al**-juh)
fibrosarcoma (fī-brō-sahr-**kō**-muh)
fibula (**fib**-ū-luh)
flexion (**flek**-shun)
fracture (**frak**-chur)
gout (gout)
hematopoiesis (hem-uh-tō-poi-**ē**-sis)
herniated disk (**hur**-nē-āt-ud disk)
humeral (**hū**-mur-ul)
humeroscapular (hū-mur-ō-**skap**-ū-lur)
humeroulnar (hū-mur-ō-**ul**-nur)
humerus (**hū**-mur-us)
hyperuricemia (hī-pur-ū-ri-**sē**-mē-uh)
iliac (**il**-ē-ak)
iliopubic (il-ē-ō-**pū**-bik)
ilium (**il**-ē-um)
intercostal (in-tur-**kos**-tul)
intervertebral (in-tur-**vur**-tuh-brul)
involuntary (in-**vol**-un-tar-ē)
ischial (**is**-kē-ul)
ischiococcygeal (is-kē-ō-kok-**sij**-ē-ul)
ischiofemoral (is-kē-ō-**fem**-uh-rul)
ischiopubic (is-kē-ō-**pū**-bik)
ischium (**is**-kē-um)
kyphosis (kī-**fō**-sis)
laminectomy (lam-i-**nek**-tuh-mē)
leukemia (l͞oo-**kē**-mē-uh)
ligament (**lig**-uh-munt)
lumbago (lum-**bā**-gō)
lumbar (**lum**-bur, **lum**-bahr)
lupus erythematosus (l͞oo-pus er-uh-them-uh-**tō**-sis)

metacarpal (met-uh-**kahr**-pul)
metatarsal (met-uh-**tahr**-sul)
multiple myeloma (**mul**-ti-pul mī-uh-**lō**-muh)
muscular dystrophy (**mus**-kū-lur **dis**-truh-fē)
musculofascial (mus-kū-lō-**fash**-ē-ul)
musculoskeletal (mus-kū-lō-**skel**-uh-tul)
myalgia (mī-**al**-juh)
myasthenia gravis (mī-us-**thē**-nē-uh **grav**-is)
myelitis (mī-uh-**lī**-tis)
myeloencephalitis (mī-uh-lō-en-sef-uh-**lī**-tis)
myelofibrosis (mī-uh-lō-fī-**brō**-sis)
myelogram (**mī**-uh-lō-gram)
myelosuppression (mī-uh-lō-suh-**presh**-un)
myocele (**mī**-ō-sēl)
myocellulitis (mī-ō-sel-ū-**lī**-tis)
myofibrosis (mī-ō-fī-**brō**-sis)
myolysis (mī-**ol**-i-sis)
myopathy (mī-**op**-uh-thē)
myoplasty (**mī**-ō-plas-tē)
nonarticular (non-ahr-**tīk**-ū-lur)
orthopedics (or-thō-**pē**-diks)
orthopedist (or-thō-**pē**-dist)
ostectomy (os-**tek**-tuh-mē)
osteectomy (os-tē-**ek**-tuh-mē)
osteitis (os-tē-**ī**-tis)
osteitis deformans (os-tē-**ī**-tis di-**for**-mans)
osteoarthritis (os-tē-ō-ahr-**thrī**-tis)
osteochondritis (os-tē-ō-kon-**drī**-tis)
osteoid (**os**-tē-oid)
osteomalacia (os-tē-ō-muh-**lā**-shuh)
osteomyelitis (os-tē-ō-mī-uh-**lī**-tis)
osteoporosis (os-tē-ō-puh-**rō**-sis)
paraparesis (par-uh-puh-**rē**-sis)
paraplegia (par-uh-**plē**-juh)
paresis (puh-**rē**-sis)
patella (puh-**tel**-uh)
patellofemoral (puh-tel-ō-**fem**-uh-rul)
pelvic (**pel**-vik)
phalanges (fuh-**lan**-jēz)
phalangitis (fal-un-**jī**-tis)
phalanx (**fā**-lanks)
polyarthritis (pol-ē-ahr-**thrī**-tis)
pubic (**pū**-bik)
pubis (**pū**-bis)
quadriparesis (kwod-ri-puh-**rē**-sis)
quadriplegia (kwod-ri-**plē**-juh)
rachialgia (rā-kē-**al**-juh)
rachiodynia (rā-kē-ō-**din**-ē-uh)
radial (**rā**-dē-ul)
radius (**rā**-dē-us)

QUICK & EASY (Q&E) LIST—cont'd

reduction (rē-**duk**-shun)
rheumatism (**roo**-muh-tiz-um)
rheumatoid arthritis (**roo**-muh-toid ahr-**thrī**-tis)
rheumatoid spondylitis (**roo**-muh-toid spon-duh-**lī**-tis)
rotation (rō-**tā**-shun)
sacral (**sā**-krul)
sacrum (**sā**-krum)
sarcoma (sahr-**kō**-muh)
scapula (**skap**-ū-luh)
scapular (**skap**-ū-lur)
scoliosis (skō-lē-**ō**-sis)
spina bifida (**spī**-nuh **bif**-i-duh)
spine (spīn)
spondylarthritis (spon-dul-ahr-**thrī**-tis)
spondylitis (spon-duh-**lī**-tis)
spondylomalacia (spon-duh-lō-muh-**lā**-shuh)
sprain (sprān)
sternal (**stur**-nul)
sternoclavicular (stur-nō-kluh-**vik**-ū-lur)
sternocostal (stur-nō-**kos**-tul)
sternum (**stur**-num)
strain (strān)
subchondral (sub-**kon**-drul)
subcostal (sub-**kos**-tul)
substernal (sub-**stur**-nul)

synovial (si-**nō**-vē-ul)
synovium (si-**nō**-vē-um)
tarsal (**tahr**-sul)
tarsoptosis (tahr-sop-**tō**-sis)
tarsus (**tahr**-sus)
tendinitis (ten-di-**nī**-tis)
tendon (**ten**-dun)
tendonitis (ten-duh-**nī**-tis)
tendoplasty (**ten**-dō-plas-tē)
tenomyoplasty (ten-ō-**mī**-ō-plas-tē)
tetraparesis (tet-ruh-puh-**rē**-sis)
tetraplegia (tet-ruh-**plē**-juh)
thoracic (thuh-**ras**-ik)
thoracic cage (thuh-**ras**-ik kāj)
thoracolumbar (thor-uh-kō-**lum**-bur)
thorax (**thor**-aks)
tibia (**tib**-ē-uh)
tibialgia (tib-ē-**al**-juh)
ulna (**ul**-nuh)
ulnar (**ul**-nur)
vertebra (**vur**-tuh-bruh)
vertebrochondral (vur-tuh-brō-**kon**-drul)
vertebrocostal (vur-tuh-brō-**kos**-tul)
vertebroplasty (**vur**-tuh-brō-plas-tē)
visceral (**vis**-ur-ul)

Don't forget the games and other activities available at http://evolve.elsevier.com/Leonard/quick.

QUICK CONNECT

Review all lists of word parts and their meanings for this chapter using the flashcards you prepared or the flashcards on the Evolve site.

MUSCULOSKELETAL: THINK OF MUSCLES AND BONES!

Functions:

- protection: Bones provide a framework for the body and protect and support internal organs.
- support: Bone marrow produces erythrocytes, leukocytes, and platelets (hematopoiesis); bones store fat and minerals, especially calcium.
- movement: Muscles move an organ or part of the body by contracting and relaxing, whether attached to bones or to internal organs and blood vessels.

SKELETAL STRUCTURES: BONES AND CARTILAGE
Know the functions of muscles, joints, tendons, and ligaments

Orthopedics: Branch of medicine involved in prevention and correction of deformities or diseases of the musculoskeletal system.
Know the common names and combining forms for the following:

cranium	ulna	patella
costa	carpals	fibula
sternum	metacarpals	tibia
vertebrae and 5 types	phalanges	tarsals
clavicle	ilium	calcaneus
scapula	ischium	metatarsals
humerus	pubis	
radius	femur	

Think of adjectives that you learned in this chapter associated with these skeletal structures (for example cranial). Know the meaning of the following terms regarding bones: osteoid, calcification vs. decalcification.

Think about the importance of calcification of bone vs. dangers of calcification occurring in soft tissue, such as the arteries.

Know the meaning of these terms regarding bones: osteoid, calcification vs. decalcification.

The skull is composed of cranial and facial bones. Newborns have soft spots called fontanels (allows for growth of the brain).

The vertebral column (backbone) encloses the spinal cord, supports the head, and serves as a place for attachment of ribs and muscles of the back; composed of 33 vertebrae. The 5 types of vertebrae are cervical, thoracic, lumbar, sacral (fuse to become the sacrum), and coccygeal vertebrae (fuse to become the coccyx). Remember the general location of the vertebrae by their name. Vertebral column protects the spinal cord (part of the nervous system).

Intervertebral disks are cushions of cartilage between adjoining vertebrae and absorb shock.

Know the meanings of these terms associated with the spine: rachiodynia/rachialgia, spondylitis, lumbago.

What structures are affected in carpal tunnel syndrome, phalangitis, and tibialgia?

What is the role of cartilage, muscles (visceral vs skeletal), tendons, articulations, and ligaments?

Articulation has more than one definition. What is the one learned in Q&E as it pertains to the musculoskeletal system? (Articulation also means the act of speaking clearly). Know the difference in these terms relating to joint motion: extension, flexion, rotation, circumduction, range of motion. What do the terms *abductors* and *adductors* have to do with joint motion?

In addition to differentiation of the types of fractures, distinguish other disease and disorders of the musculoskeletal system presented in the chapter. In addition to injuries and infections, distinguish diseases that are related to malignancies, metabolic disturbances (e.g., osteoporosis), congenital defects, or arthritis and connective tissue diseases.

Visualize the meaning of *reduction of a fracture* and why it is considered closed reduction. Consider the difference between craniotomy vs. craniectomy and other therapeutic interventions presented.

CHAPTER 7

Circulatory System

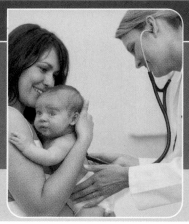

Cardiology is the study of the anatomy, normal functions, and disorders of the heart. This patient has been referred to a cardiologist by his pediatrician.

OBJECTIVES

After completing Chapter 7, you will be able to:

1. Recognize or write the functions of the circulatory system.
2. Recognize or write the meanings of Chapter 7 word parts and use them to build and analyze medical terms.
3. Write terms for selected structures of the cardiovascular and lymphatic systems or match terms with their descriptions.
4. Write the names of the diagnostic terms and pathologies related to the cardiovascular and lymphatic systems when given their descriptions or match terms with their meanings.
5. Match surgical and therapeutic interventions for the cardiovascular and lymphatic systems or write the names of the interventions when given their descriptions.
6. Spell terms for the circulatory system correctly.

Function First

The **circulatory** system consists of the **cardio**+**vascul**+**ar** system (heart and blood vessels) and the **lymphatic** system (structures involved in the conveyance of the fluid **lymph**). The circulatory system cooperates with other body systems to maintain homeostasis, or equilibrium of the internal environment of the body.

    Body cells must have a constant supply of food, oxygen, and other substances to function properly. Blood circulates through the heart and blood vessels, carrying oxygen, nutrients, vitamins, antibodies, and other substances. It carries away waste and carbon dioxide.

    The cardiovascular system supplies body cells with needed substances, transports waste products for disposal, maintains the acid-base balance of the body, prevents hemorrhage through blood clotting, protects against disease, and helps regulate body temperature.

cardi/o = heart
vascul/o = vessel

home/o = sameness
-stasis = controlling

Name the two body systems that make up the circulatory system.

1. _____   2. _____

*Use Appendix III, Answers, to check your answers to all the exercises in Chapter 7.

CARDIOVASCULAR SYSTEM

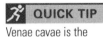 ### Structures of the Cardiovascular System

There are five anatomic types of blood vessels: arteries, arterioles, capillaries, venules, and veins. Blood that is rich in oxygen is pumped by the heart to all parts of the body. It leaves the heart by the **arteries**, which branch many times and become **arterioles**. The arterioles branch even more to become tiny vessels with one-cell-thick walls called **capillaries**.

The capillaries have the important feature of being the site where oxygen and waste carbon dioxide are exchanged. Blood leaving the capillaries returns to the heart through the **venules**, which flow into the **veins** (Fig. 7.1). The veins carry blood back to the heart by way of the **venae cavae**, the largest veins in the body. Before it is again pumped to the body cells, blood picks up a fresh supply of oxygen by passing through the lungs.

Components of the cardiovascular system include the heart and a vast network of vessels (Fig. 7.2).

> **QUICK TIP**
>
> Venae cavae is the plural of vena cava.

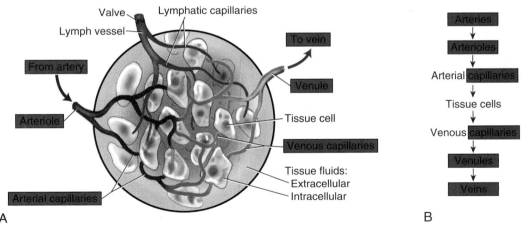

A   **B**

Fig. 7.1 Capillary Bed Showing the Relationship of Blood Vessels. A, Relationship of blood flow through blood vessels. Blood that is rich in oxygen is carried by the arteries, which branch many times to become arterioles. Arterioles branch to become capillaries, the site of oxygen and carbon dioxide exchange. Oxygen-poor blood is returned to the heart through the venules, which flow into the veins. The veins carry the blood to the two largest veins, the superior and inferior venae cavae, which empty into the heart. **B,** Schematic showing relationship of blood flow through vessels. Main types of vessels are highlighted. **arter/o** = artery; **-ole** = little; **lymphat/o** = lymphatic

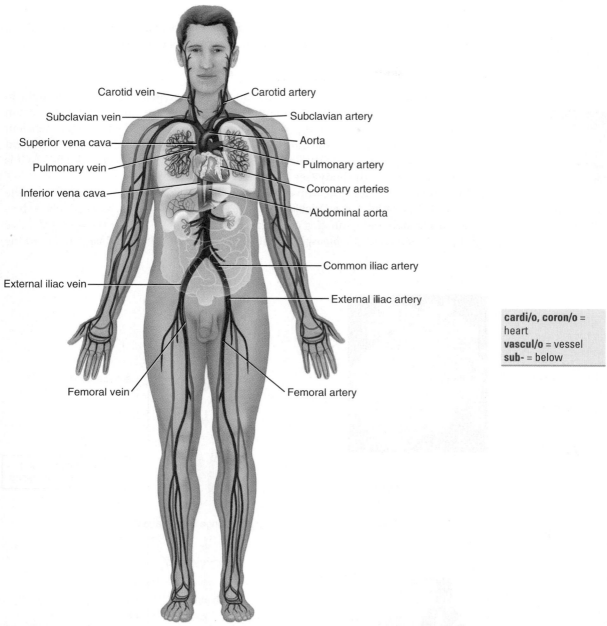

Fig. 7.2 Cardiovascular System: the Heart and Blood Vessels. Two major components of the vascular network are shown, the arteries *(red)* and the veins *(blue)*. Only the larger or more common blood vessels are labeled.

Carotid vein
Subclavian vein
Superior vena cava
Pulmonary vein
Inferior vena cava
External iliac vein
Femoral vein

Carotid artery
Subclavian artery
Aorta
Pulmonary artery
Coronary arteries
Abdominal aorta
Common iliac artery
External iliac artery
Femoral artery

cardi/o, coron/o = heart
vascul/o = vessel
sub- = below

WRITE IT!
EXERCISE 2

List the five anatomical types of blood vessels (in any order).

1. _____   4. _____
2. _____   5. _____
3. _____

Heart

The heart is a muscular cone-shaped organ, about the size of a clenched fist (Fig. 7.3, *A*). Study Fig. 7.3, *B*, a cross section of the heart, and note its four chambers:

- Right **atrium**
- Right **ventricle**
- Left atrium
- Left ventricle

Deoxygenated blood, which has had much of its oxygen removed, is brought to the right atrium by the body's two largest veins, the venae cavae. The right atrium contracts and forces blood through a valve to the right ventricle. The oxygen-deficient blood is then transported to the lungs, where it absorbs oxygen. This oxygenated blood is transported back to the heart (left atrium, then pumped to left ventricle) before it is pumped throughout the body (see Fig. 7.3, *B*).

In normal heart function, valves close and prevent backflow of blood when the heart contracts. **Atrial** and **ventricular** pertain to atrium or ventricle, respectively. Valves between the **atria** and ventricles are **atrio+ventricul+ar** (AV) valves: the **tricuspid** valve on the right side and the **bicuspid** or **mitral** valve on the left side. **Cuspid** refers to the

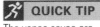
QUICK TIP

The venae cavae are the inferior vena cava and the superior vena cava.

tri- = three
bi- = two

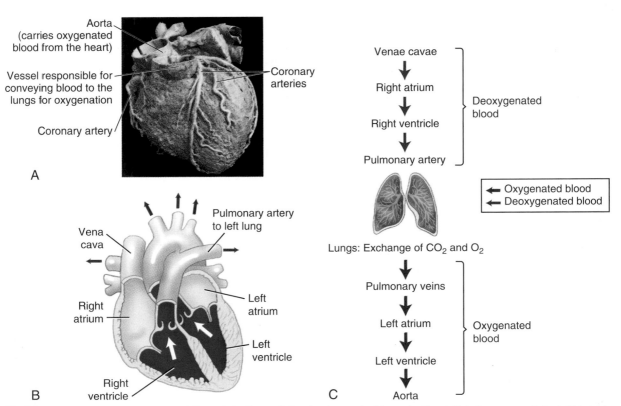

Fig. 7.3 Anatomy and Circulation of Blood Through the Heart. **A,** Anterior photograph of the external heart. Note the coronary arteries (which supply blood to all of the heart), the aorta (which carries oxygenated blood from the heart), and the vessel which conveys blood away from the heart to the lungs for oxygenation. **B,** Anterior cross section showing the heart chambers. The arrows indicate the direction of blood flow from the ventricles. **C,** Schematic representation of deoxygenated or oxygenated status of the blood as it flows through the heart.

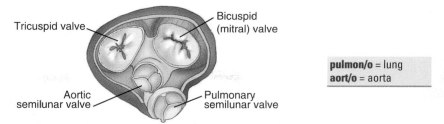

Fig. 7.4 Valves of the Heart. The valves between the atria and the ventricles are the tricuspid valve on the right side of the heart and the bicuspid, or mitral, valve on the left side. Cuspid refers to the little flaps of tissue that make up the valve. Mitral indicates the mitered appearance of the bicuspid valve.

small flaps that make up the atrioventricular valves (Fig. 7.4). The pulmonary (or pulmonic) valve regulates the flow of blood to the lungs and the aortic valve regulates the flow of blood into the **aorta**, the artery by which blood leaves the heart to be routed throughout the body. The pulmonary and aortic valves are called **semilunar** because of their half-moon appearance when the valves are closed.

The **peri+card+ium**, a sac made up of a double membrane, encloses the heart. Notice that one *i* is dropped when cardi/o and -ium are joined (to facilitate pronunciation). The innermost layer of the pericardium is the **visceral** pericardium, or **epicardium**.

Another membrane, the **endocardium**, forms the lining inside the heart (Fig. 7.5, *inset*). The heart muscle itself is called the **myocardium**. This is the thickest tissue of the heart and is composed of muscle fibers that contract, resulting in the squeezing of blood from the heart with each heartbeat.

Blood vessels that supply oxygen to the heart are coronary arteries (see Fig. 7.5). **Coronary** means encircling, in the manner of a crown, and refers to the way in which coronary arteries encircle the heart in a crownlike fashion.

> **pulmon/o** = lung
> **aort/o** = aorta

> 🏃 **QUICK TIP**
> To remember blood flow through valves: "Tri before you Bi."

> **peri-** = around
> **cardi/o** = heart
> **-ium** = membrane

> **endo-** = inside
> **my/o** = muscle

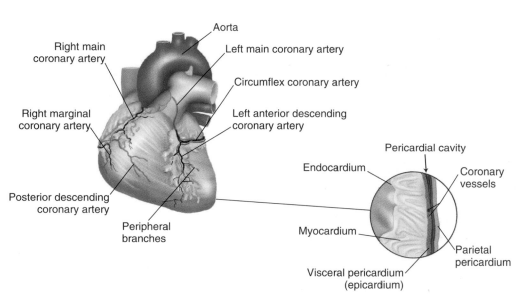

Fig. 7.5 Coronary Arteries and Heart Tissues. The two main coronary arteries are the left coronary artery and right coronary artery. The three layers of the heart, beginning with the innermost layer, are the endocardium, myocardium, and epicardium (also called the visceral pericardium).

MATCH IT!
EXERCISE 3

Match the types of heart tissue in the left column with their meanings in the right column.

_____ 1. endocardium
_____ 2. myocardium
_____ 3. pericardium

A. muscular middle layer of the heart
B. lining of the heart
C. sac that encloses the heart

Blood Vessels

Five types of blood vessels are shown in Fig. 7.1: arteries, smaller arteries called arterioles, veins, smaller veins called venules, and capillaries.

Blood pressure is the pressure exerted by the blood on the wall of an artery. Indirect blood pressure readings generally consist of two numbers expressed as a fraction (see Fig. 4.3). A healthy young person has a blood pressure of approximately 120/80 mm Hg. Recall that the first number represents the maximum pressure on the artery (systolic pressure), and the second number is the amount of pressure that still exists when the heart is relaxed (i.e., not contracting), the diastolic pressure.

Commit the meanings of the combining forms in the following table to memory.

COMBINING FORMS: BLOOD VESSELS	
Combining Form	**Meaning**
angi/o, vas/o,* vascul/o	vessel
aort/o	aorta
arter/o, arteri/o	artery
arteriol/o	arteriole
ather/o	yellow fatty plaque
phleb/o, ven/o	vein
venul/o	venule

Use the electronic flashcards on the Evolve site or make your own set of flashcards using the above list. Select the word parts just presented, and study them until you know their meanings. Do this each time a set of word parts is presented.

*Sometimes vas/o means vas deferens, a duct in the male reproductive system.

MATCH IT!
EXERCISE 4

Match the combining forms in the left column with their meanings in the right column (a choice may be used more than once).

_____ 1. angi/o
_____ 2. arteri/o
_____ 3. arteriol/o
_____ 4. ather/o
_____ 5. phleb/o
_____ 6. vas/o
_____ 7. vascul/o
_____ 8. venul/o

A. arteriole
B. artery
C. vessel (in general)
D. vein
E. venule
F. yellow fatty plaque

FIND IT!
EXERCISE 5

Write the combining forms and meanings in the following new terms. A short definition is provided.

1. **aortic** _____ pertaining to the aorta
2. **arterial** _____ pertaining to an artery or arteries
3. **arteriovenous** _____ pertaining to both arteries and veins
4. **vascular** _____ pertaining to blood vessels in general
5. **venous** _____ pertaining to a vein or veins

Diseases, Disorders, and Diagnostic Terms

Heart

Cardiomyopathy is a general diagnostic term that designates primary disease of the heart muscle itself (Fig. 7.6). An example of a cardiomyopathy is **myocarditis**, inflammation of the heart muscle. Each layer of the heart can become inflamed. **Endocarditis** is often caused by infective microorganisms that invade the endocardium, and the heart valves are frequently affected. Inflammation of the pericardium is **pericarditis**, which can be caused by infectious microorganisms, by a cancerous growth, or by other problems.

cardi/o = heart
my/o = muscle
-pathy = disease
-itis = inflammation

Stress tests measure the function of the heart when it is subjected to carefully controlled amounts of physiologic stress, usually using exercise but sometimes specific drugs. In a treadmill stress test, often performed when blockage of coronary arteries is suspected, an **electrocardiogram** and other measurements are taken while the patient walks on a treadmill at varying speeds and inclines. The electrical currents of the heart muscle are recorded by an **electrocardiograph** in **electrocardiography** (see Fig. 3.15).

electr/o = electrical
cardi/o = heart
-gram = a record

Echocardiography (echo) is the term generally associated with the use of ultrasonography in diagnosing heart disease. The **echocardiogram** is a record of the heart obtained by directing ultrasonic waves through the chest wall (Fig. 7.7). Cardiac magnetic resonance imaging (MRI) may be performed, in addition to computed tomography (CT).

echo- = sound
-graphy = process of recording

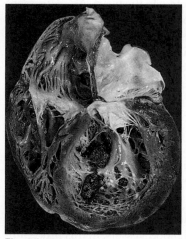

Fig. 7.6 Cardiomyopathy. Any disease of the myocardium is also called myocardiopathy. **cardi/o** = heart; **my/o** = muscle; **-pathy** = disease

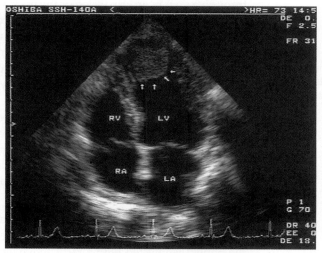

Fig. 7.7 Echocardiogram. The heart is viewed from the top, and the four chambers are labeled: *RV*, right ventricle; *RA*, right atrium; *LV*, left ventricle; and *LA*, left atrium. A large thrombus, a blood clot, is indicated by the arrows. **echo-** = sound; **cardi/o** = heart; **-gram** = a record

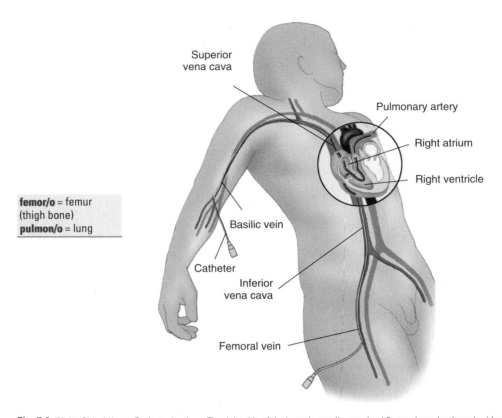

femor/o = femur
(thigh bone)
pulmon/o = lung

Fig. 7.8 Right-Sided Heart Catheterization. The right side of the heart is usually examined first and may be the only side examined because examination of the left side presents more risks to the patient. The catheter is inserted into the femoral vein, a large vein in the thigh, or the basilic vein in the arm. The catheter is then advanced to the right atrium, the right ventricle, and into the pulmonary artery.

Cardiac catheterization is the passage of a long, flexible tube into the heart chambers through a vein in an arm or leg or the neck. Cardi+ac refers to the heart. An instrument called a **catheter** is used. This allows the collection of blood samples from different parts of the heart and determines pressure differences in various chambers (Fig. 7.8). Combined with special endoscopic equipment, cardiac catheterization allows internal parts of the heart to be viewed. An endoscopic examination uses an endoscope, a device consisting of a tube and an optical system that allows observation of the inside of a hollow organ or cavity.

endo- = inside
scop/o = to view
-ic = pertaining to

Noninvasive procedures such as electrocardiography do not require entering the body or puncturing the skin and therefore are less hazardous for the patient than invasive procedures. Several noninvasive procedures are available for the diagnosis of heart disease. Conventional x-ray procedures provide information about heart size and gross abnormalities, but newer methods have contributed greatly to information about the heart.

Positron emission tomography (PET) is used in other areas of the body but is especially helpful in examining blood flow in the heart and blood vessels. In this procedure the patient is injected with a radioactive element, which becomes concentrated in the heart, and color-coded images are produced. Additional diseases and disorders that affect the heart are described in the following list.

angina pectoris Severe chest pain and constriction about the heart caused by an insufficient supply of blood to the heart itself. (Angina is frequently used with other terms and refers to pain of that particular part. Pectoris refers to the chest and is derived from the Latin word *pectora*, meaning chest.)

arrhythmia (a-, without) Irregularity or loss of rhythm of the heartbeat. Although this term is often used, **dysrhythmia** is more technically correct.

asystole absence of a heartbeat

cardiomegaly (cardi/o, heart + -megaly, enlargement) Enlarged size of the heart.

congenital heart defects Abnormalities present in the heart at birth (congenital means existing at birth). These defects often involve the septum, a partition that divides the right and left chambers of the heart. Atrial septal defects and ventricular septal defects involve abnormal openings between the atria and ventricles, respectively (Fig. 7.9).

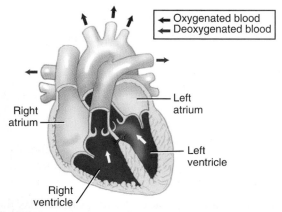

Fig. 7.9 Ventricular Septal Defect. Compare this illustration with Fig. 7.3, *B.* Note the abnormal opening in the septal wall *(yellow arrow)* that divides the left and right ventricles. The direction of abnormal blood flow (left to right or right to left) depends on the stage of the septal defect. Dilution of oxygenated blood results in cyanosis, or a bluish discoloration of the skin.

congestive heart failure (CHF) Condition characterized by weakness, breathlessness, and edema in lower portions of the body; the work demanded of the heart is greater than its ability to perform; also called congestive heart disease or **heart failure**.

coronary artery disease (CAD) Abnormal condition that affects the heart's arteries and produces various pathologic effects, especially the reduced flow of blood to the myocardium.

coronary heart disease (CHD) Heart damage resulting from insufficient oxygen caused by pathologic changes in the coronary arteries.

fibrillation Severe cardiac arrhythmia in which contractions are too rapid and uncoordinated for effective blood circulation. It can sometimes be reversed by the use of a **defibrillator**, an electronic apparatus that delivers a shock to the heart, often through the placement of electrodes on the chest (de- means down, from, or reversing). **Defibrillation** may also be used to slow the heart or restore its normal rhythm.

heart murmur Soft blowing or rasping sound that may be heard when listening to the heart with a stethoscope; it is not necessarily pathologic.

hyperlipidemia (hyper-, excessive + -emia, blood) Excessive lipids (fats) in the blood. An elevated blood level of one type of lipid, cholesterol, is associated with an increased risk of developing coronary heart disease in most individuals.

hypertension (hyper-, excessive or above normal) Elevated blood pressure above the normal values of 120/80 mm Hg in an adult over 18 years of age. A person with hypertension is said to be hypertensive.

hypotension (hypo-, below normal) Low blood pressure. A blood pressure of 95/60 indicates hypotension, but each person's reading must be interpreted individually.

infarction Necrosis of a localized area of tissue caused by lack of blood supply to that area. Necrosis means death of tissue. It can result from **occlusion** (obstruction) or **stenosis** (narrowing) of the artery that supplies blood to that tissue. **Myocardial infarction** (MI) is the death of an area of the heart muscle that occurs as a result of oxygen deprivation; also called acute myocardial infarction (AMI) (Fig. 7.10).

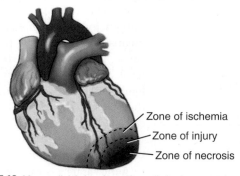

Fig. 7.10 Myocardial Infarction. Also called a heart attack, myocardial infarction (MI) is necrosis of a portion of cardiac muscle. MI is usually caused by an obstruction in a coronary artery.

myocardial ischemia Deficiency of blood supply to the myocardium. The word *ischemia* refers to a temporary deficiency of blood supply to any body part.

septal defect Defect in the wall separating the left and right sides of the heart. The defect is usually congenital and is either an atrial septal defect (ASD) or a ventricular septal defect (VSD).

shock Serious condition in which blood flow to the heart is reduced to such an extent that body tissues do not receive enough blood. This condition can result in death. Shock may have various causes, including hemorrhage, infection, drug reaction, injury, poisoning, MI, and excessive emotional stress.

MATCH IT!   EXERCISE 6

Match the following diseases, disorders, and diagnostic terms pertaining to the heart in the left column with their meanings in the right column.

_____ 1. angina pectoris
_____ 2. cardiomegaly
_____ 3. cardiomyopathy
_____ 4. congenital heart defect
_____ 5. congestive heart failure
_____ 6. fibrillation
_____ 7. heart murmur
_____ 8. myocardial infarction
_____ 9. myocardial ischemia
_____ 10. hypertension

A. death of an area of the heart muscle
B. abnormality present in the heart at birth
C. soft blowing or rasping heart sound
D. contractions that are too rapid and uncoordinated for effective blood circulation
E. elevated blood pressure
F. severe chest pain caused by insufficient blood supply
G. condition characterized by weakness, shortness of breath, and edema of the lower portions of the body
H. deficiency of blood supply to the heart
I. general designation for primary myocardial disease
J. enlarged heart

Blood Vessels

Vasodilation is an increase in the diameter of a blood vessel. **Vasoconstriction** has the opposite meaning of vasodilation. The dilation and constriction of blood vessels influence blood pressure and distribution of blood to various parts of the body. The vasomotor center located in the brain regulates vasoconstriction and vasodilation, thus influencing the diameter of the blood vessels. You already know that hypertension means elevated blood pressure. The most common type has no single identifiable cause, but risk for the disorder is increased by obesity, a high blood level of cholesterol, and a family history of high blood pressure. Both **cholesterol** and **triglycerides** are **lipids**. High levels of these two lipids are associated with greater risk of hardening of the arteries. Laboratory tests for cardiovascular disorders include testing for lipids and cardiac enzymes in the blood.

Angi+omas are tumors consisting principally of blood vessels (**hemangioma**) or lymph vessels (**lymphangioma**). Such tumors are usually benign (not malignant).

Aorto+graphy is radiography of the aorta after the injection of a contrast medium to enhance the visibility of the aorta on an x-ray image. The record produced from this procedure is an **aortogram**. **Aortic stenosis** is narrowing of the aortic valve (Fig. 7.11).

🏃 QUICK TIP

Lipids are fatty substances in the body.

angi/o = vessel
-oma = tumor
hem/a or hem/o = blood

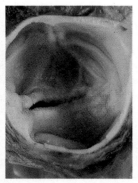

Fig. 7.11 Aortic stenosis. Narrowing of the aortic valve.
aort/o = aorta;   **-stenosis** = narrowing, stricture.

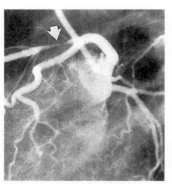

Fig. 7.12 Arteriogram. Radiographic image after injection of a radiopaque contrast medium reveals blockage of an artery *(arrow)*.
arteri/o = artery;   **-gram** = a record

Arterio+graphy is radiography of arteries after injection of radiopaque material into the bloodstream. The image produced is an **arteriogram** (Fig. 7.12).

Angio+cardio+graphy is radiography of the heart and great vessels after intravenous injection of a radiopaque solution. **Angiography** is a general term for radiography of vessels.

QUICK CASE STUDY | EXERCISE 7

Define the terms as indicated.

Marshall is seen in the emergency department with pain in the chest and left arm. He has shortness of breath, tachycardia, hypotension, dysrhythmia, elevation of the S-T segment on the electrocardiogram, and a normal chest x-ray, except for moderate cardiomegaly. Marshall is placed on heparin and admitted for further testing in the AM.

1. tachycardia _____
2. hypotension _____
3. dysrhythmia _____
4. electrocardiogram _____
5. cardiomegaly _____

PROGRAMMED LEARNING

Remember to cover the answers (left column) with folded paper or the bookmark. Write an answer in each blank, and then check your answer before proceeding to the next frame.

arteriopathy	1. Remembering that -pathy means disease, write a word that means any disease of the arteries: _____.
artery	2. **Arter+itis** is inflammation of an _____. (Notice that one *i* in arteritis is omitted to make pronunciation easier.)
arteries	3. **Arterio+scler+osis** is hardening of the _____.

arteries	4. Arteriosclerosis is a thickening and loss of elasticity of the walls of the arteries. This is a major cause of hypertension. **Athero+sclerosis**, a form of arteriosclerosis, is characterized by the formation of fatty, cholesterol-like deposits on the walls of the _____. Ather/o means yellow fatty plaque. Atherosclerosis is a common cause of coronary artery disease.
aort/o	5. Arteries carry blood away from the heart. The aorta, the largest artery in the body, is approximately 3 cm in diameter at its origin in the left side of the heart. The aorta has many branches, and early divisions of this vessel supply the heart, head, and upper part of the body. The combining form for aorta is _____.
aortitis	6. Write a word that means inflammation of the aorta: _____.
aorta	7. An **aneurysm** is a ballooning out of the wall of a vessel, usually an artery, caused by a congenital defect or weakness of the wall of the vessel. Fig. 7.13, *A*, shows common sites of arterial aneurysms. Aortic aneurysms can affect any part of which vessel? _____. A potentially dangerous effect of an aneurysm is rupture of the vessel and resulting **hemorrhage** (loss of a large amount of blood in a short time). An aortic aneurysm can be repaired by surgery.
aortography	8. Aneurysms are often clinically silent, but abdominal aneurysms may be discovered during a thorough physical examination. They are often associated with atherosclerosis, especially in older persons. A term that means radiographic study of the abdominal aorta after introduction of a contrast medium through a catheter is abdominal _____ (see Fig. 7.13, B). These aneurysms can usually be corrected surgically by replacing the diseased area with an artificial plastic vessel.

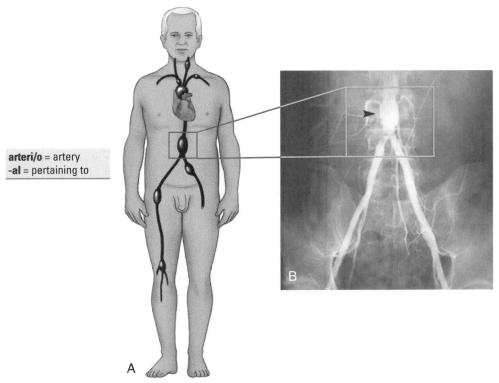

arteri/o = artery
-al = pertaining to

Fig. 7.13 A, Common anatomic sites of arterial aneurysms. **B,** Arteriogram of an abnormal aortic aneurysm. Note the abnormal dilation (bulging out) of the site indicated by the arrow.

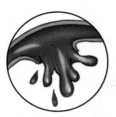
A Hemorrhagic
stroke

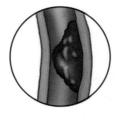
B Thrombotic
stroke

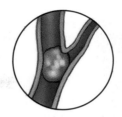
C Embolic
stroke

Fig. 7.14 Types of Stroke. **A,** Hemorrhagic stroke. A blood vessel bursts and allows blood to seep into brain tissue until clotting stops the seepage. **B,** Thrombotic stroke. Plaque can cause a clot to form that blocks blood flow. **C,** Embolic stroke. A blood clot or other embolus reaches an artery in the brain, lodges there, and blocks the flow of blood.

vessel	9. A cerebral aneurysm is a ballooning out of a blood _____ in the brain. **Cerebr+al** (cerebr/o + -al, pertaining to) refers to the cerebrum or brain. Cerebral aneurysms pose a danger of rupture and hemorrhage within the skull. An aneurysm may rupture to produce a hemorrhagic cerebrovascular accident. In a **cerebro+vascular accident** (CVA, stroke, or stroke syndrome), blood vessels in the brain have become diseased or damaged. CVAs may also be caused by blockage of a cerebral artery by either a thrombus or an embolus (Fig. 7.14).
thrombus	10. A **thrombus** is an internal blood clot, and a cerebral thrombus can cause a thrombotic stroke. **Thrombotic** means pertaining to a _____. Another cause of blockage is an embolism.
thrombotic	11. An **embolism** is the sudden blocking of an artery or lymph vessel by foreign material that has been brought to the site of blockage by the circulating blood. The foreign material brought to the vessel is called an **embolus**. Emboli (plural of embolus) can be bits of tissue, tumor cells, globules of fat, air bubbles, clumps of bacteria, blood clots, or other material. If the embolus is a blood clot, it is called a _____ embolus.
clot	12. A thrombotic embolus is a blood _____ that has broken loose from its place of origin and has been brought to an artery or lymph vessel by the circulating blood.
	13. Use -itis to write a term that means inflammation of an artery:
arteritis	_____.
many	14. **Poly+arter+itis** is a disease that involves inflammation of _____ arteries. It leads to diminished flow of blood to areas normally supplied by these arteries.
	15. A disease that involves inflammation of several arteries is called
polyarteritis	_____.
	16. Arteries are used to measure the pulse rate. The **pulse** is the periodic thrust felt over the arteries; it is consistent with the heartbeat. The pulse, the rhythmic expansion of the
artery (arteries)	_____, can be felt with a finger (see Fig. 4.1, *A*).

bradycardia	17. The normal pulse rate of an adult in a resting state is approximately 70 to 80 beats per minute. An increased pulse rate is called **tachy+cardia** (tachy-, fast + cardi/o + -ia). Use brady- to form a word that means decreased pulse rate: _____.
arterioles	18. You read earlier that arteries branch out to form what type of vessels? _____.
capillaries	19. Arterioles carry blood to the smallest blood vessels, the _____. where exchange of oxygen and carbon dioxide occurs.
venules	20. Small vessels that collect blood from the capillaries are _____.
phleb/o	21. Veins carry blood back to the heart. Write the two combining forms that mean vein: ven/o and _____.
phlebitis	22. Use phleb/o to write a word that means inflammation of a vein: _____.
vein	23. **Thrombo+phleb+itis** is inflammation of a _____ associated with a blood clot. Thromb/o is a combining form for thrombus, or blood clot. Be aware that some specialists differentiate between the type of blood clot that occurs to prevent hemorrhage and a thrombus, a blood clot that occurs internally. Thus, it is preferable to refer to the latter as a thrombus.
vein	24. Venous **thromb+osis** is a blood clot in a _____. This can be caused by an injury to the leg or by prolonged bed confinement, or it can be a complication of phlebitis.
coronary	25. Remember that coronary arteries supply blood to the heart. Formation of a blood clot in a coronary artery, which then leads to occlusion of the vessel, is called _____ thrombosis. This is a common cause of myocardial infarction.
varicose	26. **Varicose** veins are swollen and knotted veins that occur most often in the legs. Sluggish blood flow, weakened walls, and incompetent valves contribute to varicose veins (Fig. 7.15). A varicose vein is also called a **varicosity**. Swollen and knotted veins are called _____ veins. **Hemorrhoids** are masses of dilated varicose veins in the **anal** canal. Hemorrhoids are often accompanied by pain, itching, and bleeding.

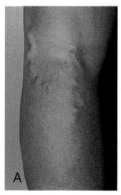
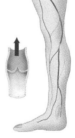
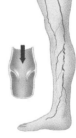

NORMAL VEINS
Functional valves aid
in flow of venous blood
back to heart

VARICOSE VEINS
Failure of valves and
pooling of blood in
superficial veins

A   B

Fig. 7.15 Varicose Veins. **A,** The appearance of superficial varicose veins in the legs, a common location. **B,** Comparison of normal veins and varicose veins. Note the large and tortuous (twisted) veins.

BUILD IT!
EXERCISE 8

Combine the word parts to write terms for these descriptions.

1. hardening of the arteries (arteri/o + -sclerosis)   _____
2. inflammation of the aorta (aort/o + -itis)   _____
3. pertaining to vessels of the brain (cerebr/o + vascul/o + -ar)   _____
4. inflammation of a vein associated with a blood clot   _____
   (thromb/o + phleb/o + -itis)
5. inflammation of many arteries (poly- + arter/o + -itis)   _____

MATCH IT!
EXERCISE 9

Match the definitions with the appropriate term in the right column (not all selections will be used).

_____ 1. ballooning out of the wall of a vessel
_____ 2. condition of a blood clot in a vessel or the heart cavity
_____ 3. increased blood pressure
_____ 4. increased pulse rate

A. aneurysm
B. bradycardia
C. hypertension
D. hypotension
E. tachycardia
F. thrombosis

Surgical and Therapeutic Interventions

Heart

The treatment of heart disease has seen major advances, including heart transplantation, the replacement of a diseased heart with a donor organ. Open heart surgery refers to operative procedures on the heart after it has been exposed through incision of the chest wall. Atrial or ventricular septal defects usually require surgical closure of the abnormal opening.

Cardiopulmonary means pertaining to the heart and lungs. **Cardiopulmonary bypass** is the method used to divert blood away from the heart and lungs temporarily when surgery of the heart and major vessels is performed. A heart-lung machine collects the blood, replenishes it with oxygen, and returns it to the body (Fig. 7.16). The term *bypass* is also used to mean bypass surgery.

Recent research is providing early evidence that stem cells may be able to replace damaged heart muscle cells and establish new blood vessels to supply them. This

cardi/o = heart
pulmon/o = lungs
-ary = pertaining to

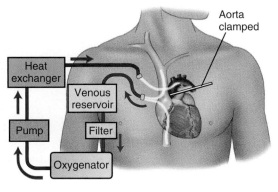

cardi/o = heart
pulmon/o = lungs
ven/o = vein

Fig. 7.16 Cardiopulmonary Bypass. Components of a cardiopulmonary bypass system used during heart surgery.

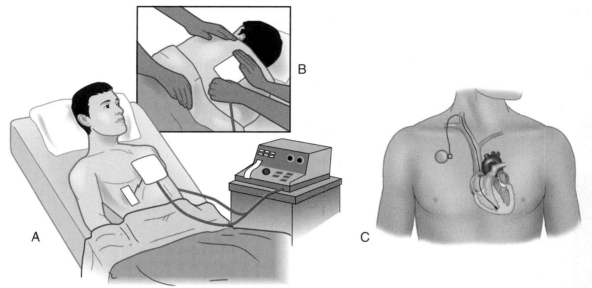

Fig. 7.17 Artificial Cardiac Pacemaker. An *external* (trancutaneous) pacemaker is used temporarily in a hospital setting to deliver electric current through the skin. Electrodes are placed on the patient's anterior (**A**) and posterior (**B**) chest walls and attached to an external pacing unit. **C,** An *internal* artificial cardiac pacemaker provides an electric current that travels from the battery through a conducting wire to the myocardium and stimulates the heart to beat.

revolutionary treatment may become the most efficient means of treating cardiovascular diseases, especially congestive heart disease.

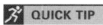

QUICK TIP

The SA and AV nodes are involved in the heart's electrical activity.

The heart has a natural pacemaker called the **sinoatrial** (SA) **node**. The use of the term *pacemaker* in reference to the heart often implies an artificial cardiac pacemaker, a small battery-powered device generally used to increase the heart rate by electrically stimulating the heart muscle. Depending on the patient's need, a cardiac pacemaker may be permanent or temporary, may send an impulse to the atrium, ventricle, or both, and may fire only on demand or at a constant rate (Fig. 7.17). **Cardio+version**, restoring the heart's normal rhythm using electrical shock, may be used when drug therapy is ineffective in treating a cardiac dysrhythmia. An automatic implanted **cardioverter defibrillator** (ICD) is a device that detects sustained ventricular tachycardia or fibrillation and delivers a low energy shock to the heart, restoring the normal rhythm (Fig. 7.18).

Cardiopulmonary resuscitation (CPR) is recommended as an emergency first-aid procedure to reestablish heart and lung action if breathing or heart action has stopped. It consists of closed heart massage and artificial respiration (mouth-to-mouth breathing

Fig. 7.18 Implanted Cardioverter-Defibrillator. This surgically implanted electric device automatically terminates arrhythmias by delivering low-energy shocks to the heart, restoring proper rhythm when the heart begins beating too fast or erratically. It is generally attached to the chest wall and has a wire lead embedded in the heart.

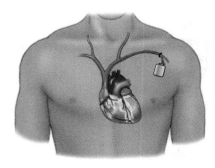

or a mechanical means; hands-only CPR is recommended for the untrained). CPR provides basic life support until it is no longer needed or until more advanced life support equipment is available.

Antiarrhythmic drugs are used to prevent, alleviate, or correct an abnormal heart rhythm. **Digoxin** is a well-known drug that is prescribed in the treatment of congestive heart failure and certain arrhythmias. Beta blockers are often given after a myocardial infarction to allow the heart to work less. The pain of angina pectoris is often relieved by rest and vasodilation of the coronary arteries with **nitroglycerin**, a coronary vasodilator.

WRITE IT!   EXERCISE 10

Write the correct term in the blanks to complete each sentence.

1. Drugs used to correct abnormal heart rhythms are _____ drugs.
2. Operative procedures on the heart after incision of the chest wall are called _____ heart surgeries.
3. A word that refers to the lungs and heart is _____.
4. Medications that are given after a myocardial infarction to allow the heart to work less are _____ blockers.
5. An electrical device that can keep the heart rhythm within a desirable range is a cardiac _____.

MATCH IT!   EXERCISE 11

Match the medical terms in the left column with their meanings in the right column.

_____ 1. cardioversion
_____ 2. cardiopulmonary bypass
_____ 3. cardiopulmonary resuscitation
_____ 4. digoxin
_____ 5. nitroglycerin

A. vasodilator often used in angina pectoris
B. drug often used in CHF and certain arrhythmias
C. method used to divert blood away from the heart and lungs during heart surgery
D. emergency first-aid procedure used to reestablish heart and lung action
E. restoring the heart's normal rhythm using electrical shock

---

Blood Vessels

Nonsurgical Vascular Treatments. In some cases, blood flow through vessels can be increased by using methods that do not require surgery. A blood clot is sometimes treated with a **thrombolytic** agent administered through a catheter to dissolve the clot. Oral anticoagulants such as warfarin (Coumadin) and heparin, as well as newer medication such as Eliquis are prescribed in the treatment and prevention of a variety of **thrombo**+**embol**+**ic** disorders.

thromb/o = clot
-lytic = capable of destroying
embol/o = embolus
-ic = pertaining to

Vasodilators are medications that cause dilation of blood vessels. Calcium channel blockers are drugs that help diminish muscle spasms, particularly those of the coronary artery.

Antihypertensives are agents that are used to reduce high blood pressure. **Diuretics** are also used and act to reduce the blood volume through greater excretion of water by the kidneys.

anti- = against
-emic = pertaining to blood

Antilipidemic drugs are prescribed to lower cholesterol levels in the blood, which is generally considered to coincide with a lower incidence of coronary heart disease. However, the best way to prevent hyperlipidemia is to eat a low-fat diet, to exercise, and to maintain a proper weight.

Surgical Treatments of Vascular Problems. **Angioplasty** is surgical repair of blood vessels that have become damaged by disease or injury. Balloon angioplasty uses a balloon catheter that is inflated inside an artery to flatten the plaque against the arterial wall; a stent is sometimes inserted. This procedure may be necessary in coronary artery disease (Fig. 7.19). If blockage is too severe, a **coronary artery bypass graft** (CABG) using venous or arterial grafts may be necessary (Fig. 7.20).

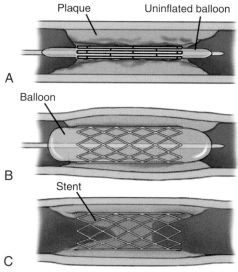

Fig. 7.19 Balloon Angioplasty and Placement of a Coronary Artery Stent. A small, balloon-tipped catheter is threaded into a coronary artery and inflated to compress the plaque. A stent, an expandable meshlike structure, is placed over the angioplasty site to keep the coronary artery open. **A,** The stent and uninflated balloon catheter are positioned in the artery. **B,** The stent expands as the balloon is inflated. **C,** The balloon is then deflated and removed, leaving the implanted stent. **angi/o =** vessel; **-plasty =** surgical repair

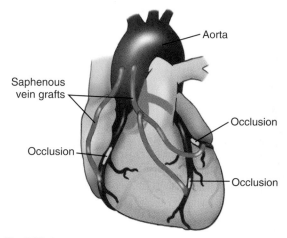

Fig. 7.20 Coronary Artery Bypass Graft. Sections of blood vessels (such as the saphenous veins from the patient's leg) are grafted onto the coronary arteries to bypass the blocked coronary arteries.

per- = through
cutane/o = skin
-ous = pertaining to

Other per+cutane+ous procedures to remove blockage include laser or a specially designed catheter for cutting away plaque from the lining of an artery (**atherectomy**). **Intravascular thrombolysis** incorporates a thrombolytic agent delivered through a catheter to a clot.

ather/o = yellow, fatty plaque
-ectomy = excision

Cardiopulmonary bypass is generally required to perform **aorto+plasty**; however, the aorta can sometimes be repaired percutaneously. In the latter case, the physician threads a catheter mounted with a compressed replacement valve on a tiny balloon through an incision in a vein in the groin.

Surgical excision of a vein, or a segment of vein, is called **phleb+ectomy**. A **hemorrhoid+ectomy** is surgical excision of a hemorrhoid.

WRITE IT!
EXERCISE 12

Write a term in each blank to complete these sentences.

1. The initials of the surgery that uses venous or arterial grafts to bypass blocked coronary arteries are

   _____.

2. A term for surgical repair of the aorta is _____.

3. Flattening plaque against the arterial wall with a balloon catheter is called balloon

   _____.

4. Surgical excision of a vein or a segment of vein is called _____.

5. Agents used to reduce high blood pressure are called _____.

6. Agents used to lower cholesterol levels in the blood are called _____.

LYMPHATIC SYSTEM

Structures of the Lymphatic System

The lymphatic system is also called "the lymphatics." The primary function of the lymphatic system is to collect fluid that escapes from the blood capillaries and return it to the circulation. As blood circulates, some of the fluid leaves the capillaries to bathe the tissue cells. Thin-walled lymphatic vessels, distributed throughout the body, collect the escaped fluid. This fluid, **lymph**, is transported by the lymphatic vessels (Fig. 7.21). The system depends on muscular contraction because there is no pump, just valves that carry the fluid away from the tissue.

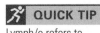 **QUICK TIP**

Lymph/o refers to either the lymphatics or the fluid lymph.

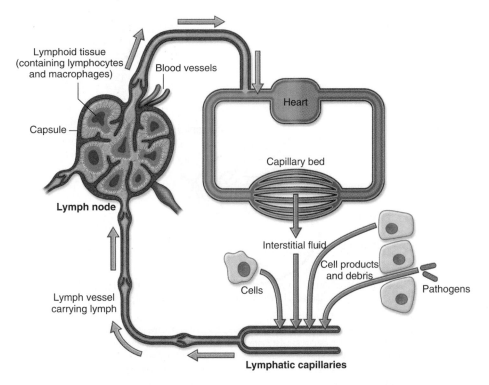

Fig. 7.21 Circulation of Lymph in the Lymphatic System. Macrophages, large phagocytes, engulf foreign materials.

The lymph vessels, lymph nodes, lymph, tonsils, **thymus**, and **spleen** compose the lymphatic system (Fig. 7.22). Small knots of tissue found at intervals along the course of the lymphatic vessels are called the lymph nodes. The **tonsils** are masses of lymphatic tissue located in depressions of the mucous membranes of the pharynx. We usually think of tonsils as the small masses located at the back of the throat, but these are just one type of tonsil, the **palatine tonsils**. The combining form tonsill/o generally refers to the palatine tonsil. **Pharyngeal** tonsils are commonly called **adenoids**. When the component parts of the term *adenoid* are analyzed, they are seen to mean "resembling a gland." Thus, pharyngeal tonsil is a more appropriate name.

aden/o = gland
-oid = resembling

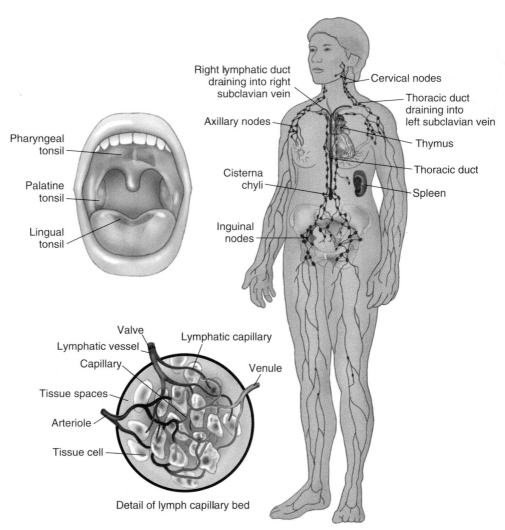

Fig. 7.22 Lymphatic System. Only a few of the lymph nodes are shown: cervical lymph nodes in the neck, axillary lymph nodes in the armpit, and inguinal lymph nodes in the groin. The close relationship to the cardiovascular system is shown in the detailed drawing. Lymph capillaries merge to form lymphatic vessels that join other vessels to become trunks that drain large regions of the body. The right lymphatic duct receives fluid from the upper right quadrant of the body and empties into the right subclavian vein. The thoracic duct, which begins with the cisterna chyli, collects fluid from the rest of the body and empties it into the left subclavian vein. Also shown are the lymphatic organs: tonsils, thymus, and spleen.

Commit the following combining forms and meanings to memory.

ADDITIONAL WORD PARTS AND THEIR MEANINGS

Word Part	Meaning	Word Part	Meaning
adenoid/o	adenoids	lymphat/o	lymphatics
cervic/o	neck (or the uterine cervix)	splen/o	spleen
home/o	sameness	thromb/o	thrombus, blood clot

Diseases, Disorders, and Diagnostic Terms

The lymphatic system frequently becomes involved in metastasis, the spread of cancer cells from their origin to other parts of the body. When cancer cells enter a lymphatic vessel, the cells may be trapped by the lymph nodes and begin growing there, or the cells may be carried to sites far from their origin. Lymphatic carcinoma is cancer that has spread to the lymphatics from another site. **Lymph+oma** is a general term for cancer that originates in the lymphatic system.

> **lymph/o** = lymphatic
> **-oma** = tumor

Lymph+ang+itis is an acute or a chronic inflammation of lymphatic vessels and can be caused by various microorganisms (Fig. 7.23). **Lymphangiography** is radiography of the lymphatic vessels and nodes after injection of a radiopaque substance has made them visible on x-ray images. Accumulation of lymph in tissue and the resultant swelling are called **lymphedema** (see Fig. 2.21). **Lymphangiograms** are useful for checking the integrity of the lymphatic system in lymphedema and for investigating the spread of malignant tumors.

> **angi/o** = vessel
> **-itis** = inflammation
> **lymph/o** = lymphatics
> **-edema** = swelling

One example of edema is seen in the late stages of **elephantiasis,** a parasitic disease generally seen in the tropics (Fig. 7.24). The excessive swelling, usually of the external reproductive organs and the legs, is caused by obstruction of the lymphatic vessels by parasites.

> **WORD ORIGIN**
> *elephas* (G.), elephant

The lymph nodes were once considered to be glands, so the word part aden/o often appears in terms related to lymph nodes. **Lymphadenitis** is inflammation of the

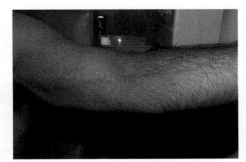

Fig. 7.23 Streptococcal Lymphangitis. This type of inflammatory condition of the lymph nodes is caused by streptococcal bacteria. Examination of the area distal to the affected node usually reveals the source of the infection. **lymph/o** = lymph or lymphatics; **angi/o** = vessel; **-itis** = inflammation; **dist/o** = distant

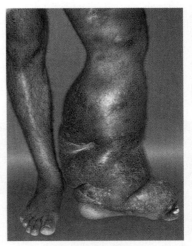

Fig. 7.24 Lymphedema. Extensive swelling, caused by chronic obstruction of the lymphatic vessels, occurs in the late stages of elephantiasis.

lymph/o = lymph or lymphatics
aden/o = gland
-itis = inflammation
cervic/o = neck
-al = pertaining to

Fig. 7.25 Lymphadenitis. The cervical lymph node is enlarged, firm, painless, and freely movable. The node may resolve without treatment or may eventually rupture and drain.

-oma = swelling
splen/o = spleen
-megaly = enlargement

lymph nodes (Fig. 7.25), **lymphadenopathy** refers to any disease of the lymph nodes, and **lymphadenoma** is a tumor of a lymph node. **Tonsillitis** is inflammation of the tonsils. **Spleno+megaly** means enlarged spleen, which has many causes.

Surgical and Therapeutic Interventions

Infected lymph nodes or lymph vessels often respond to antibiotic therapy or resolve on their own.

Lymph nodes are frequently biopsied to determine whether cancer has spread from an internal organ. **Lymph+aden+ectomy** is excision of a lymph node. Treatment of lymphoma is determined by the type of lymphoma and can include intensive radiotherapy, chemotherapy, and biologic therapies, including interferon.

A ruptured spleen often requires a **splenectomy**. Excision of the tonsils is a **tonsillectomy**. An **adenoidectomy** is performed because the adenoids are enlarged, chronically infected, or causing obstruction. Adenoids are sometimes removed at the same time as a tonsillectomy; this combined procedure is abbreviated T&A.

MATCH IT!
EXERCISE 13

Match the meanings in the left column with the medical terms in the right column.

_____ 1. swelling caused by obstruction of a lymphatic tissue

_____ 2. general term for cancer originating in the lymphatic system

_____ 3. inflammation of the lymphatic vessels

_____ 4. radiograph of lymph vessels

_____ 5. any disease of the lymph nodes

A. lymphadenopathy
B. lymphangiogram of the lymphatic vessels and nodes
C. lymphangitis
D. lymphedema
E. lymphoma

A Career as an Echocardiographer

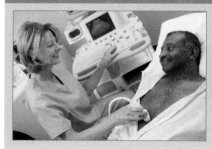

Meet Marsha Brown, an echocardiographer. She is a radiologic technologist who has specialized in echocardiography (echo). Echo is a type of ultrasonography that shows video of the heart's contractions. An ECG is done at the same time to compare the heart's physical motion and electrical activity. For more information on this career, visit http:/www.asecho.org or see https://www.asrt.org/main/careers/careers-in-radiologic-technology/who-are-radiologic-technologists.

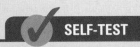
SELF-TEST

Work the following exercises to test your understanding of the material in Chapter 7. It is best to do all the exercises before checking your answers against the answers in Appendix III. Pay particular attention to spelling.

A. LABELING!   Using this illustration of a capillary bed, write combining forms for the structures that are indicated. (Line 1 is done as an example.) Write two combining forms for line 2 (artery) and line 4 (vein), as indicated on the drawing.

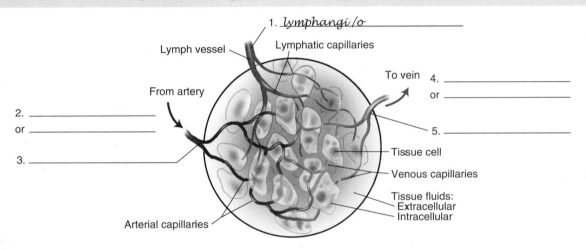

1. *lymphangi/o*

Lymph vessel

Lymphatic capillaries

To vein   4. _____

or _____

From artery

2. _____

or _____

5. _____

3. _____

Tissue cell

Venous capillaries

Tissue fluids:
Extracellular
Intracellular

Arterial capillaries

B. CHOOSING!   Circle the one correct answer (A, B, C, or D) for each question.

1. Charlie is told that he has a form of arteriosclerosis in which yellowish plaque has accumulated on the walls of the arteries. What is the name of this form of arteriosclerosis?
   (A) aortostenosis   **(B)** atherosclerosis   **(C)** cardiomyopathy   **(D)** coarctation

2. Which of these surgeries can be used to correct coronary occlusion?
   (A) cardioversion   **(B)** coronary artery bypass   **(C)** defibrillation   **(D)** lymphadenectomy

3. Kristen, a 28-year-old woman, is told she has inflammation of the lining of the heart. What is the medical term for this heart pathology?   **(A)** coronary heart disease   **(B)** endocarditis   **(C)** myocarditis   **(D)** pericarditis

4. Jayne had ventricular fibrillation during coronary angiography. What procedure did the physician use to stop fibrillation?
   (A) atherectomy   **(B)** endarterectomy   **(C)** cardiopulmonary resuscitation   **(D)** defibrillation

5. Jim developed a blood clot in a coronary artery. What is Jim's condition called?
   (A) myocardial infarction   **(B)** coronary artery bypass   **(C)** coronary thrombosis   **(D)** fibrillation

6. Baby Seth is born with cyanosis and a heart murmur. Which congenital heart disease does the neonatologist think is most likely?   **(A)** atrial septal defect   **(B)** atrioventricular block   **(C)** megalocardia   **(D)** pericarditis

7. Angie has an angiogram that shows a ballooning out of the wall of a cerebrovascular artery. Which condition does Angie have?   **(A)** aneurysm   **(B)** angioma   **(C)** arteriosclerosis   **(D)** coronary thrombosis

8. Mary has a varicose vein that must be excised. What is the name of the surgery?
   (A) arterectomy   **(B)** balloon angioplasty   **(C)** phlebectomy   **(D)** resuscitation

9. Sixteen-year-old Jason has an inflamed cervical lymph node. What is the name of his condition?
    (A) lymphadenitis   **(B)** lymphangitis   **(C)** lymphedema   **(D)** lymphoma

10. Mr. Smith has angina pectoris and uses a coronary vasodilator when he has chest pain. Which of the following is a coronary vasodilator?   **(A)** antiarrhythmic   **(B)** antilipidemic   **(C)** heparin   **(D)** nitroglycerin

C. WRITING!   *Write words in the blanks to complete the sentences.*

Oxygen-rich blood is pumped from the heart into the (1) _____ and is routed to arteries, which branch to become (2) _____, which branch to become capillaries. The capillaries are the site of (3) _____ and carbon dioxide exchange. Blood leaving the capillaries returns to the heart through the venules, which flow into the (4) _____. Blood returns to the heart by way of the superior and inferior venae cavae. The chamber of the heart that receives the oxygen-poor blood is the right (5) _____. Blood is reoxygenated by the lungs. A primary function of the (6) _____ system is to collect fluid that escapes from the blood capillaries and return it to the circulation.

   Arteries that provide oxygen and nutrients to the heart itself are called (7) _____ arteries.

   The three layers of the heart, beginning with the innermost layer, are (8) _____, (9) _____, and (10) _____ (also called the visceral pericardium).

D. SPELLING AND PRONOUNCING!   *Circle all incorrectly spelled terms and write the correct spellings.* Then pronounce the terms.

adenoidektomy   colesterol   cardiovascular   defibrillater   infarktion

E. READING HEALTH CARE REPORTS   *Read the case study and define the five underlined terms listed after the report.*

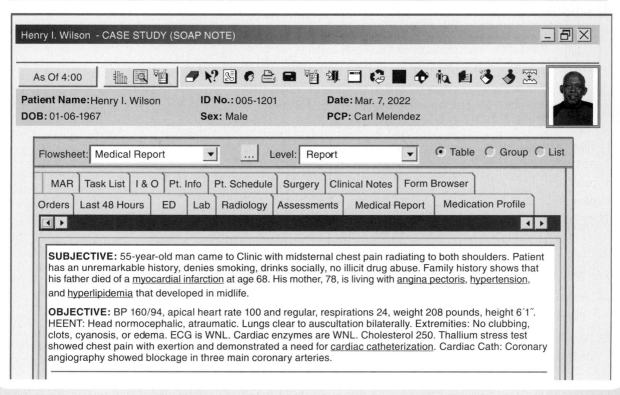

Henry I. Wilson - CASE STUDY (SOAP NOTE)

As Of 4:00

Patient Name: Henry I. Wilson   **ID No.:** 005-1201   **Date:** Mar. 7, 2022
DOB: 01-06-1967   **Sex:** Male   **PCP:** Carl Melendez

Flowsheet: Medical Report   …   Level: Report   ⊙ Table ○ Group ○ List

MAR | Task List | I & O | Pt. Info | Pt. Schedule | Surgery | Clinical Notes | Form Browser
Orders | Last 48 Hours | ED | Lab | Radiology | Assessments | Medical Report | Medication Profile

SUBJECTIVE: 55-year-old man came to Clinic with midsternal chest pain radiating to both shoulders. Patient has an unremarkable history, denies smoking, drinks socially, no illicit drug abuse. Family history shows that his father died of a <u>myocardial infarction</u> at age 68. His mother, 78, is living with <u>angina pectoris</u>, <u>hypertension</u>, and <u>hyperlipidemia</u> that developed in midlife.

OBJECTIVE: BP 160/94, apical heart rate 100 and regular, respirations 24, weight 208 pounds, height 6′1″. HEENT: Head normocephalic, atraumatic. Lungs clear to auscultation bilaterally. Extremities: No clubbing, clots, cyanosis, or edema. ECG is WNL. Cardiac enzymes are WNL. Cholesterol 250. Thallium stress test showed chest pain with exertion and demonstrated a need for <u>cardiac catheterization</u>. Cardiac Cath: Coronary angiography showed blockage in three main coronary arteries.

1. myocardial infarction   _____
2. hypertension   _____
3. hyperlipidemia   _____
4. cardiac catheterization   _____
5. angina pectoris   _____

F.   *Read the following partial Emergency Treatment Record; then write the terms from the report that are described.*

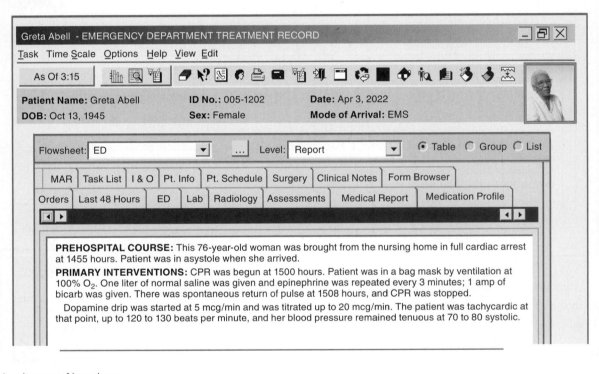

Greta Abell - EMERGENCY DEPARTMENT TREATMENT RECORD

Task Time Scale Options Help View Edit

As Of 3:15

Patient Name: Greta Abell   **ID No.:** 005-1202   **Date:** Apr 3, 2022
DOB: Oct 13, 1945   **Sex:** Female   **Mode of Arrival:** EMS

Flowsheet: ED   ...   Level: Report   ⊙ Table ○ Group ○ List

MAR Task List I & O Pt. Info Pt. Schedule Surgery Clinical Notes Form Browser

Orders Last 48 Hours ED Lab Radiology Assessments Medical Report Medication Profile

PREHOSPITAL COURSE: This 76-year-old woman was brought from the nursing home in full cardiac arrest at 1455 hours. Patient was in asystole when she arrived.

PRIMARY INTERVENTIONS: CPR was begun at 1500 hours. Patient was in a bag mask by ventilation at 100% O_2. One liter of normal saline was given and epinephrine was repeated every 3 minutes; 1 amp of bicarb was given. There was spontaneous return of pulse at 1508 hours, and CPR was stopped.

Dopamine drip was started at 5 mcg/min and was titrated up to 20 mcg/min. The patient was tachycardic at that point, up to 120 to 130 beats per minute, and her blood pressure remained tenuous at 70 to 80 systolic.

1. absence of heartbeat   _____
2. pertaining to an increased pulse rate   _____
3. pertaining to the heart   _____
4. pertaining to the higher number in a blood pressure reading   _____
5. the rhythmic expansion and contraction of an artery   _____

G.   *Read the Office Visit Note and circle the correct answers.*

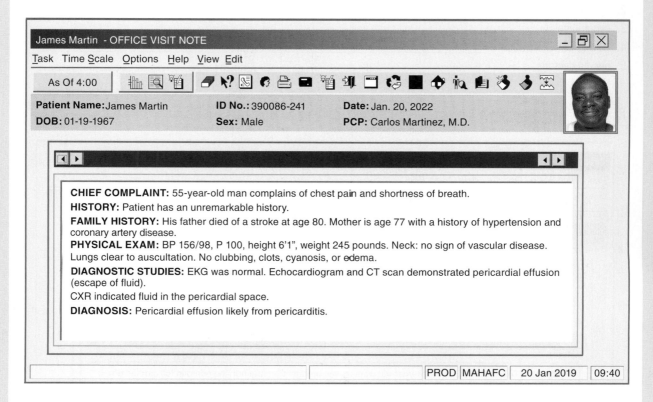

James Martin - OFFICE VISIT NOTE

Task   Time Scale   Options   Help   View   Edit

As Of 4:00

Patient Name: James Martin   **ID No.:**390086-241   **Date:** Jan. 20, 2022
DOB: 01-19-1967   **Sex:** Male   **PCP:** Carlos Martinez, M.D.

CHIEF COMPLAINT: 55-year-old man complains of chest pain and shortness of breath.
HISTORY: Patient has an unremarkable history.
FAMILY HISTORY: His father died of a stroke at age 80. Mother is age 77 with a history of hypertension and coronary artery disease.
PHYSICAL EXAM: BP 156/98, P 100, height 6'1", weight 245 pounds. Neck: no sign of vascular disease. Lungs clear to auscultation. No clubbing, clots, cyanosis, or edema.
DIAGNOSTIC STUDIES: EKG was normal. Echocardiogram and CT scan demonstrated pericardial effusion (escape of fluid).
CXR indicated fluid in the pericardial space.
DIAGNOSIS: Pericardial effusion likely from pericarditis.

PROD | MAHAFC | 20 Jan 2019 | 09:40

1. Which layer of the patient's heart tissue was affected by disease? (inner layer, middle layer, outer layer)
2. The mother's history indicates (fibrillation, heart murmur, high blood pressure, hyperlipidemia).
3. Which term in the report means pertaining to the "pericardium?" (coronary, effusion, pericardial, pericarditis)

H. WRITING!   *Write a one-word term for each of these meanings.*

1. abnormally low blood pressure   _____
2. agent used to reduce blood pressure   _____
3. an enlarged spleen   _____
4. any disease of the lymph nodes   _____
5. excision of the tonsils   _____
6. increased pulse rate   _____
7. fatty substances such as triglycerides   _____
8. radiography of the heart and great vessels _____
9. the lining of the heart   _____
10. the smallest blood vessels   _____

I. IDENTIFYING!   *Label these illustrations using one of the following: aortography, arteriogram, aneurysm, angiography, embolus, thrombus.*

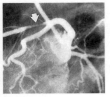

1. image produced in arteriography

_____

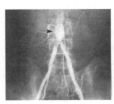

2. abnormality indicated by the arrow

_____

J. QUICK CHALLENGE!   *Find an incorrect term in each sentence and write the correct term.*

1. Electrocardiography is the use of ultrasonography (echography) in diagnosing heart disease. _____
2. Cardiomegaly designates primary disease of the heart muscle itself. _____
3. Myocardial vasodilation is deficiency of myocardial blood supply. _____
4. A fat thrombus can block an artery or lymph vessel. _____
5. Antihypertensives are medications that cause dilation of blood vessels. _____

Q&E LIST

Use the Evolve website (http://evolve.elsevier.com/Leonard/quick) to review the terms. Look closely at spelling!

adenoidectomy (ad-uh-noid-**ek**-tuh-mē)
adenoids (**ad**-uh-noidz)
anal (**ā**-nul)
aneurysm (**an**-ū-riz-um)
angina pectoris (an-**jī**-nuh **pek**-tuh-ris)
angiocardiography (an-jē-ō-kahr-dē-**og**-ruh-fē)
angiography (an-jē-**og**-ruh-fē)
angioma (an-jē-**ō**-muh)
angioplasty (**an**-jē-ō-plas-tē)
antiarrhythmic (an-tē-uh-**rith**-mik)
antihypertensive (an-tē-hī-pur-**ten**-siv)
antilipidemic (an-tē-lip-i-**dē**-mik)
aorta (ā-**or**-tuh)
aortic (ā-**or**-tik)
aortic stenosis (ā-**or**-tik stuh- **nō** -sis)
aortitis (ā-or-**tī**-tis)
aortogram (ā-**or**-tō-gram)
aortography (ā-or-**tog**-ruh-fē)
aortoplasty (ā-**or**-tō-plas-tē)

arrhythmia (uh-**rith**-mē-uh)
arterial (ahr-**tē**-rē-ul)
arteriogram (ahr-**tēr**-ē-ō-gram)
arteriography (ahr-tēr-ē-**og**-ruh-fē)
arteriole (ahr-**tēr**-ē-ōl)
arteriopathy (ahr-tēr-ē-**op**-uh-thē)
arteriosclerosis (ahr-tēr-ē-ō-skluh-**rō**-sis)
arteriovenous (ahr-tēr-ē-ō-**vē**-nus)
arteritis (ahr-tuh-**rī**-tis)
artery (**ahr**-tuh-rē)
asystole (ā-**sis**-tō-lē)
atherectomy (ath-er-**ek**-tuh-mē)
atherosclerosis (ath-ur-ō-skluh-**rō**-sis)
atria (**ā**-trē-uh)
atrial (**ā**-trē-ul)
atrioventricular (ā-trē-ō-ven-**trik**-ū-lur)
atrium (**ā**-trē-um)
bicuspid (bī-**kus**-pid)
bradycardia (brad-ē-**kahr**-dē-uh)

QUICK & EASY (Q&E) LIST—cont'd

capillaries *(kap-i-lar-ēz)*
cardiac catheterization *(kahr-dē-ak kath-uh-tur-i-zā-shun)*
cardiomegaly *(kahr-dē-ō-meg-uh-lē)*
cardiomyopathy *(kahr-dē-ō-mī-op-uh-thē)*
cardiopulmonary *(kahr-dē-ō-pool-muh-nar-ē)*
cardiopulmonary bypass *(kahr-dē-ō-pool-muh-nar-ē bī-pas)*
cardiopulmonary resuscitation *(kahr-dē-ō-pool-muh-nar-ē rē-sus-i-tā-shun)*
cardiovascular *(kahr-dē-ō-vas-kū-lur)*
cardioversion *(kahr-dē-ō-vur-zhun)*
cardioverter-defibrillator *(kahr-dē-ō-vur-tur dē-fib-ri-lā-tur)*
catheter *(kath-uh-tur)*
cerebral *(suh-rē-brul, ser-uh-brul)*
cerebrovascular accident *(ser-uh-brō-vas-kū-lur ak-si-dunt)*
cholesterol *(kuh-les-tur-ol)*
circulatory *(sur-kū-luh-tor-ē)*
congenital heart defects *(kun-jen-i-tul hahrt dē-fekts)*
congestive heart failure *(kun-jes-tiv hahrt fāl-yur)*
coronary *(kor-uh-nar-ē)*
coronary artery bypass graft *(kor-uh-nar-ē ahr-tuh-rē bī-pas graft)*
coronary artery disease *(kor-uh-nar-ē ahr-tuh-rē di-zēz)*
coronary heart disease *(kor-uh-nar-ē hahrt di-zēz)*
cuspid *(kus-pid)*
defibrillation *(dē-fib-ri-lā-shun)*
defibrillator *(dē-fib-ri-lā-tur)*
digoxin *(di-jok-sin)*
diuretic *(dī-ū-ret-ik)*
dysrhythmia *(dis-rith-mē-uh)*
echocardiogram *(ek-ō-kahr-dē-ō-gram)*
echocardiography *(ek-ō-kahr-dē-og-ruh-fē)*
electrocardiogram *(ē-lek-trō-kahr-dē-ō-gram)*
electrocardiograph *(ē-lek-trō-kahr-dē-ō-graf)*
electrocardiography *(ē-lek-trō-kahr-dē-og-ruh-fē)*
elephantiasis *(el-uh-fun-tī-uh-sis)*
embolism *(em-buh-liz-um)*
embolus *(em-bō-lus)*
endocarditis *(en-dō-kahr-dī-tis)*
endocardium *(en-dō-kahr-dē-um)*
epicardium *(ep-i-kahr-dē-um)*
fibrillation *(fib-ri-lā-shun)*
heart failure *(hahrt fāl-yur)*
heart murmur *(hahrt mur-mur)*
hemangioma *(hē-man-jē-ō-muh)*
hemorrhage *(hem-uh-ruj)*
hemorrhoidectomy *(hem-uh-roid-ek-tuh-mē)*
hemorrhoids *(hem-uh-roidz)*
heparin *(hep-uh-rin)*
hyperlipidemia *(hī-pur-lip-i-dē-mē-uh)*
hypertension *(hī-pur-ten-shun)*
hypotension *(hī-pō-ten-shun)*
infarction *(in-fahrk-shun)*

intravascular thrombolysis *(in-truh-vas-kyū-lur throm-bol-i-sis)*
lipid *(lip-id)*
lymph *(limf)*
lymphadenectomy *(lim-fad-uh-nek-tuh-mē)*
lymphadenitis *(lim-fad-uh-nī-tis)*
lymphadenoma *(lim-fad-uh-nō-muh)*
lymphadenopathy *(lim-fad-uh-nop-uh-thē)*
lymphangiogram *(lim-fan-jē-ō-gram)*
lymphangiography *(lim-fan-jē-og-ruh-fē)*
lymphangioma *(lim-fan-jē-ō-muh)*
lymphangitis *(lim-fan-jī-tis)*
lymphatic *(lim-fat-ik)*
lymphedema *(lim-fuh-dē-muh)*
lymphoma *(lim-fō-muh)*
mitral *(mī-trul)*
myocardial infarction *(mī-ō-kahr-dē-ul in-fahrk-shun)*
myocardial ischemia *(mī-ō-kahr-dē-ul is-kē-mē-uh)*
myocarditis *(mī-ō-kahr-dī-tis)*
myocardium *(mī-ō-kahr-dē-um)*
nitroglycerin *(nī-trō-glis-ur-in)*
occlusion *(ō-kloo-zhun)*
palatine tonsil *(pal-uh-tīn ton-sil)*
pericarditis *(per-i-kahr-dī-tis)*
pericardium *(per-i-kahr-dē-um)*
pharyngeal *(fuh-rin-jē-ul)*
phlebectomy *(fluh-bek-tuh-mē)*
phlebitis *(fluh-bī-tis)*
polyarteritis *(pol-ē-ahr-tuh-rī-tis)*
pulse *(puls)*
semilunar *(sem-ē-loo-nur)*
septal defect *(sep-tul dē-fekt)*
shock *(shok)*
sinoatrial node *(sī-nō-ā-trē-ul nōd)*
spleen *(splēn)*
splenectomy *(splē-nek-tuh-mē)*
splenomegaly *(splē-nō-meg-uh-lē)*
stenosis *(stuh-nō-sis)*
tachycardia *(tak-i-kahr-dē-uh)*
thromboembolic *(throm-bō-em-bol-ik)*
thrombolytic *(throm-bō-lit-ik)*
thrombophlebitis *(throm-bō-fluh-bī-tis)*
thrombosis *(throm-bō-sis)*
thrombotic *(throm-bot-ik)*
thrombus *(throm-bus)*
thymus *(thī-mus)*
tonsil *(ton-sil)*
tonsillectomy *(ton-si-lek-tuh-mē)*
tonsillitis *(ton-si-lī-tis)*
tricuspid *(trī-kus-pid)*
triglyceride *(trī-glis-ur-īd)*
varicose *(var-i-kōs)*

QUICK & EASY (Q&E) LIST—cont'd

varicosity *(var-i-**kos**-i-tē)*
vascular *(**vas**-kū-lur)*
vasoconstriction *(vā-zō-kun-**strik**-shun)*
vasodilation *(vā-zō-dī-**lā**-shun)*
vasodilator *(vā-zō-**dī**-lā-tur)*
vein *(vān)*

vena cava *(**vē**-nuh **kā**-vuh)*
venous *(**vē**-nus)*
ventricle *(**ven**-tri-kul)*
ventricular *(ven-**trik**-ū-lur)*
venule *(**ven**-ūl)*
visceral *(**vis**-ur-ul)*

Don't forget the games and other activities available at http://evolve.elsevier.com/Leonard/quick.

 QUICK CONNECT

Review all lists of word parts and their meanings for this chapter using the flashcards you prepared or the flashcards on the Evolve site.

CIRCULATORY SYSTEM:

- The cardiovascular system (heart and blood vessels) carries oxygen, food, and other substances to body cells, carrying away waste products and carbon dioxide, prevents hemorrhage through blood clotting, protects against disease, and helps regulate body temperature.
- The lymphatic system (vessels, nodes, and organs) produces various blood cells and helps protect and maintain the internal fluid environment by collecting and restoring fluids to the cardiovascular system.

THE CARDIOVASCULAR SYSTEM:

The blood flow through blood vessels: arteries (rich in oxygen and nutrients), arterioles, capillaries (where oxygen and waste carbon dioxide are exchanged), venules, and veins (carry blood back to the heart).

The heart (muscular organ that pumps blood) enters the right atrium via the venae cavae. Blood flow through the heart:

- right atrium
- right ventricle (pulmonary artery to the lungs where exchange of carbon dioxide and oxygen occurs, then returns to heart via pulmonary veins)
- left atrium
- left ventricle (aorta, the largest artery where blood leaves the heart to travel throughout the body)

Septum divides the right and left sides of the heart.

Heart valves: atrioventricular valves (tricuspid) and (bicuspid, mitral)

Tissue layers of the heart, starting from the outside: epicardium, myocardium and endocardium

Diagnostic tests: pulse rate, blood pressure (diastolic pressure and systolic pressure), ECG, stress tests (treadmill vs. thallium), radiology (cardiac CT, cardiac MRI, echocardiography, positron emission tomography, arteriography, cardiac catheterization, coronary angiography, electrophysiology studies); arteriography vs. angiography.

Other diagnostic terms: hypertension vs. hypotension, arrhythmia, dysrhythmia, arrhythmia, asystole.

Diseases and Disorders of the heart: Cardiomyopathy designates primary disease of the heart muscle itself. Distinguish between endocarditis and pericarditis. Know the meanings of angina pectoris, asystole, cardiomegaly, congenital heart vs, congestive heart, coronary artery vs. coronary heart disease, fibrillation, hypotension vs. hypertension, myocardial ischemia vs. infarction, septal defect, shock.

Terms related to the blood vessels: vasodilation vs. vasoconstriction. How does aortography help diagnose aortic stenosis? Name at least two types of angiomas. Know these terms: arteritis, arteriosclerosis., atherosclerosis, aneurysm, hemorrhage, CVA, thrombus vs. embolus, polyarteritis, thrombophlebitis, bradycardia vs. tachycardia, venous thrombosis, varicosity, hemorrhoids.

Heart surgical terms: cardiopulmonary bypass, cardiopulmonary resuscitation, cardioversion, cardioverter defibrillator

Surgical terms related to blood vessels: angioplasty, CABG, atherectomy, intravascular thrombolysis, aortoplasty, phlebectomy, hemorrhoidectomy

Therapeutic cardiac interventions: antiarrhythmic drugs, digoxin, nitroglycerin

Nonsurgical vascular treatments: thrombolytic agents (preventatives: warfarin, heparin or Eliquis); vasodilators, antihypertensives, diuretics, antilipidemics

LYMPHATIC SYSTEM

The lymphatics are composed of lymphatic vessels, lymph, lymph nodes, and three main organs (spleen, thymus, and tonsils). Remember two types of tonsils (palatine tonsils and pharyngeal tonsils, adenoids).

Function: Collect fluid (lymph) that escapes from the blood capillaries and return it to the circulatory system

Diagnostic tests: lymphangiography, biopsy

Selected pathologies: lymphangitis, lymphoma, lymphedema, elephantiasis, lymphadenitis, lymphadenopathy, lymphadenoma, tonsillitis, splenomegaly, splenectomy, adenoidectomy

Surgical interventions: lymphadenectomy, tonsillectomy, adenoidectomy, thymectomy, tonsilloadenoidectomy

CHAPTER 8

Respiratory System

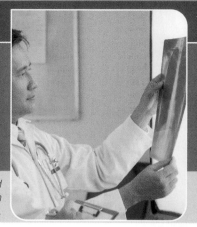

The specialist in pulmonary medicine, a pulmonologist, depends on observation and diagnostic tests to evaluate the individual's respiratory functions. He or she is often assisted by a pulmonary function technologist.

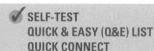
OBJECTIVES

After completing Chapter 8, you will be able to:

1. Recognize or write the functions of the respiratory system.
2. Recognize or write the meanings of Chapter 8 word parts and use them to build and analyze terms.
3. Write terms for selected structures of the respiratory system, or match terms with their descriptions.
4. Write the names of the diagnostic terms and pathologies related to the respiratory system when

given their descriptions, or match terms with their meanings.
5. Match surgical and therapeutic interventions for the respiratory system, or write the names of the interventions when given their descriptions.
6. Spell terms for the respiratory system correctly.

 Function First

Respiration is the combined activity of various processes that supply oxygen to all body cells and remove carbon dioxide. Breathing is external respiration, the absorption of oxygen from the air and the removal of carbon dioxide by the lungs. Breathing is often called pulmonary ventilation or simply ventilation. The **respiratory** system consists of a series of passages that bring outside air in contact with special structures that lie close to blood capillaries. Oxygen and carbon dioxide are exchanged at the interface between these special structures and the capillaries (internal respiration). This exchange of gases is part of **homeo+stasis,** a state of equilibrium of the internal environment of the body.

WORD ORIGIN
ventilare (L.), to fan

EXTERNAL VS. INTERNAL RESPIRATION

External respiration moves oxygen from the air into the blood; internal respiration moves oxygen from the blood to the tissues.

Breathing consists of the **inspiration** of air into and the **expiration** of air out of the lungs. Inspiration is also called **inhalation**, and expiration is called **exhalation**. (Another meaning of expiration is termination or death.)

A **pulmonologist** is a physician who specializes in the anatomy, physiology, and pathology of the lungs.

in- = in
spir/o = to breathe
ex- = out

pulmon/o = lung
-logist = specialist

WRITE IT! EXERCISE 1

Write a term for each clue.

1. state of equilibrium of the body's internal environment _____
2. another term for inhalation _____
3. another term for exhalation _____
4. the essential gas supplied by respiration _____

Structures of the Respiratory System

The respiratory system consists of the organs involved in the exchange of gases between an organism and the atmosphere. Fig. 8.1 shows the major organs of the respiratory system. The conducting passages of this system are known as the upper respiratory tract and the lower respiratory tract. Label the numbered blanks as you read the information that accompanies the drawing.

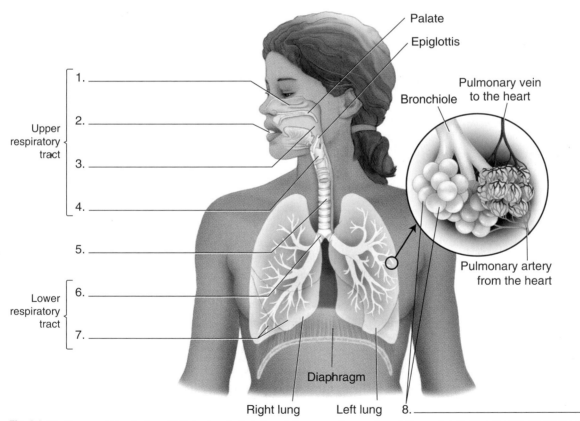

Fig. 8.1 The Organs of Respiration. Air first enters the body through the nose and passes through the nasal cavity (*1*), or it enters through the mouth (*2*) and passes through the oral cavity. The nasal and oral cavities are separated by the palate. The air reaches the pharynx (*3*) and passes to the larynx (*4*) and the trachea (*5*). The trachea divides into a left and a right bronchus (*6*). Each bronchus divides into smaller tubes called bronchioles (*7*). At the end of each bronchiole are clusters of air sacs called alveoli (*8*), where oxygen is exchanged for waste carbon dioxide. Normal quiet breathing is accomplished almost entirely by movement of the diaphragm. The epiglottis (not part of the respiratory system) covers the larynx during swallowing to prevent food from entering the larynx and trachea.

The **diaphragm** is a muscular wall that separates the abdomen from the **thorac+ic** cavity. The diaphragm contracts and relaxes with each inspiration and expiration. **Phren+ic** means pertaining to the diaphragm, but it sometimes means pertaining to the mind (as in schizophrenic). If the meaning is unclear, use a dictionary to determine it.

thorac/o = chest
phren/o = mind or diaphragm **-ic** = pertaining to

Looking again at Fig. 8.1, note that the right lung has three lobes (rounded parts), and the left lung has two lobes. The lungs are pinkish white at birth and darken in later life, due to deposition of carbon granules near their surface. Each lung is surrounded by a membrane called the **pleura**. The walls of the chest cavity are also lined with pleura. The space between the pleura that covers the lungs and the pleura that lines the thoracic cavity is called the **pleural** cavity (filled with fluid to ease friction).

Within the body, the lungs are separated from each other by other organs in the chest, especially the heart. You are able to recognize the trachea (windpipe), the two branches (bronchi), and the spongy lungs in the illustration (Fig. 8.2). We are totally dependent on the exchange of waste carbon dioxide for oxygen by millions of tiny alveoli within the lungs.

The nose, nasal cavity, **para+nasal sinuses** (air-filled paired cavities in various bones around the nose [Fig. 8.3]), pharynx (throat), and larynx (voice box) comprise the upper respiratory tract (URT). The sinuses lighten the weight of the skull, and those located in various bones around the nose contribute to sound production by serving as resonant spaces. The mucous membranes of the paranasal sinuses also produce mucus, which helps moisten the air as it enters the nose. The trachea, bronchi, bronchioles, alveoli (air sacs), and lungs belong to the lower respiratory tract (LRT). A lidlike structure, the epiglottis (see Fig. 8.1), covers the larynx during swallowing.

para- = beside **nas/o** = nose **-al** = pertaining to

THE NOSE IS RESPONSIBLE FOR THE SENSE OF SMELL

The special sense of smell enables us to not only detect different scents but also experience different tastes of food. Advancing age may bring about reduced sense of smell.

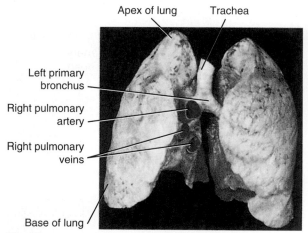

Fig. 8.2 Lungs, Bronchi, and Trachea (removed from the body). Descriptions often include the apex (top) and base of the lung. The pulmonary artery and vein (part of the cardiovascular system) are involved in oxygenation of the blood by the lungs.

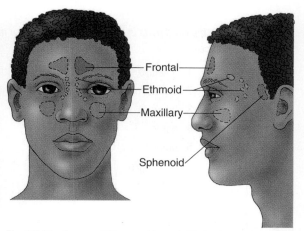

Fig. 8.3 The Paranasal Sinuses. These air-filled, paired cavities in various bones around the nose are lined with mucous membranes. Their openings into the nasal cavity are easily obstructed.
para- = beside; **nas/o** = nose

Commit to memory the word parts and their meanings in the following table. After you have studied the list, cover the left column and check to make sure that you know the combining form or forms for each structure before working Exercise 2.

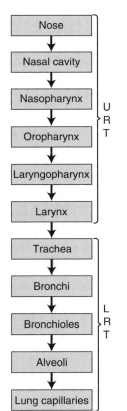

COMBINING FORMS: RESPIRATORY STRUCTURES

Combining Form	Meaning
alveol/o	alveolus (pl. alveoli)
bronch/o, bronchi/o	bronchus (pl. bronchi)
bronchiol/o	bronchiole
epiglott/o	epiglottis
laryng/o	larynx (voice box)
lob/o	lobe
nas/o, rhin/o	nose
phren/o*	diaphragm
pleur/o	pleura
pharyng/o	pharynx (throat)
pneum/o,† pneumon/o, pulm/o, pulmon/o	lung
trache/o	trachea (windpipe)

Use the electronic flashcards on the Evolve site, or make your own set of flashcards. Select the word parts just presented, and study them until you know their meanings. Do this each time a set of word parts is presented.

*phren/o sometimes means mind.
†pneum/o sometimes means air.

QUICK REVIEW!

Note the pathway of air through the upper respiratory tract and lower respiratory tract (see blue diagram on the right).

MATCH IT!*   **EXERCISE 2**

Match the word parts in the left column with their meanings in the right column (some answers will be used more than once).

_____ 1. alveol/o
_____ 2. bronch/o
_____ 3. laryng/o
_____ 4. nas/o
_____ 5. phren/o
_____ 6. pharyng/o
_____ 7. pneum/o
_____ 8. pulm/o
_____ 9. rhin/o
_____ 10. trache/o

A. air sacs of the lungs
B. branch of the trachea
C. diaphragm
D. lung
E. nose
F. throat
G. voice box
H. windpipe

*Use Appendix III, Answers, to check your answers to all the exercises in Chapter 8.

Write the combining forms and their meanings for these new terms. A short definition is provided.

Term/Meaning	Combining Form(s)	Meaning
1. **alveolar** pertaining to the alveoli	_____	_____
2. **bronchial** pertaining to the bronchi	_____	_____
3. **laryngeal** pertaining to the larynx	_____	_____
4. **nasal** pertaining to the nose	_____	_____
5. **nasopharyngeal** pertaining to the nose and pharynx	_____	_____
6. **pharyngeal** pertaining to the pharynx	_____	_____
7. **pneumatic** pertaining to respiration or air (Sometimes pertains to rarefied or compressed air, as in pneumatic tires)	_____	_____
8. **pneumocardial** pertaining to the lungs and heart	_____	_____
9. **pulmonary, pulmonic** pertaining to the lungs	_____	_____
10. **tracheal** pertaining to the trachea	_____	_____

Diseases, Disorders, and Diagnostic Terms

Oximetry is a noninvasive photo+diagnostic method of monitoring blood oxygen saturation in the arteries. Common sites for measurement using an **oximeter** are either the earlobe or finger (Fig. 8.4). Oxygen saturation is the percent of hemoglobin molecules that are saturated with oxygen in standardized testing.

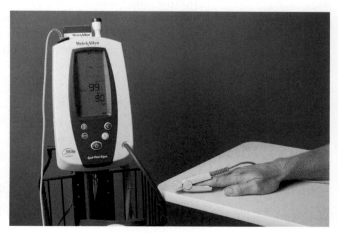

Fig. 8.4 Oximetry: Noninvasive Monitoring of Oxygen Saturation. The oximeter shows an oxygen (O_2) saturation of 99%. The finger probe is usually used for stationary measurements. **ox/o** = oxygen; **-metry** = measurement; **-meter** = device that measures

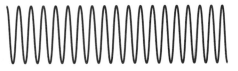

Normal (eupnea)

Regular at a rate
of 12-20 breaths per minute

Bradypnea

Slower than 12 breaths
per minute

Tachypnea

Faster than 20 breaths
per minute

Hyperpnea

Deep breathing, faster than
20 breaths per minute

Fig. 8.5 Select Patterns of Respiration. Pattern of normal respiration compared with respiratory patterns seen in bradypnea, tachypnea, and hyperpnea. **eu-** = normal; **-pnea** = breathing; **brady-** = slow; **tachy-** = fast; **hyper-** = more than normal

eu- = normal
dys- = difficult
-pnea = breathing
orth/o = straight

Normal respiration in an adult consists of 15 to 20 breaths per minute. **Eu+pnea** means normal respiration. **Dys+pnea** is labored or difficult breathing, and the patient often complains of shortness of breath (SOB). **A+pnea** means temporary absence of breathing. Perhaps you have heard of sleep apnea, a condition in which brief absences of breathing are most pronounced while a person is sleeping. **Ortho+pnea** is a condition in which breathing is uncomfortable in any position except sitting erect or standing.

Abnormally slow breathing is **brady+pnea** (less than 12 breaths per minute). Respiration that exceeds 20 breaths per minute is **tachy+pnea**; it may be the result of exercise or physical exertion, but it also frequently occurs in disease. **Hyper+pnea** is an increased respiratory rate or breathing that is deeper than normal. A certain degree of hyperpnea is normal after exercise, but it can also result from pain, respiratory or heart disease, or several other conditions. Hyperpnea may lead to **hyper+ventilation**, increased aeration of the lungs, which reduces carbon dioxide levels in the body and can disrupt homeostasis. Compare the patterns of respiration shown in Fig. 8.5.

brady- = slow
tachy- = fast
hyper- = more than normal

HEALTH CARE CONNECTION

Carbon monoxide poisoning, most often from inhalation of automobile exhaust fumes, is a toxic condition in which carbon monoxide gas has been inhaled and binds to hemoglobin molecules. Carbon monoxide displaces oxygen from the erythrocytes and decreases the capacity of the blood to carry oxygen to the body cells. Early symptoms are often described as flu-like and commonly include headache, dizziness, weakness, drowsiness, and confusion, followed by apnea if early signs are ignored.

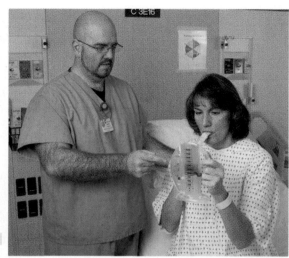

Fig. 8.6 Spirometry. A spirometer is used to evaluate the air capacity of the lungs. It measures and records the volume of inhaled and exhaled air.
spir/o = to breathe (sometimes, spiral);   **-metry** = process of measuring;
-meter = instrument used to measure

Spiro+metry is measurement of the amount of air taken into and expelled from the lungs (Fig. 8.6). The largest volume of air that can be exhaled after maximum inspiration is the vital capacity (VC). A reduction in vital capacity often indicates a loss of functioning lung tissue. Inability of the lungs to perform their ventilatory function is acute respiratory failure. This leads to **hyp+ox+ia** or to **an+ox+ia**. Both terms mean a deficiency of oxygen, which can be caused by respiratory disorders but can occur under other conditions as well. Hypoxia can result from reduced oxygen concentration in the air at high altitudes or from anemia (decrease in hemoglobin or in number of erythrocytes in the blood, or both).

spir/o = to breathe
-metry = measurement

CAUTION

Note that in hypoxia (hypo- + -oxia), one *o* is dropped.

MATCH IT!
EXERCISE 4

Match the terms in the right column with their meanings in the left column.

_____ 1. breathing air into the lungs
_____ 2. breathing out
_____ 3. labored or difficult breathing
_____ 4. abnormally slow breathing
_____ 5. acceleration in the number of breaths per minute
_____ 6. normal respiration

A. bradypnea
B. dyspnea
C. eupnea
D. expiration
E. inspiration
F. tachypnea

PROGRAMMED LEARNING

Remember to cover the answers (left column) with folded paper or the bookmark. Write an answer in each blank, and then check your answer before proceeding to the next frame.

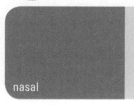

nasal

1. Air usually first enters the respiratory passageway through the nose, which refers both to the external nose and to the nasal cavity. The **nares** (singular, naris), or nostrils, are the external openings of the nose. These openings lead into two nasal cavities separated by the **nasal septum**. The partition between the two nasal cavities is the _____ septum.

nose	2. The para+nasal sinuses open into the nasal cavities. The term *sinus* has several meanings, including canal, passage, and cavity within a bone. The paranasal sinuses are cavities within the bones of the face. Fluids from the paranasal sinuses are discharged into the _____.
sinus	3. **Sinus+itis** is inflammation of a _____, especially of a paranasal sinus.
rhinitis	4. Use rhin/o to build a term that means inflammation of the nasal membrane: _____. **Rhino+rrhea** is a watery discharge from the nose.
nose	5. Air from the nose passes to the **pharynx**, commonly called the throat. **Naso+pharyng+eal** means pertaining to the _____ and pharynx.
inflammation	6. **Pharyng+itis** is _____ of the pharynx.
pharynx	7. The **eustachian tube**, or **auditory tube**, extends from the middle ear to the pharynx. It is sometimes called the **oto+pharyng+eal** tube, meaning a tube that connects the ear with the _____.
larynx	8. The lower part of the pharynx is also called the **laryngopharynx** because it is here that the pharynx divides into the **larynx** and the **esophagus**. Air passes to the _____, and food passes to the esophagus.
laryngitis	9. Inflammation of the larynx is _____. This condition can be caused by infectious microorganisms, allergies, irritants, or overuse of the voice.
aphonia	10. Laryngitis can result in absence of voice. In **a+phon+ia**, absence of voice, sounds cannot be produced from the larynx (phon/o means voice). Laryngitis can cause absence of voice, which is called _____.
voice	11. **Dys+phonia** means difficulty in speaking or a weak _____. Dysphonia is the same as hoarseness and may precede aphonia.
speech	12. **A+phasia** is the inability to communicate through speech, writing, or signs. It is caused by improper functioning of the brain. The combining form phas/o means speech. The term *aphasia* describes only one aspect of the condition, which is the absence of _____.
aphasia	13. An **a+phasic** individual is one affected by _____. Remember that in aphasia the problem does not arise in the larynx, but in the brain.
speech	14. **Dys+phasia** is a speech impairment resulting from a brain lesion. There is a lack of coordination and an inability to arrange words in their proper order. In dysphasia there is difficulty in _____.
aphonia	15. Be sure that you know the difference between aphasia and aphonia. Both can produce an absence of speech sound. Aphasia is caused by a brain dysfunction; however, aphonia is loss of audible voice. In laryngitis, for example, which is more likely to occur, aphasia or aphonia? _____.
pain	16. Laryngitis can cause only minor discomfort, or the condition can become painful. **Laryng+algia** is _____ of the larynx.

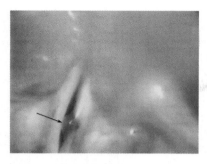

Fig. 8.7 Laryngeal Polyp. This hemorrhagic polyp *(arrow)* on the vocal cord occurs most often in adults who smoke, have many allergies, live in dry climates, or abuse their voice.
laryng/o = larynx; **hem/o** = blood; **-rrhagia** = hemorrhage

glottis

17. The larynx is commonly called the voice box. The vocal apparatus of the larynx is the **glottis**, which consists of the vocal cords (or folds) and the openings between them. Muscles open and close the glottis during breathing and also regulate the vocal cords during the production of sound. Examine the structure of the larynx in Fig. 8.7. This illustration also shows a **laryngeal polyp**, a small tumorlike growth on the vocal cords that can cause hoarseness. The lidlike structure that covers the larynx during the act of swallowing is called the **epiglottis** (epi-, above). The epiglottis lies above the

_____.

bronchitis

18. Air passes from the larynx to the **trachea**, or windpipe. The trachea divides into two **bronchi** (singular, **bronchus**), one leading to each lung. Use bronch/o to write a word that means inflammation of the mucous membrane of the bronchi:

_____.

sputum

19. Mucous membranes secrete mucus. Inflammation of the mucous membranes in bronchitis usually leads to the production of **sputum**, which can be expelled by coughing or clearing the throat. Material raised from inflamed mucous membranes of the respiratory tract and expelled by coughing is called _____.

bronchi

20. The bronchi are examined in a **broncho+scopic** examination. **Tracheo+bronchial** means pertaining to both the trachea and the _____. The appearance of the trachea and bronchi in radiography (Fig. 8.8) probably led to the use of the term *tracheobronchial tree*.

Trachea

Clavicle

Aortic arch

Heart

Breast shadows

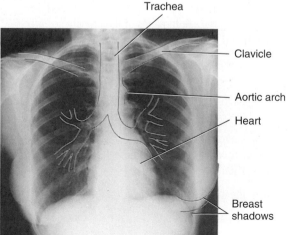

Fig. 8.8 Normal Radiograph of the Chest With the Tracheobronchial Tube Outlined. Do not be concerned about the meanings of all the terms in the chest x-ray image. The clavicle is the collarbone.
radi/o = radiant energy; **-gram** = a record;
trache/o = trachea; **bronchi/o** = bronchus; **-al** = pertaining to

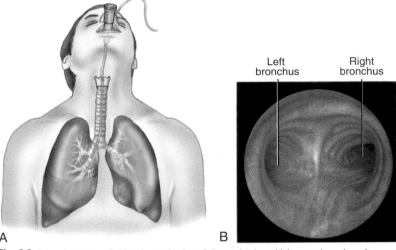

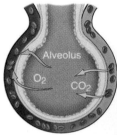

Fig. 8.9 Bronchoscopy. **A,** Visual examination of the tracheobronchial tree using a bronchoscope. Other uses for this procedure include suctioning, obtaining a biopsy specimen or fluid, or removing foreign bodies. **B,** Endoscopic view of the lower end of the trachea and the beginning of the bronchi.
bronch/o = bronchus;   **-scopy** = visual examination;   **trache/o** = trachea

Fig. 8.10 Alveolus. A diagram of the exchange of gases between an alveolus and a lung capillary.

bronchoscopy	21. Add a suffix to bronch/o to write a word that means a bronchoscopic examination using a **bronchoscope**: _____. This procedure may be used for obtaining a biopsy specimen, for suctioning, or for removing foreign bodies (Fig. 8.9).
larynx	22. Both **bronchoscopy** and **laryngoscopy** are endoscopic examinations, procedures that allow visualization of organs and cavities of the body using an endoscope. In a laryngoscopy, the _____ is examined.
lungs	23. **Broncho+pulmon+ary** means pertaining to the bronchi and the _____.
bronchi	24. **Bronchi+oles** literally means "little bronchi." You see that -ole means little. Bronchioles are subdivisions of the _____. At the ends of the bronchioles are tiny air sacs called alveoli (singular, **alveolus** (Fig. 8.10).
alveoli	25. In certain diseases, such as emphysema, destructive changes occur in the alveolar walls. These changes interfere with the exchange of oxygen and carbon dioxide. This gas exchange takes place by diffusion across the walls of blood capillaries and the _____.
lungs	26. **Pneumon+ia** or **pneumon+itis** means inflammation of the _____. There are many causes of pneumonia, but it is caused primarily by bacteria, viruses, or chemical irritants.
bronchi	27. **Broncho+pneumonia** is inflammation of the lungs and of the _____.

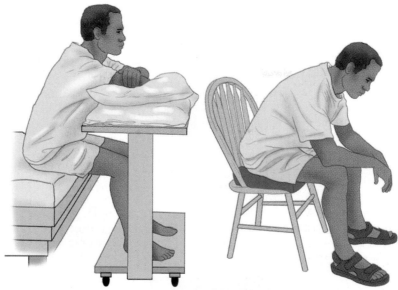

Fig. 8.11 Two Positions for the Orthopneic Patient. These positions ease the work of breathing for persons with chronic airflow limitation (CAL). This "tripod position" is often assumed by the patient with respiratory insufficiency. **orth/o** = straight;   **-pnea** = breathing

lungs	28. **Pulmonary edema** is **effusion** (escape) of fluid into the air spaces and tissue spaces of the _____ (edema is abnormal accumulation of fluid in the interstitial spaces of the tissue). Although pulmonary edema can have other causes, a major cause is insufficient cardiac activity. Remember that cardi/o means heart, so cardi+ac refers to the heart.
breathing	29. Dyspnea on exertion is one of the earliest symptoms of pulmonary edema. As the condition becomes more advanced, the patient can become **ortho+pne+ic** (-pnea + -ic is shortened to -pneic), which means that _____ is difficult except when the patient is sitting erect or standing (Fig. 8.11).
air	30. **Thorax** means chest. **Pneumo+thorax** refers to air or gas in the chest cavity, specifically the pleural cavity. **Hemo+thorax** means blood in the pleural cavity (Fig. 8.12). **Pneumo+hemo+thorax** means the presence of _____ and blood in the pleural cavity.
pulmonary	31. Pulmonary arteries carry blood from the heart to the lungs so carbon dioxide can be exchanged for oxygen. A pulmonary embolus is an obstruction of the _____ artery or one of its branches.
pulmonary	32. Embolism is the sudden blocking of an artery by foreign material that has been brought to its site of blockage by the circulating blood. An **embolus** is often a blood clot, called a **thrombus**. The pulmonary artery is obstructed in _____ **embolism** (Fig. 8.13).

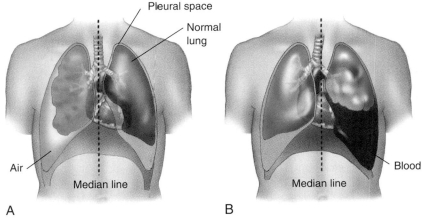

pneum/o = air or lung
hem/o = blood
medi/o = middle

Fig. 8.12 Two Abnormal Conditions of the Chest Cavity. **A,** Pneumothorax is air or gas in the chest cavity, usually caused by blunt injury or an open wound in the chest wall. A normal left lung is shown for comparison. **B,** Hemothorax, or blood in the pleural cavity, may be associated with pneumothorax and is a common problem associated with chest trauma or penetrating injuries.

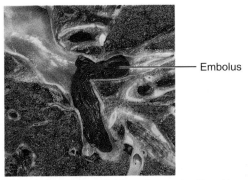

Fig. 8.13 Pulmonary Embolism. This blood clot broke loose and traveled from a lower extremity and is now located in a branch of the pulmonary artery.
pulmon/o = lung;   **embol/o** = embolus

"Vaping" can cause deadly lung diseases, including cancer and damage to unborn babies. These devices deliver an aerosol by heating a liquid that contains nicotine (e-cigarettes), flavorings, marijuana, or other chemicals.

QUICK CASE STUDY | EXERCISE 5

Define the terms listed after the case study.
Valesca Morales, age 2, is seen by Dr. Wong in the ED. She presents with fever, tachycardia, hyperpnea, severe coughing, and dyspnea. Radiography indicates bronchopneumonia. Antibiotics and oxygen therapy are initiated, and the patient is admitted, transferred immediately to an isolation unit, and referred to Dr. Walter Smith, a pulmonologist.

1. tachycardia _____
2. hyperpnea _____
3. dyspnea _____
4. bronchopneumonia _____
5. pulmonologist _____

WRITE IT! **EXERCISE 6**

Write one-word terms for each of these meanings.

1. growth protruding from a mucous membrane _____
2. pertaining to the pharynx _____
3. pertaining to the larynx _____
4. painful larynx _____
5. loss of voice _____
6. loss of the power of expression of speech _____
7. pertaining to the alveoli _____
8. inflammation of the mucous membranes of the nose _____
9. inflammation of a sinus _____
10. material coughed up from the trachea, bronchi, and lungs _____

Review the following new word parts.

ADDITIONAL WORD PARTS

Word Part	Meaning
atel/o	imperfect
coni/o	a relationship to dust
embol/o	embolus
home/o	sameness
-ole	little
ox/o	oxygen
-pnea	breathing
silic/o	silica
spir/o	to breathe (sometimes, spiral)

WRITE IT! **EXERCISE 7**

Write the combining forms for these terms.

1. a relationship to dust _____
2. imperfect _____
3. oxygen _____
4. sameness _____
5. silica _____
6. to breathe _____

Additional diseases and disorders that affect the respiratory system are described in the following glossary list.

adult respiratory distress syndrome (ARDS) Disorder characterized by respiratory insufficiency and hypoxemia.

asthma Paroxysmal dyspnea accompanied by wheezing; asthma is brought about by a spasm of the bronchial tubes or by swelling of their mucous membranes. A **wheeze** is a whistling sound made during respiration. **Paroxysmal** means occurring in sudden, periodic attacks or recurrence of symptoms.

atelectasis (atel/o, imperfect + -ectasis, stretching) Incomplete expansion of a lung or a portion of it; airlessness or collapse of a lung that had once been expanded.

bronchiectasis (bronchi/o + -ectasis) Chronic dilation of a bronchus or the bronchi accompanied by a secondary infection that usually involves the lower part of the lung.

bronchography (-graphy, recording) Radiography of the bronchi after injection of a radiopaque contrast medium. The record of the bronchi and lungs produced by bronchography is a **bronchogram**. This procedure has generally been replaced by computed tomography.

carcinoma of the lung Lung cancer, the leading cause of cancer-related death. Research has consistently confirmed that smoking plays a predominant role in the development of lung cancer. Compare healthy lung tissue with that of a smoker (Fig. 8.14).

chronic obstructive pulmonary disease (COPD) Disease process that decreases the lungs' ability to perform their ventilatory function. This process can result from chronic bronchitis, emphysema, chronic asthma, or chronic **bronchiolitis**. COPD, characterized by chronic airflow limitation (CAL), is also called chronic obstructive lung disease (COLD).

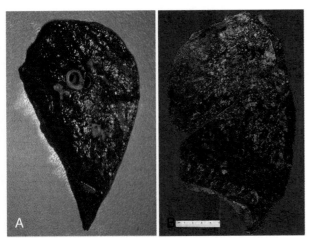

Fig. 8.14 Healthy Lung Tissue (sectioned) and the Lungs of a Smoker. **A,** Healthy lung tissue is pink and highly elastic. **B,** A lung damaged by cigarette smoking is scarred, dark, and has lost much of its elasticity.

emphysema Chronic pulmonary disease characterized by an increase in the size of alveoli and by destructive changes in their walls, resulting in difficulty in breathing, hypoventilation, and hypoxemia.

hypoventilation Reduced air entering the alveoli

hypoxemia Deficient oxygen in the blood

influenza Acute, contagious respiratory infection characterized by sudden onset, chills, headache, fever, and muscular discomfort; it is caused by several different types of viruses. The H1N1 flu virus, like most influenza viruses, spreads mainly from person to person. This disease was originally called "swine flu" because the viral genetic makeup is similar to influenza viruses that normally occur in pigs.

nasal polyp Abnormal, protruding growth from the nasal mucosa (Fig. 8.15).

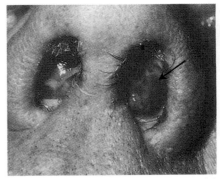

Fig. 8.15 Nasal Polyp. Note the rounded tumorlike growth (arrow) projecting into the nasal cavity.

pleuritis (pleur/o, pleura) Inflammation of the pleura. It can be caused by infection, injury, or a tumor, or it can be a complication of certain lung diseases. It is characterized by a sharp pain on inspiration; it is also called **pleurisy**.

pneumoconiosis (pneum/o, lung + coni/o, dust) Respiratory condition caused by inhalation of dust particles; frequently seen in people involved in occupations such as mining and stonecutting.

pulmonary embolism Blockage of a pulmonary artery by foreign matter such as fat, air, tumor tissue, or a blood clot.

severe acute respiratory syndrome (SARS) Infectious respiratory disease spread by close contact with an infected person and caused by a coronavirus. It is reported to have a fatality rate of approximately 3%.

silicosis (silic/o, silica) Form of pneumoconiosis resulting from inhalation of the dust of stone, sand, quartz, or flint that contains silica. (Workers are frequently exposed to silica powder that is used in manufacturing processes.)

sudden infant death syndrome (SIDS) Sudden, unexpected death of an apparently normal and healthy infant that occurs during sleep and with no physical or autopsy evidence of disease.

tuberculosis (TB) Infectious disease caused by the bacterium *Mycobacterium tuberculosis*. It is often chronic in nature and usually affects the lungs, although it can occur elsewhere in the body. The disease is named for the **tubercles** (small, round nodules) that are produced in the lungs by the bacteria.

WRITE IT!   **EXERCISE 8**

Write the correct term in each blank to complete these sentences.

1. Another name for pneumonia is _____.
2. Inflammation of the lungs and the bronchi is _____.
3. A collapsed condition of the lung is called _____.
4. Inability to communicate through speech, writing, or signs because of a brain dysfunction is _____.
5. An infectious, sometimes fatal respiratory disease caused by a coronavirus is called severe acute respiratory _____.
6. A chronic disease that is characterized by an increased size and destructive changes to the alveoli is _____.
7. A condition characterized by dyspnea and wheezing is _____.
8. A respiratory condition caused by inhalation of dust particles is _____.

 Surgical and Therapeutic Interventions

Asphyxiation requires immediate corrective measures to prevent loss of consciousness and, if not corrected, death. Removal of a foreign body in the airway may be needed before oxygen and artificial respiration are administered. One method of dislodging food or other obstructions from the windpipe is the **Heimlich maneuver** (Fig. 8.16). In

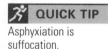 **QUICK TIP**
Asphyxiation is suffocation.

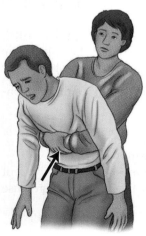

Fig. 8.16 Heimlich Maneuver. The rescuer grasps the choking person from behind, placing the thumb side of the fist against the victim's abdomen, in the midline, slightly above the navel and well below the breastbone. Abruptly pulling the fist firmly upward will often force the obstruction up the windpipe.

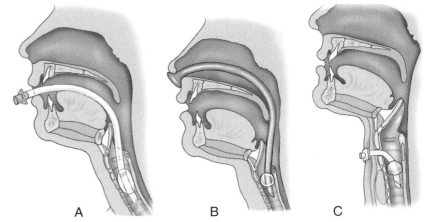

trache/o = trachea
(windpipe)
or/o = mouth
nas/o = nose

Fig. 8.17 Comparison of an Endotracheal Intubation and a Tracheostomy Tube. **A,** Orotracheal intubation for short-term airway management. **B,** Nasotracheal intubation for short-term airway management. **C,** Tracheostomy tube for long-term airway maintenance.

asphyxiation, oxygen and artificial ventilation need to be promptly administered to prevent damage to the brain. An emergency **tracheostomy** may be necessary in upper airway obstruction. A tracheostomy requires a **tracheotomy**, an incision of the trachea through the skin and muscles of the neck overlying the trachea (usually performed for insertion of a tube to relieve tracheal obstruction). A tracheostomy is also required when prolonged mechanical ventilation is needed. A **ventilator** is a machine that is used for prolonged artificial ventilation of the lungs.

trache/o = windpipe
-stomy = opening
-tomy = incision

Endotracheal intubation is the insertion of an airway tube through the mouth or nose into the trachea. It may be used to keep an airway open, prevent aspiration of material from the digestive tract in an unconscious or paralyzed patient, permit suctioning of secretions, or provide ventilation that cannot be accomplished with a mask. **Nasotracheal intubation** and **orotracheal intubation** refer to insertion of a tube into the trachea through the nose or mouth, respectively. Compare these two types of intubation with a tracheostomy tube used for prolonged airway management (Fig. 8.17).

endo- = inside
nas/o = nose
or/o = mouth
trans- = across

Respiratory infections are often treated with antibiotics. Smoking cessation drugs aid in quitting smoking or the use of other tobacco products. Several other medications are used in treating respiratory disorders:

- **Antiasthmatics**: Prevent or treat the symptoms of asthma
- **Decongestants**: Eliminate or reduce swelling or congestion

de- = reversing

- **Anti+tussives**: Prevent or relieve coughing
- **Anti+histamines**: Used to treat colds and allergies
- **Broncho+dilators**: Agents that cause dilation of the bronchi; used in respiratory conditions such as asthma
- **Expectorants**: Improve expulsion of mucus from lungs
- **Inhalers**: Devices used to administer medications that are breathed in
- **Muco+lytics**: Destroy or dissolve mucus; help open the breathing passages

Seasonal influenza vaccine is recommended each year for most individuals, except for those with certain allergies. A vaccine that protects against the most common cause of bacterial pneumonia is recommended for older persons, those with a chronic lung disease, or those who are immunodeficient.

In COPD or other problems in hypoxic patients, oxygen therapy may be prescribed by the physician. Oxygen is also administered during general surgery. In patients who can breathe, oxygen is often delivered through tubing using a simple face mask or nasal prongs. **Transtracheal** oxygen is more efficient and is sometimes preferred to the administration of oxygen through a mask or **nasal cannula**. Compare the three types of oxygen administration (Fig. 8.18).

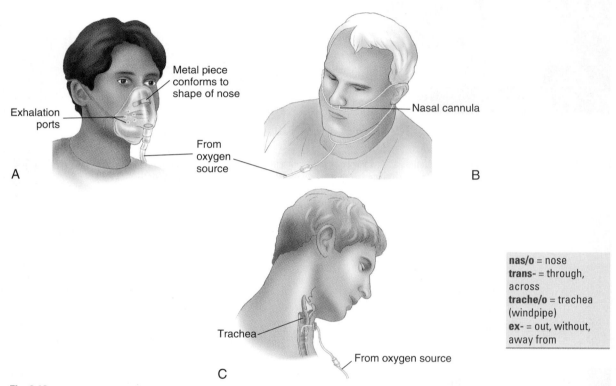

nas/o = nose
trans- = through, across
trache/o = trachea (windpipe)
ex- = out, without, away from

Fig. 8.18 Administration of Oxygen. **A,** Simple oxygen mask is used for short-term oxygen therapy or in an emergency. **B,** Nasal cannula delivers oxygen by way of two small tubes that are inserted into the nostrils and is frequently used for long-term oxygen maintenance. **C,** Transtracheal oxygen is a more efficient long-term method of delivering oxygen and is an alternative to the nasal cannula.

Read about the following surgical procedures.

lung biopsy Removal of small pieces of lung tissue for the purpose of diagnosis. In an open lung biopsy, a segment of the lung is removed through an incision in the chest. In a **percutaneous** (per-, through + cutane/o, skin) **biopsy**, tissue is obtained by puncturing the suspected lesion through the skin. Depending on the location of the lesion, a biopsy specimen can sometimes be obtained during bronchoscopy.

pneumocentesis Surgical puncture of a lung to drain fluid that has accumulated.

pneumonectomy (pneumon/o, lung + -ectomy, excision) Surgical removal of all or part of a lung; **pneumectomy**. If a lobe of the lung is removed, it is called a pulmonary **lobectomy**.

rhinoplasty (rhin/o, nose + -plasty, surgical repair) Plastic surgery of the nose; usually performed for cosmetic reasons but may also be necessary to provide a passage for respiration.

thoracocentesis (thorac/o, chest + -centesis, surgical puncture) Surgical puncture of the chest cavity to remove fluid; also called **thoracentesis** or thoracic **paracentesis** (Fig. 8.19).

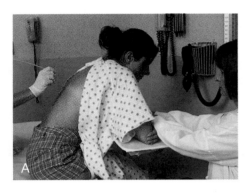

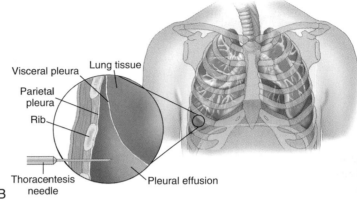

Visceral pleura
Lung tissue
Parietal pleura
Rib
Thoracentesis needle
Pleural effusion

A

B

Fig. 8.19 Insertion of the Needle in Thoracentesis. **A,** Common position for thoracentesis. **B,** The insertion site depends on the location of the fluid. The term *thoracocentesis* is frequently shortened to thoracentesis. **thorac/o** = chest; **-centesis** = surgical puncture

MATCH IT!
EXERCISE 9

Match the word parts in the left column with their meanings in the right column.

_____ 1. atel/o   A. breathing
_____ 2. coni/o   B. dust
_____ 3. home/o   C. imperfect
_____ 4. -ole   D. little
_____ 5. -pnea   E. sameness

BUILD IT!
EXERCISE 10

Combine the word parts to write terms for these descriptions.

1. plastic surgery of the nose (rhin/o + -plasty): _____

2. surgical puncture of the chest cavity (thorac/o + -centesis): _____

3. incision of the windpipe (trache/o + -tomy) _____

4. surgical removal of all or part of the lung (pneum/o + -ectomy) _____

5. agent that causes bronchial dilation (bronch/o + dilator) _____

6. agent that dissolves mucus (muc/o + -lytic) _____

> ! **Be Careful With These!**
>
> *aphonia* (loss of audible voice; a vocal dysfunction) versus *aphasia* (inability to communicate through speech, writing, or signs; a brain dysfunction)
> *phren/o* (diaphragm or mind) versus *pleur/o* (pleura)
> pronunciation of *larynx* (**lar**-inks) and *pharynx* (**far**-inks)

A Career as a Respiratory Therapist

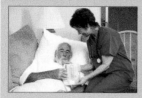

Donna Robertson, a respiratory therapist in a hospital, works with physicians to establish and evaluate breathing therapies. She combines technologic information with a patient's physiologic data to develop an individualized respiratory therapy program. Donna's work is rewarding because she can see the success of her efforts as patients improve. She had the option of working in the intensive care unit or in the emergency department, but Donna prefers helping patients who have asthma, are recovering from infections, or who have COPD. For more information on careers in this field, visit the website of the American Association for Respiratory Care: www.aarc.org/career/what-is-an-rt/.

 SELF-TEST

Work the following exercises to test your understanding of the material in Chapter 8. It is best to do all the exercises before checking your answers against the answers in Appendix III. Pay particular attention to spelling.

A. MATCHING!   *Match the structures in the left column with their characteristics or functions in the right column.*

_____ 1.	alveolus	A. branch of the trachea
_____ 2.	bronchus	B. muscular partition that facilitates breathing
_____ 3.	diaphragm	C. commonly called the throat
_____ 4.	larynx	D. commonly called the windpipe
_____ 5.	nose	E. connected with the paranasal sinuses
_____ 6.	pharynx	F. contains the vocal cords
_____ 7.	trachea	G. where oxygen and carbon dioxide exchange occurs

B. WRITING!   *Write one-word terms for each of these meanings.*

1. agent that dissolves mucus   _____
2. agent used to control coughing   _____
3. difficult or weak voice   _____
4. direct visualization of the bronchi _____
5. incision of the trachea   _____
6. inflammation of the throat   _____
7. pertaining to the air sacs of the lung _____
8. record produced in bronchography _____
9. surgical repair of the nose   _____
10. within the trachea   _____

C. CHOOSING!   *Circle the one correct answer (A, B, C, or D) for each question.*

1. Mrs. Smith's doctor tells her that she has pneumonia. What is another name for her diagnosis?
   (A) congestive heart disease   **(B)** pneumonitis   **(C)** pulmonary edema   **(D)** pulmonary insufficiency

2. John R. is told that he has periodic absence of breathing. What is the name of his condition?
   (A) apnea   **(B)** dyspnea   **(C)** hyperpnea   **(D)** hypopnea

3. What is the name of the serous membrane that lines the walls of the thoracic cavity?
   (A) emphysema   **(B)** pleura   **(C)** rhinorrhea   **(D)** thrombus

4. Mrs. Sema has difficulty breathing except when sitting in an upright position. What is the term for her condition?
   (A) anoxia   **(B)** hyperventilation   **(C)** inspiration   **(D)** orthopnea

5. The pulmonary specialist orders a test to measure the amount of air taken into and expelled from the lungs. What is the name of the test?
   (A) laryngoscopy   **(B)** mediastinoscopy   **(C)** spirometry   **(D)** thoracometry

6. Which term means a lack of oxygen in body tissues?
   (A) anoxia   **(B)** dyspnea   **(C)** effusion   **(D)** orthopnea

7. Which term is another term for inspiration?
   (A) exhalation   **(B)** homeostasis   **(C)** inhalation   **(D)** pertussis

8. Which term means pertaining to the diaphragm?
   (A) aphasic   **(B)** pharyngeal   **(C)** phrenic   **(D)** thoracic

9. Which term means inflammation of the air-filled cavities in various bones around the nose?
   (A) laryngitis   **(B)** pleuritis   **(C)** tracheitis   **(D)** sinusitis

10. Which term means incomplete expansion of a lung or a portion of a lung?
    (A) atelectasis   **(B)** pneumoconiosis   **(C)** pulmonary edema   **(D)** silicosis

D. IDENTIFYING!   *Label these illustrations using one of the following: bronchography, bronchoscopy, embolism, eupnea, hemothorax, phrenic, rhinorrhea.*

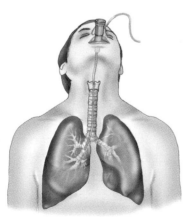

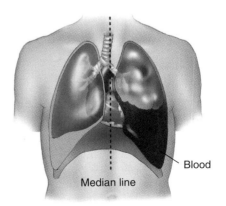

Blood

Median line

1. visual examination of the tracheobronchial tree

   _____

2. an accumulation of blood in the pleural cavity

   _____

E. READING HEALTH CARE REPORTS   *Write the terms from the report that correspond to each of these descriptions.*

Margaret Ann Gordon - BRIEF HISTORY AND PHYSICAL EXAMINATION   ☐ ⧉ ✕

Task   Time Scale   Options   Help   View   Edit

As Of 6:20		

Patient Name: Margaret Ann Gordon   **ID No.:** 009-3002   **Date:** May 4, 2022
DOB: 09-21-1959   **Sex:** Female   **PCP: Simon Rubenstein, MD**

Flowsheet: Clinical Notes ▼   ...   Level: Physical Exam ▼   ⦿ Table ○ Group ○ List

MAR	Task List	I & O	Pt. Info	Pt. Schedule	Surgery	Clinical Notes	Form Browser

Orders	Last 48 Hours	ED	Lab	Radiology	Assessments	Medical Report	Medication Profile

CHIEF COMPLAINT: Fever with mild dyspnea. Productive cough. Malaise and loss of appetite.

PAST HISTORY: This 62-year-old female patient, well known to me, has a history of bronchitis, myocardial infarction (status post CABG one year ago), and deep venous thrombosis with pulmonary embolism.

FAMILY HISTORY: Mother is living at age 85 with bronchiectasis. Father deceased with a history of emphysema.

PHYSICAL EXAM: Vital signs show T 100.8, P 98, R 28, BP 160/94. O_2 saturation level 92% on 2 L oxygen. Exam limited to chest: Fine crackles at bilateral lung bases with some wheezes. Increased dyspnea on exertion.

DIAGNOSTIC DATA: WBCs 24.6. Chest x-ray with increased right lung density. No pneumothorax or pleural effusion. Increasing right lung infiltrate with masslike density, right hilum. Sputum collected for culture.

DIAGNOSIS: Community-acquired pneumonia.

TREATMENT PLAN: IV antibiotics pending sputum culture results. Bronchodilator, such as Alupent. Expectorant, such as guaifenesin.

Ruth Wong, MD
Ruth Wong, MD
Pulmonologist

			PROD	MAHAFC	04 May 2022	07:00

---

1. abnormal accumulation of fluid in the pleural space   _____

2. chronic dilation of the bronchi accompanied by secondary infection   _____

3. chronic pulmonary disease characterized by destructive changes in alveoli   _____

4. inflammation of the bronchi   _____

5. inflammation of the lungs   _____

6. labored or difficult breathing   _____

7. material coughed up from the bronchi or lungs   _____

8. blockage of a pulmonary artery by a substance brought by the circulating blood   _____

9. presence of air or gas in the pleural space   _____

10. therapeutic agent that relaxes the bronchioles   _____

F.　SPELLING AND PRONOUNCIATION! *Circle all incorrectly spelled terms, and write their correct spellings. Then pronounce the terms.*

asfixiation	embalis	larinkgitis	numocardial	pulmonik

G.　READING HEALTH CARE REPORTS　*Write terms from the report that correspond to each of the six descriptions.*

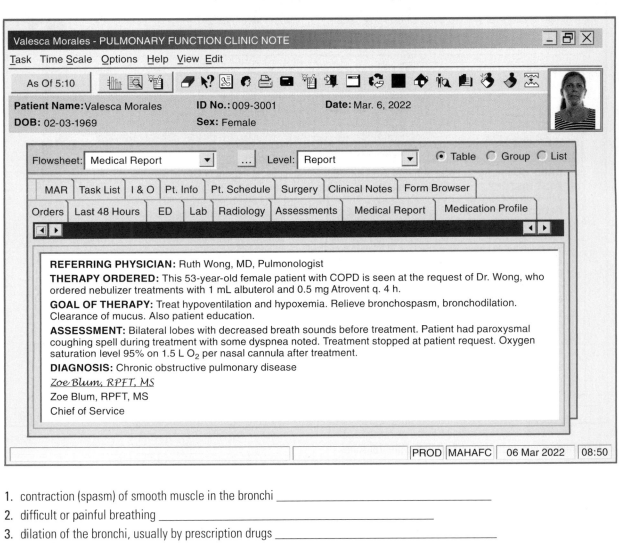

Valesca Morales - PULMONARY FUNCTION CLINIC NOTE

Task　Time Scale　Options　Help　View　Edit

As Of 5:10

Patient Name: Valesca Morales　**ID No.:** 009-3001　**Date:** Mar. 6, 2022
DOB: 02-03-1969　**Sex:** Female

Flowsheet: Medical Report ▾ ... Level: Report ▾ ⦿ Table ◯ Group ◯ List

| MAR | Task List | I & O | Pt. Info | Pt. Schedule | Surgery | Clinical Notes | Form Browser |
| Orders | Last 48 Hours | ED | Lab | Radiology | Assessments | Medical Report | Medication Profile |

REFERRING PHYSICIAN: Ruth Wong, MD, Pulmonologist

THERAPY ORDERED: This 53-year-old female patient with COPD is seen at the request of Dr. Wong, who ordered nebulizer treatments with 1 mL albuterol and 0.5 mg Atrovent q. 4 h.

GOAL OF THERAPY: Treat hypoventilation and hypoxemia. Relieve bronchospasm, bronchodilation. Clearance of mucus. Also patient education.

ASSESSMENT: Bilateral lobes with decreased breath sounds before treatment. Patient had paroxysmal coughing spell during treatment with some dyspnea noted. Treatment stopped at patient request. Oxygen saturation level 95% on 1.5 L O_2 per nasal cannula after treatment.

DIAGNOSIS: Chronic obstructive pulmonary disease

Zoe Blum, RPFT, MS

Zoe Blum, RPFT, MS

Chief of Service

| | | PROD | MAHAFC | 06 Mar 2022 | 08:50 |

1.　contraction (spasm) of smooth muscle in the bronchi _____

2.　difficult or painful breathing _____

3.　dilation of the bronchi, usually by prescription drugs _____

4.　referring to a marked, episodic increase in symptoms _____

5.　reduced respiration _____

6.　low levels of oxygen in arterial blood _____

H. HEALTH CARE REPORT EXERCISE
Read the following note from an Office Visit, then circle the correct answers in the statements that follow the report.

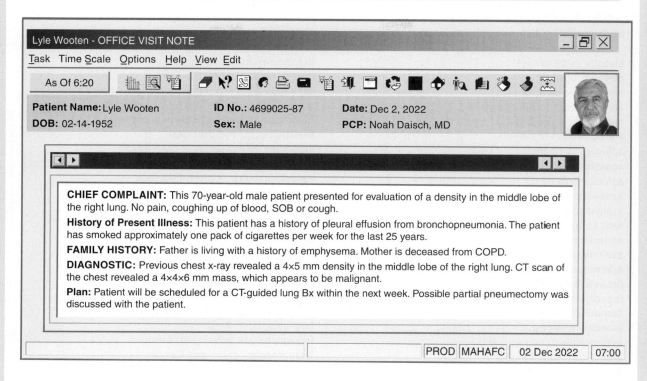

Lyle Wooten - OFFICE VISIT NOTE

Task Time Scale Options Help View Edit

As Of 6:20

Patient Name: Lyle Wooten   **ID No.:** 4699025-87   **Date:** Dec 2, 2022
DOB: 02-14-1952   **Sex:** Male   **PCP:** Noah Daisch, MD

CHIEF COMPLAINT: This 70-year-old male patient presented for evaluation of a density in the middle lobe of the right lung. No pain, coughing up of blood, SOB or cough.

History of Present Illness: This patient has a history of pleural effusion from bronchopneumonia. The patient has smoked approximately one pack of cigarettes per week for the last 25 years.

FAMILY HISTORY: Father is living with a history of emphysema. Mother is deceased from COPD.

DIAGNOSTIC: Previous chest x-ray revealed a 4×5 mm density in the middle lobe of the right lung. CT scan of the chest revealed a 4×4×6 mm mass, which appears to be malignant.

Plan: Patient will be scheduled for a CT-guided lung Bx within the next week. Possible partial pneumectomy was discussed with the patient.

PROD MAHAFC   02 Dec 2022   07:00

1. Effusion refers to an abnormal amount of (air, blood, fluid, infection).
2. A pneumectomy indicates a complete or partial portion of a lung is (surgically incised, surgically punctured, surgically removed, surgically repaired).
3. A pulmonary disease characterized by destruction of many of the alveolar walls is indicated by (hemoptysis, effusion, bronchopneumonia, emphysema).

I. QUICK CHALLENGE!   *Find an incorrect term in each sentence and write the correct term.*

1. Drugs that are used to eliminate or reduce congestion are antihistamines. _____
2. Thoracentesis means the same as thoracic expiration. _____
3. Bronchogenic means pertaining to the lungs and bronchi. _____
4. Dysphonia means occurring in sudden, periodic attacks. _____
5. Escape of fluid into air spaces or tissue spaces of the lungs is pulmonary edema or hypoxia.
_____

*Use Appendix III to check your answers.

QUICK & EASY (Q&E) LIST

Use the Evolve website (http://evolve.elsevier.com/Leonard/quick) to review the terms presented in Chapter 8. Look closely at the spelling of each term as it is pronounced.

adult respiratory distress syndrome (uh-**dult** res-pi-ruh-tor-ē dis-**tres** sin-drōm)
alveolar (al-**vē**-uh-lur)
alveolus (al-**vē**-uh-lus)
anoxia (uh-**nok**-se-uh)
antiasthmatics (an-tē-az-**mat**-iks)
antihistamine (an-tē-**his**-tuh-mēn)
antitussive (an-tē-**tus**-iv)
aphasia (uh-**fā**-zhuh)
aphasic (uh-**fā**-zik)
aphonia (ā-**fō**-nē-uh)
apnea (**ap**-nē-uh)
asphyxiation (as-fik-sē-**ā**-shun)
asthma (**az**-muh)
atelectasis (at-uh-**lek**-tuh-sis)
auditory tube (**aw**-di-tor-ē tōōb)
bradypnea (brad-ē-**nē**-uh, brad-**ip**-nē-uh)
bronchi (**brong**-kī)
bronchial (**brong**-kē-ul)
bronchiectasis (brong-kē-**ek**-tuh-sis)
bronchiole (**brong**-kē-ōl)
bronchiolitis (brong-kē-ō-**lī**-tis)
bronchitis (brong-**kī**-tis)
bronchodilator (brong-kō-**dī**-lā-tur)
bronchogram (**brong**-kō-gram)
bronchography (brong-**kog**-ruh-fē)
bronchopneumonia (brong-kō-noo-**mō**-nyuh)
bronchopulmonary (brong-kō-**pool**-muh-nar-ē)
bronchoscope (**brong**-kō-skōp)
bronchoscopic (brong-kō-**skop**-ik)
bronchoscopy (brong-**kos**-kuh-pē)
bronchus (**brong**-kus)
carcinoma of the lung (kar-si-**nō**-muh uv thuh lung)
chronic obstructive pulmonary disease (**kron**-ik ob-**struk**-tiv **pool**-mō-nar-ē di-**zēz**)
decongestant (dē-kun-**jes**-tunt)
diaphragm (**dī**-uh-fram)
dysphasia (dis-**fā**-zhuh)
dysphonia (dis-**fō**-nē-uh)
dyspnea (disp-**nē**-uh)
effusion (uh-**fū**-zhun)
embolism (**em**-buh-liz-um)
embolus (**em**-bō-lus)
emphysema (em-fuh-**sē**-muh)
endotracheal intubation (en-dō-**trā**-kē-ul in-tōō-**bā**-shun)
epiglottis (ep-i-**glot**-is)
esophagus (uh-**sof**-uh-gus)

eupnea (yōōp-**nē**-uh)
eustachian tube (ū-**stā**-kē-un tōōb)
exhalation (eks-huh-**lā**-shun)
expectorants (ek-**spek**-tuh-runts)
expiration (ek-spi-**rā**-shun)
glottis (**glot**-is)
Heimlich maneuver (**hīm**-lik muh-**nōō**-vur)
hemothorax (hē-mō-**thor**-aks)
hyperpnea (hī-pur-**nē**-uh, hī-purp-**nē**-uh)
hyperventilation (hī-pur-ven-ti-**lā**-shun)
hypoventilation (hī-pō-ven-ti-**lā**-shun)
hypoxemia (hī-pok-**sē**-mē-uh)
hypoxia (hī-**pok**-sē-uh)
influenza (in-flōō-**en**-zuh)
inhalation (in-huh-**lā**-shun)
inhalers (in-**hāl**-urz)
inspiration (in-spi-**rā**-shun)
laryngalgia (lar-in-**gal**-juh)
laryngeal (luh-**rin**-jē-ul)
laryngeal polyp (luh-**rin**-jē-ul **pol**-ip)
laryngitis (lar-in-**jī**-tis)
laryngopharynx (luh-ring-gō-**far**-inks)
laryngoscopy (lar-ing-**gos**-kuh-pē)
larynx (**lar**-inks)
lobectomy (lō-**bek**-tuh-mē)
lung biopsy (lung **bī**-op-sē)
mucolytic (mū-kō-**lit**-ik)
nares (**nā**-rēz)
nasal (**nā**-zul)
nasal cannula (**nā**-zul kan-ū-luh)
nasal polyp (**nā**-zul **pol**-ip)
nasal septum (**nā**-zul **sep**-tum)
nasopharyngeal (nā-zō-fuh-**rin**-jē-ul)
nasotracheal intubation (nā-zō-**trā**-kē-ul in-tōō-**bā**-shun)
orotracheal intubation (or-ō-**trā**-kē-ul in-tōō-**bā**-shun)
orthopnea (or-thop-**nē**-uh)
orthopneic (or-thop-**nē**-ik)
otopharyngeal (ō-tō-fuh-**rin**-jē-ul)
oximeter (ok-**sim**-uh-tur)
oximetry (ok-**sim**-uh-trē)
paracentesis (par-uh-sen-**tē**-sis)
paranasal sinuses (par-uh-**nā**-zul **sī**-nus-uz)
paroxysmal (par-ok-**siz**-mul)
percutaneous biopsy (pur-kū-**tā**-nē-us **bī**-op-sē)
pharyngeal (fuh-**rin**-jē-ul)
pharyngitis (far-in-**jī**-tis)
pharynx (**far**-inks)

QUICK & EASY (Q&E) LIST—cont'd

phrenic (*fren*-ik)
pleura (*ploor*-uh)
pleural (*ploor*-ul)
pleurisy (*ploor*-i-sē)
pleuritis (ploo-*rī*-tis)
pneumatic (noo̅-*mat*-ik)
pneumectomy (noo̅-*mek*-tuh-mē)
pneumocardial (noo̅-mō-*kahr*-dē-ul)
pneumocentesis (noo̅-mō-sen-*tē*-sis)
pneumoconiosis (noo̅-mō-kō-nē-*ō*-sis)
pneumohemothorax (noo̅-mō-hē-mō-*thor*-aks)
pneumonectomy (noo̅-mō-*nek*-tuh-mē)
pneumonia (noo̅-*mōn*-yuh)
pneumonitis (noo̅-mō-*nī*-tis)
pneumothorax (noo̅-mō-*thor*-aks)
pulmonary (*pool*-mō-nar-ē)
pulmonary edema (*pool*-mō-nar-ē uh-*dē*-muh)
pulmonary embolism (*pool*-mō-nar-ē *em*-buh-liz-um)
pulmonic (pul-*mon*-ik)
pulmonologist (pool-muh-*nol*-uh-jist)
respiration (res-pi-*rā*-shun)
respiratory (*res*-pur-uh-tor-ē)
rhinitis (rī-*nī*-tis)
rhinoplasty (*rī*-nō-plas-tē)
rhinorrhea (rī-nō-*rē*-uh)

severe acute respiratory syndrome (suh-*vēr* uh-*kūt* res-pur-uh-tor-ē *sin*-drōm)
silicosis (sil-i-*kō*-sis)
sinusitis (sī-nus-*ī*-tis)
spirometry (spī-*rom*-uh-trē)
sputum (*spū*-tum)
sudden infant death syndrome (*sud*-un *in*-funt deth *sin*-drōm)
tachypnea (tak-ip-*nē*-uh, tak-ē-*nē*-uh)
thoracentesis (thor-uh-sen-*tē*-sis)
thoracic (thuh-*ras*-ik)
thoracocentesis (thor-uh-kō-sen-*tē*-sis)
thorax (*thor*-aks)
thrombus (*throm*-bus)
trachea (*trā*-kē-uh)
tracheal (*trā*-kē-ul)
tracheobronchial (trā-kē-ō-*brong*-kē-ul)
tracheostomy (trā-kē-*os*-tuh-mē)
tracheotomy (trā-kē-*ot*-uh-mē)
transtracheal (trans-*trā*-kē-ul)
tubercle (*too̅*-bur-kul)
tuberculosis (too̅-bur-kū-*lō*-sis)
ventilator (*ven*-ti-lā-tur)
wheeze (hwēz)

Don't forget the games and other activities available at http://evolve.elsevier.com/Leonard/quick.

 QUICK CONNECT

Review all lists of word parts and their meanings for Chapter 8, using the flashcards you prepared or the flashcards on the Evolve site.

A pulmonologist is a physician who specializes in the anatomy physiology, and pathology of the lungs.

Respiration is the process of moving air into and out of the lungs, as well as the exchange of oxygen and carbon dioxide within the body's tissues. External respiration moves oxygen from the air into the blood; internal respiration moves oxygen from the blood to the tissues.

Breathing consists of inhalation (inspiration) and exhalation (expiration).

The respiratory tract also warms the air passing into the body and assists in speech by providing air for the larynx and vocal cords.

MAJOR ORGANS OF RESPIRATION

Upper respiratory tract: nose, nasal cavity, nasopharynx, oropharynx, larynx, and trachea (Know their order; be aware that sometimes air enters through the mouth and passes through the oral cavity.) The palate separates the nasal and oral cavities.

Lower respiratory tract: left and right bronchi, bronchioles, and alveoli. (The lungs' surfaces are partially concave, with a cardiac impression that cradles the heart. Right lung has 3 lobes; left lung has 2 lobes. The walls of the chest cavity as well as each lung is surrounded by a membrane, the pleura.)

A muscular wall, the diaphragm, separates the abdomen from the thoracic cavity. Phrenic can mean either pertaining to the diaphragm or pertaining to the mind.

The paranasal sinuses are air-filled cavities in various bones around the nose.

Recall the adjectives that mean pertaining to these structures: alveoli, bronchi, larynx, nose, nasopharynx pharynx, lungs, lungs and heart, trachea.

Distinguish these terms: nares, nasal septum, paranasal sinuses.

Diseases, Disorders, and Diagnostic Terms:

Distinguish these terms: dyspnea, eupnea , orthopnea, apnea, bradypnea, tachypnea, hyperpnea, hyperventilation, hypoxia, anoxia.

Know the structures to which these terms refer: nasopharyngeal, eustachian vs. otopharyngeal vs. auditory tube, glottis vs. epiglottis, alveoli,

Remember the meaning of these diagnostic terms: bronchography, oximetry (oximeter), spirometry, atelectasis.

Diseases/disorders or other diagnostic terms: sinusitis, rhinitis, rhinorrhea, pharyngitis, laryngitis, aphonia vs. dysphonia, aphasia vs. dysphasia, laryngalgia vs. laryngeal polyp, bronchitis, sputum, bronchoscopic, tracheobronchial, bronchoscope vs. bronchoscopy vs. laryngoscopy; bronchopulmonary, pneumonitis vs. bronchopneumonia' pulmonary edema, effusion, orthopneic, pneumothorax vs. hemothorax vs. pneumohemothorax; thrombus vs. embolism; embolus, ARDS, asthma, wheeze, atelectasis vs. bronchiectasis, COPD, emphysema, hyperventilation, hypoxemia, influenza, nasal polyp, pleuritis, pneumoconiosis, pulmonary embolism, SARS, silicosis, SIDS, TB, asphyxiation;

Surgical and Therapeutic Interventions:

Heimlich maneuver, endotracheal vs. orotracheal vs. nasotracheal intubation, transtracheal oxygen, nasal cannula

Pharmacology: antiasthmatics, decongestants, antitussives, antihistamine, bronchodilators, expectorants, inhalers, mucolytics.

Surgical procedures: lung biopsy (open vs. percutaneous), pneumocentesis, pneumonectomy (pneumectomy) vs. lobectomy, rhinoplasty, thoracentesis (also called thoracentesis or thoracic paracentesis).

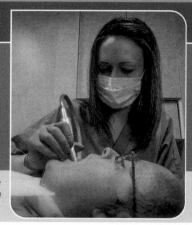

CHAPTER **9**

Digestive System

Dental hygienists work under the supervision of dentists and provide dental prophylaxis (protection against dental disease) by cleaning the teeth and inspecting the mouth and gums, radiography, administration of medications, and dental education.

OBJECTIVES

After completing Chapter 9, you will be able to:

1. Recognize or write the functions of the digestive system.
2. Recognize or write the meanings of Chapter 9 word parts and use them to build and analyze terms.
3. Write terms for selected structures of the digestive system, or match them with their descriptions.
4. Write the names of the diagnostic terms and pathologies related to the digestive system when

given their descriptions, or match terms with their meanings.
5. Match surgical and therapeutic interventions for the digestive system, or write the names of the interventions when given their descriptions.
6. Spell terms for the digestive system correctly.

 Function First

The digestive system provides the body with water, nutrients, and minerals. **Alimentation** is the process of providing **nutrition** for the body. After becoming available to the body cells, nutrients are used for growth, generation of energy, and elimination of wastes, all of which result from this process (**metabolism**).

The digestive system accomplishes its role through the following activities:

- ingestion
- absorption
- digestion
- elimination

The activities begin with **ingestion**, which in humans is the oral intake of substances into the body. Ingestion is followed by **digestion**, the mechanical and chemical conversion of food into substances that can eventually be absorbed by cells. The mechanical breakdown of food is accomplished by chewing. Chemical breakdown begins in the mouth and is completed in the stomach. **Absorption** is the process in which the digested food molecules pass through the lining of the small intestine into the blood or lymph capillaries. The final activity, **elimination**, is removal of undigested food particles. The elimination of wastes through the anus in the form of feces is called **defecation**.

> **WORD ORIGIN**
>
> *alimentum* (L.), to nourish
>
> **-ation** = process

> **QUICK TIP**
>
> Digestion consists of both mechanical and chemical processes.

WRITE IT! EXERCISE 1

In the order in which they occur, write the names of the four digestive activities.

1. _____   3. _____

2. _____   4. _____

*Use Appendix III, Answers, to check your answers to all the exercises in Chapter 9.

Carbohydrates, **proteins**, and **lipids** (fats) are the three major classes of nutrients. Carbohydrates, the basic source of energy for human cells, include sugars and starches. The chemical breaking down of nutrients into simpler substances requires **enzymes**. Specific enzymes act on different types of sugars and other organic substances. The suffixes -ose (meaning sugar) and -ase (meaning enzyme) are generally used in the terms referring to the sugars and the enzymes that act on them. For example, **lact+ase** breaks down **lact+ose**. The eventual product of the digestion of sugars as well as starches is **glucose**, a simple sugar that is the major source of energy for the body. The enzyme that breaks down starch is **amyl+ase**. The effective enzyme that breaks down protein is called **prote+ase** or **protein+ase**. The effective enzyme that breaks down a lipid (fat) is a **lip+ase**. Lipids serve as an energy reserve.

lact/o = milk
-ose = sugar
-ase = enzyme

amyl/o = starch
prote/o, protein/o = protein
lip/o = fat
-ase = enzyme

WRITE IT! EXERCISE 2

List the three major classes of nutrients.

1. _____   3. _____

2. _____

WRITE IT! EXERCISE 3

Write the name of the enzyme that breaks down the following nutrients.

1. lactose _____   3. protein (2 answers) _____

2. lipid _____   4. starch _____

The following table contains several word parts introduced in the material you just read, in addition to some new ones often associated with the digestive tract. Word parts for structures of the digestive system are included in the next section. Commit the following word parts to memory.

WORD PARTS: DIGESTION AND NUTRITION

Word Part	Meaning	Word Part	Meaning
-ation	action or process	-orexia	appetite
bil/i, chol/e	bile	-pepsia	digestion
cirrh/o	orange-yellow	vag/o	vagus nerve
de-	down, from, reversing, or removing	viscer/o	viscera
glycos/o	sugar		

Use the electronic flashcards on the Evolve site or make your own set of flashcards using the above list Select the word parts just presented, and study them until you know their meanings. Do this each time a set of word parts is presented.

Structures of the Digestive System

The digestive system is traditionally divided into the **alimentary** canal and several organs that are considered "accessory" organs because they produce substances needed for proper digestion and absorption of nutrients. Homeostasis is maintained even though the amounts of water and food substances that we take in vary. The alimentary canal is often called the digestive tract or the **alimentary tract**.

Alimentary Tract

The digestive tract, basically a long, muscular tube, is lined with mucous membrane, begins at the mouth and ends at the anus. **Intestinal** means pertaining to the intestine; **gastrointestinal** refers to the stomach and the intestines.

> **gastr/o** = stomach
> **intestin/o** = intestines
> **-al** = pertaining to

THE ADULT ALIMENTARY CANAL IS ABOUT 9 METERS (29 FEET) LONG

The upper gastrointestinal tract (UGI) consists of the mouth, pharynx, esophagus, and stomach. The lower gastrointestinal tract (LGI) is made up of the small and large intestines.

Become familiar with the names of the digestive organs and recognize the parts that make up the small and large intestines. Commit the meanings of the following word parts to memory.

WORD PARTS: DIGESTIVE ORGANS

Word Part	Meaning	
cheil/o	lips	⎱
dent/i, dent/o, odont/o	teeth	
gingiv/o	gums	⎰ mouth and teeth
gloss/o, lingu/o	tongue	
or/o, stomat/o	mouth	⎰
esophag/o	esophagus	
gastr/o	stomach	
intestin/o, enter/o*	intestines	
duoden/o	duodenum	⎱
jejun/o	jejunum	⎰ divisions of small intestine
ile/o	ileum	⎰
col/o, colon/o	colon or large intestine†	⎱
append/o, appendic/o	appendix	
cec/o	cecum	
sigmoid/o	sigmoid colon	⎰ large intestine
proct/o	anus or rectum	
rect/o	rectum	⎰
an/o	anus	

*enter/o sometimes refers only to the small intestine.
†The colon makes up most of the large intestine. Therefore the word "colon" is sometimes used inaccurately as a synonym for the entire large intestine. In words containing col/o, the distinction between the colon and large intestine is usually not significant.

The major organs of digestion are shown in Fig. 9.1. Label the numbered blanks as you read the information that accompanies the drawing.

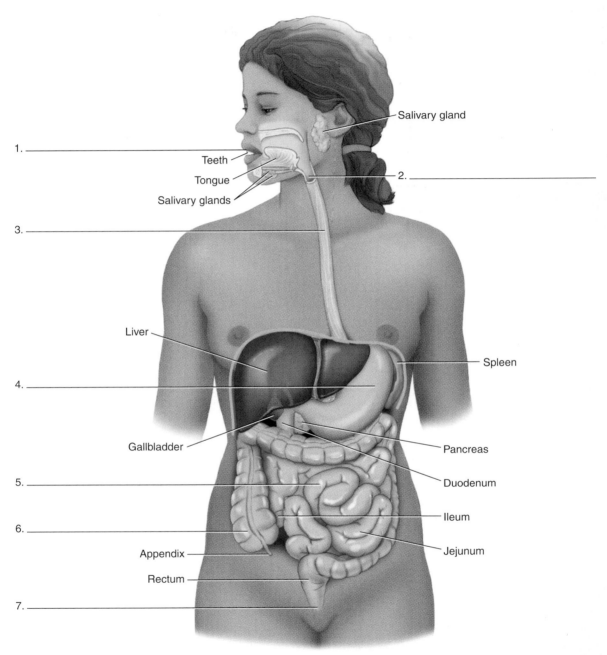

1. _____

2. _____

3. _____

4. _____

5. _____

6. _____

7. _____

Salivary gland

Teeth

Tongue

Salivary glands

Liver

Spleen

Gallbladder

Pancreas

Duodenum

Ileum

Jejunum

Appendix

Rectum

Fig. 9.1 Structures of the Digestive System. The alimentary tract, beginning at the mouth and ending at the anus, is basically a long, muscular tube. Several accessory organs (salivary glands, liver, gallbladder, pancreas) are also shown. Label the drawing as you read the following explanation. Digestion begins in the mouth *(1)*, or oral cavity. The teeth grind and chew the food before it is swallowed. The pharynx *(2)*, or throat, passes the chewed food to the esophagus *(3)*, which leads to the stomach *(4)*, where food is churned and broken down chemically and mechanically. The liquid mass is passed to the small intestine *(5)*, where digestion continues and absorption of nutrients occurs. The three parts of the small intestine are shown: duodenum, jejunum, and ileum. Undigested food passes to the large intestine *(6)*, where much of the water is absorbed. It is then excreted from the anus *(7)*, the opening of the rectum on the body surface.

MATCH IT!   EXERCISE 4

Match the word parts in the left column with their meanings in the right column (a choice may be used more than once).

_____ 1. bil/i
_____ 2. chol/e
_____ 3. de-
_____ 4. cirrh/o
_____ 5. glycos/o
_____ 6. -orexia
_____ 7. -pepsia
_____ 8. viscer/o

A. appetite
B. bile
C. digestion
D. down, from, reversing, or removing
E. orange-yellow
F. sugar
G. viscera

MATCH IT!   EXERCISE 5

Match the word parts in the left column with their meanings in the right column (a choice may be used more than once).

_____ 1. cheil/o
_____ 2. enter/o
_____ 3. gastr/o
_____ 4. gingiv/o
_____ 5. gloss/o
_____ 6. lingu/o
_____ 7. odont/o
_____ 8. proct/o

A. anus or rectum
B. gums
C. intestines
D. lips
E. stomach
F. teeth
G. tongue

PROGRAMMED LEARNING

Remember to cover the answers (left column) with folded paper or the bookmark. Write an answer in each blank, and then check your answer before proceeding to the next frame.

mouth	1. The mouth, or **oral** cavity, is the beginning of the digestive tract. An oral surgeon is one who specializes in surgery of the _____.
gum	2. **Gingiva** is another name for the gum, the mucous membrane that surrounds the teeth. **Gingiv+al** means pertaining to the _____.
under	3. You have learned that combining forms for the tongue are gloss/o and lingu/o. **Hypo+glossal** means _____ the tongue.
sublingual	4. Certain medications are placed under the tongue, where the medicine dissolves. **Lingual** means pertaining to the tongue. Use sub- + lingu/o + -al to write an adjective that describes the use of this type of medication: _____.

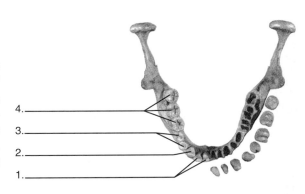

Fig. 9.2 Designations of Permanent Teeth of the Lower Jaw (Mandibular Arch). Half of the teeth are removed to demonstrate the sockets. Label the teeth in one dental quadrant (1 to 4) as you read this explanation. There are two incisors *(1)*, one cuspid or canine *(2)*, two bicuspids *(3)*, and three molars *(4)*.

| mandibul/o = mandible (lower jaw) |
| -ar = pertaining to |
| bi- = two |

4.———
3.———
2.———
1.———

---

teeth

5. An adult has 32 permanent teeth in a full set, 8 in each dental quadrant. **Dental** means pertaining to the teeth. Label the teeth of the lower jaw (**mandible**), called the **mandibular** arch, in Fig. 9.2. The combining forms dent/i, dent/o, and odont/o all mean _____.

   Permanent teeth are named **incisors**, **cuspids** (or canines), **bicuspids**, and **molars**. The last teeth on each side of the upper and lower jaw (the third molars) are called the "wisdom teeth" because they usually erupt between 17 and 25 years of age.

6. Dentists care for the teeth and associated structures of the oral cavity. Or+al means pertaining to the mouth. The word part odont/o is used to write the names of most of the dental specialties:
   endodontics: Diagnosis and treatment of diseases of the dental pulp, tooth root, and surrounding tissues and the practice of root canal therapy.
   orthodontics: Diagnosis and treatment of problems with tooth alignment and associated facial problems.
   pedodontics: Devoted to the care of children's teeth and mouth; pediatric dentistry.
   periodontics: The study and treatment of the **peri+odont+ium**, the tissue that supports the teeth and keeps them firmly anchored.
   A specialist in orthodontics is an _____.

orthodontist

7. Use -al to form a word that means pertaining to the periodontium: _____.

periodontal

8. Food that is swallowed passes from the mouth to the **pharynx** (throat) and then to a long tube called the _____.

esophagus

9. The **esophagus** carries food to the stomach. Washing out of the stomach is called **gastric lavage.** Lavage means the irrigation or washing out of an organ, such as the stomach or bowel. Gastric lavage specifically refers to washing out of the _____. This procedure might be performed to remove poisonous material or to clean the stomach before gastric surgery.

stomach

10. Pain associated with digestive problems often involves examination of the abdomen. Abdominal quadrants are useful to describe location of pain in the abdomen (see Fig. 5.16). **Gastric** means pertaining to the stomach. **Gastr+algia** and **gastro+dynia** both mean _____ of the stomach.

pain

11. Gastro+intestinal (GI) means pertaining to the _____ and the intestines.

stomach

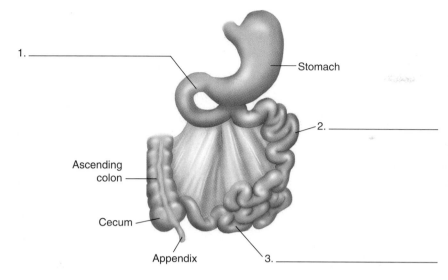

1. _____

— Stomach

2. _____

Ascending colon

Cecum

Appendix

3. _____

dist/o = distant, far
-al = pertaining to

Fig. 9.3 The Three Divisions of the Small Intestine. Label the three parts of the small intestine (1 to 3) as you read. The first portion, the duodenum *(1),* begins at the opening from the stomach and is the shorter section. The second section is the jejunum *(2),* which is continuous with the third portion, the ileum *(3).* The ileum, the distal part of the small intestine, joins with the cecum (the beginning of the large intestine).

ileum

12. Label the three divisions of the small intestine as you read the material that accompanies Fig. 9.3. The three divisions of the small intestine are the **duodenum**, the **jejunum**, and the _____.

ileum

13. The large intestine is much broader and shorter than the small intestine. It is composed of the **cecum**, **colon**, **rectum**, and anal canal (Fig. 9.4). The first part of the large intestine is a blind pouch only a few inches long called the cecum. The **vermiform appendix**, a wormlike structure extending from the cecum, is best known for becoming inflamed. The **ileo+cecal** valve is a group of muscles that are located between the _____ and the cecum.

WORD ORIGIN
sigma (G), the letter S

sigmoid

14. The colon makes up the major portion of the large intestine. The colon consists of four distinct parts: **ascending colon**, **transverse colon**, **descending colon**, and **sigmoid colon**. Locate the four parts of the colon using Fig. 9.4. The latter part of the colon is S-shaped and thus is called the _____ colon.

col/o

15. The colon makes up most of the large intestine. Thus, when speaking of the colon, one is often referring to the large intestine in general. The combining form that means colon or large intestine is _____.

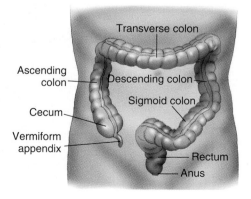

Transverse colon

Ascending colon
Descending colon
Cecum
Sigmoid colon
Vermiform appendix
Rectum
Anus

an/o = anus
-al = pertaining to
trans- = through, across

Fig. 9.4 Divisions of the Large Intestine. The large intestine is composed of the cecum, colon, rectum, and anal canal. Note the four parts of the colon: ascending colon, transverse colon, descending colon, and sigmoid colon.

rectum

16. The lower part of the large intestine, the rectum, ends in a narrow anal canal, which opens to the exterior at the **anus**. The combining form proct/o refers to the anus or the rectum. A **procto+logist** is a physician who specializes in diseases of the anus and _____, in addition to disorders of the colon.

17. Rhythmic muscular contraction forces food through the digestive tract. This is aided by **mucus**, secreted by the inner lining of the digestive tract, and bile (which is discussed in the next section). The slimy material, mucus, is produced by all **mucous** membranes. Remember that muc/o means _____.

mucus

18. **Gastro+entero+logy** is the study of the stomach, intestines, and associated structures. Write the term for a physician who specializes in gastroenterology: _____.

gastroenterologist

QUICK REVIEW!

Note the pathway of food as it travels through the digestive tract. Accessory organs are shown in purple, green, and blue.

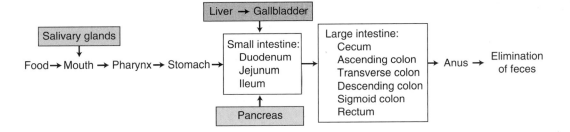

FIND IT!   **EXERCISE 6**

Write the combining forms and their meanings for each of these new terms. A short definition is provided for each term.

Term/Meaning	Combining Form	Meaning
1. **anal** pertaining to the anus	_____	_____
2. **duodenal** pertaining to the duodenum	_____	_____
3. **endogastric** pertaining to the interior of the stomach	_____	_____
4. **enteral** pertaining to the small intestine	_____	_____
5. **esophageal** pertaining to the esophagus	_____	_____
6. **glossal** pertaining to the tongue	_____	_____
7. **rectal** pertaining to the rectum	_____	_____

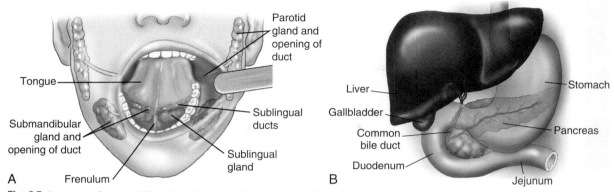

Fig. 9.5 Accessory Organs of Digestion. **A,** Mouth with raised tongue. The salivary glands (paired parotid, sublingual, and submandibular glands) consist of numerous lobes connected by vessels and ducts. **B,** The liver, gallbladder, and pancreas.

Accessory Organs of Digestion

The accessory organs of digestion produce substances that are needed for proper digestion and absorption of nutrients. The liver, gallbladder, pancreas, and salivary glands are accessory organs to the digestive system (Fig. 9.5). Both the liver and pancreas have additional functions in other body systems.

Commit to memory the meanings of the following word parts.

WORD PARTS: ACCESSORY ORGANS OF DIGESTION			
Word Part	**Meaning**	**Word Part**	**Meaning**
bil/i, chol/e	bile	hepat/o	liver
cholecyst/o	gallbladder	pancreat/o	pancreas
choledoch/o	common bile duct	sial/o	salivary gland

The **salivary** glands are located in the oral cavity. **Saliva** is produced by these glands. Saliva moistens the oral cavity and contains amy+lase, the enzyme responsible for the breakdown of starch. Because amylase is contained in saliva, starch digestion begins in the mouth.

The liver is the largest internal organ. It performs so many vital functions that you cannot live without it. The liver produces **bile**, which breaks down fats before absorption by the small intestine. **Biliary** means pertaining to bile. Bile is continuously produced by the liver and is either stored by the gallbladder or transported to the small intestine for immediate use. **Cholecystic** means pertaining to the gallbladder. The main duct that conveys bile to the duodenum is the common bile duct. **Choledoch+al** means pertaining to the common bile duct.

bil/i = bile
-ary = pertaining to

choledoch/o = common bile duct
-al = pertaining to

The pancreas has two important functions. It produces pancreatic juice, which is important in the digestion of food. The pancreas also produces **insulin**, a hormone that regulates the blood sugar level.

The first letter of each word part is given after its meaning. Use this clue to write the combining form indicated for each term.

Meaning	First Letter	Combining Form
1. common bile duct	c	_____
2. pancreas	p	_____
3. liver	h	_____
4. gallbladder	c	_____
5. salivary gland	s	_____

Diseases, Disorders, and Diagnostic Terms

> **QUICK TIP**
>
> Barium sulfate is a radiopaque medium used in radiographic imaging.

Assessment of the intestinal tract has been greatly facilitated by radiology and endoscopy, revealing abnormalities such as masses, tumors, and obstructions. An **esophagram** (or **esophagogram**) is an x-ray image of the esophagus taken while the patient swallows a liquid barium suspension. This procedure is also called a **barium swallow**. A barium suspension is ingested in an upper gastrointestinal (GI) series (esophagus, stomach, and duodenum) as well as a small bowel series of the small intestine, either occurring as a stand alone exam. The lower intestinal tract is studied with a **barium enema**, a rectal infusion of barium sulfate to diagnose obstructions or other abnormalities.

The **biliary tract** is the pathway for bile flow from the liver to the bile duct and into the duodenum. A biliary calculus (**gallstone**) is a stone formed in the biliary tract, varying in size from very small to 4 or 5 cm in diameter (Fig. 9.6). Biliary stones may cause **jaundice** (see Fig. 3.14), right upper quadrant pain, obstruction, and inflammation of the gallbladder (cholecystitis). Common locations of biliary stones are illustrated in Fig. 9.7. The presence of stones in the gallbladder is **chole+lith+iasis**. Stones also can become lodged in the common bile duct (**choledocho+lith+iasis**).

> **chol/e** = bile
> **angi/o** = vessel
> **pancreat/o** = pancreas
> **-graphy** = process of recording

The presence of a pancreatic stone is **pancreatolithiasis**. Other causes of obstructions include tumors. Endoscopic retrograde chol+angio+pancreato+graphy (ERCP) is an endoscopic test that provides radiographic visualization of the bile ducts and pancreatic ducts. An endoscope is placed into the common bile duct, a radiopaque substance is instilled directly into the duct, and x-ray images are taken.

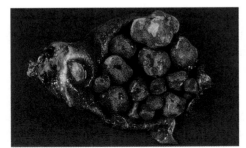

Fig. 9.6 Cholelithiasis, the Presence of Gallstones. This photograph of an opened gallbladder, taken after cholecystectomy, shows several stones of different sizes.
chol/e = bile;   **lith/o** = stone;   **-iasis** = condition

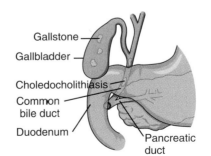

Gallstone
Gallbladder
Choledocholithiasis
Common bile duct
Duodenum
Pancreatic duct

> **choledoch/o** = common bile duct
> **lith/o** = stone
> **-iasis** = condition

Fig. 9.7 Common Locations of Biliary Calculi. Tiny stones may pass spontaneously into the duodenum. Very large stones remain in the gallbladder (cholelithiasis). Smaller stones can become lodged in the common bile duct (choledocholithiasis).

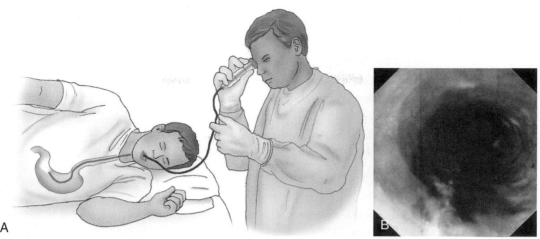

Fig. 9.8 Upper Gastrointestinal (GI) Endoscopy. **A,** Upper GI endoscopy is visual examination of the esophagus, stomach, and duodenum. **B,** Endoscopic view of the gastroesophageal junction shows a mucosal tear at about 6 o'clock. The patient was admitted to the hospital with hematemesis after an alcohol binge. **gastr/o** = stomach; **intestin/o** = intestine; **-scopy** = visual examination; **duoden/o** = duodenum

The salivary ducts can be studied by injecting radiopaque substances into the ducts in a procedure called **sialography**, which may be used to demonstrate the presence of calculi in the ducts.

Upper gastrointestinal endoscopy is visual examination of the esophagus, stomach, and duodenum (Fig. 9.8). If the focus of the examination is the esophagus, the procedure is called **esophagoscopy**. If the stomach is the focus, the procedure is called **gastroscopy**.

Colono+scopy is the endoscopic examination of the lining of the colon with a **colonoscope**. **Coloscopy**, used less often, has the same meaning. The physician may also obtain tissue biopsy specimens or remove polyps during this procedure (Fig. 9.9). **Sigmoidoscopy** is inspection of the rectum and sigmoid colon with an endoscope, and **proctoscopy** is endoscopic examination of the rectum with a **proctoscope**.

proct/o = anus or rectum

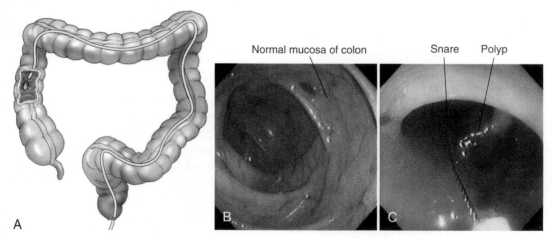

Normal mucosa of colon   Snare   Polyp

Fig. 9.9 Colonoscopy. **A,** Endoscopic examination of the colon using a flexible colonoscope. **B,** View of a normal colon through a colonoscope. **C,** Colonic polyps can often be removed with the use of a snare (wire noose) that fits through the colonoscope.
colon/o = colon; **-scopy** = visual examination; **-scope** = instrument used for visually examining

BUILD IT!

EXERCISE 8

Combine the word parts to write terms for these descriptions.

1. radiographic image of the esophagus (esophag/o + -gram): _____
2. presence of stones in the gallbladder (chol/e + -lith/o + -iasis): _____
3. presence of stones in the common bile duct (choledoch/o + lith/o + -iasis): _____
4. presence of a pancreatic stone (pancreat/o + lith/o + -iasis): _____
5. radiography of the salivary ducts (sial/o + -graphy): _____
6. visual examination of the esophagus (esophag/o + -scopy): _____
7. endoscopic examination of the colon (colon/o + -scopy): _____
8. inspection of the rectum and sigmoid colon (sigmoid/o + -scopy): _____

Several blood tests, urine tests, and stool examinations are useful in assessing the organs of the digestive system, particularly liver function tests and tests for diabetes. To be accurate when referring to diabetes mellitus, it is better not to shorten the term to **diabetes** alone, although this is often done. **Diabetes mellitus** (DM) is primarily a result of resistance to insulin or lack of insulin secretion by the insulin-secreting cells of the pancreas.

hyper- = increased
glyc/o = sugar
-emia = blood

-phagia = eating
-uria = urination
-dipsia = thirst

glyc/o = sugar

Without insulin, glucose builds up in the blood and results in **hyper+glycemia**, an increased glucose level in the blood. Hyperglycemia ultimately results in the classic symptoms of diabetes mellitus:

- **poly+phagia**: excessive hunger and uncontrolled eating
- **poly+uria**: excessive urination
- **poly+dipsia**: excessive thirst.

The urine sometimes contains glucose (**glycosuria**).

HEALTH CARE CONNECTION

The term "diabetes" is derived from a Greek word that means "to pass through," named for polyuria, the large quantity of urine produced. "Mellitus" was added to indicate that the urine was sweet (*mellus* [L.], honey). Ancient physicians tested urine by dipping their fingers in the patient's urine and tasting it for sweetness. If the urine wasn't sweet, the disease was called diabetes insipidus (*insipidus* [L.], without taste). Read more about both of these metabolic diseases in Chapter 15.

Broad classifications of DM are type 1, type 2, gestational, and other types. Type 1 diabetes is genetically determined and results in absolute insulin deficiency; however, most people with this gene never develop type 1 diabetes. The specific genetic link and development of type 2 diabetes is unclear, but genetics, environmental factors, aging, and obesity may contribute to its development. Type 2 diabetes is characterized by insulin resistance rather than insufficient secretion. **Gestational diabetes mellitus**, first recognized during pregnancy, is carbohydrate intolerance, usually caused by a deficiency of insulin. It disappears after delivery of the infant; but in a significant number of cases, it returns years later. A fourth subclass called **prediabetes** includes persons whose blood glucose levels are abnormal but not sufficiently above the normal range to be diagnosed as having diabetes.

In another dysfunction, the pancreas produces too much insulin and causes **hypo+glycemia**. In hypoglycemia the blood contains less than the normal amount of sugar.

hypo- = less than normal

Carcinoma can occur in almost any organ of the gastrointestinal system, but cancers of the colon, rectum, and the oral cavity are more common. Pancreatic cancer, although uncommon, has a high mortality rate.

You are probably familiar with cholesterol, a type of lipid that generally is elevated in **hyper+lip+emia**. Sometimes the combining form, lip/o, is not used, and **hyperlipidemia** is also used to mean an increased amount of fat or lipids in the blood.

hyper- = excessive
lip/o = lipid
-emia = blood

Obesity is an abnormal increase in the proportion of fat cells of the body. A person is regarded as medically obese if he or she is 20% above the desirable body weight for the person's age, gender, height, and body type.

Hyper+emesis and **dia+rrhea** can also interfere with proper nutrition. **Emesis** is also used as a word that means vomiting. Hyperemesis or diarrhea can lead to **de+hydr+ation**. Dehydration occurs when the output of body fluid exceeds fluid intake.

-emesis = vomiting
de- = remove
hydr/o = water
-ation = process

Emaciation is excessive leanness caused by disease or lack of nutrition. **An+orexia** is loss of appetite for food. **Anorexia nervosa**, often associated with psychologic stress or conflict, is a disorder characterized by prolonged refusal to eat that results in emaciation. **Bulimia** is episodic binge eating, usually followed by behavior designed to rid the body of excessive intake of food, most commonly self-induced vomiting or laxative abuse.

an- = without
-orexia = appetite

Either prolonged anorexia or bulimia leads to depletion of nutrients for body cells and results in **mal+nutrition**. Malnutrition can also be caused by malabsorption, the improper absorption of nutrients into the bloodstream from the intestines. **Malabsorption syndrome** is a complex of symptoms that include anorexia, weight loss, **flatulence** (excessive gas in the stomach and intestinal tract that leads to bloating), muscle cramps, and bone pain.

WRITE IT! EXERCISE 9

Write the correct term in the blanks to complete each sentence.

1. A disorder that results from a resistance to or lack of insulin is diabetes _____.
2. The term for increased glucose in the blood is _____.
3. The term for excessive urination is _____.
4. The term for excessive thirst is _____.
5. Glucose in the urine is called _____.
6. A type of diabetes that sometimes occurs first during pregnancy is called _____ diabetes mellitus.
7. Less than the normal amount of sugar in the blood is called _____.
8. Hyperlipidemia is an increased amount of _____ in the blood.
9. Excessive vomiting is _____.
10. Excessive leanness is _____.
11. A disorder characterized by prolonged refusal to eat is _____ nervosa.
12. Binge eating often terminating in self-induced vomiting is _____.
13. Excessive hunger and uncontrolled eating is _____.
14. The result of depletion of nutrients for body cells is _____.

PROGRAMMED LEARNING

Remember to cover the answers (left column) with folded paper or the bookmark. Write an answer in each blank, and then check your answer before proceeding to the next frame.

appendix	1. The vermiform (worm-shaped) appendix is attached to the cecum (see Fig. 9.3). **Appendic+itis** is inflammation of the vermiform _____ (Fig. 9.10). It is characterized by abdominal pain followed by nausea and vomiting.
hepatitis	2. Inflammation of the liver is _____, which is frequently accompanied by jaundice (Fig. 9.11). Causes of this condition include bacterial or viral infection, parasites, drugs, and toxins. The liver is usually able to regenerate its tissue, but severe hepatitis may lead to chronic liver dysfunction.
hepatomegaly	3. When the liver becomes inflamed, it is not unusual for it also to become enlarged. Use a suffix you learned earlier to write a word that means enlargement of the liver: _____.
liver	4. **Hepatic** means pertaining to the liver. **Cirrhosis** is a chronic liver disease characterized by marked degeneration of liver cells. It might be more difficult for you to remember the meaning of cirrhosis because it does not use a familiar word part. The combining form cirrh/o is derived from a Greek word meaning orange-yellow, but you need to remember that cirrh+osis is a chronic disease of the _____.
cirrhosis	5. There are other causes of cirrhosis, but a common cause is alcohol abuse. The term for chronic liver disease characterized by marked degeneration of liver cells is _____.
liver	6. **Hepato+toxic** means toxic or destructive to the _____. Hepatotoxic agents, usually a drug or alcohol, can damage the liver.

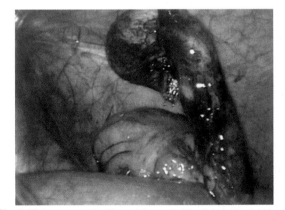

Fig. 9.10 Laparoscopic View of Appendicitis. Pain in the right lower quadrant prompted this patient to see the physician. Laparoscopy revealed acute appendicitis, and the appendix was easily removed laparoscopically.

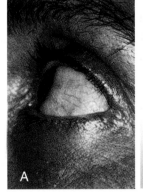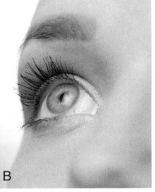

Fig. 9.11 Jaundice. Note the yellow discoloration of the skin, mucous membranes, and sclerae (white parts of the eyes) is characteristic of hepatitis. Compare **A,** person with jaundice and **B,** the skin and sclera of a person without jaundice.

gallbladder	7. Bile is produced by the liver but stored in the _____. (*Gall* is another term for bile; thus the use of the term *gallbladder*.) Bile breaks down fats, preparing them for further digestion and absorption in the small intestine.
vessel	8. **Chol+ang+itis** is inflammation of the bile ducts, the vessels that transport bile. The combining form chol/e, meaning bile, is used to write *cholangitis*. The combining form angi/o means _____. (In cholangitis, the *i* in angi/o is omitted to make pronunciation easier.)
cholangiogram	9. **Cholangio+graphy** is x-ray examination of the bile ducts, usually using a contrast agent. The record of the bile ducts produced in cholangiography is called a _____.
cholecystitis	10. The combining form cyst/o means bladder or sac. Whenever you see *cholecyst* in a word, you will know that it means gallbladder. Inflammation of the gallbladder is _____.
pancreatolith	11. Stones can form in the pancreas as well as the gallbladder. Write a word that means pancreatic stone: _____.
stone	12. Saliva is produced by the salivary glands. **Sialo+lith+iasis** is the presence of a salivary _____.
"bad," poor, or abnormal	13. If **eu+pepsia** is good or normal digestion, **dys+pepsia** is _____ digestion.
viscera	14. The term **viscera** (singular, viscus) refers to large internal organs enclosed within a body cavity, including the chest, pelvic, and abdominal cavities, but especially the abdominal organs. **Visceral** means pertaining to the large internal organs in the abdominal cavity. Thus, many of the digestive organs are viscera. Write the term that means large internal organs within the abdominal cavity: _____.
peritonitis	15. **Peritoneum** (periton/o + -eum, membrane) is the membrane that surrounds the viscera and lines the abdominal cavity. The peritoneum holds the viscera in position. Inflammation of the peritoneum is _____.
hernia	16. A hernia is protrusion of an organ through an abnormal opening in the muscle wall of the cavity that surrounds it. A weakness in the abdominal wall can result in various hernias, including umbilical hernias (those near the umbilicus), incisional hernias (herniation through inadequately healed surgery), and inguinal hernias (those in which a loop of intestine enters the **inguinal** canal, an opening in the abdominal wall for passage of the spermatic cord in males and a ligament of the uterus in females). A protrusion of an organ through an abnormal opening in the muscle wall of the cavity that contains it is called a _____. Common types of abdominal hernias are shown in Fig. 5.19.

The following sections define additional diseases and disorders affecting alimentary structures and organs of digestion.

Mouth

canker sores Ulcers, chiefly of the mouth and lips.

cheilitis (cheil/o, lip + -itis, inflammation) Inflammation of the lip.

gingivitis (gingiv/o, gum) Inflammation of the gums.

glossitis (gloss/o, tongue) Inflammation of the tongue. The tongue is painful, sometimes covered with ulcers, and swallowing is difficult.

stomatitis (stomat/o, mouth) Inflammation of the mouth.

Esophagus

dysphagia (dys-, painful or difficult + phag/o, eat + -ia, condition) Inability to swallow or difficulty in swallowing. This condition is often associated with disorders such as paralysis, constriction, and spasm of the esophageal muscles.

esophageal varices (esophag/o, esophagus) A complex of enlarged and swollen veins at the lower end of the esophagus that are susceptible to hemorrhage.

esophagitis Inflammation of the esophagus.

gastroesophageal reflux disease (GERD) Condition resulting from a backflow of the stomach contents into the esophagus. The acidic gastric juices cause burning pain in the esophagus. Repeated episodes of reflux can result in esophagitis, narrowing of the esophagus, or an esophageal ulcer. Treatment is elevation of the head of the bed, avoidance of acid-stimulating foods, and use of **antacids** (ant-, against) or antiulcer medications.

Stomach

gastritis (gastr/o, stomach) Inflammation of the stomach.

gastrocele (-cele, hernia) Herniation of the stomach. A common type of gastrocele is a **hiatal hernia**, protrusion of a structure through the opening in the diaphragm that allows passage of the esophagus. Often the protruding structure is part of the stomach (Fig. 9.12).

gastroenteritis (enter/o, intestine) Inflammation of the stomach and the intestinal tract.

hyperacidity Excessive amount of acid in the stomach. The condition may lead to ulceration of the stomach and is treated with antacids or anti-ulcer medications. Antibiotics are also effective in some patients.

ulcer Lesion of the mucous membrane, accompanied by the sloughing (shedding) of dead tissue.

upper gastrointestinal bleeding Bleeding of the upper digestive structures, sometimes evidenced by hematemesis, blood in the vomit (Fig. 9.13).

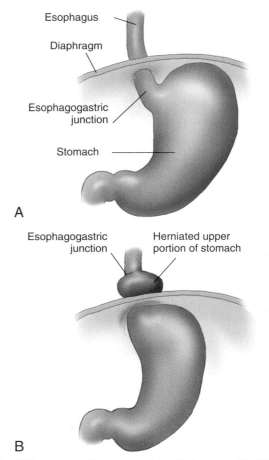

Fig. 9.12 Structural Abnormality of the Diaphragm in Hiatal Hernia. **A,** Normally, muscles in the diaphragm encircle the esophagogastric junction and prevent the stomach from ascending into the thoracic cavity. **B,** Hiatal hernia, in which the upper portion of the stomach slides up and down through the opening in the diaphragm. **esophag/o** = esophagus; **gastr/o** = stomach; **thorac/o** = thorax (chest)

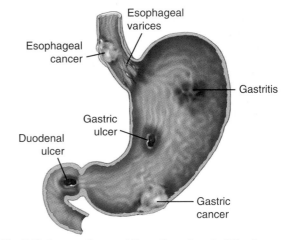

Fig. 9.13 Common Causes of Upper Gastrointestinal Bleeding.

Intestines

appendicitis (appendic/o, appendix) Inflammation of the vermiform appendix.

colitis (col/o, colon) Inflammation of the colon.

diverticulitis (diverticul/o, diverticulum) Inflammation of a diverticulum in the intestinal tract, especially in the colon, causing stagnation, or lack of movement, of feces, and pain. If diverticulitis is severe, a **diverticulectomy** is performed. A **diverticulum** (plural, diverticula) is a small sac or pouch in the wall of an organ. **Diverticulosis** is the presence of diverticula without inflammation, a condition that affects a number of people older than 50 years and may cause few symptoms.

duodenal ulcer (duoden/o, duodenum + -al, pertaining to) An ulcer of the duodenum. Bleeding is sometimes present with this type of ulcer. Perforation can occur, which can lead to peritonitis (periton/o, peritoneum).

duodenitis Inflammation of the duodenum.

dysentery (dys-, bad + enter/o, intestine + -y, condition) Inflammation of the intestine, especially the colon. The most common types are caused by bacteria or protozoa, characterized by frequent and bloody feces. Diarrhea, the frequent passage of loose, watery stools, is an important symptom of dysentery as well as several other disorders.

enterostasis (enter/o, intestine + -stasis, stopping) Stoppage or delay in the passage of food through the intestine.

hemorrhoids Masses of veins in the anal canal that are unnaturally distended and lie just inside or outside the rectum. They are often accompanied by pain, itching, and bleeding.

irritable bowel syndrome (IBS) Abnormally increased motility of the small and large intestines of unknown origin. Most of those affected are young adults who report diarrhea and occasionally pain in the abdomen, usually relieved by passing gas or stool. Also called functional bowel syndrome, mucous colitis, or spastic colon. This is a noninflammatory condition and no specific treatment is required; however, more serious conditions such as dysentery, lactose intolerance (sensitivity disorder resulting in the inability to digest lactose from milk products), and the inflammatory bowel

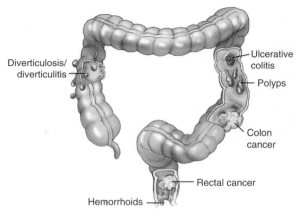

Fig. 9.14 Common Causes of Lower Gastrointestinal Bleeding.

diseases (for example, Crohn's disease) must be ruled out.

lower gastrointestinal bleeding Bleeding of the lower digestive structures (see Fig. 9.14).

Gallbladder

cholecystitis (cholecyst/o, gallbladder) Inflammation of the gallbladder.

cholelithiasis (chol/e, gall or bile + lith/o, stone + -iasis, condition) Formation or presence of gallstones in the gallbladder or common bile duct (see Fig. 9.6).

cholestasis Stoppage of bile excretion.

Liver

cirrhosis Chronic liver disease characterized by marked degeneration of liver cells.

hepatitis (hepat/o, liver) Inflammation of the liver.

hepatomegaly (-megaly, enlargement) Enlargement of the liver.

Pancreas

diabetes General term for diseases characterized by excessive urination; the term usually refers to diabetes mellitus.

hypoglycemia (hypo-, below normal + glyc/o, sugar + -emia, blood) Condition in which the blood glucose level is abnormally low. It can be caused by excessive production of insulin by the pancreas or by excessive injection of insulin.

pancreatitis (pancreat/o, pancreas) Inflammation of the pancreas.

CHOOSE IT!
EXERCISE 10

Choose the correct answer to complete each sentence.

1. The presence of gallstones in the gallbladder or common bile duct is (cholecystitis, cholecystography, cholelithiasis, cholestasis).
2. One type of liver disease is (cirrhosis, diverticulitis, dysphagia, splenomegaly).
3. A lesion of a mucous membrane accompanied by sloughing of dead tissue is (dysphagia, diverticulitis, a hemorrhoid, an ulcer).
4. A hiatal hernia is one type of (enterostasis, esophagitis, gastrocele, peptic ulcer).
5. Inflammation of the tongue is (cheilitis, gingivitis, glossitis, stomatitis).
6. Varicose veins of the anal canal are called (diverticula, hemorrhoids, hepatitis, hepatomegaly).

WRITE IT!
EXERCISE 11

Write a term for each description.

1. inflammation of the esophagus   _____
2. inflammation of the stomach and intestinal tract   _____
3. stoppage or delay in the passage of food through the intestine   _____
4. endoscopic inspection of the stomach   _____
5. inflammation of the gallbladder   _____
6. chronic liver disease with marked degeneration of liver cells   _____

Surgical and Therapeutic Interventions

Conservative approaches to weight loss for obese individuals include restricted food intake and increased exercise. An appetite-suppressing drug is an **anorexiant**. Surgical approaches for treating extreme obesity, generally used when conservative methods have failed, limit food intake or absorption by either **gastro+plasty** or **gastric bypass**. These surgeries reduce the stomach's capacity.

Several pharmaceuticals are helpful in the treatment of gastrointestinal problems, in addition to antibiotics that are used to treat infections. **Anti+diarrheals** are used to treat diarrhea, and **anti+emetics** to relieve or prevent vomiting. To induce (cause) vomiting in an individual in the emergency treatment of drug overdose or certain cases of poisoning, **emetics** are used. **Laxatives** cause evacuation of the bowel and may be prescribed to correct constipation. **Purgatives** or **cathartics** are strong medications used to promote full evacuation of the bowel, as in preparation for diagnostic studies or surgery of the digestive tract.

Some forms of diabetes are treated with diet, exercise, and weight control, and other forms require glucose-lowering agents (oral agents or insulin by injection). Individuals with type 1 diabetes, and some with type 2 diabetes, require an outside source of insulin.

Patients who can digest and absorb nutrients but need nutritional support may receive enteral nutrition, in which nutrients are introduced directly into the gastrointestinal tract when the patient cannot chew, ingest, or swallow food. This is accomplished by using an enteral feeding tube, including a **nasogastric** tube, a **nasoduodenal** tube, or a **nasojejunal** tube. In some patients the tube is inserted through a new opening made in the esophagus, stomach, or jejunum (**esophagostomy**, **gastrostomy**, or **jejunostomy**, respectively). Note the location of these types of enteral feeding tubes in Fig. 9.15.

enter/o = intestine
nas/o = nose
gastr/o = stomach

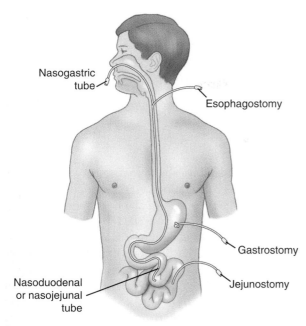

Fig. 9.15 Common Locations for Placement of Enteral Feeding Tubes. **enter/o** = intestine;   **nas/o** = nose;   **gastr/o** = stomach; **esophag/o** = esophagus;   **-stomy** = formation of an opening; **duoden/o** = duodenum;   **jejun/o** = jejunum

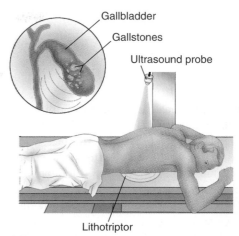

Fig. 9.16 Biliary Lithotripsy. The gallbladder is positioned over the lithotriptor. The lithotriptor is then fired, and particles slough off the gallstones until they are fragmented and can pass through the biliary ducts.

bil/i = bile;   **lith/o** = stone;   **-triptor** = instrument used for crushing;   **ultra-** = beyond, excess

Gallstones are a common disorder of the gallbladder, and nonsurgical treatments include oral drugs that dissolve stones, **laser lithotripsy**, and **shock wave lithotripsy** (Fig. 9.16).

Although these procedures are called lithotripsy, there is no surgical incision. The methods rely on laser or a high-energy shock wave to disintegrate the stone, and the particles pass through the biliary ducts and are eliminated. If these methods fail, cholecystectomy may be necessary. When possible, **laparoscopic cholecystectomy** is performed. In the latter procedure, the gallbladder is excised with a laser and removed through a small incision in the abdominal wall.

Additional information about surgical procedures of the digestive organs follows:

lith/o = stone
-tripsy = surgical crushing
lapar/o = abdominal wall
cholecyst/o = gallbladder
-ectomy = excision

appendectomy (append/o, appendix + -ectomy, excision) Removal of the vermiform appendix. It is removed when it is acutely infected to prevent peritonitis, which can occur if the appendix ruptures.

cholecystectomy (cholecyst/o, gallbladder) Surgical removal of the gallbladder. Exploration of the common bile duct is often performed during cholecystectomy. In this situation, cholangiography (chol/e, bile + angi/o, vessel + -graphy, recording) is performed. Biliary vessels are injected with contrast medium; x-ray images can show stones or other obstruction.

colostomy (col/o, colon + -stomy, artificial opening) Creation of an artificial anus on the abdominal wall by incising the colon and drawing it out to the surface. It is performed when the feces cannot pass through the colon and out through the anus.

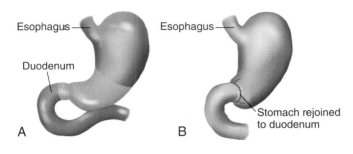

Esophagus

Duodenum

A

Esophagus

Stomach rejoined
to duodenum

B

Fig. 9.17 Partial Gastrectomy. **A,** The stomach before surgery, showing the distal acid-secreting portion *(tan)*. **B,** The stomach after surgery. A new opening has been made between the stomach and the duodenum, the first part of the small intestine. This type of surgery, gastroduodenostomy, might be performed for severe chronic gastric ulcers.

gastrectomy (gastr/o, stomach) Surgical removal of all or part of the stomach (Fig. 9.17). When the remaining portion of the stomach is joined to the duodenum, the procedure is called **gastroduodenostomy**. This is a type of duodenal anastomosis. Translated literally, anastomosis (from the Greek word *anastomoien*) means "to provide a mouth." An **anastomosis** is the joining of two organs, vessels, or ducts that are normally separate. The opening created between the stomach and the duodenum in Fig. 9.17, *B*, is an anastomosis.

gastrostomy Surgical creation of a new opening into the stomach through the abdominal wall. This allows the insertion of a synthetic feeding tube and is performed when the patient cannot eat normally.

hemorrhoidectomy (hemorrhoid/o, hemorrhoid) Removal of hemorrhoids by any of several means, including surgery.

ileostomy (ile/o, ileum) Creation of a surgical passage through the abdominal wall into the ileum. An ileostomy is necessary when the large intestine has been removed. Fecal material from the ileum drains through an opening called a **stoma** into a bag worn on the abdomen (Fig. 9.18).

laparoscopy (lapar/o, abdominal wall + -scopy, visual examination) Examination of the abdominal cavity with a laparoscope through one or more small incisions in the abdominal wall. The procedure is done for inspection of abdominal organs, particularly the ovaries and uterine tubes, and also for laparoscopic surgeries, such as a laparoscopic cholecystectomy.

liver biopsy Removal of tissue from the liver for pathologic examination. A **percutaneous liver biopsy** is removal of liver tissue by using a needle to puncture the skin overlying the liver. This is considered to be a closed biopsy. (Percutaneous is derived from per-, through + cutane/o, skin + -ous, pertaining to.) An open liver biopsy involves incision of the abdominal wall to remove liver tissue for pathologic examination.

pancreatolithectomy (pancreat/o, pancreas + -lith, stone + -ectomy, excision) Excision of a pancreatic stone.

vagotomy (vag/o, vagus nerve + -tomy, incision) Resection (partial excision) of portions of the vagus nerve near the stomach. This procedure is performed to decrease the amount of gastric juices by severing the nerve (vagus nerve) that controls their release.

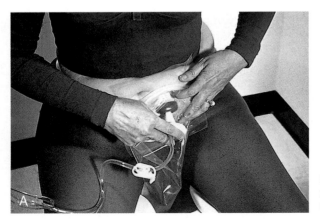

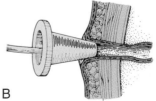

B

Fig. 9.18 Colostomy Irrigation. **A,** Patient places an irrigation cone in the stomal opening. **B,** Cone with irrigation tubing in place and instillation of fluid to promote evacuation of feces.

Match the procedures in the left column with their descriptions.

_____ 1. appendectomy
_____ 2. cholecystectomy
_____ 3. colostomy
_____ 4. esophagostomy
_____ 5. gastrectomy
_____ 6. gastric bypass
_____ 7. gastrostomy
_____ 8. laparoscopy

A. an opening from the colon through the abdominal wall
B. examination of the abdominal cavity through a small incision in the abdominal wall
C. excision of the gallbladder
D. new opening into the esophagus
E. new opening into the stomach
F. removal of the vermiform appendix
G. surgery performed to reduce the stomach's capacity
H. surgical removal of the stomach

QUICK CASE STUDY | EXERCISE 13

Define the underlined terms.

Gregory Harper is examined by Dr. Harry Malone, a <u>gastroenterologist</u>. Mr. Harper underwent an endoscopy last May that showed active <u>colitis</u>. His mother, deceased, had hemorrhoids, <u>gastrocele</u>, and <u>diabetes mellitus</u>. Rectal exam: Good tone, but painful. Assessment: Toxic colitis.

1. gastroenterologist _____
2. colitis _____
3. gastrocele _____
4. diabetes mellitus _____

! Be Careful With These!

-orexia (appetite) versus *-pepsia* (digestion)
choledoch/o (common bile duct) versus *cholecyst/o* (gallbladder)
elimination vs. emaciation
mucus vs. mucous
periodontics vs. periodontium
sialolithiasis vs. cholelithiasis

A Career as a Registered Dietician

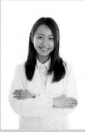

Maggie Sage is a registered dietician who works in a hospital. Maggie counsels patients about how the foods they eat affect disease processes such as diabetes and heart disease. She worked in food service management previously but decided she prefers the higher level of patient contact in clinical dietetics. Some of her friends work in sports dietetics; others counsel patients online. Maggie knows her work is vital to management of patients' conditions and that eating right is its own reward. For more information, visit the American Dietetic Association's website: www.eatright.org.

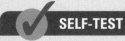 **SELF-TEST**

Work the following exercises to test your understanding of the material in Chapter 9. It is best to do all the exercises before checking your answers against the answers in Appendix III. Pay particular attention to spelling.

A. MATCHING!   Match the diagnostic test or procedure in the left column with the digestive structure in the right column that is the focus of study.

_____ 1. cholangiography   A. bile ducts
_____ 2. esophagram   B. esophagus
_____ 3. gastroscopy   C. rectum
_____ 4. proctoscopy   D. salivary ducts
_____ 5. sialography   E. stomach

B. MATCHING!   Match activities of the digestive system with their meanings.

_____ 1. absorption   A. mechanical and chemical breakdown of food
_____ 2. digestion   B. oral taking of substances into the body
_____ 3. elimination   C. passage of food molecules through the lining of the small intestine
_____ 4. ingestion   D. removal of undigested food particles

C. CHOOSING!   Circle the one correct answer (A, B, C, or D) for each question.

1. Mrs. Vogel's physician tells her that she needs to see a specialist for the problem that she's been having with her colon. What is the name of the specialty practiced by the physician Mrs. Vogel should see?
   (A) cardiology   (B) gastroenterology   (C) gynecology   (D) urology

2. Tests show that Cal S. has a gallstone in the common bile duct. Which of the following is a noninvasive conservative procedure to alleviate Cal's problem?
   (A) cholecystostomy   (B) choledochostomy   (C) choledochojejunostomy   (D) shock wave lithotripsy

3. Linda M., a 16-year-old girl, is diagnosed as having self-induced starvation. What is the name of the disorder associated with Linda's problem?
   (A) anorexia nervosa   (B) aphagia   (C) malaise   (D) polyphagia

4. Unless there is intervention for Linda's self-induced starvation, which condition will result?
   (A) adipsia   (B) atresia   (C) emaciation   (D) volvulus

5. Mary suffers from GERD. The physician explains to her that radiography indicates that a portion of the stomach is protruding upward through the diaphragm. What is the name of this disorder?
   (A) anorexia nervosa   (B) caries   (C) cholelith   (D) hiatal hernia

6. A 70-year-old woman has an obstruction that has led to stagnation of the normal movement of food in the intestinal tract. What is the name of this condition?
   (A) duodenitis   (B) enterostasis   (C) peptic ulcer   (D) peristalsis

7. Which term means a procedure that provides radiographic visualization of the bile and pancreatic ducts?
   (A) barium enema   (B) cholangiopancreatography   (C) gastrostomy   (D) sigmoidoscopy

8. Which of the following is the main source of energy for body cells?
   (A) fats   (B) glucose   (C) lactose   (D) starches

9. Which of the following is a disorder characterized by episodes of binge eating that are terminated by abdominal pain, sleep, self-induced vomiting, or purging with laxatives?
   (A) anorexia nervosa   (B) bulimia   (C) Crohn disease   (D) malabsorption syndrome

10. Which of the following is the name of the procedure in which the stomach is anastomosed with the duodenum?
    (A) gastrectasis   (B) gastrotomy   (C) gastroduodenostomy   (D) lithotripsy

D. WRITING!   *Write one-word terms for each of these meanings.*

1. a new opening into the jejunum _____

2. an appetite-suppressing drug _____

3. enzyme that breaks down starch _____

4. excessive vomiting _____

5. excision of a pancreatic stone _____

6. incision of the vagus nerve _____

7. inflammation of the stomach _____

8. pertaining to the esophagus _____

9. poor digestion _____

10. presence of a gallstone _____

E. SPELLING AND PRONUNCATION!   *Circle the incorrectly spelled terms, and write the correct spelling. Then pronounce the terms.*

cholangiograpfy   enterel   hepatik   nazojejunal   proctascope

_____

F. WRITING!   *Name the three major classes of nutrients and at least one example of an enzyme involved in breaking them down.*

1. _____
2. _____
3. _____

G. READING HEALTH CARE REPORTS

Read the medical report and answer the questions that follow it. Although you may be unfamiliar with some of the terms, you should be able to decide their meanings by determining the word parts.

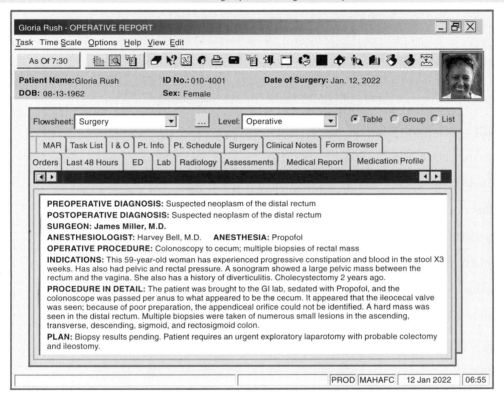

Circle the correct answer for each question.

1. To which body structure does the diagnosis pertain?
   (A) gallbladder   **(B)** large intestine   **(C)** small intestine   **(D)** stomach

2. Which of the following describes the rectum in the preoperative diagnosis?
   (A) abnormal new growth   **(B)** enlarged   **(C)** inflamed   **(D)** impacted with feces

3. The patient has a history of cholecystectomy. Which organ is removed in a cholecystectomy?
   (A) colon   **(B)** gallbladder   **(C)** liver   **(D)** small intestine

4. What structure is incised in a laparotomy?
   (A) abdominal wall   **(B)** cecum   **(C)** ileum   **(D)** umbilicus

5. All or part of which structure is excised in a colectomy?
   (A) large intestine   **(B)** small intestine   **(C)** stomach   **(D)** umbilicus

6. Where is the stoma created in an ileostomy?
   (A) abdomen   **(B)** anus   **(C)** colon   **(D)** umbilicus

7. Which of the following procedures is performed in a colonoscopy?
   (A) barium enema   **(B)** endoscopic examination   **(C)** liver function test   **(D)** radiographic examination

8. Which term in the report means inflammation of small pouches in the intestinal wall?
   (A) appendiceal orifice   **(B)** diverticulitis   **(C)** neoplasm   **(D)** rectal mass

H.   *Read the gastrointestinal consult and circle the correct answer in questions 1 through 4.*

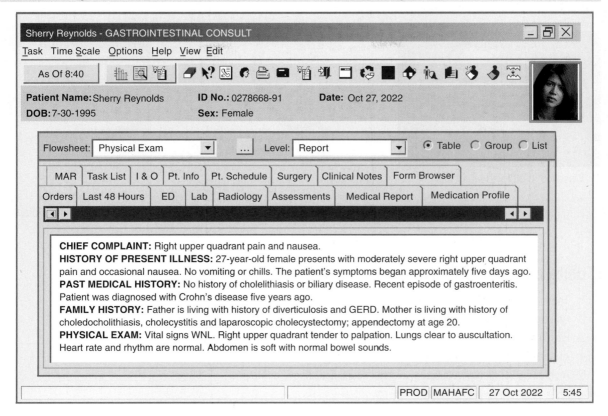

Sherry Reynolds - GASTROINTESTINAL CONSULT   — ⊡ ✕

Task Time Scale Options Help View Edit

As Of 8:40

Patient Name: Sherry Reynolds   **ID No.:** 0278668-91   **Date:** Oct 27, 2022
DOB: 7-30-1995   **Sex:** Female

Flowsheet: Physical Exam ▼ ... Level: Report ▼ ⦿ Table ○ Group ○ List

MAR | Task List | I & O | Pt. Info | Pt. Schedule | Surgery | Clinical Notes | Form Browser

Orders | Last 48 Hours | ED | Lab | Radiology | Assessments | Medical Report | Medication Profile

CHIEF COMPLAINT: Right upper quadrant pain and nausea.
HISTORY OF PRESENT ILLNESS: 27-year-old female presents with moderately severe right upper quadrant pain and occasional nausea. No vomiting or chills. The patient's symptoms began approximately five days ago.
PAST MEDICAL HISTORY: No history of cholelithiasis or biliary disease. Recent episode of gastroenteritis. Patient was diagnosed with Crohn's disease five years ago.
FAMILY HISTORY: Father is living with history of diverticulosis and GERD. Mother is living with history of choledocholithiasis, cholecystitis and laparoscopic cholecystectomy; appendectomy at age 20.
PHYSICAL EXAM: Vital signs WNL. Right upper quadrant tender to palpation. Lungs clear to auscultation. Heart rate and rhythm are normal. Abdomen is soft with normal bowel sounds.

PROD | MAHAFC | 27 Oct 2022 | 5:45

Circle the correct answer.

1. GERD indicates the patient's father suffered from a backflow of contents from the
   (A) esophagus   **(B)** small intestine   **(C)** stomach   **(D)** colon

2. Which term means pertaining to bile?
   (A) biliary   **(B)** cholecystitis   **(C)** diverticulosis   **(D)** quadrant

3. The term in the report that refers to a stone in the gallbladder is
   (A) cholecystectomy   **(B)** cholecystitis   **(C)** choledocholithiasis   **(D)** cholelithiasis

4. The term *gastroenteritis* indicates a disease involving the stomach and the
   (A) esophagus   **(B)** liver   **(C)** mouth   **(D)** small intestine

5. Which term means the presence of small sacs in the wall of an organ without inflammation?
   (A) Crohn's   **(B)** diverticulosis   **(C)** palpation   **(D)** quadrant

6. Cholecystitis is inflammation of the
   (A) duodenum   **(B)** gallbladder   **(C)** large intestine   **(D)** small intestine

7. What does the suffix in "appendectomy" mean?
   (A) excision   **(B)** inflammation   **(C)** incision   **(D)** ulceration

8. Which organ is excised in a cholecystectomy?
   (A) colon   **(B)** gallbladder   **(C)** liver   **(D)** pancreas

I. IDENTIFYING!   *Label these illustrations using one of the following: cholelithiasis, diverticulitis, hemorrhoidectomy, gastroduodenostomy, hiatal hernia*

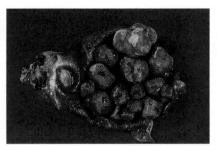

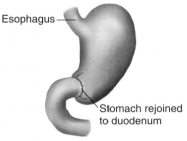

Esophagus

Stomach rejoined to duodenum

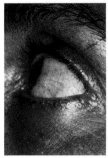

1. Presence of gallbladder stones

    _____

2. Anastomosis of the stomach and duodenum _____

3. A yellow discoloration of the skin, mucous membranes, and sclerae is _____

J. QUICK CHALLENGE!   *Find an incorrect term in each sentence and write the correct term.*

1. The mechanical and chemical breakdown of food is alimentation. _____

2. An enzyme that breaks down fat is a lipid._____

3. Pertaining to the membrane that surrounds the teeth is periodontal or glossal._____

4. An increased amount of fat in the blood is hypoglycemia._____

5. A chronic liver disease caused by alcohol abuse is alcoholic peritonitis._____

*Use Appendix III to check your answers.

🔊) QUICK & EASY (Q&E) LIST

Use the Evolve website (http://evolve.elsevier.com/Leonard/quick) to review the terms presented in Chapter 9. Look closely at the spelling of each term as it is pronounced.

absorption (ab-**sorp**-shun)
alimentary (al-uh-**men**-tur-ē)
alimentary tract (al-uh-**men**-tur-ē trakt)
alimentation (al-uh-men-**tā**-shun)
amylase (**am**-uh-lās)
anal (**ā**-nul)
anastomosis (uh-nas-tuh-**mō**-sis)
anorexia (an-ō-**rek**-sē-uh)
anorexia nervosa (an-ō-**rek**-sē-uh ner-**vō**-suh)
anorexiant (an-ō-**rek**-sē-unt)
antacid (ant-**as**-id)
antidiarrheal (an-tē-dī-uh-**rē**-ul)

antiemetic (an-tē-uh-**met**-ik)
anus (**ā**-nus)
appendectomy (ap-en-**dek**-tuh-mē)
appendicitis (uh-pen-di-**sī**-tis)
ascending colon (uh-**send**-ing **kō**-lun)
barium enema (**bar**-ē-um **en**-uh-muh)
barium swallow (**bar**-ē-um **swahl**-ō)
bicuspids (bī-**kus**-pids)
bile (bīl)
biliary (**bil**-ē-ar-ē)
biliary tract (**bil**-ē-ar-ē trakt)
bulimia (boo-**lē**-mē-uh)

QUICK & EASY (Q&E) LIST—cont'd

canker sores (*kang*-kur sorz)
carbohydrates (kahr-bō-*hī*-drāts)
cathartic (kuh-*thahr*-tik)
cecum (*sē*-kum)
cheilitis (kī-*lī*-tis)
cholangiogram (kō-*lan*-jē-ō-gram)
cholangiography (kō-lan-jē-*og*-ruh-fē)
cholangitis (kō-lan-*jī*-tis)
cholecystectomy (kō-luh-sis-*tek*-tuh-mē)
cholecystic (kō-luh-*sis*-tik)
cholecystitis (kō-luh-sis-*tī*-tis)
choledochal (kō-*led*-uh-kul)
choledocholithiasis (kō-led-uh-kō-li-*thī*-uh-sis)
cholelithiasis (kō-luh-li-*thī*-uh-sis)
cholestasis (kō-luh-*stā*-sis)
cirrhosis (si-*rō*-sis)
colitis (kō-*lī*-tis)
colon (*kō*-lun)
colonoscope (kō-*lon*-ō-skōp)
colonoscopy (kō-lun-*os*-kuh-pē)
coloscopy (kō-*los*-kō-pē)
colostomy (kuh-*los*-tuh-mē)
cuspids (*kus*-pids)
defecation (def-uh-*kā*-shun)
dehydration (dē-hī-*drā*-shun)
dental (*den*-tul)
descending colon (dē-*send*-ing *kō*-lun)
diabetes (dī-uh-*bē*-tēz)
diabetes mellitus (dī-uh-*bē*-tēz *mel*-luh-tus, muh-*lī*-tis)
diarrhea (dī-uh-*rē*-uh)
digestion (dī-*jes*-chun)
diverticulectomy (dī-vur-tik-ū-*lek*-tuh-mē)
diverticulitis (dī-vur-tik-ū-*lī*-tis)
diverticulosis (dī-vur-tik-ū-*lō*-sis)
diverticulum (dī-vur-*tik*-ū-lum)
duodenal (dōō-ō-*dē*-nul, dōō-*od*-uh-nul)
duodenal ulcer (dōō-ō-*dē*-nul, dōō-*od*-uh-nul *ul*-sur)
duodenitis (dōō-od-uh-*nī*-tis)
duodenum (dōō-ō-*dē*-num, dōō-*od*-uh-num)
dysentery (*dis*-un-ter-ē)
dyspepsia (dis-*pep*-sē-uh)
dysphagia (dis-*fā*-jē-uh)
elimination (ē-lim-i-*nā*-shun)
emaciation (ē-mā-shē-*ā*-shun)
emesis (*em*-uh-sis)
emetics (uh-*met*-iks)
endodontics (en-dō-*don*-tiks)
endogastric (en-dō-*gas*-trik)
enteral (*en*-tur-ul)
enterostasis (en-tur-ō-*stā*-sis)

enzymes (*en*-zīms)
esophageal (uh-sof-uh-*jē*-ul)
esophageal varices (uh-sof-uh-*jē*-ul *var*-i-sēz)
esophagitis (uh-sof-uh-*jī*-tis)
esophagogram (uh-*sof*-uh-gō-gram)
esophagoscopy (uh-sof-uh-*gos*-kuh-pē)
esophagostomy (uh-sof-uh-*gos*-tuh-mē)
esophagram (uh-*sof*-uh-gram)
esophagus (uh-*sof*-uh-gus)
eupepsia (ū-*pep*-sē-uh)
flatulence (*flat*-ū-luns)
gallstone (*gawl*-stōn)
gastralgia (gas-*tral*-juh)
gastrectomy (gas-*trek*-tuh-mē)
gastric (*gas*-trik)
gastric bypass (*gas*-trik *bī*-pas)
gastric lavage (*gas*-trik lah-*vahzh*)
gastritis (gas-*trī*-tis)
gastrocele (*gas*-trō-sēl)
gastroduodenostomy (gas-trō-dōō-ō-duh-*nos*-tuh-mē)
gastrodynia (gas-trō-*din*-ē-uh)
gastroenteritis (gas-trō-en-tur-*ī*-tis)
gastroenterologist (gas-trō-en-tur-*ol*-uh-jist)
gastroenterology (gas-trō-en-tur-*ol*-uh-jē)
gastroesophageal reflux disease (gas-trō-e-sof-uh-*jē*-ul rē-fluks di-*zēz*)
gastrointestinal (gas-trō-in-*tes*-ti-nul)
gastroplasty (*gas*-trō-plas-tē)
gastroscopy (gas-*tros*-kuh-pē)
gastrostomy (gas-*tros*-tuh-mē)
gestational diabetes mellitus (jes-*tā*-shun-ul dī-uh-*bē*-tēz *mel*-luh-tus, muh-*lī*-tis)
gingiva (*jin*-ji-vuh)
gingival (*jin*-ji-vul)
gingivitis (jin-ji-*vī*-tis)
glossal (*glos*-ul)
glossitis (glos-*ī*-tis)
glucose (*glōō*-kōs)
glycosuria (glī-kō-*sū*-rē-uh)
hemorrhoid (*hem*-uh-roid)
hemorrhoidectomy (hem-uh-roid-*ek*-tuh-mē)
hepatic (huh-*pat*-ik)
hepatitis (hep-uh-*tī*-tis)
hepatomegaly (hep-uh-tō-*meg*-uh-lē)
hepatotoxic (*hep*-uh-tō-tok-sik)
hiatal hernia (hī-*ā*-tul *hur*-nē-uh)
hyperacidity (hī-pur-uh-*sid*-i-tē)
hyperemesis (hī-pur-*em*-uh-sis)
hyperglycemia (hī-pur-glī-*sē*-mē-uh)
hyperlipemia (hī-pur-li-*pē*-mē-uh)

QUICK & EASY (Q&E) LIST—cont'd

hyperlipidemia *(hī-pur-lip-i-**dē**-mē-uh)*
hypoglossal *(hī-pō-**glos**-ul)*
hypoglycemia *(hī-pō-glī-**sē**-mē-uh)*
ileocecal *(il-ē-ō-**sē**-kul)*
ileostomy *(il-ē-**os**-tuh-mē)*
ileum *(**il**-ē-um)*
incisors *(in-**sī**-zurs)*
ingestion *(in-**jes**-chun)*
inguinal *(**ing**-gwi-nul)*
insulin *(**in**-suh-lin)*
intestinal *(in-**tes**-ti-nul)*
irritable bowel syndrome *(**ir**-i-tuh-bul **bou**-ul **sin**-drōm)*
jaundice *(**jawn**-dis)*
jejunostomy *(je-jō̄ō-**nos**-tuh-mē)*
jejunum *(juh-**jō̄ō**-num)*
lactase *(**lak**-tās)*
lactose *(**lak**-tōs)*
laparoscopic cholecystectomy *(lap-uh-rō-**skop**-ik kō-luh-sis-**tek**-tuh-mē)*
laparoscopy *(lap-uh-**ros**-kuh-pē)*
laser lithotripsy *(**lā**-zur **lith**-ō-trip-sē)*
laxative *(**lak**-suh-tiv)*
lingual *(**ling**-gwul)*
lipase *(**lip**-ās, **lī**-pās)*
lipid *(**lip**-id)*
liver biopsy *(**liv**-ur **bī**-op-sē)*
lower gastrointestinal bleeding *(**lō**-ur gas-trō-in-**tes**-ti-nul **blēd**-ing)*
malabsorption syndrome *(mal-ub-**sorp**-shun **sin**-drōm)*
malnutrition *(mal-nō̄ō-**trish**-un)*
mandible *(**man**-di-bul)*
mandibular *(man-**dib**-ū-lur)*
metabolism *(muh-**tab**-uh-liz-um)*
molars *(**mō**-lurz)*
mucous *(**mū**-kus)*
mucus *(**mū**-kus)*
nasoduodenal *(nā-zō-dō̄ō-ō-**dē**-nul)*
nasogastric *(nā-zō-**gas**-trik)*
nasojejunal *(nā-zō-juh-**jō̄ō**-nul)*
nutrition *(nō̄ō-**tri**-shun)*
obesity *(ō-**bēs**-i-tē)*
oral *(**or**-ul)*
orthodontics *(or-thō-**don**-tiks)*

orthodontist *(or-thō-**don**-tist)*
pancreatitis *(pan-krē-uh-**tī**-tis)*
pancreatolith *(pan-krē-**at**-ō-lith)*
pancreatolithectomy *(pan-krē-uh-tō-li-**thek**-tuh-mē)*
pancreatolithiasis *(pan-krē-uh-tō-li-**thī**-uh-sis)*
pedodontics *(pē-dō-**don**-tiks)*
percutaneous liver biopsy *(pur-kū-**tā**-nē-us **liv**-ur **bī**-op-sē)*
periodontal *(per-ē-ō-**don**-tul)*
periodontics *(per-ē-ō-**don**-tiks)*
periodontium *(per-ē-ō-**don**-shē-um)*
peritoneum *(per-i-tō-**nē**-um)*
peritonitis *(per-i-tō-**nī**-tis)*
pharynx *(**far**-inks)*
polydipsia *(pol-ē-**dip**-sē-uh)*
polyphagia *(pol-ē-**fā**-juh)*
polyuria *(pol-ē-**ū**-rē-uh)*
proctologist *(prok-**tol**-uh-jist)*
proctoscope *(**prok**-tō-skōp)*
proctoscopy *(prok-**tos**-kuh-pē)*
protease *(**prō**-tē-ās)*
protein *(**prō**-tēn)*
proteinase *(**prō**-tēn-ās)*
purgative *(**pur**-guh-tiv)*
rectal *(**rek**-tul)*
rectum *(**rek**-tum)*
saliva *(suh-**lī**-vuh)*
salivary *(**sal**-i-var-ē)*
shock wave lithotripsy *(shok wāv **lith**-ō-trip-sē)*
sialography *(sī-uh-**log**-ruh-fē)*
sialolithiasis *(sī-uh-lō-li-**thī**-uh-sis)*
sigmoid colon *(**sig**-moid **kō**-lun)*
sigmoidoscopy *(sig-moi-**dos**-kuh-pē)*
stoma *(**stō**-muh)*
stomatitis *(stō-muh-**tī**-tis)*
sublingual *(sub-**ling**-gwul)*
transverse colon *(trans-**vurs kō**-lon)*
ulcer *(**ul**-sur)*
upper gastrointestinal bleeding *(**up**-ur gas-trō-in-**tes**-ti-nul **blēd**-ing)*
vagotomy *(vā-**got**-uh-mē)*
vermiform appendix *(**vur**-mi-form uh-**pen**-diks)*
viscera *(**vis**-ur-uh)*
visceral *(**vis**-ur-ul)*

Don't forget the games and other activities available at http://evolve.elsevier.com/Leonard/quick.

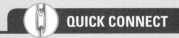

Review all lists of word parts and their meanings for this chapter using the flashcards you prepared or the flashcards on the Evolve site.

Function: To provide the body with water, nutrients, and minerals. Alimentation provides nutrition (nourishment) for the body that is used for metabolism (growth, energy, and elimination of wastes). Activities of the digestive system include ingestion, absorption, digestion, and elimination.

Three major classes of nutrients: carbohydrates, proteins and lipids (fats), all requiring enzymes (-ase) to break them down into simpler substances.

Carbohydrates (mainly sugars and starches) are the basic source of energy for cells. Know the enzyme responsible for breaking down lactose, glucose, starch, protein, and fats.

THE DIGESTIVE TRACT (ALIMENTARY TRACT AND SEVERAL ACCESSORY ORGANS):

Alimentary tract: mouth, pharynx, esophagus, stomach, small intestine (duodenum, jejunum, and ileum), and large intestine (cecum, colon, rectum, anal canal ending at he anus for excretion of wastes). Vermiform appendix extends from the cecum. Differentiate these two terms: gastroenterologist vs. proctologist.

Mouth: know the meaning of gingival, glossal/lingual, and dental. Permanent teeth are incisors, cuspids, bicuspids, and molars). Differentiate dental specialties: endodontics, orthodontics, pedodontics, and periodontics.

Accessory organs of digestion: salivary glands, liver, gallbladder, and pancreas. Adjectives relating to these organs are salivary, hepatic, cholecystic (for storage of bile), and pancreatic. Related secretions of the salivary glands, liver, and pancreas plus the substances they break down are, respectively: amylase (starch into sugars), bile (fats) and pancreatic juice (digestive enzymes), and insulin (regulates blood sugar).

Diseases, disorders, and diagnostic terms: Know the meanings and differentiate the names of disorders vs. diagnostic procedures: esophagram, barium swallow and barium enema, jaundice, cholelithiasis, choledocholithiasis, pancreatolithiasis, cholangiopancreatography, sialography, esophagoscopy, gastroscopy, colonoscopy, sigmoidoscopy, diabetes mellitus vs. gestational diabetes mellitus, hyperglycemia, polyphagia, polyuria, polydipsia, glycosuria, hypoglycemia, hyperlipemia, obesity, hyperemesis, dehydration, emaciation, anorexia nervosa, bulimia, malnutrition, malabsorption syndrome, flatulence.

Know the meanings of appendicitis, hepatitis, cirrhosis, jaundice, cholangitis, pancreatolith, sialolithiasis, eupepsia vs. dyspepsia, viscera, peritoneum, peritonitis, hernias including umbilical and inguinal hernias).

Can you differentiate these terms pertaining to the mouth? canker sores vs. gingivitis; glossitis vs. cheilitis vs. stomatitis.

Understand these terms as they relate to the esophagus? dysphagia, varices, esophagitis, GERD.

Do you know the difference in these terms related to the stomach? gastritis, gastrocele, gastroenteritis, hiatal hernia, hyperacidity, ulcer, upper intestinal bleeding.

Differentiate these terms related to the intestines: appendicitis, colitis, diverticulitis, diverticulum, diverticulosis, duodenal ulcer, duodenitis, dysentery, enterostasis, hemorrhoids, irritable bowel syndrome, lower intestinal bleeding (hemorrhoids, diverticulosis vs. diverticulitis, ulcerative colitis, polyps, colon cancer).

Know the difference in cholecystitis, cholelithiasis, and cholestasis.

Do you understand the difference in cirrhosis and hepatitis? How does the term *hepatomegaly* relate to these disorders?

Understand the relationship of the pancreas to diabetes, hypoglycemia, and pancreatitis.

Know the meanings of these approaches to weight loss and which are conservative and which are extreme (including surgery): restricted food intake, increased exercise, anorexiant, gastroplasty, gastric bypass, diverticulectomy.

Understand the meaning of the following: anorexiant, antidiarrheals, antiemetics, emetics, insulin, laxatives, purgatives or cathartics.

Differentiate these surgical procedures: Gastroplasty repairs any stomach defect, while gastric bypass is used for weight loss to reduce the stomach capacity.

Know the difference in a nasogastric, nasoduodenal, or nasojejunal tube vs. esophagostomy, gastrostomy, or jejunostomy. Differentiate shock wave lithotripsy vs. laparoscopic cholecystectomy.

Know the meanings of appendectomy, cholecystectomy, colostomy,

What is the difference between gastrectomy and gastrostomy? What is the relationship of a gastrectomy to gastroduodenostomy? How is anastomosis related to these terms?

Differentiate these terms: hemorrhoidectomy, ileostomy, laparoscopy, percutaneous liver biopsy, pancreatolithectomy, stoma, and vagotomy.

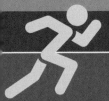

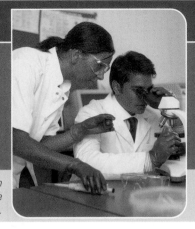

CHAPTER 10

Urinary System

Medical laboratory technicians (MLTs) work under the supervision of a medical technologist or physician. Analyzing urine is just one of the many tasks they perform.

OBJECTIVES

After completing Chapter 10, you will be able to:

1. Recognize or write the functions of the urinary system.
2. Recognize or write the meanings of Chapter 10 word parts and use them to build and analyze terms.
3. Write terms for selected structures of the urinary system or match them with their descriptions.
4. Write the names of the diagnostic terms and pathologies related to the urinary system when

given their descriptions, or match terms with their meanings.
5. Match surgical and therapeutic interventions for the urinary system, or write the interventions when given their descriptions.
6. Spell terms for the urinary system correctly.

 Function First

The body produces wastes that are eliminated by the process of **excretion**. The body eliminates waste in several ways. The lungs and other parts of the respiratory system eliminate carbon dioxide; the digestive system rids the body of solid waste; and the skin eliminates wastes through perspiration. Through urination, the urinary system eliminates waste products that accumulate as a result of cellular metabolism. **Urin+ation** is the act of voiding.

Excretion of wastes to maintain the volume and chemical composition of blood is only one function of the urinary system. Most of the work of this body system takes place in the kidneys. The functions of the kidneys include the following:

- Maintenance of an appropriate blood volume by varying the excretion of water in the urine
- Maintenance of the chemical composition of blood by selecting certain chemicals to excrete
- Maintenance of blood pH
- Excretion of waste products of protein metabolism
- Regulation of blood pressure
- Stimulation of erythrocyte production by secretion of **erythro+poietin**

 QUICK TIP

pH, "potential" hydrogen (hydrogen ion concentration) of a solution is its relative acidity or alkalinity.

erythr/o = red
-poietin = substance that causes production

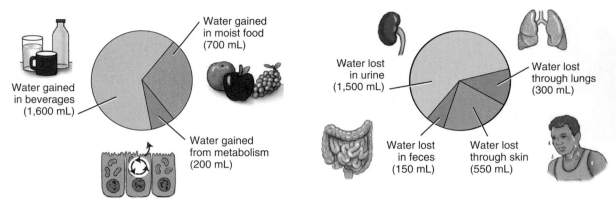

Fig. 10.1 Fluid Intake and Output. Generally, fluid intake equals fluid output, so the total amount of body fluid remains constant.

Excretion of waste products by the kidneys is vital for good health. **Urea** is the final product of protein metabolism and the major nitrogenous waste product in urine.

Fluid intake generally equals output (Fig. 10.1). The kidneys are the main regulators of fluid loss. Water is the most important constituent of the body and essential to every process. Depriving the body of needed water eventually leads to dehydration.

ur/o = urinary tract
-logy = science of

Uro+logy is the branch of medicine concerned with the male genital tract and the urinary tracts of both genders, and the specialist is a **urologist**.

WRITE IT!* EXERCISE 1

Write a word in each blank to complete the functions of the urinary system.

1. excretion of _____ in urine to maintain blood volume
2. maintaining the chemical composition of _____ by selecting certain chemicals to excrete
3. maintaining the blood pH, also called the "potential" _____
4. excretion of _____ products of protein metabolism
5. regulation of blood _____
6. secretion of _____ to stimulate erythrocyte production

*Use Appendix III, Answers, to check your answers to all the exercises in Chapter 10.

Many word parts in the following table are used to write terms about the urinary system. Commit to memory the word parts and their meanings.

WORD PARTS ASSOCIATED WITH THE URINARY SYSTEM

Word Part	Meaning	Word Part	Meaning
albumin/o	albumin	olig/o	few, scanty
-ation	process	ur/o	urine or urinary tract
-esis	action, process, or result of	urin/o	urine
glycos/o	sugar	-uria	urine or urination

Use the electronic flashcards on the Evolve site or make your own set of flashcards using the above list. Select the word parts just presented, and study them until you know their meanings. Do this each time a set of word parts is presented.

MATCH IT!
EXERCISE 2

Match the word parts in the left column with their meanings.

_____ 1. -ation   **A.** action, process, or result of
_____ 2. -esis   **B.** few, scanty
_____ 3. glycos/o   **C.** process
_____ 4. olig/o   **D.** sugar
_____ 5. ur/o   **E.** urine or urination
_____ 6. -uria   **F.** urine or urinary tract

Structures of the Urinary Tract

The urinary system is frequently called the urinary tract because its parts are arranged in a series and serve a common function to produce and eliminate urine. **Urin+ary** means pertaining to urine or the formation of urine. The urinary tract is composed of two kidneys, a ureter for each kidney, a bladder and a urethra. Label these structures as you read the legend for Fig. 10.2.

The bean-shaped, purplish-brown kidneys are located in the dorsal part of the abdomen, one on each side of the spinal column. Each kidney functions independently of the other.

Urine leaves the kidneys by way of the **ureters**. Both ureters lead to the urinary bladder, where urine is stored. The filling of the bladder with urine stimulates receptors, producing the urge to urinate. Voluntary control prevents urine from being released. When this control is removed, urine is expelled through a canal called the **urethra**. The external opening of the urethra is the urinary meatus.

> **urin/o** = urine
> **-ary** = pertaining to

>  **QUICK TIP**
> Kidneys and kidney beans have similar shapes.

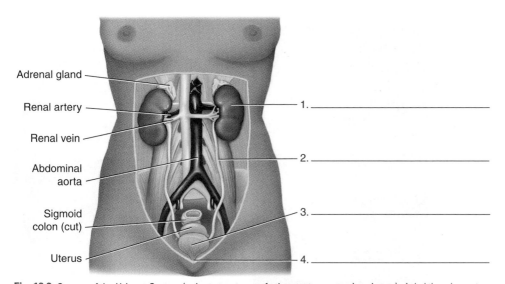

Adrenal gland
Renal artery
Renal vein
Abdominal aorta
Sigmoid colon (cut)
Uterus

1. _____
2. _____
3. _____
4. _____

Fig. 10.2 Organs of the Urinary System (select structures of other systems are also shown). Label the urinary structures as you read this explanation. Urine, formed in the right kidney and left kidney *(1)*, leaves by way of the ureters. Label the left ureter *(2)*. The bladder *(3)* is a temporary reservoir for the urine until it is excreted through the urethra *(4)*.

> **urin/o** = urine
> **-ary** = pertaining to

Combining forms for major structures of the urinary system are presented in the following table.

WORD PARTS: STRUCTURES OF THE URINARY SYSTEM	
Combining Form	**Name of Structure**
cyst/o	bladder (sometimes cyst or sac)
glomerul/o	glomerulus (filtering structure of the kidney)
nephr/o, ren/o	kidney
pyel/o	renal pelvis (reservoir in the kidney that collects the urine)
ureter/o	ureter
urethr/o	urethra

The adjectives **ren+al**, **ureter+al**, and **urethr+al** mean pertaining to the kidney, ureter, and urethra, respectively. **Cyst+ic** has several meanings, including pertaining to a cyst, pertaining to the gallbladder, and pertaining to the urinary bladder. The rest of the sentence must usually be read to determine the intended meaning of the word *cystic*. Used alone, bladder usually refers to the urinary bladder.

Most of the work of the urinary system takes place in the kidneys. The other components serve to save some substances and eliminate urine from the body. Anatomic features of the kidney are shown in Fig. 10.3. A kidney is encased in a fibrous capsule, which provides protection for the delicate internal parts of the kidney. The ribs and muscle also provide protection from direct trauma. The renal pelvis is a funnel-shaped structure located in the center of each kidney. Each renal pelvis drains urine from the kidney to its particular ureter. Blood enters a kidney via the renal artery and leaves through the renal vein.

cyst/o = urinary bladder or a cyst or a sac

fibr/o = fiber
-ous = characterized by

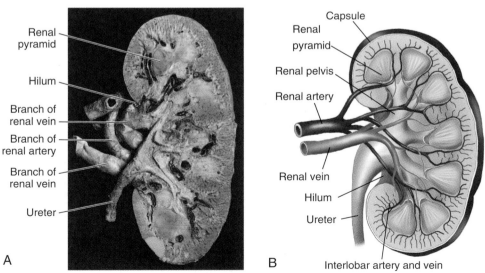

Fig. 10.3 Longitudinal Section Through the Kidney. **A,** Cross section of an excised kidney. **B,** Longitudinal drawing of a kidney.

Match the word parts in the two left columns with their meanings (choices may be used more than once).

_____ 1. cyst/o　　　_____ 4. ren/o
_____ 2. nephr/o　　_____ 5. ureter/o
_____ 3. pyel/o　　　_____ 6. urethr/o

A. bladder
B. kidney
C. renal pelvis
D. ureter
E. urethra

Match the terms in the left column with their meanings.

_____ 1. urinary bladder
_____ 2. renal pelvis
_____ 3. ureter
_____ 4. urethra

A. funnel-shaped structure located in the center of each kidney
B. where urine is stored until urination
C. tube through which urine passes from the kidney
D. tubular passage by which urine is discharged from the bladder

A kidney contains approximately 1 million microscopic **nephrons**, its functional unit. Each nephron resembles a microscopic funnel with a long stem and tubular sections, called the **tubules** (Fig. 10.4). A **glomerulus** is a cluster of blood vessels surrounded by a structure called Bowman's capsule. The proxim+al tubule is that part of the tubule nearer the glomerulus. Follow the long twisting tubule. Notice that a tubule consists of a proximal tubule, the loop of Henle, and a dist+al tubule that opens into a collecting duct.

glomerul/o = glomerulus

proxim/o = near
dist/o = far

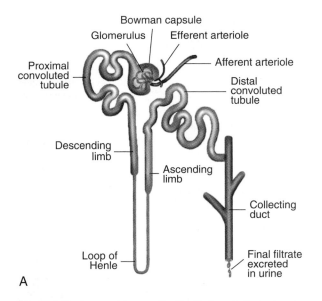
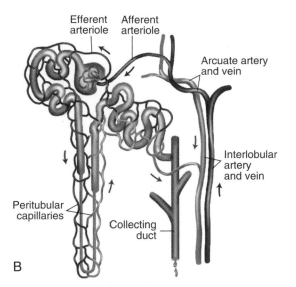

Fig. 10.4 Nephron and Surrounding Capillaries. **A,** The nephron is composed of a glomerulus and tubules. **B,** As the filtrate passes through the tubular portion of the nephron, reabsorption of variable quantities of water, electrolytes, and other substances occurs across the tubule walls into blood capillaries nearby.

inter- = between
peri- = around

QUICK TIP

Filtering System
1. Filter
2. Reabsorb
3. Secrete

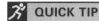

QUICK TIP

reabsorption, the process of being absorbed back into the blood

The kidneys constantly filter the blood, selectively reabsorb some substances, and secrete waste into the urine. These functions directly relate to urine formation:

- Filtering of the blood = **glomerular filtration**, the initial process in the formation of urine. The glomerulus allows water, salts, wastes, and most other substances, except blood cells and proteins, to pass through its thin walls.
- Selective reabsorption of some substances = **tubular reabsorption**. Bowman's capsule collects the substances that filter through the glomerular walls and passes them to a long, twisted tube called a tubule. As fluid passes through the tubules, substances that the body conserves, such as sugar and much of the water, are reabsorbed into the blood vessels surrounding the tubules. The water and other substances remaining in the tubule become urine.
- Secretion of substances into the urine = **tubular secretion**. The third process in urine formation is the secretion of some substances from the bloodstream into the renal tubule (waste products of metabolism that become toxic if they are not excreted and certain drugs, such as penicillin). These three processes—glomerular filtration, tubular reabsorption, and tubular secretion—are summarized in Fig. 10.5.

Waste products and some of the water remaining in the tubules after reabsorption combine to become urine, which passes to the collecting duct. Thousands of collecting ducts deposit urine in the renal pelvis, the large central reservoir of the kidney, where it drains to the bladder by way of the ureters. The bladder is a collapsible muscular bag that stores the urine until it is expelled by urination, also called voiding.

Anti+diuretic hormone (ADH) increases the reabsorption of water by the renal tubules, thus decreasing the amount of urine produced. ADH is secreted by special brain cells and released as needed.

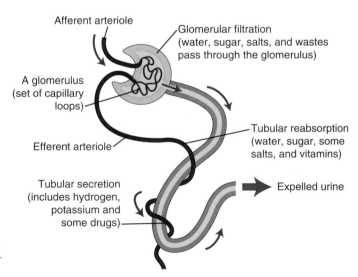

Fig. 10.5 Functions of the Nephron. Glomerular filtration *(upper right)*, tubular reabsorption, and tubular secretion *(lower left.)*

QUICK REVIEW!

Primary structures of the urinary system are the right and left kidneys, right and left ureters, the bladder, and the urethra (review Fig. 10.2). Functions of the nephrons within the kidneys include:
1. glomerular filtration   2. tubular reabsorption   3. tubular secretion

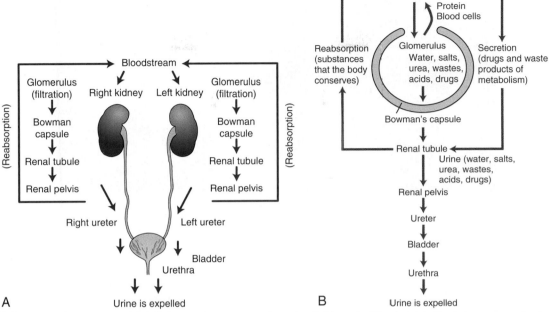

Fig. 10.6 Forming and Expelling Urine. **A,** Diagram of forming and expelling urine. **B,** Schematic of filtration of the blood, the processes of reabsorption and secretion, and expelling urine.

All the blood in the body passes through the kidneys several times every hour, but only about one-fifth is routed through the nephrons (Fig. 10.6).

WRITE IT! EXERCISE 5

List the three processes in urine formation.

1. _____

2. _____

3. _____

Diseases, Disorders, and Diagnostic Terms

Several urine tests are used to evaluate the status of the urinary system. A **urinalysis** (U/A, UA) is usually part of a physical examination but is particularly useful for patients with suspected urologic disorders. The complete urinalysis generally includes physical, chemical, and microscopic examinations performed in the clinical laboratory. Simple urine tests can provide valuable information about a person's health (Fig. 10.7). Many substances for which urine is tested are not found in a normal urine specimen (e.g., sugar, protein, and blood). The presence of one of these substances in urine is called **glycos+uria**, **protein+uria**, or **hemat+uria**, respectively. The term **albumin+uria** is sometimes used instead of proteinuria when there is a very high concentration of albumin, a type of protein, in the urine. **Py+uria** is the presence of pus in the urine.

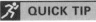

QUICK TIP

A urinalysis was originally called a urine analysis.

glycos/o = sugar
hemat/o = blood
py/o = pus
-uria = urine

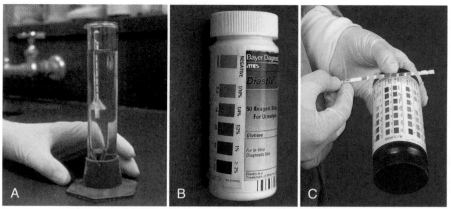

Fig. 10.7 Simple Urine Tests. **A,** A urinometer is used to determine the specific gravity (density) of a sample of urine. **B,** Glucose test strips screen for the presence of glucose in the urine. **C,** Testing urine with a Multistix, a plastic strip with reagent areas for testing various chemical constituents that may be present in the urine. These reagent strips are considered qualitative tests, and a positive result for an abnormal substance in the urine generally requires further testing.

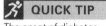

QUICK TIP

The onset of diabetes mellitus is sudden in children.

Ketone bodies are end products of lipid (fat) metabolism in the body. Excessive production of ketone bodies, however, leads to **keton+uria**, the presence of ketones in the urine. Ketones are found in the urine when the body's fat stores are metabolized for energy, thus providing an excess of metabolic end products. This can occur in uncontrolled diabetes mellitus because of a deficiency of insulin. **Diabetes mellitus** is an endocrine disorder characterized by glycosuria and hyperglycemia (increased level of glucose in the blood) and results from inadequate production or use of insulin.

The microscopic study of a healthy urine sample sometimes shows a few red blood cells and white blood cells. Except in a menstruating woman, the presence of many red blood cells is abnormal (Fig. 10.8, *A*). The presence of a large number of white blood cells may be indicative of an infectious or inflammatory process somewhere in the urinary tract (Fig. 10.8, *B*).

There are normally very few bacteria in freshly collected urine. The presence of many bacteria may indicate a urinary tract infection (UTI). If the patient has symptoms of a UTI, the physician often orders a urine culture and an antibiotic sensitivity test to determine which drugs are effective in killing or stopping growth of the bacteria.

Specific instructions determine the collection of urine specimens.

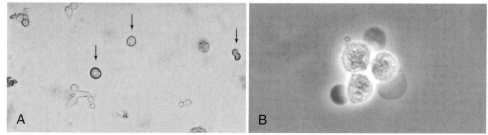

Fig. 10.8 Increased Number of Red Blood Cells and White Blood Cells in a Microscopic Examination of Urine. **A,** Red blood cells *(arrows).* **B,** White blood cells (nucleated cells are shown).

- A *voided* specimen is one in which the patient voids (urinates) into a container supplied by the laboratory or physician's office. Because improperly collected urine may yield incorrect test results, voided urine should always be collected by using the "clean-catch midstream" technique. This technique is based on the concept that the tissues adjacent to the urethral opening must be cleansed before collection to avoid contamination of the specimen, and only the middle portion of the urine stream is collected.
- A catheterized urine specimen is obtained by placing a catheter in the bladder and withdrawing urine. This may be necessary to obtain an uncontaminated urine specimen. In urinary catheterization, a catheter is inserted through the urethra and into the bladder for temporary or longer-term drainage of urine. Urinary catheterization may be done to collect a urine specimen and for other reasons, including urinary testing, instillation of medications into the bladder, and drainage of the bladder during many types of surgeries or in cases of urinary obstruction or paralysis.

Blood urea nitrogen (BUN), a measure of the amount of urea in the blood, is directly related to the metabolic function of the liver and the excretory function of the kidneys. A critically elevated BUN level indicates serious impairment of renal function. Another substance, creatinine, is measured in blood and urine as an indicator of kidney function.

Adequate blood circulation is essential for normal renal function, and anything that interferes with the normal circulation significantly reduces renal capabilities. **Renal angiography (renal arteriography)** is a radiographic study to assess the arterial blood supply to the kidneys. This procedure requires injection of a radiopaque contrast agent into the renal arteries by a catheter; the record produced is a **renal arteriogram**. An example of **stenosis** (constriction or narrowing) of the right renal artery is shown in Fig. 10.9. A kidney scan also provides information about renal blood flow. In this procedure, radioactive material is intravenously injected and is absorbed by kidney tissue. Special equipment measures, records, and produces an image of the low-level radioactivity that is emitted.

Nephro+**tomo**+**graphy**, sectional radiographic examination of the kidneys, generally using contrast dyes, provides images called **nephrotomograms** (Fig. 10.10); however,

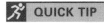

QUICK TIP

catheter = an instrument
catheterize (a verb)
catheterization (a noun)
catheterized (an adjective)

QUICK TIP

Complete renal failure, without treatment, leads to death.

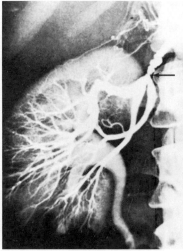

Fig. 10.9 Renal arteriogram showing stenosis *(red arrow)* of the right renal artery.
ren/o = kidney;   **arteri/o** = artery

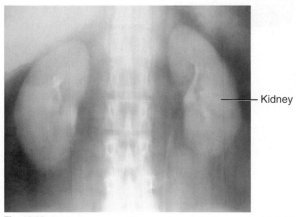

Fig. 10.10 Nephrotomogram. The procedure, nephrotomography, is helpful in assessing various frontal planes of kidney tissue for tumors, cysts, or stones.
nephr/o = kidney;   **tom/o** = to cut;   **-gram** = a record;   **-graphy** = process of recording

Kidney

these have generally been replaced by CT and nephrosonography. Other radiologic and endoscopic procedures are described in the programmed learning section that follows and in the listings on pp. 281 and 282.

WRITE IT! **EXERCISE 6**

Write a term for each description.

1. presence of albumin in the urine _____
2. presence of blood in the urine _____
3. presence of ketones in the urine _____
4. presence of pus in the urine _____
5. presence of sugar in the urine _____
6. sectional radiographic examination of kidneys _____
7. act of obtaining a catheterized urine specimen _____
8. analysis of urine _____

Programmed Learning

Remember to cover the answers (left column) with folded paper or the bookmark. Write an answer in each blank, and then check your answer before proceeding to the next frame.

kidney	1. **Nephro+malacia** is softening of the _____.
enlargement	2. **Nephro+megaly** is _____ of one or both kidneys. Bilateral nephromegaly is enlargement of both kidneys. Lateral pertains to a side. Bi+lateral (bi-, two) means pertaining to two sides—in other words, both sides. Nephromegaly and many other structural abnormalities of the kidneys (e.g., tumors or cancer) can be observed by **nephro+sonography**, which is ultrasonic scanning of the kidneys.
many	3. **Poly/cyst/ic kidney disease**, one of the more common hereditary renal disorders, is characterized by enlarged kidneys containing many fluid-filled cysts. Poly/cystic means containing _____ cysts. See Fig. 10.11 for comparison of a polycystic kidney and a normal kidney.

poly- = many
cyst/o = cyst or bladder

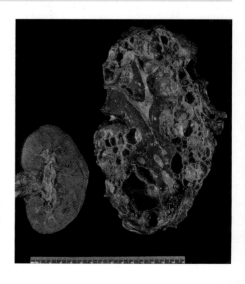

Fig. 10.11 Normal Sectioned Kidney Compared With Polycystic Kidney. The kidney on the left side of the photograph is from a transplant kidney of normal size. The kidney on the right is the native kidney from a patient with adult-onset polycystic kidney disease. The diseased kidney is greatly enlarged (nephromegaly) because of the replacement of normal kidney tissue by cysts of varying sizes.

nephroptosis

4. Remembering that -ptosis means sagging or prolapse, use nephr/o to write a word that means prolapse of a kidney: _____. This is also called a hypermobile (hyper-, excessive) or floating kidney. Nephroptosis can occur when the kidney supports are weakened by a sudden strain or blow, or it can be present at birth.

stones

5. **Urolithiasis** is the presence of urinary stones, most often found in the renal pelvis or the urinary bladder. **Cystolithiasis** is the presence of a stone or stones in the urinary bladder (Fig. 10.12). **Nephro+lith+iasis** is a condition marked by the presence of kidney _____. Stones and an enlarged prostate gland are common causes of urinary tract obstructions.

renal

6. **Nephro+lith** is a word, but kidney stones are usually called **renal calculi**. Notice that nephr/o is used more often in building medical terms, but ren/o is used to write an adjective that means pertaining to the kidney. Write that adjective: _____.

kidney

7. In a renal transplant, the recipient receives a _____ from a donor.

renal

8. Pelvis means any basin-shaped structure or cavity. Standing alone, pelvis usually refers to the bony structure that serves as a support for the spinal column. When referring to the funnel-shaped cavity of the kidney, it is called the _____ pelvis.

pyelitis

9. Write a word that means inflammation of the renal pelvis: _____.

glomeruli

10. **Nephritis**, also called Bright disease, is inflammation of the kidney. The most common form of acute nephritis is **glomerulo+nephritis**, in which _____ (plural of glomerulus) of the kidney are inflamed.

urogram

11. In **intravenous uro+graphy**, a contrast medium is injected intravenously, and serial x-ray films are taken as the medium passes through the urinary structures. This provides information about the structure and function of the kidney, ureters, and bladder (Fig. 10.13). The image produced in urography is a _____.

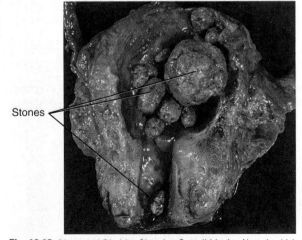

Stones

Fig. 10.12 Dissected Bladder Showing Cystolithiasis. Note the thickening of the bladder wall (signifying inflammation) and the presence of numerous stones in the urinary bladder; one stone has moved to the urethra.

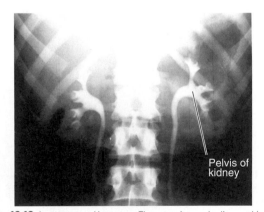

Pelvis of kidney

Fig. 10.13 Intravenous Urogram. The x-ray image (radio+graph) was taken as the contrast medium was cleared from the blood by the kidneys. The renal pelvis and ureters are clearly visible and indicate normal findings. **ur/o** = urinary tract;   **-gram** = record

pyelogram	12. Intravenous urography was formerly called intravenous **pyelography** (IVP), and the image produced was called a _____.
bladder	13. Used alone, bladder usually refers to the urinary bladder. **Cysto+scopy** is examination of the urinary bladder. In this procedure, an instrument is passed through the urethra and into the _____ (Fig. 10.14). The lining of the bladder is examined by special lenses, mirrors, and a light. The instrument used in cystoscopy is a **cystoscope. Urethro+scopy** is visual examination of the urethra.
cystitis	14. Inflammation of the bladder is _____.
nephritis	15. Sometimes people say they have a kidney infection when they actually have cystitis, a bladder infection, and a more common type of urinary tract infection. Inflammation of the kidney is _____.
difficult	16. Discomfort during urination and unexplained change in the volume of urine are sometimes the earliest indications of a urinary problem. **Dys+uria** is _____ or painful urination and can be caused by a bacterial infection or a urinary tract obstruction. **Urgency** (a sudden onset of the need to urinate immediately), **frequency** (greater number of urinations than expected in a given time), and **hesitancy** (difficulty in beginning the urinary flow) are terms often used to describe urination patterns.
many	17. **Poly+uria** is excretion of an abnormally large quantity of urine. Literal translation of polyuria is "_____ urines or urinations." You will need to remember that polyuria means excretion of an abnormally large quantity of urine. This is also called **di+ur+esis** (dia-, through + ur/o, urine + -esis, action) and can be brought about by excessive intake of fluids, the use of medications, or disease. **Nocturia** (noct/i, night) is excessive urination at night, either in people who drink excessive amounts of fluids before bedtime or when nearby structures put pressure on the bladder.

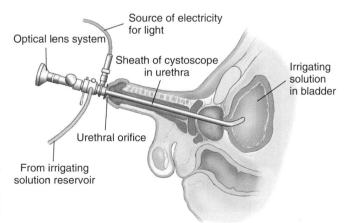

Fig. 10.14 Cystoscope Inside the Male Bladder. In cystoscopy, the cystoscope is passed through the urethra and into the bladder, which is examined using a special lens and a light. (This is an example of rigid cystoscopy, but flexible cystoscopy is more common in males.)

cyst/o = bladder; **-scope** = instrument for viewing

urination

18. The literal translation of **an+uria** is absence of _____. The precise meaning of anuria is a urine output of less than 100 mL per day. This may be caused by a kidney dysfunction, a very low blood pressure, or an obstruction in the urinary passages.

19. Compare the meanings of anuria and **olig+uria.** The latter means diminished capacity to form urine, or excreting less than 500 mL of urine per day. The combining form olig/o means few or scanty. Write the term that means diminished urine production of less than 500 mL per day: _____.

oliguria

20. **Uremia** (ur/o + -emia, blood condition) is a toxic condition associated with renal insufficiency or renal failure. Urea, the chief nitrogen-containing waste product of protein metabolism, is not properly removed from the blood by the kidneys in uremia. Write the term that refers to the presence of nitrogen-containing wastes in the blood: _____. The meaning of uremia cannot be interpreted literally from its word parts, so pay particular attention to its meaning! (It might help to think of "urea in the blood," but you also need to remember that uremia is a toxic condition associated with renal insufficiency or failure.)

uremia

WRITE IT!
EXERCISE 7

Write a term for each description.

1. examination of the urinary bladder _____
2. excretion of large quantities of urine _____
3. excretion of less than 100 mL of urine per day _____
4. excretion of less than 500 mL of urine per day _____
5. kidney enlargement _____
6. inflammation of the renal glomeruli _____
7. inflammation of the renal pelvis _____
8. prolapsed kidney _____
9. softening of the kidney _____
10. presence of kidney stones _____
11. toxic blood condition associated with renal failure _____
12. ultrasonic scanning of the kidneys _____

QUICK CASE STUDY | EXERCISE 8

Define the terms as indicated.

Prem Chadry's catheterized urine specimen was tested and he is found to have <u>glycosuria</u>, <u>proteinuria</u>, and <u>hematuria</u>. <u>Ketones</u> were not detected. He has been tested and treated in the past for diabetes mellitus.

1. glycosuria _____
2. proteinuria _____
3. hematuria _____
4. ketones _____

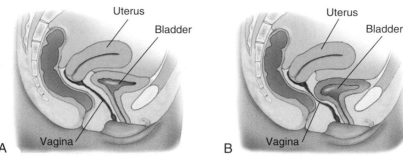

Fig. 10.15 Normal Female Bladder Compared With Cystocele. **A,** Normal position of the bladder in relation to other pelvic structures. **B,** A cystocele, herniation of the bladder. Note how the bladder sags and protrudes into the vagina.

Study the terms in this list to learn more about pathologic conditions and diagnostic procedures.

cystocele (-cele, hernia) Bladder hernia that protrudes into the vagina (Fig. 10.15).

nephrosis (-osis, condition) Condition in which there are degenerative changes in the kidneys but no inflammation.

nephrotoxic (tox/o, poison) Destructive to kidney tissue.

polyp Tumor found on a mucosal surface, such as the inner lining of the bladder.

renal cell carcinoma A malignant neoplasm of the kidney; kidney cancer (Fig. 10.16).

renal failure Failure of the kidney to perform its essential functions. Acute renal failure (ARF) is a critical situation.

renal insufficiency (in-, not) Reduced ability of the kidney to perform its functions.

retrograde urography X-ray examination of the renal pelvis and ureter after injection of a contrast medium into the renal pelvis. In this procedure the contrast material is injected through catheters that are introduced into the ureters. (The prefix retro- means behind or backward. The use of retrograde urography provides an alternative to intravenous urography [IVU] for viewing the renal pelvis and ureters. In IVU, the contrast medium flows through the renal pelvis and ureters after reaching the kidney by way of the bloodstream. In retrograde urography, contrast medium is introduced through the ureter and could be considered backward or in the opposite manner of IVU.)

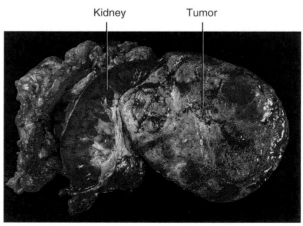

Fig. 10.16 Renal Cell Carcinoma. Macroscopic appearance of an excised kidney with a large tumor.

urinary incontinence (in-, not) Inability to hold urine in the bladder.

urinary retention Inability to empty the bladder.

urinary tract infection (UTI) An infection of the urinary tract.

voiding cystourethrogram (cyst/o, bladder + urethr/o, urethra) Radiographic record of the bladder and urethra. After the bladder has been filled with a contrast medium, radiographs are taken while the patient is expelling urine.

CHOOSE IT!

EXERCISE 9

Choose the correct answer (A, B, C, or D) for each question.

1. What term means herniation of the bladder so that it protrudes into the vagina?
   (A) cystocele   **(B)** polyp   **(C)** nephromalacia   **(D)** nephroptosis

2. Which term means degenerative changes in the kidneys without inflammation?
   (A) nephritis   **(B)** nephromegaly   **(C)** nephrosclerosis   **(D)** nephrosis

3. Which of the following means an inability to hold urine in the bladder?
   (A) catheterization   **(B)** incontinence   **(C)** urinary failure   **(D)** urinary insufficiency

4. Which term means a tumor found on a mucosal surface?
   (A) cystocele   **(B)** polycystic kidney disease   **(C)** polyp   **(D)** urinary tract infection

5. Which of these terms means a radiographic record of the bladder and urethra?
   (A) cystourethrogram   **(B)** nephrotomogram   **(C)** renal angiogram   **(D)** urography

---

Surgical and Therapeutic Interventions

Urinary catheterization may be used for obtaining a sterile urine sample, for instilling medication in the bladder, or for continuous drainage of the bladder, such as during surgery. Four methods (urethral, ureteral, and suprapubic catheterization as well as percutaneous nephrostomy) are used for urinary diversion. **Urethral catheterization** is the most common. An indwelling catheter (held securely in place by a balloon tip filled with water) is left in place for a longer period.

In **ureteral catheterization**, catheters are passed into the distal ends of the ureters from the bladder and threaded up the ureters into the renal pelves. If necessary, a ureteral catheter may be surgically inserted through the abdominal wall into the ureter.

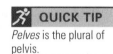

QUICK TIP

Pelves is the plural of pelvis.

If disease or obstruction is present, a **suprapubic catheter** can be placed in the bladder through a small incision or puncture of the abdominal wall approximately 1 inch above the symphysis pubis, the bony eminence that lies beneath the pubic hair.

The fourth means of urinary diversion is **percutaneous nephrostomy**, in which a tube is inserted on a temporary basis into the renal pelvis when a complete obstruction of the ureter is present. In a nephrostomy, a new opening is made into the renal pelvis through the overlying skin. Compare the four methods shown in Fig. 10.17.

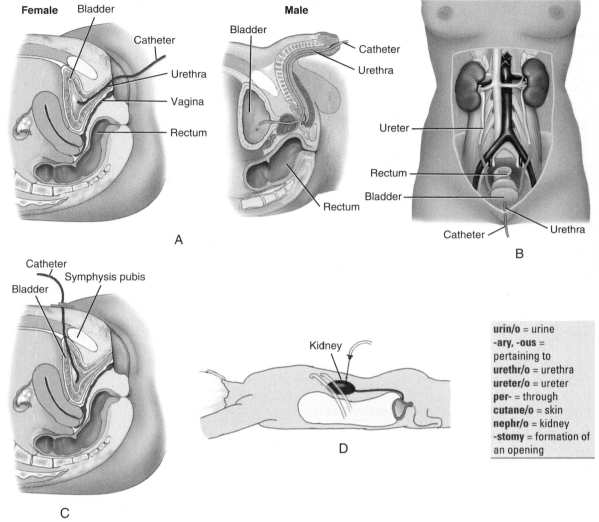

Fig. 10.17 Urinary Diversion. **A,** Urethral catheterization (female and male). **B,** Ureteral catheterization. **C,** Suprapubic catheterization. **D,** Percutaneous nephrostomy.

urin/o = urine
-ary, -ous = pertaining to
urethr/o = urethra
ureter/o = ureter
per- = through
cutane/o = skin
nephr/o = kidney
-stomy = formation of an opening

hem/o = blood
dia- = through
-lysis = freeing or destroying

periton/o = peritoneum
-eal = pertaining to

Kidney dialysis or **hemo+dia+lysis** is required if the kidneys fail to remove waste products from the blood. Kidney dialysis is the process of diffusing blood through a membrane to remove toxic materials and maintain proper chemical balance. **Peritoneal dialysis** is an alternative to hemodialysis. The peritoneum is the membrane that covers the large internal organs of the abdominal cavity and lines that cavity. In peritoneal dialysis the dialyzing solution is introduced into and removed from the peritoneal cavity.

Diuretic means increasing urination or an agent that causes increased urination. Common substances such as tea, coffee, alcohol, and water act as diuretics.

Stones in the urinary tract are sometimes passed through the urethra, but many are too large, may be trapped, do not dissolve, or for another reason are impassable. Stones can cause urinary obstruction, which interferes with function and can be very painful.

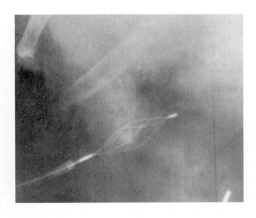

Fig. 10.18 Removal of a Kidney Stone. This radiograph shows a renal calculus that has been caught in a stone basket and is ready for removal. After percutaneous nephrostomy, the stone basket was maneuvered to engage the renal calculus; both then were removed through the cannula.

per- = through;   **cutane/o** = skin;   **-ous** = pertaining to;
nephr/o = kidney;   **-stomy** = artificial opening

There are several methods of treating stones, including noninvasive **litho+tripsy** (high-energy shock wave or laser to break the stone into fragments; see Fig. 2.14), crushing of a ureteral stone often using laser introduced via the bladder, or "catching" the stone in a basket that has been introduced through the ureter or percutaneous nephrostomy (Fig. 10.18).

In renal transplantation the patient (recipient) receives a kidney from a suitable donor, often a living sibling or close relative (Fig. 10.19). Surgical removal of the donated kidney is a **nephrectomy**. Selected situations may allow **laparoscopic nephrectomy**, removal of the kidney through several small incisions in the abdominal wall, rather than an open surgical excision (Fig. 10.20). **Immunosuppressive** therapy, the administration of agents that significantly interfere with the immune response of the recipient, are provided after renal transplantation to prevent rejection of the donor kidney.

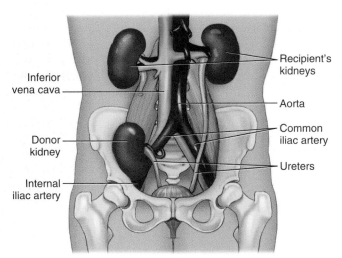

Fig. 10.19 Renal Transplantation (anterior view of the body). In kidney transplantation, a complete kidney from a donor is transferred to a recipient whose kidneys have failed. Note the location of the donated kidney; the diseased kidneys are left in place.

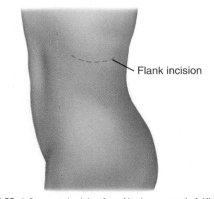

Fig. 10.20 A Common Incision for a Nephrectomy, Left Kidney. This is called a *flank incision*.

Trans+urethral means through the urethra. Transurethral surgery is performed by inserting an instrument through or across the wall of the urethra, which makes it possible to perform surgery on certain organs that lie near the urethra without an abdominal incision. In **transurethral resection** (TUR), small pieces of tissue from a nearby structure are removed through the wall of the urethra. One surgery of this type is a transurethral resection of the prostate (TURP). In TURP, surgery is performed on the **prostate** gland in men by means of an instrument passed through the wall of the urethra and is sometimes done to alleviate urinary problems of benign prostatic hyperplasia.

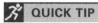
trans- = through or across

> **QUICK TIP**
> Note the difference in spelling of prostate and prostrate, which means lying in a facedown, horizontal position.

Treatment for bladder cancer depends on several factors, including the size of the lesion. Radiation therapy, laser eradication of small lesions, chemotherapy, and **cystectomy** (surgical excision of the bladder) may be used. Various surgical procedures may be performed for urinary diversion if the bladder is removed. The ureters must be diverted into some type of collecting reservoir, either opening onto the abdomen or into the large intestine so that urine is expelled with bowel movements.

The following list provides more information about surgical procedures performed on urinary structures.

cystostomy (cyst/o, bladder + -stomy, new opening) Surgical creation of a new opening into the bladder.

lithotripsy (lith/o, stone + -tripsy, surgical crushing) Crushing of a stone. The stone may be crushed surgically or by using high-energy shock waves or a laser (see Fig. 2.14). A **lithotrite** is an instrument used for surgically crushing bladder stones. Renal lithotripsy using shock waves is called **extra+corpor+eal** (extra-, outside + corpor/o, body + -eal, pertaining to) shock wave lithotripsy (ESWL). After lithotripsy, the stone fragments may be expelled or washed out. A **nephroscope** is sometimes used when small stones are broken up by ESWL. The nephroscope is a fiberoptic instrument that is inserted through the skin (Fig. 10.21). The stone is located through the use of x-ray imaging, and its fragments are removed by suction through the scope. The use of the nephroscope to eliminate renal calculi or to examine the kidney visually is called **nephroscopy**.

nephrolithotomy (nephr/o, kidney + -tomy, incision) Incision of the kidney (**nephrotomy**) for removal of a kidney stone (removal of the stone is implied in this term).

nephropexy (-pexy, surgical fixation) Surgical attachment of a prolapsed kidney.

nephrostomy, pyelostomy Creation of a new opening into the renal pelvis of the kidney (the opening into the renal pelvis is implied in nephrostomy). This procedure is usually done to drain urine from the kidney (see Fig. 10.17, *D*).

percutaneous bladder biopsy Removal of tissue from the bladder by using a needle inserted through the skin overlying the bladder; done for diagnostic purposes (percutaneous is derived from per-, through + cutane/o, skin + -ous, pertaining to).

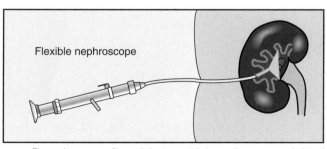

nephr/o = kidney
-scope = instrument for viewing
per- = through
cutane/o = skin

Flexible nephroscope

Fig. 10.21 One Type of Nephroscope. The nephroscope, a fiberoptic instrument, is inserted percutaneously into the kidney. When stones are present, an ultrasonic probe can be added that emits high-frequency sound waves, which break up the calculi.

percutaneous renal biopsy Removal of tissue from the kidney using needle puncture of the skin and tissue overlying the kidney; done for diagnostic purposes.

pyelolithotomy (pyel/o, renal pelvis) Surgical incision of the kidney to remove a stone from the renal pelvis (removal of the stone is implied).

ureteroplasty Surgical repair of a ureter.

WRITE IT!
EXERCISE 10

Write a term for each description.

1. agent that causes increased urination _____
2. excision of a kidney _____
3. inflammation of the bladder _____
4. kidney dialysis _____
5. nephrostomy _____

! Be Careful With These!

cyt/o (cell) versus *cyst/o* (bladder or sac)
ureter/o (ureter) versus *urethr/o* (urethra)
-esis (action, process, or result of) versus *-stasis* (controlling)

A Career as a Radiologist Assistant

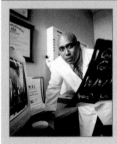

Thomas Clark, a radiologist assistant (RA), is a registered radiographer who has obtained additional education and certification that qualifies him to serve as a radiology extender, working under the supervision of a radiologist to provide patient care in diagnostic imaging. Radiologist assistants take a leading role in patient management and assessment and perform selected radiology procedures. The RA also may be responsible for evaluating image quality, making initial image observations, and forwarding those observations to the supervising radiologist. Radiologist assistants complete an academic program and a radiologist-supervised clinical internship and must be certified by the American Registry of Radiologic Technologists. For more information, visit www.arrt.org.

✓ SELF-TEST

Work the following exercises to test your understanding of the material in Chapter 10. It is best to do all the exercises before checking your answers against the answers in Appendix III. Pay particular attention to spelling.

A. MATCHING!   *Match structures in the left column with their functions in the right column*

_____ 1. bladder
_____ 2. nephron
_____ 3. renal pelvis
_____ 4. ureter
_____ 5. urethra

A. cavity in the kidney that collects urine from many collecting ducts
B. carries urine from the bladder
C. carries urine to the bladder
D. functional unit of the kidney
E. reservoir for urine until it is expelled

B. MATCHING!

Choose A or B from the right column to classify the urinary substances as those normally detected in urine or as those not normally detected.

_____ 1. blood   _____ 4. sugar   **A.** normally detected in urine

_____ 2. ketones   _____ 5. urea   **B.** not normally detected in urine

_____ 3. protein

C. READING HEALTH CARE REPORTS

Read the report, and answer the questions that follow. Although some terms are new, you will be able to determine their meanings by analyzing the word parts.

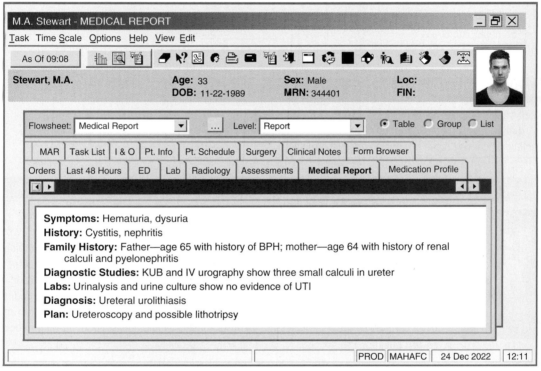

M.A. Stewart - MEDICAL REPORT

Task Time Scale Options Help View Edit

As Of 09:08

Stewart, M.A.   **Age:** 33   **Sex:** Male   **Loc:**
                    DOB: 11-22-1989 **MRN:** 344401   **FIN:**

Flowsheet: Medical Report   …   Level: Report   ⦿ Table ○ Group ○ List

MAR | Task List | I & O | Pt. Info | Pt. Schedule | Surgery | Clinical Notes | Form Browser
Orders | Last 48 Hours | ED | Lab | Radiology | Assessments | **Medical Report** | Medication Profile

Symptoms: Hematuria, dysuria
History: Cystitis, nephritis
Family History: Father—age 65 with history of BPH; mother—age 64 with history of renal calculi and pyelonephritis
Diagnostic Studies: KUB and IV urography show three small calculi in ureter
Labs: Urinalysis and urine culture show no evidence of UTI
Diagnosis: Ureteral urolithiasis
Plan: Ureteroscopy and possible lithotripsy

PROD MAHAFC 24 Dec 2022 12:11

Circle the correct answer (A, B, C, or D) for each question.

1. Mr. Stewart's symptom of dysuria indicates which characteristic of urine or urination?
   (A) blood **(B)** decreased output **(C)** difficult or painful **(D)** protein

2. Which of the following conditions does his history indicate?
   (A) inflammation caused by trauma **(B)** inflammation of the bladder and kidney **(C)** bladder and kidney stones
   (D) frequent urinary infections

3. Which of the following is indicated in his mother's history?
   (A) kidney stones **(B)** polycystic kidney **(C)** renal stenosis **(D)** uremia

4. Which of the following is Mr. Stewart's diagnosis?
   (A) narrowing of the ureter **(B)** obstruction of the ureter **(C)** stone in the ureter **(D)** urinary infection

5. Which procedure is indicated by a ureteroscopy?
   (A) surgical fixation **(B)** renal angiography **(C)** ureteral resection **(D)** visual examination

D. *Read the following report and circle an answer to the multiple-choice questions.*

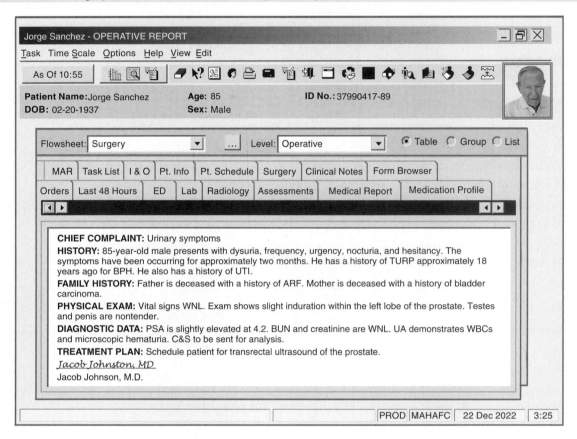

Jorge Sanchez - OPERATIVE REPORT

Task Time Scale Options Help View Edit

As Of 10:55

Patient Name: Jorge Sanchez   **Age:** 85   **ID No.:** 37990417-89
DOB: 02-20-1937   **Sex:** Male

Flowsheet: Surgery   ...   Level: Operative   ● Table ○ Group ○ List

MAR | Task List | I & O | Pt. Info | Pt. Schedule | Surgery | Clinical Notes | Form Browser

Orders | Last 48 Hours | ED | Lab | Radiology | Assessments | Medical Report | Medication Profile

CHIEF COMPLAINT: Urinary symptoms
HISTORY: 85-year-old male presents with dysuria, frequency, urgency, nocturia, and hesitancy. The symptoms have been occurring for approximately two months. He has a history of TURP approximately 18 years ago for BPH. He also has a history of UTI.
FAMILY HISTORY: Father is deceased with a history of ARF. Mother is deceased with a history of bladder carcinoma.
PHYSICAL EXAM: Vital signs WNL. Exam shows slight induration within the left lobe of the prostate. Testes and penis are nontender.
DIAGNOSTIC DATA: PSA is slightly elevated at 4.2. BUN and creatinine are WNL. UA demonstrates WBCs and microscopic hematuria. C&S to be sent for analysis.
TREATMENT PLAN: Schedule patient for transrectal ultrasound of the prostate.
Jacob Johnston, MD
Jacob Johnson, M.D.

PROD | MAHAFC | 22 Dec 2022 | 3:25

1. Difficulty in beginning the urinary flow is **(A)** frequency **(B)** hematuria **(C)** hesitancy **(D)** nocturia
2. The term in the report that indicates urination at night is **(A)** frequency **(B)** hesitancy **(C)** nocturia **(D)** urgency
3. The abbreviation that describes testing of the patient's urine sample is **(A)** BUN **(B)** DRE **(C)** PSA **(D)** UA
4. The patient's father suffered from a disease that primarily affected the
   (A) kidneys **(B)** ureters **(C)** urethra **(D)** urinary bladder
5. The term that means blood in the urine is **(A)** dysuria **(B)** frequency **(C)** hematuria **(D)** hesitancy

E. WRITING! *Write one-word terms for these meanings.*

1. frequent urination   _____
2. functional unit of the kidney   _____
3. examination of the bladder   _____
4. inflammation of the renal pelvis   _____
5. kidney dialysis   _____
6. new opening into the renal pelvis   _____
7. pertaining to the urethra   _____

8. presence of kidney stones
   _____
9. surgical fixation of a prolapsed kidney
   _____
10. surgical repair of a ureter
    _____

F. SPELLING AND PRONUNCIATION!   *Circle all incorrectly spelled terms, and write the correct spelling. Then pronounce the terms.*

cistosel   nefrectomy   oliguria   suprapubik   urinery

G. CHOOSING!   *Circle the one correct answer (A, B, C, or D) for each question.*

1. Which of the following means the same as nephromegaly?
   (A) kidney dialysis   **(B)** kidney failure   **(C)** renal enlargement   **(D)** renal stone

2. Which of the following is an instrument used for surgically crushing a stone?
   (A) lithotripsy   **(B)** lithotrite   **(C)** pyelogram   **(D)** pyelolithotomy

3. Which term means passage of a tubular, flexible instrument into a body channel or cavity for withdrawal of fluid or introduction of fluid?   (A) catheterization   (B) cystostomy   (C) lithotripsy   (D) tracheotomy

4. Which of the following means excision of a calculus from the renal pelvis?
   (A) cystectomy   **(B)** lithotripsy   **(C)** pyelolithotomy   **(D)** tomography

5. Which term means absence of urination or production of less than 100 mL of urine per day?
   (A) anuria   **(B)** diuresis   **(C)** polyuria   **(D)** renal failure

6. Which of the following means sugar in the urine?   (A) glycosuria   (B) ketonuria   (C) pyuria   (D) uremia

7. Which term means inflammation of the kidney?   (A) cystitis   (B) nephritis   (C) nephrosis   (D) pyelolithiasis

8. Which term means an inability to control urination?   (A) excretion   (B) incontinence   (C) stenosis   (D) uremia

9. What is the name of the instrument used in cystoscopy?
   (A) cystogram   **(B)** cystograph   **(C)** cystoscope   **(D)** nephroscope

10. Which of the following means ultrasonic scanning of the kidney?
    (A) nephroscopy   **(B)** nephrosonography   **(C)** pyelogram   **(D)** pyelography

H. IDENTIFYING!   *Label these illustrations with the appropriate terms.*

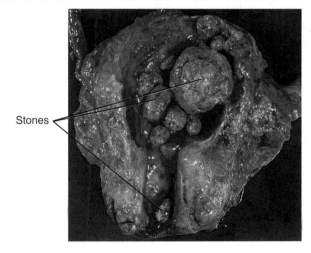

Stones

1. _____
   Presence of stones in the bladder

2. _____ kidney disease
   Kidney disorder with many cysts

I. QUICK CHALLENGE!   *Find an incorrect term in each sentence and write the correct term.*

1. A toxic condition associated with renal insufficiency or renal failure is pyelitis. _____

2. Diminished capacity to form urine (less than 500 mL per day) is polyuria. _____

3. The initial process of filtering of the blood is called glomerular reabsorption. _____

4. Hundreds of fluid-filled sacs throughout both kidneys is nephrotoxic kidney disease. _____

5. Lithotripsy is surgical removal of a donated kidney. _____

*Use Appendix III to check your answers.

QUICK & EASY (Q&E) LIST

Use the Evolve website (http://evolve.elsevier.com/Leonard/quick) to review the terms presented in Chapter 10. Look closely at the spelling of each term as it is pronounced.

albuminuria *(al-bū-mi-**nū**-rē-uh)*
anuria *(an-**ū**-rē-uh)*
cystectomy *(sis-**tek**-tuh-mē)*
cystic *(**sis**-tik)*
cystitis *(sis-**tī**-tis)*
cystocele *(**sis**-tō-sēl)*
cystolithiasis *(sis-tō-li-**thī**-uh-sis)*
cystoscope *(**sis**-tō-skōp)*
cystoscopy *(sis-**tos**-kuh-pē)*
cystostomy *(sis-**tos**-tuh-mē)*
diabetes mellitus *(dī-uh-**bē**-tēz **mel**-luh-tus, muh-**lī**-tis)*
diuresis *(dī-ū-**rē**-sis)*
diuretic *(dī-ū-**ret**-ik)*
dysuria *(dis-**ū**-rē-uh)*
erythropoietin *(uh-rith-rō-**poi**-uh-tin)*
excretion *(eks-**krē**-shun)*
extracorporeal *(eks-truh-kor-**por**-ē-ul)*
frequency *(**frē**-kwun-sē)*
glomerular filtration *(glō-**mer**-ū-lar fil-**trā**-shun)*
glomerulonephritis *(glō-mer-ū-lō-nuh-**frī**-tis)*
glomerulus *(glō-**mer**-ū-lus)*
glycosuria *(glī-kō-**sū**-rē-uh)*
hematuria *(hē-muh-**tū**-rē-uh)*
hemodialysis *(hē-mō-dī-**al**-uh-sis)*
hesitancy *(**he**-zuh-tun-sē)*
immunosuppressive *(im-ū-nō-suh-**pres**-iv)*
intravenous urography *(in-truh-**vē**-nus ū-**rog**-ruh-fē)*
ketonuria *(kē-tō-**nū**-rē-uh)*
laparoscopic nephrectomy *(lap-uh-rō-**skop**-ik nuh-**frek**-tuh-mē)*
lithotripsy *(**lith**-ō-trip-sē)*

lithotrite *(**lith**-ō-trīt)*
nephrectomy *(nuh-**frek**-tuh-mē)*
nephritis *(nuh-**frī**-tis)*
nephrolith *(**nef**-rō-lith)*
nephrolithiasis *(nef-rō-li-**thī**-uh-sis)*
nephrolithotomy *(nef-rō-li-**thot**-uh-mē)*
nephromalacia *(nef-rō-muh-**lā**-shuh)*
nephromegaly *(nef-rō-**meg**-uh-lē)*
nephron *(**nef**-ron)*
nephropexy *(**nef**-rō-pek-sē)*
nephroptosis *(nef-rop-**tō**-sis)*
nephroscope *(**nef**-rō-skōp)*
nephroscopy *(nuh-**fros**-kuh-pē)*
nephrosis *(ne-**frō**-sis)*
nephrosonography *(nef-rō-sō-**nog**-ruh-fē)*
nephrotoxic *(**nef**-rō-tok-sik)*
nephrostomy *(nuh-**fros**-tuh-mē)*
nephrotomogram *(nef-rō-**tō**-mō-gram)*
nephrotomography *(nef-rō-tō-**mog**-ruh-fē)*
nephrotomy *(nuh-**frot**-uh-mē)*
nocturia *(nok-**tū**-rē-uh)*
oliguria *(ol-i-**gū**-rē-uh)*
percutaneous bladder biopsy *(pur-kū-**tā**-nē-us **blad**-ur **bī**-op-sē)*
percutaneous nephrostomy *(pur-kū-**tā**-nē-us nuh-**fros**-tuh-mē)*
percutaneous renal biopsy *(pur-kū-**tā**-nē-us **rē**-nul **bī**-op-sē)*
peritoneal dialysis *(per-i-tō-**nē**-ul dī-**al**-uh-sis)*
polycystic kidney disease *(pol-ē-**sis**-tik **kid**-nē di-**zēz**)*
polyp *(**pol**-ip)*
polyuria *(pol-ē-**ū**-rē-uh)*

QUICK & EASY (Q&E) LIST—cont'd

prostate (**pros**-tāt)
proteinuria (prŏ-tē-**nū**-rē-uh)
pyelitis (pī-uh-**lī**-tis)
pyelogram (**pī**-uh-lō-gram)
pyelography (pī-uh-**log**-ruh-fē)
pyelolithotomy (pī-uh-lō-li-**thot**-uh-mē)
pyelostomy (pī-uh-**los**-tuh-mē)
pyuria (pī-**ū**-rē-uh)
renal (**rē**-nul)
renal angiography (**rē**-nul an-jē-**og**-ruh-fē)
renal arteriogram (**rē**-nul ahr-**tēr**-ē-ō-gram)
renal arteriography (**rē**-nul ahr-tēr-ē-**og**-ruh-fē)
renal calculi (**rē**-nul **kal**-kū-lī)
renal cell carcinoma (**rē**-nul sel kahr-si-**nō**-muh)
renal failure (**rē**-nul **fāl**-yur)
renal insufficiency (**rē**-nul in-suh-**fish**-un-sē)
retrograde urography (**ret**-rō-grād ū-**rog**-ruh-fē)
stenosis (stuh-**nō**-sis)
suprapubic catheter (s $\overline{oo}$ --pruh-**pū**-bik **kath**-uh-tur)
transurethral resection (trans-ū-**rē**-thrul rē-**sek**-shun)
tubular reabsorption (t $\overline{too}$ -bū-lur rē-ab-**sorp**-shun)
tubular secretion (t $\overline{too}$ -bū-lur sē-**krē**-shun)
tubule (t $\overline{too}$ -būl)

urea (ū-**rē**-uh)
uremia (ū-**rē**-mē-uh)
ureter (ū-**rē**-tur, **ū**-ruh-tur)
ureteral (ū-**rē**-tur-ul)
ureteral catheterization (ū-**rē**-tur-ul kath-uh-tur-i-**zā**-shun)
ureteroplasty (ū-**rē**-tur-ō-plas-tē)
urethra (ū-**rē**-thruh)
urethral (ū-**rē**-thrul)
urethral catheterization (ū-**rē**-thrul kath-uh-tur-i-**zā**-shun)
urethroscopy (ū-ruh-**thros**-kuh-pē)
urgency (**ur**-jun-sē)
urinalysis (ū-ri-**nal**-i-sis)
urinary (**ū**-ri-nar-ē)
urinary incontinence (**ū**-ri-nar-ē in-**kon**-ti-nuns)
urinary retention (**ū**-ri-nar-ē rē-**ten**-shun)
urinary tract infection (**ū**-ri-nar-ē trakt in-**fek**-shun)
urination (ū-ri-**nā**-shun)
urogram (**ū**-rō-gram)
urolithiasis (ū-rō-li-**thī**-uh-sis)
urologist (ū-**rol**-uh-jist)
urology (ū-**rol**-uh-jē)
voiding cystourethrogram (**void**-ing sis-tō-ū-**rē**-thrō-gram)

Don't forget the games and other activities available at http://evolve.elsevier.com/Leonard/quick.

QUICK CONNECT

Review all lists of word parts and their meanings for this chapter using the flashcards you prepared or the flashcards on the Evolve site.

Urology is the branch of medicine concerned with the male genital tract and the urinary tracts of both genders.

Urination (voiding), the act of passing urine, excretes wastes to maintain the volume and chemical composition of blood (takes place mainly in the kidneys). The functions of the kidneys include maintenance of an appropriate blood volume by varying the excretion of water, maintenance of the chemical composition of blood by selecting the excretion of certain chemicals, maintenance of blood pH, excretion of waste products (urea) of protein metabolism, regulation of blood pressure, and stimulation of erythrocyte production by secretion of erythropoietin.

Filtration of blood and expelling urine depends on a healthy blood pressure: Blood flows from the bloodstream, entering each kidney via the glomerulus (filtration of the blood). Water, salts, urea, wastes, acids and drugs are collected by Bowman's capsule, which passes it on to the tubules. Tubular secretion is reabsorption of substances that the body preserves (sugar and much of the water). The filtrate flows then to the renal pelvis, ureter, bladder, and is then excreted via the urethral opening.

Remember adjectives that mean pertaining these structures: kidney(s), ureter, urethra, bladder,

A complete urinalysis generally includes physical (appearance as well as other qualities), chemical (sugar, ketones, protein, and blood), and microscopic examinations (blood cells, for example). Remember the meanings of glycosuria, proteinuria, hematuria, ketonuria, and pyuria. Know the difference in a voided specimen vs. a catheterized specimen.

Radiography: Renal angiography/arteriography is the radiographic study of the kidneys. The record is a renal arteriogram. Nephrotomography uses contrast dyes and provides images called a nephrotomogram; however, these are largely replaced by CT and nephrosonography, ultrasonic scanning of the kidneys, retrograde urography (formerly intravenous pyelography), and voiding cystourethrogram.

Differentiate these terms: nephromalacia, nephromegaly, polycystic kidney disease, nephritis, urolithiasis vs. cystolithiasis vs. nephrolithiasis.

Know the difference in these endoscopic procedures: cystoscopy and urethroscopy. Know the difference in cystoscopy and a cystoscope.

Distinguish these diagnostic terms: dysuria, urgency, frequency, hesitancy, polyuria, diuresis, nocturia, and uremia. Differentiate anuria, oliguria, cystocele, nephrosis, nephrotoxic, bladder polyp, renal cell carcinoma, renal insufficiency vs. renal failure, urinary incontinence, urinary retention, urinary tract infection.

Differentiate these methods of urinary catheterization: urethral, ureteral, suprapubic; percutaneous nephrostomy.

Know the difference in hemodialysis vs. peritoneal dialysis. Know these terms: diuretic and immunosuppressive agents.

Differentiate these terms: lithotripsy using a lithotrite vs. extracorporeal shock wave lithotripsy, nephrectomy, transurethral resection, cystectomy vs. cystostomy, nephrostomy, nephroscopy, nephrolithotomy, nephropexy, nephrostomy, percutaneous bladder biopsy vs. percutaneous renal biopsy, pyelolithotomy, and ureteroplasty.

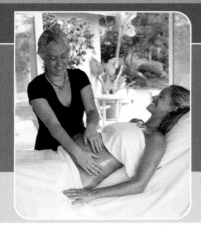

CHAPTER 11

Reproductive System

(A certified prenatal massage therapist addresses specific pregnancy needs (such as relaxation), relieving muscle aches and joint pains to improve the labor outcome and newborn's health.)

CONTENTS

Function First
FEMALE REPRODUCTIVE SYSTEM
  Structures
  Diseases, Disorders, and Diagnostic Terms
  Surgical and Therapeutic Interventions
Pregnancy and Childbirth
Female Breasts

MALE REPRODUCTIVE SYSTEM
  Structures
  Diseases, Disorders, and Diagnostic Terms
  Surgical and Therapeutic Interventions
Sexually Transmitted Diseases or Infections
SELF-TEST
QUICK & EASY (Q&E) LIST
QUICK CONNECT

OBJECTIVES

After completing Chapter 11, you will be able to:

1. Recognize or write the functions of the reproductive system.
2. Recognize or write the meanings of Chapter 11 word parts and use them to build and analyze terms.
3. Write terms for selected structures of the female and male reproductive systems and their associated functions or match them with their descriptions.
4. Write the names of the diagnostic terms and pathologies related to the female and male reproductive systems when given their descriptions or match terms with their meanings.

5. Match surgical and therapeutic interventions for the female and male reproductive systems or write the names of the interventions when given their descriptions.
6. Write selected terms related to pregnancy and childbirth or match them with their descriptions.
7. Write selected terms related to the female breasts or match them with their descriptions.
8. Write terms for sexually transmitted diseases or match them with their causative agents.
9. Spell terms for the reproductive system and sexually transmitted diseases correctly.

 Function First

Reproduction is the process by which genetic material is passed from one generation to the next. The major function of the reproductive system is to produce offspring. The male and female reproductive systems can be broadly organized by organs with different functions. For example, the testes and ovaries are called the **gonads**, and they function in the production of reproductive cells: spermatozoa (sperm) or ova (eggs). Singular terms for spermatozoa and ova are **spermatozoon** and **ovum**, respectively. The gonads also secrete important hormones. Ducts transport and receive eggs or sperm and important fluids. Still other reproductive organs produce materials that support the sperm and ova. Reproductive organs, whether male or female, particularly those external to the body, are called the genitals or **genitalia**.

 QUICK TIP
Singular form: testis *or* testicle

gon/o = genital *or* reproduction

WRITE IT!*
EXERCISE 1

Find the terms in the material you just read and write them for these meanings.

1. another term for genitals _____
2. organs that produce either sperm or ova _____
3. singular form of ova _____
4. singular form of spermatozoa _____
5. the female gonad _____
6. the male gonad _____
7. process by which genetic material is passed from one generation to the next _____

*Use Appendix III, Answers, to check your answers to all the exercises in Chapter 11.

FEMALE REPRODUCTIVE SYSTEM

 Structures

The female reproductive system aids in the creation of new life and provides an environment and support for the developing child. After birth, the female breasts produce milk to feed the infant and are thus often considered part of the female reproductive system (see later section).

Gyneco+**logy** is the study of diseases of the female reproductive organs, and a **gyneco**+**logist** is a specialist in the study of these diseases. Female genitalia include both external and internal structures.

gynec/o = female
-logy = study of

The word parts in the following table refer to female reproductive structures and are frequently used when reproduction is discussed. Commit to memory the word parts and their meanings.

WORD PARTS: FEMALE REPRODUCTIVE SYSTEM

Female Genitalia	Meaning	Other Word Parts	Meaning
cervic/o*	cervix	-cidal	killing
colp/o, vagin/o	vagina	cyst/o, vesic/o	bladder, cyst, or sac
gynec/o	female	genit/o	genitals
hyster/o, uter/o	uterus	gonad/o	genitals or reproduction
metr/o (occasionally metr/i)†	uterine tissue	men/o	month
oophor/o, ovar/o	ovary	-plasia	development or formation
salping/o	uterine tube (fallopian tube)	rect/o	rectum
vulv/o	vulva (external genitalia)	urethr/o	urethra
		urin/o	urine

Use the electronic flashcards on the Evolve site or make your own set of flashcards using the above list. Select the word parts just presented, and study them until you know their meanings. Do this each time a set of word parts is presented.

*Sometimes *cervic/o* means the neck.

†Sometimes *metr/o* and *metr/i* mean measure.

Match the word parts in #s 1-8 with their meanings in the right columns.

_____ **1.** -cidal   _____ **5.** metr/o   A. bladder, cyst, or sac   E. uterine tissue

_____ **2.** colp/o   _____ **6.** oophor/o   B. killing   F. uterine tube

_____ **3.** hyster/o   _____ **7.** salping/o   C. month   G. uterus

_____ **4.** men/o   _____ **8.** vesic/o   D. ovary   H. vagina

External Structures. The external genitalia are called the **vulva**, which includes the following structures:

- **mons pubis**
- **labia majora** (labium majus, singular)
- **labia minora** (labium minus, singular)
- **clitoris**
- openings for glands

Label these structures as you read the legend for Fig. 11.1. The two pairs of skinfolds protect the vaginal opening.

WORD ORIGIN

labium (L.), lip
majora (L.), major
minora (L.), minor, small

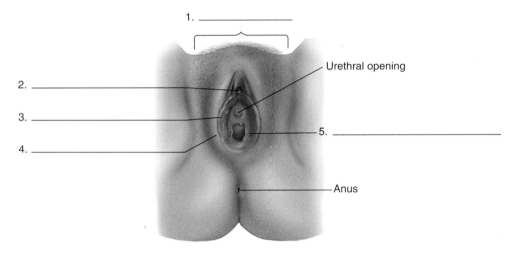

Fig. 11.1 Female External Genitalia. These structures are external to the vagina and are also called the vulva. The mons pubis *(1)* is a pad of fatty tissue and thick skin that overlies the front of the pubic bone. The pubic bone is the anterior portion of the hip bones. The mons pubis is covered with hair after puberty. The clitoris *(2)* is a small mass of erectile tissue and nerves that has similarities to the male penis. Two pairs of skinfolds protect the vaginal opening. The smaller pair is called the labia minora *(3)*, and the larger pair is called the labia majora *(4)*. Small glands secrete mucus for lubrication. Openings for the glands lie near the vagina; label one of them *(5)*. **urethr/o** = urethra; **vagin/o** = vagina

Match these female external structures with their descriptions.

_____ **1.** clitoris   A. general term for external genitalia

_____ **2.** labia majora   B. larger pair of skin folds

_____ **3.** labia minora   C. pad of fatty tissue overlying the pubic bone

_____ **4.** mons pubis   D. small mass of erectile tissue

_____ **5.** vulva   E. smaller pair of skin folds

Internal Structures. The following structures are internal genitalia:

- Left ovary and associated left uterine tube
- Right ovary and associated right uterine tube
- Uterus
- Vagina
- Special glands

Label the structures of the internal genitalia as you read the legend for Fig. 11.2. The ovaries produce ova. The uterine tubes (also called **fallopian** tubes or oviducts) transport the ova to the uterus (womb). The **vagina**, commonly called the "birth canal," receives the sperm during intercourse. The **uterus** provides nourishment from the time the fertilized egg is implanted until birth.

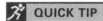

QUICK TIP

A membrane called the hymen sometimes covers the entrance to the vagina.

vagin/o = vagina

A HUMAN EMBRYO IS THE PERIOD OF TIME FROM FERTILIZATION UNTIL THE END OF THE 8TH WEEK

A **fetus** is the latter stages of developing offspring and, in humans, is that time *in utero* after the first 8 weeks. **In utero** means within the uterus. Uterine is the adjective that means pertaining to the uterus.

---

1. _____
2. _____
3. _____
4. _____
5. _____

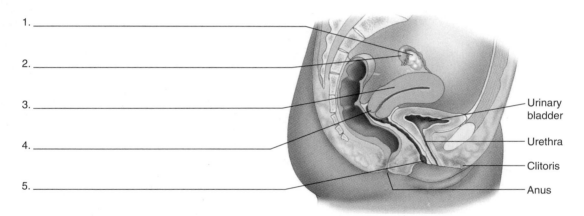

Urinary bladder

Urethra

Clitoris

Anus

Fig. 11.2 Female Genitalia, Midsagittal View. Write the names of the structures on the numbered lines as you read the following. Each ovary *(1)* produces ova and hormones. One uterine tube *(2)* is associated with each ovary. The uterus *(3)* is the muscular organ that prepares to receive and nurture the fertilized ovum. The lower and narrower part protrudes into the vagina and has the outlet, the cervix uteri *(4)*. The vagina *(5)* is the canal that connects the internal and external genitalia.

MATCH IT! **EXERCISE 4**

Match the terms in the left column with their descriptions.

_____ 1. ovary
_____ 2. ovum
_____ 3. uterine tube
_____ 4. uterus
_____ 5. vagina

A. a gonad
B. receives and nurtures the fertilized ovum
C. receives the sperm during intercourse
D. reproductive cell
E. transports ova to the uterus

Locate the vagina, uterus, and the left and right ovaries (Fig. 11.3). The cavity of the uterus has upper openings for the uterine tubes (at the uterine horns) and a lower opening into the vagina (**cervix uteri**, commonly called the cervix). The cervix is the lowermost cylindric part of the uterus (cervic/o means the neck or the cervix uteri). The adjective **cervical** pertains either to the neck itself or to the cervix, which is the neck of the uterus. Other parts of the word, or the way in which it is used, usually indicate whether cervical refers to the neck itself or the cervix.

metr/o = measurement *or* uterine tissue (latter usage here)
endo- = inside
-ium = membrane
my/o = muscle
peri- = around

The uterus consists of three layers of tissue. From the innermost layer to the outermost layer, the layers are called the endometrium, myometrium, and perimetrium. Find these three layers of tissue in Fig. 11.3, *B*, and compare their locations. The tissue that forms the lining of the uterus is called the **endo+metr+ium**. The **myometrium** is the thick muscular tissue of the uterus, and the **perimetrium** is the membrane that surrounds the uterus.

ovar/o = ovary

The **ovaries** are located on each side of the uterus. Ovaries function in **ovulation** (the release of ova) and in the production of two important hormones, **estrogen** and **progesterone**. These hormones are responsible for the development and maintenance of secondary sexual characteristics, preparation of the uterus for pregnancy, and development of the mammary glands.

mamm/o = breast

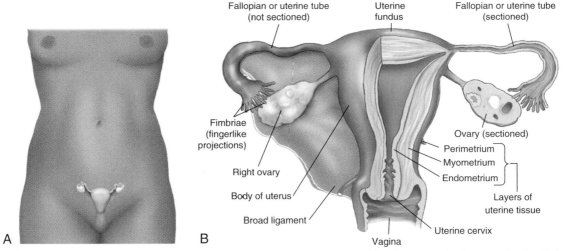

A   B

Fig. 11.3 Anterior View of Female Reproductive Structures. **A,** Anterior view of the internal female structures in reference to location. **B,** Anterior view of the internal organs of the female reproductive system. The left ovary, the left uterine tube, and the left side of the uterus are sectioned to show their internal structure. **endo-** = inside; **metr/o** = uterine tissue; **uter/o** = uterus

---

QUICK REVIEW!

Internal Structures	*External Structures*
Left ovary and associated left uterine tube	Mons pubis
Right ovary and associated left uterine tube	Labia majora
Uterus	Labia minora
Vagina	Clitoris
Special glands	Openings for glands

Maturation. Puberty is the period of life at which the capability of reproduction begins (Fig. 11.4). Genitalia mature and secondary sex characteristics appear (in females, these include adult distribution of hair, development of the breasts, and the start of menstruation). **Menstruation** is the discharge of a bloody fluid from the uterus at fairly regular intervals, approximately once each month, from puberty to menopause. The monthly cycles are brought about by the secretion of female reproductive hormones. The **climacteric**, or **menopause**, marks the end of a woman's reproductive period. Menstruation, also called **menses**, is the sloughing off of the endometrium that has been prepared to receive a fertilized ovum but is not needed. Menstruation ceases temporarily during pregnancy and breastfeeding and permanently with the onset of menopause (unless hormones are administered).

men/o = month

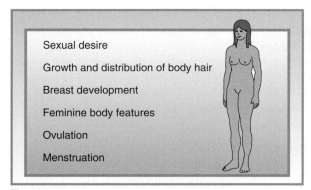

Sexual desire

Growth and distribution of body hair

Breast development

Feminine body features

Ovulation

Menstruation

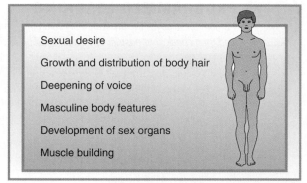

Sexual desire

Growth and distribution of body hair

Deepening of voice

Masculine body features

Development of sex organs

Muscle building

Fig. 11.4 Secondary Female and Male Sexual Characteristics. The changes that occur at puberty are brought about by the hypothalamus and the anterior pituitary of the brain.

FIND IT!
EXERCISE 5

Write the combining forms and meanings for the following new terms. A short definition is provided.

1. **extrauterine** _____ occurring or located outside the uterus
2. **intrauterine** _____ pertaining to inside of the uterus
3. **ovarian** _____ pertaining to the ovary
4. **vaginal** _____ pertaining to the vagina
5. **vulval, vulvar** _____ pertaining to the vulva

WRITE IT!
EXERCISE 6

Write terms for these descriptions.

1. pertaining to the cervix _____
2. pertaining to the uterus _____
3. inner lining of the uterus _____
4. membrane that surrounds the uterus _____
5. muscular tissue of the uterus _____
6. the release of ova by the ovaries _____
7. another term for menses _____
8. another term for menopause _____
9. a developing human after 8 weeks in utero _____
10. another important female hormone besides estrogen _____

Diseases, Disorders, and Diagnostic Terms

The physical assessment of the female reproductive system includes examination of the breasts, the external genitalia, and the pelvis. A pelvic examination is a diagnostic procedure in which the external and internal genitalia are examined. Gynecologic and obstetric care accounts for one-fifth of all visits by female patients to physicians. Throughout a female's life, annual assessment and screening for cancers of the reproductive system increase the chances that problems are detected and often corrected in their early stages. Many diagnostic procedures and treatments are available.

PROGRAMMED LEARNING

Remember to cover the answers (left column) with folded paper or the bookmark. Write an answer in each blank, and then check your answer before proceeding to the next frame.

vaginal	1. A vaginal **speculum** is an instrument that can be pushed apart after it is inserted into the vagina to allow examination of the cervix and the walls of the vagina (Fig. 11.5, *A*). A speculum is an instrument for examining body orifices (openings) or cavities. A speculum that is used to examine the vagina is a _____ speculum.
cells	2. Specimens (scrapings) for cytology can be collected during the pelvic examination. **Cyto+logy** means the study of _____.
cytology	3. **Pap smear** is an abbreviated way of saying Papanicolaou smear or test. In a Pap smear, material is collected from areas of the body that shed cells. The cells are then studied microscopically. The study of cells is called _____.
Pap	4. The term *Pap smear* usually refers to collection and examination of cells from the vagina and cervix (Fig. 11.5, *B and C*), but the term may refer to collection of material from other surfaces that shed cells. Both _____ smears and biopsies are performed to detect cancer of the cervix, and a vaginal speculum is used for both. The external surface of a normal cervix should not show lesions, tears, or signs of inflammation.

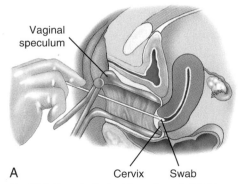
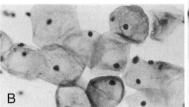
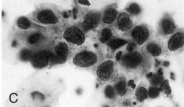

A — Vaginal speculum, Cervix, Swab
B
C

Fig. 11.5 Use of a Vaginal Speculum. **A,** Obtaining a cervical Pap smear. **B** and **C,** The appearance of cervical cells in a Pap smear. **B,** Normal cells; **C,** cervical cancer cells.

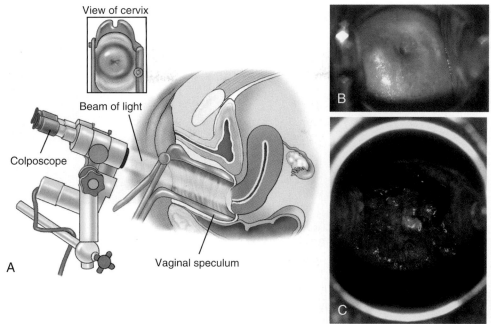

Fig. 11.6 Colposcopy. **A,** The vagina and cervix are examined with a colposcope. **B,** The appearance of a normal uterine cervix. **C,** The colposcopic appearance of an abnormal cervix, which was followed up with a biopsy and determined to be cervical cancer.
colp/o = vagina;   **-scopy** = visual examination;   **cervic/o** = cervix

	5. It is standard practice to grade Pap smears as class I, II, III, IV, or V. Class I is normal, and class V is definitely cancer. Early diagnosis of cervical cancer is possible with the Pap test. When the Pap smear is examined microscopically, malignant cells have a characteristic appearance that indicates cancer, sometimes before symptoms appear. It may begin with **dys+plasia**, a change in the shape, growth, and number of cells. This finding is not cancer, but cells of this type tend to become malignant. Write the term for this abnormality in the shape, growth, and number of cells that may be seen in a Pap
dysplasia	smear: _____.
colposcope	6. **Colpo+scopy** involves the use of a low-power microscope to magnify the mucosa of the vagina and cervix (Fig. 11.6). The instrument used is a _____.
uterus	7. Suspicious cervical or vaginal lesions may be seen during colposcopy. Some findings indicate the need for a cervical or endometrial biopsy. A cervical biopsy is removal of tissue from the cervix, and an endometrial biopsy requires collection of tissue from the lining of the _____.
laparoscope	8. Computed tomography and pelvic ultrasonography may be helpful in detecting abdominal masses. **Laparo+scopy** is the examination of the abdominal cavity through one or more small incisions in the abdominal wall. This surgical procedure is especially useful for inspection of structures within the pelvic cavity and for collection of biopsy specimens and in certain types of surgery (Fig. 11.7). The name of the instrument used in laparoscopy is a _____. Laparotomy is an abdominal incision.

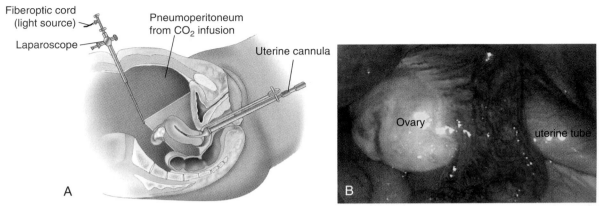

Fig. 11.7 Laparoscopy. **A,** Using the laparoscope with a fiberoptic light source, the surgeon can see the pelvic cavity and the reproductive organs. Additional procedures, such as tubal sterilization or removal of the uterus or ovaries, are performed through a second small abdominal incision. **B,** Laparoscopic view of the right uterine tube and the right ovary. **lapar/o** = abdominal wall;   **-scopy** = visual examination

hysteroscope	9. **Hystero+scopy** is direct visual inspection of the cervical canal and uterine cavity, using an endoscope passed through the vagina (Fig. 11.8). Change the suffix of hysteroscopy to write the name of the endoscope: _____.
hysterosalpin-gography	10. A **hystero+salpingo+gram** is an x-ray image of the uterus and uterine tubes using a radiopaque substance introduced through the cervix (Fig. 11.9). Write the name of the procedure in which a hysterosalpingogram is produced: _____.

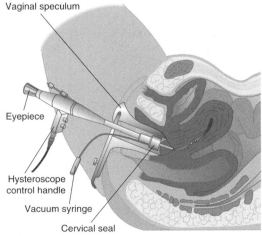

Fig. 11.8 Hysteroscopy. Direct visual examination of the cervical canal and uterine cavity using a hysteroscope is performed to examine the endometrium, to obtain a specimen for biopsy, to excise cervical polyps, or to remove an intrauterine device. **cervic/o** = cervix;   **hyster/o** = uterus;   **-scopy** = visual examination

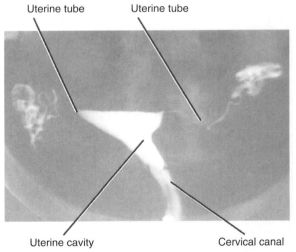

Fig. 11.9 Hysterosalpingogram. This x-ray image of the uterus and uterine tubes was taken after the introduction of a radiopaque substance through the cervix. **hyster/o** = uterus;   **salping/o** = uterine tube

WRITE IT!
EXERCISE 7

Write a term in the blanks to complete each sentence.

1. A vaginal _____ is an instrument that can be pushed apart after its insertion to allow examination of the cervix and walls of the vagina.

2. Material is collected from the vagina and cervix and then studied microscopically in a _____ smear.

3. An abnormality in the shape, growth, and number of cervical cells that often tends to become malignant is called _____.

4. The procedure in which a colposcope is used to magnify the vaginal mucosa and the cervix is _____.

5. Using a hysteroscope for direct visual inspection of the cervical canal and uterine cavity is _____.

6. An x-ray image of the uterus and uterine tubes after a radiopaque substance has been injected into them is called _____.

Common reasons for seeking gynecologic care are pain, vaginal discharge, bleeding, annual gynecologic examinations, and the prevention of pregnancy. A less common problem is infertility, the condition of being unable to produce offspring after a reasonable period of regular intercourse without **contraception** (prevention of pregnancy). Infertility may be caused by female, male, or combined factors, and sometimes the cause cannot be identified. In women the risk for infertility increases with age.

Menstrual irregularities include the following:
- **amenorrhea**: Absence of menstrual flow when it is normally expected.
- **dysmenorrhea**: Painful menstruation.
- **menorrhagia**: Excessive flow during menstruation.
- **metrorrhagia**: Bleeding from the uterus at any time other than during the menstrual period.

Metrorrhagia literally means "hemorrhage from the uterus." Menstruation, normal menstrual flow, contains the word part men/o, which means month. You will need to remember that metrorrhagia is abnormal bleeding that is not associated with menstruation.

men/o = month
-rrhea = discharge
-rrhagia = hemorrhage
metr/o = uterine tissue

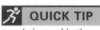 **QUICK TIP**

men/o is used in the words *menses* and *menstruation*.

MATCH IT!
EXERCISE 8

Match the menstrual disorders with their descriptions.

_____ 1. amenorrhea
_____ 2. dysmenorrhea
_____ 3. menorrhagia
_____ 4. metrorrhagia

A. abnormally heavy or long menstrual periods
B. absence of menstruation
C. painful or difficult menstruation
D. uterine bleeding other than menstruation

The following list provides additional diseases and disorders of female reproduction.

cervical polyp Fibrous or mucous stalked tumor of the cervical mucosa (lining) (*polyp* is a general term for tumors that bleed easily and are found on mucous membranes).

cervicocolpitis Inflammation of the cervix and vagina.

colpitis (colp/o, vagina + -itis, inflammation) Inflammation of the vagina; same as **vaginitis**.

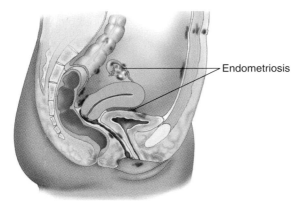

Fig. 11.10 Common Sites of Endometriosis. This abnormal location of endometrial tissue is often the ovaries and, less frequently, other pelvic structures.

metr/i = uterine tissue;   **pelv/i** = pelvis

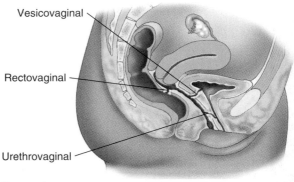

Fig. 11.11 Sites of Vaginal Fistulas. Abnormal openings between the vagina and the bladder, rectum, and urethra are shown. These abnormal openings are called a vesicovaginal fistula, rectovaginal fistula, and urethrovaginal fistula, respectively.

rect/o = rectum;   **urethr/o** = urethra;   **vagin/o** = vagina;   **vesic/o** = bladder

cystocele (cyst/o, bladder + -cele, hernia) Herniation or protrusion of the urinary bladder through the wall of the vagina (see Fig. 10.15, *B*).

endometriosis (endo-, inside + metr/i, uterine tissue + -osis, condition) Condition in which tissue that somewhat resembles the endometrium is found abnormally in various locations in the pelvic cavity (Fig. 11.10). Endometriosis has an unusual spelling, so be careful!

endometritis Inflammation of the endometrium.

fistula Abnormal, tubelike passage between two internal organs or between an internal organ and the body surface. A **rectovaginal** (rect/o, rectum) fistula is an abnormal opening between the rectum and the vagina. A **vesicovaginal** (vesic/o, bladder) fistula is an abnormal opening between the bladder and the vagina (Fig. 11.11).

hysteroptosis (hyster/o, uterus + -ptosis, sagging) Prolapse of the uterus (Fig. 11.12).

myoma Common benign fibroid tumor of the uterine muscle.

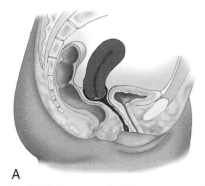
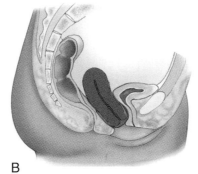
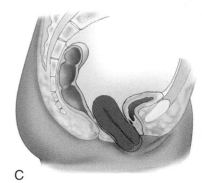

A   B   C

Fig. 11.12 Hysteroptosis. Three stages of uterine prolapse. **A,** Grade I: The uterus bulges into the vagina but does not protrude through the entrance. **B,** Grade II: The cervix is visible within the vagina. **C,** Grade III: The body of the uterus and the cervix protrude through the vaginal orifice.

hyster/o, uter/o = uterus;   **-ptosis** = prolapse, sagging

oophoritis (oophor/o, ovary) An inflamed condition of an ovary.

oophorosalpingitis (salping/o, uterine tube) Inflammation of an ovary and its uterine tube.

ovarian carcinoma Cancer of an ovary, a malignancy that is rarely detected in the early stage and usually is far advanced when diagnosed (Fig. 11.13, *A*).

ovarian cyst Sac filled with fluid or semisolid material that develops in or on the ovary and is usually benign. Compare ovarian cancer (see Fig. 11.13, *A*) with a benign ovarian cyst (Fig. 11.13, *B*).

pelvic inflammatory disease (PID) Infection of the upper genital organs beyond the cervix, often involving the peritoneum and intestines.

premenstrual syndrome (PMS) Syndrome of nervous tension, irritability, weight gain, edema, headache, painful breasts, sleep changes, and other symptoms occurring a few days before the onset of menstruation.

salpingitis Inflammation of a uterine tube.

salpingocele (-cele, hernia) Hernial protrusion of a uterine tube.

uterine cancer Any malignancy of the uterus, including the cervix or endometrium. The extent of tumor spread is described, ranging from stage 0 (limited to the cervical mucosa) to stage IV (tumor has spread beyond the pelvis or to the adjacent organs).

uterine fibroid The most common benign tumor occurring within the uterus, and may cause general enlargement of the lower abdomen, also called **leiomyoma** (lei/o refers to the smooth muscle cells) (Fig. 11.14).

vulvitis (vulv/o, vulva) Inflammation of the vulva.

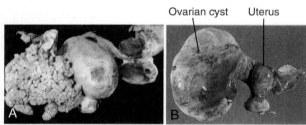

Ovarian cyst   Uterus

Fig. 11.13 Ovarian Carcinoma and Ovarian Cyst. A, Carcinoma of the ovary. The ovary is enormously enlarged by this far-advanced cancerous tumor. **B,** Ovarian cyst. This large, benign cyst is soft and surrounded by a thin capsule. Ovarian masses, both cancerous and benign, are often asymptomatic until large enough to cause pressure in the pelvis. **carcin/o** = cancer; **-oma** = tumor

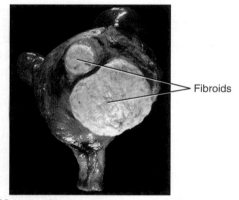

Fibroids

Fig. 11.14 Uterine Fibroids. Surgical removal of this uterus was necessary because of the large myoma. **my/o** = muscle; **-oma** = tumor

MATCH IT!
EXERCISE 9

Match the terms with their meanings.

_____ 1. abnormal passage between two internal organs or between an internal organ and body surface

_____ 2. prevention of pregnancy

_____ 3. sagging of an organ

_____ 4. tumor occurring on a mucous membrane

A. contraception
B. fistula
C. polyp
D. prolapse

CHOOSE IT! **EXERCISE 10**

Choose the correct answer to complete each sentence.

1. A word that means the same as vaginitis is (cervicitis, colpitis, salpingitis, vulvitis).
2. A condition in which tissue that somewhat resembles endometrium is found in an abnormal location in the pelvic cavity is called (endometritis, endometriosis, pelvic inflammatory disease, peritubal adhesions).
3. An examination using an instrument that magnifies the vaginal mucosa is called (colpitis, colposcopy, endometriosis, hysteroptosis).
4. Prolapse of the uterus is (extrauterine, hysterectomy, hysteroptosis, intrauterine).
5. Inflammation of the inner lining of the uterus is (colpitis, endometritis, salpingitis, vulvitis).

Surgical and Therapeutic Interventions

QUICK TIP

IVF increases the chance of multiple births.

Administration of hormones, use of vaginal medications, surgery, and counseling are some of the treatments used in correcting infertility, depending on the cause. **In vitro fertilization** (IVF) is a method of fertilizing the ova outside the body by collecting mature ova and uniting them in a dish with spermatozoa before placing them in the uterus for implantation. IVF may be successful when failure to conceive is caused by insufficient numbers of sperm.

After the cause of amenorrhea (absence of menstrual flow) is established, it is treated by surgical and pharmaceutical means (e.g., hormone replacement therapy [HRT], stimulation of ovaries).

Refraining from sexual contact (abstinence) prevents pregnancy and sexually transmitted diseases. Contraception (contra-, against) is any process or technique for preventing pregnancy in sexually active persons. Conception cannot occur after a hysterectomy, or removal of both ovaries; however, the purpose (e.g., cancer) of these surgeries is not related to contraception.

Coitus is the sexual union of opposite genders in which the penis is introduced into the vagina; it is also called copulation or sexual intercourse. A **contraceptive** is used to prevent conception or pregnancy. A douche is introduction of water or a cleaning agent into the vagina under low pressure; this is a poor contraceptive, even when used immediately after intercourse. The same is true for coitus interruptus, which is withdrawal of the penis before ejaculation.

The U.S. Food and Drug Administration (FDA) has approved a number of birth control methods or contraceptives, used to prevent conception, or pregnancy (Table 11.1). **Spermi+cides** are placed in the vagina to kill sperm but are not as effective as several other contraceptive methods. Oral contraceptives (OCs), contraceptive implants, contraceptive patches, and injectable contraceptives are methods that use hormones to prevent ovulation. An intra+uterine device (IUD) is a contraceptive device that is inserted into the uterus by the physician. Postcoital contraceptive pills or IUDs must be used within a given time after unprotected intercourse (72 hours and 7 days, respectively), but their effectiveness rate is less than that of an IUD inserted in the prescribed manner before intercourse.

TABLE 11.1   SELECTED CONTRACEPTIVE METHODS AND THEIR EFFECTIVENESS

	Method	Action
Most Effective ↑	Subdermal implant	Capsule implanted under the skin slowly releases a hormone that blocks the release of ova; surgical implant is considered permanent.
	Intrauterine device (IUD)	Small plastic or metal device placed in the uterus (some release hormones); mode of action is not known, but device is believed to prevent fertilization or implantation (Fig. 11.15).
	Injectable contraceptive	Hormonal injection on a specific schedule prevents ovulation.
	Oral contraceptive	"Pill" that contains hormones, usually progestin and estrogen, that prevent ovulation (Fig. 11.16).
	Contraceptive patch	Skin patch that releases the hormones progestin and estrogen in the bloodstream; one patch is applied weekly for 3 weeks, then the patch is not applied for 1 week.
	Vaginal contraceptive ring	Ring that is inserted into the vagina, where it releases progestin and estrogen; worn 3 out of every 4 weeks.
	Diaphragm with spermicide	Soft rubber cup that covers the uterine cervix, designed to prevent sperm from entering the cervical canal
	Sponge with spermicide*	Acts as a barrier to sperm and releases spermicide.
	Cervical cap with spermicide*	Small cup that fits over the cervix to prevent sperm from entering the cervical canal.
	Male condom	Thin sheath (usually latex) worn over the penis to collect semen; informally called a rubber. Other than abstinence, latex condoms are the best protection against sexually transmitted diseases (STDs).
	Female condom	Thin sheath (usually latex) worn in the vagina to collect semen.
	Vaginal spermicide	Foam, cream, or jelly that is inserted into the vagina before intercourse to destroy sperm.
Least Effective	Natural family planning methods	Any of several methods of conception control that do not rely on a medication or physical device for effectiveness. The calendar, or rhythm, method of natural family planning relies on determination of the fertile period and abstinence during "unsafe" days. The basal body temperature method determines ovulation by a drop and subsequent rise in the basal body temperature. The ovulation method uses observation of changes in the cervical mucus to determine ovulation. The symptothermal method incorporates the ovulation and basal body temperature methods.

*The cervical cap and sponge with spermicide methods are more effective in females who have not given birth than in those who have given birth.
Data from www.fda.gov and www.emedicinehealth.com.

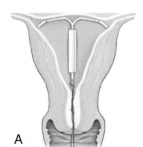

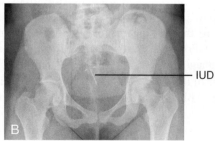

IUD

Fig. 11.15 Intrauterine Hormone-Releasing Device. **A,** A T-shaped flexible plastic device (inserted by a physician) releases hormone on a regular schedule. **B,** Pelvic x-ray showing IUD in place.

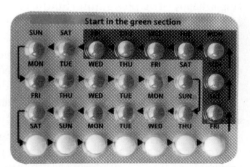

Fig. 11.16 Oral Contraceptive (Birth Control) Pill. An oral contraceptive contains estrogen and progestin. The "pill" is sometimes prescribed to help regulate irregular or heavy periods. Skipping a day increases the risk of pregnancy.

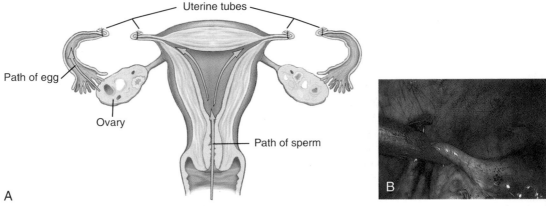

A

B

Fig. 11.17 Tubal Ligation. **A,** Note the severing of both uterine tubes. **B,** Laparoscopic view of a clip being applied to a uterine tube.

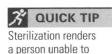
QUICK TIP

Sterilization renders a person unable to produce children.

Female and male **sterilization** are called **tubal ligation** and vasectomy, respectively. In a tubal ligation (Fig. 11.17), both uterine tubes are blocked. A vasectomy is bilateral excision of the vas deferens. Both are highly effective and are recommended as a contraceptive option for people who do not want additional children. They should be considered permanent, because reversal is not always successful.

WRITE IT!   EXERCISE 11

Write a term in each blank space to complete the sentence.

1. Refraining from sexual intercourse is called _____.
2. A small plastic or metal device placed within the uterus to prevent contraception is an _____ device.
3. Vaginal foams, creams, or jellies that are used to destroy the sperm are _____.
4. Withdrawal of the penis before ejaculation is _____ interruptus.
5. A method of practicing abstinence during fertile periods is called the calendar or _____ method.

The following list describes several surgical interventions.

colpoplasty (colp/o, vagina + -plasty, surgical repair) Plastic surgery of the vagina.

colporrhaphy (-rrhaphy, suture) Suture of the vagina.

conization of the cervix Excision of a cone of tissue from the cervix, performed to remove a lesion from the cervix or to obtain tissue for biopsy.

dilation and curettage (D&C) Surgical procedure that expands the cervical opening (dilation or dilatation) so that the uterine wall can be scraped (**curettage**).

endometrial ablation Destruction of a thin layer of the uterus to stop heavy menstrual bleeding. Ablation means removal or destruction of a part.

hysterectomy (hyster/o, uterus + -ectomy, excision) Surgical removal of the uterus. Removal of the uterus through the abdominal wall is called an abdominal hysterectomy, or **laparohysterectomy** (lapar/o, abdominal wall). Removal of the uterus through the vagina is called a vaginal hysterectomy. In a **radical hysterectomy**, the uterus, cervix, ovaries, uterine tubes, and nearby lymph nodes and lymph channels are removed.

laparoscopy (lapar/o, abdominal wall + -scopy, visually examining) Abdominal exploration using a lighted instrument, the laparoscope, which allows direct visualization of the abdominal contents (see Fig. 11.7). Another instrument, a cannula, is inserted to allow movement of the uterus during the examination. Abdominal and uterine adhesions, scar tissue that binds anatomic surfaces that are normally separate, are often seen

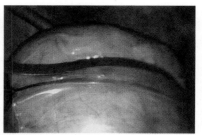

Fig. 11.18 Laparoscopic View of Uterine Adhesions. Numerous adhesions between the small bowel and uterus (shown here) were excised.

Fig. 11.19 Bagging of Excised Ovarian Cyst During Laparoscopic Surgery. Bagging the specimen prevents contamination of the peritoneal cavity or incision. Once the specimen is completely within the bag, the drawstring is closed before removal.

and can be removed during laparoscopy (Fig. 11.18), in addition to small uterine or ovarian cysts (Fig. 11.19).

oophorectomy (oophor/o, ovary) Surgical removal of one or both ovaries.

salpingectomy (salping/o, uterine tube) Surgical removal of a uterine tube.

salpingo-oophorectomy (oophor/o, ovary) Removal of an ovary and its accompanying uterine tube. Bilateral salpingo-oophorectomy is removal of both ovaries and their uterine tubes.

salpingorrhaphy Suture of a uterine tube.

vulvectomy Excision of the vulva, characteristically used to treat vulvar cancer.

WRITE IT! EXERCISE 12

Write terms in the blanks to complete each sentence.

1. Surgical removal of the uterus is a _____.
2. Plastic surgery of the vagina is _____.
3. Suture of the vagina is _____.
4. Removal of an ovary is _____.
5. Suture of a uterine tube is _____.
6. Tying or binding of a uterine tube for elective sterilization is a tubal _____.
7. Use of a lighted instrument to allow for direct visualization of the abdominal contents is _____.
8. The surgical procedure that is abbreviated D&C is dilation and _____.
9. An abdominal incision is a _____.
10. Cervical _____ is excision of a small cone of tissue from the cervix.

QUICK CASE STUDY | EXERCISE 13

Define the terms as indicated.

Mary Lou Garcia is experiencing pelvic pressure. She is <u>postmenopausal</u> and had <u>bilateral salpingo-oophorectomy</u> 1 year ago. A <u>pelvic examination</u> reveals a <u>cystocele</u>. She is scheduled for repair 1 week from today.

1. postmenopausal _____
2. bilateral salpingo-oophorectomy _____
3. pelvic examination_____
4. cystocele _____

Pregnancy and Childbirth

Fertilization is the union of an ovum and a sperm, resulting in an embryo. Fertilization of the ovum by the sperm occurs most often in the uterine tube (Fig. 11.20). **Implantation**, embedding of the fertilized ovum (called a **zygote**), usually occurs in the endometrium. Extraembryonic membranes (**amnion** and **chorion**) form around the embryo and give rise to the **placenta**, a structure through which the fetus derives nourishment during pregnancy. It is commonly called "afterbirth" because it is expelled after delivery of the baby.

In humans the developing embryo is called a fetus after 8 weeks. **Fetal** is an adjective that refers to the fetus. Within a few days after fertilization has occurred, a hormone called **human chorionic gonadotropin** (HCG) is produced and can be detected in body fluids. Testing for this hormone in urine or blood can indicate whether a woman is pregnant. HCG can be detected long before other signs of pregnancy appear.

fet/o = fetus

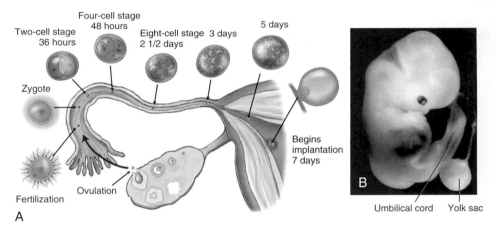

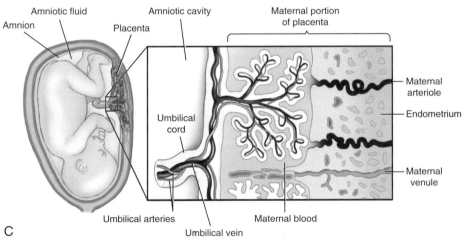

Fig. 11.20 Fertilization, Implantation, and Growth of the Embryo. **A,** A mature ovum is released in ovulation. The ovum is fertilized by a sperm, and the product of fertilization, the zygote, undergoes rapid cell division, finally implanting in the endometrium on approximately day 7. **B,** Human embryo. **C,** Drawing of a fetus at several months to show the interface between the maternal and fetal circulations.

Learn the following word parts and their meanings.

WORD PARTS: OBSTETRIC TERMS	
Word Part	**Meaning**
amni/o	amnion (fetal membrane)
fet/o	fetus
nat/i	birth
par/o	to bear offspring
-para	a woman who has given birth

WRITE IT! EXERCISE 14

Write combining forms for these terms.

1. amnion   _____
2. birth   _____
3. fetus   _____
4. to bear offspring   _____

HCG is present in the body fluids of pregnant females; blood or urine is tested to determine whether pregnancy exists (Fig. 11.21). Ultrasonography, also called ultrasound, provides an image of the developing fetus (Fig. 11.22). Ultrasonography has many uses in obstetrics, including the detection of an embryo that has implanted outside the uterus. Such abnormal implantation is called an extrauterine or **ectopic** pregnancy. The word *ectopic* means located outside the usual place.

> **ecto-** = outside
> **top/o** = location

Prenatal and **postnatal** mean occurring before birth and after birth, respectively. A **neonate** is a newborn infant up to 6 weeks of age; this period of time is known as the **neonatal** period.

> **nat/i** = birth
> **ne/o** = new

Obstetrics is the branch of medicine that specializes in the care of women during pregnancy and childbirth. The specialist is an **obstetrician**. **Gestation**, another word meaning pregnancy, is the period from conception to birth. **Parturition** is a synonym for childbirth. **Antepartum** means before childbirth, and **postpartum** means after childbirth.

> **ante-** = before
> **post-** = after

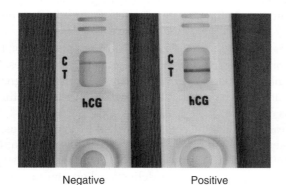

Negative   Positive

Fig. 11.21 Urine Pregnancy Test. The positive test (on the right) has a red line near the label *HCG* (human chorionic gonadotropin) and a light blue line. The negative test lacks the red band of color near the HCG.

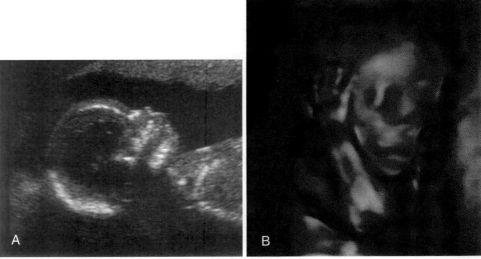

Fig. 11.22 Fetal Ultrasound Imaging. **A,** Two-dimensional ultrasound image of a fetus. **B,** Three-dimensional ultrasound image of a fetus; 3D ultrasounds allow the examiner to see width, height, and depth.

MATCH IT!
EXERCISE 15

Match the terms with their meanings.

_____ 1. antepartum   A. pregnancy

_____ 2. gestation   B. childbirth

_____ 3. parturition   C. before birth

_____ 4. postpartum   D. after birth

-para = woman who has given birth
nulli- = none

WORD ORIGIN

secundus (L.), second

The combining form par/o is often used to form words referring to the bearing of offspring. A designation showing the number of pregnancies resulting in live births is para I (or 1) or para II (or 2), but does not reflect the number of offspring in multiple births. Therefore, thinking of *para* as "birth" is acceptable if you remember that para I could represent more than one offspring. Other designations are **unipara**, **secundipara**, and **tripara**. **Nullipara** refers to a woman who has never had a viable (live) birth.

A woman who is pregnant for the first time is called **gravida** I or 1 (or **primigravida**). Gravida II or 2, III or 3, and so on designate subsequent pregnancies. Note that gravida refers only to pregnancy, whereas para designates successful pregnancies resulting in live births. A woman could be gravida III (pregnant for the third time) but para 0 (no live births, same as nullipara).

Labor, the process by which the child is expelled from the uterus, is that time from the beginning of cervical dilation to the delivery of the placenta. Cervical dilation, expulsion of the fetus, and expulsion of the placenta represent stages of labor. The postpartum stage, the hour or two after delivery when uterine tone is established, is sometimes included as a fourth stage of labor. The events just described are the stages

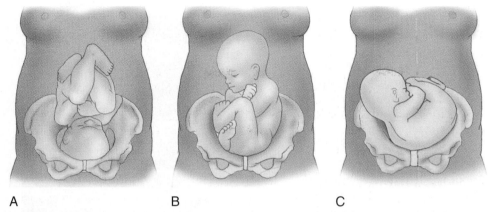

A   B   C

Fig. 11.23 Fetal Presentation. **A,** Cephalic presentation, the normal presentation of the top of the head, the brow, the face, or the chin at the cervical opening. **B,** Breech presentation. **C,** Shoulder presentation.

of a vaginal delivery. A **cesarean section** or cesarean birth, the surgical removal of the fetus from the uterus, is performed when fetal or maternal conditions make vaginal delivery hazardous.

Fetal presentation describes the part of the fetus that is touched by the examining finger through the cervix or that has entered the mother's lower pelvis during labor. **Cephalic presentation** is normal and the most common fetal presentation. In a **breech presentation** the buttocks, knees, or feet are presented. In a **shoulder presentation** the long axis of the baby's body is across the long axis of the mother's body, and the shoulder is presented at the cervical opening. This type of presentation is also called transverse presentation. Vaginal delivery is impossible unless the baby turns spontaneously or is turned in utero. Compare the three types of presentation in Fig. 11.23.

The average period of gestation (pregnancy) is 266 days from the date of fertilization, but it is clinically considered to last 280 days from the first day of the last menstrual period (LMP). The expected date of delivery (EDD) is usually calculated on the latter basis. For convenience, pregnancy is discussed in terms of the first, second, and third trimesters. A **trimester** is approximately 3 months, with the first day of the LMP to the end of 12 weeks designating the first trimester.

QUICK TIP

Cesarean section is abbreviated C-section.

cephal/o = head

QUICK TIP

Shoulder presentation is transverse presentation.

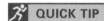

QUICK TIP

A tricycle has 3 wheels; normal pregnancy has 3 trimesters.

HEALTH CARE CONNECTION

Apgar scoring, usually performed 1 minute and again 5 minutes after birth, is an evaluation of an infant at birth. A mnemonic APGAR is helpful in remembering **A**ppearance (color), **P**ulse, **G**rimace (response to catheter in nostril), **A**ctivity (muscle tone), and **R**espiration (respiratory effort).

Study the following list of obstetric terms.

abruptio placentae Separation of the placenta from the uterine wall after 20 or more weeks of gestation or during labor; often results in pain and severe hemorrhage.

amnion The innermost of the membranes that surround the developing fetus. This transparent sac, also called the **amniotic** sac, holds the fetus suspended in amniotic fluid.

amniocentesis (amni/o, amnion + -centesis, puncture) **Transabdominal** (through the abdomen) puncture of the amniotic sac to remove amniotic fluid. The material that is removed can be studied to detect genetic disorders or other abnormalities (see Fig. 2.12).

amniotomy (-tomy, incision) Surgical rupture of the fetal membranes, performed to induce or expedite labor.

cesarean section (C-section) Incision through the walls of the abdomen and uterus for delivery of a fetus (Fig. 11.24).

chorionic villus sampling Sampling of the placental tissue for prenatal diagnosis of potential genetic defects.

Down syndrome Congenital condition characterized by mild to severe cognitive impairment and caused by an abnormality, usually the presence of three of chromosome 21, rather than the expected pair (Fig. 11.25). Ultra-Screen is a first-trimester prenatal screening test that is designed to provide specific information about the risk of Down syndrome and other chromosomal abnormalities. The test consists of a combination of ultrasound measurement and a blood test performed between 11 weeks 1 day and 13 weeks 6 days of pregnancy.

episiotomy Surgical procedure in which an incision is made to enlarge the vaginal opening for delivery.

erythroblastosis fetalis (erythr/o, red + blast/o, embryonic form + -osis, condition) Anemia of newborns characterized by premature destruction of red blood cells and resulting from maternal-fetal blood group incompatibility, specifically involving the Rh factor and the ABO blood groups. Also called hemolytic disease of the newborn.

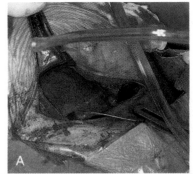

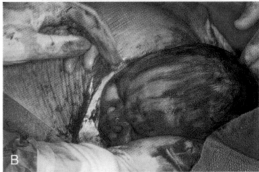

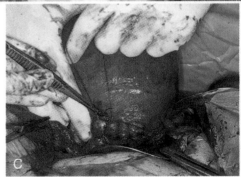

Fig. 11.24 Cesarean Section. A, The uterus is entered through a transverse incision. **B,** The fetal head is brought through the incision. **C,** The final step involves the use of heavy sutures to close the uterus.

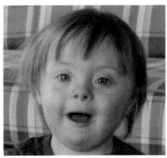

Fig. 11.25 Typical Facial Characteristics of Down Syndrome. This congenital condition, usually caused by an extra chromosome 21, is characterized by varying degrees of cognitive impairment and multiple defects. It can be diagnosed prenatally by amniocentesis and other methods that examine chromosomes.

fetal monitoring (fet/o, fetus) Assessment of the fetus in utero, usually with respect to its heartbeat (by electrocardiography).

placenta previa Abnormal implantation of the placenta in the uterus so that it impinges on or covers the opening at the upper end of the uterine cervix.

QUICK CASE STUDY | EXERCISE 16

Define the underlined terms.

Charlotte Smith, a 35-year-old <u>gravida 3</u>, visits her <u>obstetrician</u>. Both prior pregnancies were complicated by <u>breech presentations</u>, requiring a <u>cesarean section</u>.

1. gravida 3   _____
2. obstetrician   _____
3. breech presentation _____
4. cesarean section   _____

CHOOSE IT!   EXERCISE 17

Choose the correct answer for each question.

1. What is the term for a woman who has had two successful pregnancies? (nullipara, secundipara, tripara, unipara)
2. What is the correct term for an unborn 12-week-old developing human? (embryo, fetus, gestation, zygote)
3. Which term means abnormal implantation of a fertilized ovum outside the uterus? (abruptio placentae, cesarean section, ectopic pregnancy, transverse presentation)
4. Which term refers to the period covering the first 4 weeks after birth? (neonatal, obstetric, parturition, prenatal)
5. Which of the following is the normal fetal presentation? (breech, cephalic, shoulder, transverse)
6. Which term means the transparent sac that encloses the fetus in utero? (amniocentesis, amnion, congenital sac, trisomic sac)
7. Which of the following indicates a congenital condition of the newborn marked by cognitive impairment? (Down syndrome, cesarean section, ectopic pregnancy, jaundice)
8. Which term means surgical rupture of the fetal membrane? (amniocentesis, amniotomy, cesarean section, fetal monitoring)
9. What is the name of the structure through which the fetus receives nourishment? (fistula, HCG, ovary, placenta)
10. Which term means separation of the placenta from the uterine wall after 20 weeks or more of gestation or during labor? (abruptio placentae, episiotomy, labor, placenta previa)

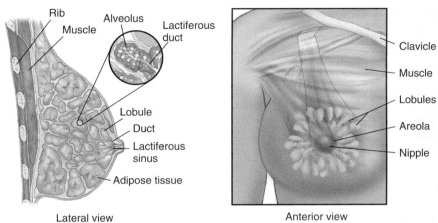

Lateral view   Anterior view

Fig. 11.26 Structure of the Adult Female Breast, Lateral and Anterior Views. The breasts are mammary glands and function as part of both the endocrine and reproductive systems. The amount of adipose tissue determines the size of the breasts, but not the amount of milk that can be produced. The nipple contains the openings of the lactiferous, or milk, ducts. Breasts are prepared for milk production during pregnancy. After childbirth, interactions between the nervous system, hormones, and the breasts result in expression of milk.

adip/o = fat
anter/o = anterior (front)
lact/o = milk

Female Breasts

The female breasts are accessory reproductive organs. Each breast contains 15 to 20 lobes of glandular tissue that radiate around the nipples, which may have many smaller sections called **lobules** (Fig. 11.26). The circular pigmented area of skin surrounding the nipple is the **areola**. The amount of adipose tissue (fat) determines the size of the breast.

The female breasts, accessory organs of the reproductive system, are milk-producing glands and are called **mamm+ary** glands. During pregnancy these glands undergo changes that prepare them for production of milk. After giving birth, hormones stimulate the secretion of milk. Each lobe is drained by a **lactiferous** duct that has openings in the nipple. **Lact+ation** is the secretion of milk. The production and secretion of milk is controlled by the endocrine (hormonal) and nervous systems.

Mammo+graphy is a diagnostic procedure that uses low-energy x-rays to study the breast (Fig. 11.27). The radiographic image produced in mammography is a **mammogram**. Breast cancer can often be diagnosed by studying a mammogram. Excluding skin cancer, breast cancer has been the most common malignancy among women in the United States for many years. Breast cancer in women is the second leading cause of cancer death, after lung cancer.

mamm/o = breast
-ary = pertaining to
lact/o = milk
-ation = process

WORD ORIGIN

lactis (L.), milk

BREAST CANCER MAY LOOK LIKE A RASH OF THE NIPPLE

A woman often may assume that a rash is a skin infection or allergy. Note the uneven, superficial red appearance of more than half of the nipple in this surgical specimen of breast cancer, which had invaded the underlying breast tissue.

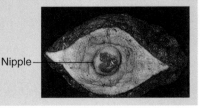

Nipple

Fig. 11.27 Mammography. A, Clinical setting for mammography. The compression device evens out breast tissue to improve the image quality. **B,** Mammogram of cancer of the breast. The arrow indicates carcinoma.

mamm/o = breast
-gram = a record
carcin/o = cancer
-oma = tumor

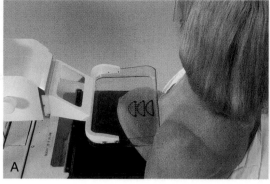
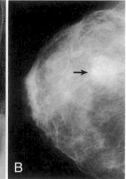

Breast masses are one of the most common disorders of the breast, and fortunately, most masses are benign. In addition to mammography, tissue and/or fluid can be examined by needle biopsy, incisional biopsy, or excisional biopsy (Fig. 11.28).

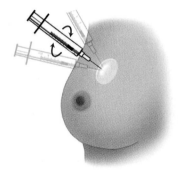
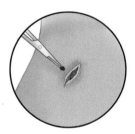
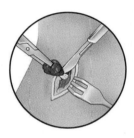

Needle biopsy and aspiration   Incisional biopsy   Excisional biopsy

Fig. 11.28 Breast Biopsy Techniques. Needle biopsy and aspiration of fluid, incisional biopsy of tissue, or excisional biopsy is used to remove all of the mass.

Treatment of breast cancer may require **lumpectomy** (removal of the lump or tumor), chemotherapy, radiation therapy, hormone therapy, or **mast+ectomy** (Fig. 15.15).

Mastalgia and **mastodynia** mean pain in the breast; **mammalgia** also means painful breast. **Mastitis** means inflammation of the breast.

Mastoptosis means sagging breasts. A surgical procedure to lift the breasts is **mastopexy**. Augmentation **mammoplasty** is plastic surgery to increase the size of the female breast (see Fig. 2.17). Reduction mammoplasty is plastic surgery to reduce the size of the breast.

mast/o = breast
-ptosis = sagging or prolapse
-pexy = surgical fixation
-plasty = surgical repair

MATCH IT!
EXERCISE 18

Match terms in the left column with those in the right column.

_____ 1. mammary
_____ 2. mastectomy
_____ 3. mammography
_____ 4. mastoptosis

A. pertaining to the breast
B. radiographic examination of the breast
C. sagging breasts
D. surgical removal of a breast

MALE REPRODUCTIVE SYSTEM

The male reproductive system produces, sustains, and transports spermatozoa; introduces sperm into the female vagina; and produces hormones. The testes, the male gonads, are responsible for production of both sperm and hormones. All other organs, ducts, and glands in this system are accessory reproductive organs that transport and sustain the sperm.

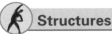 **Structures**

QUICK TIP

Gonads are either ovaries or testes.

Gonads produce ova or sperm, and the testes are the male gonads. **Testes** is the plural form of testis, which means the same as **testicle**.

Write the names of the structures in the blank lines (*1* to *12*) on Fig. 11.29 as you read the following information. The **penis** *(1)* transfers sperm to the vagina. The **prepuce** *(2)*, a loose fold of skin, covers the **glans penis** *(3)*.

Only one **testis** *(4)* is shown in Fig. 11.29. After sperm are produced by the testis, they are stored in the **epididymis** *(5)*. The testes and epididymis are contained in a pouch of skin called the **scrotum** *(6)*.

Each **ductus deferens** *(7)*, also called the **vas deferens**, begins at the epididymis, continues upward, and enters the abdominopelvic cavity. Each ductus deferens joins a duct from the **seminal vesicle** *(8)* to form a short **ejaculatory duct** *(9)*, which passes through the **prostate gland** *(10)*. Ejaculation is the expulsion of semen from the urethra *(11)*. Paired **bulbourethral glands** *(12)* contribute an alkaline, mucuslike fluid to the semen.

Several important word parts refer to male reproductive organs. Commit to memory the meanings of the word parts in the table on the next page.

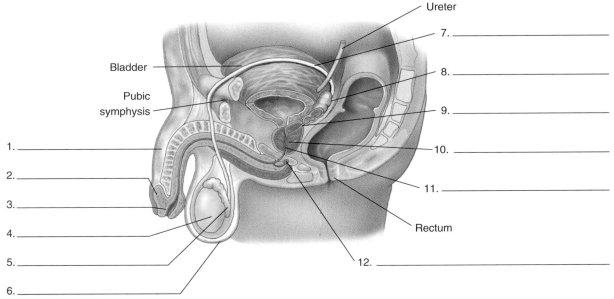

Fig. 11.29 Structures of the Male Reproductive System. Lateral view of the internal structures. The structures that are already labeled lie near, but are not part of, the male reproductive system. **pub/o** = pubis;   **semin/o** = semen;   **urethr/o** = urethra

WORD PARTS: MALE REPRODUCTIVE ORGANS

Word Part	Meaning
gon/o	genitals or reproduction
orchi/o, orchid/o, test/o, testicul/o	testes
pen/o*	penis
prostat/o	prostate
scrot/o	scrotum, bag
semin/o	semen
ser/o	serum
spermat/o	spermatozoa (sperm)
urethr/o	urethra
vas/o	vessel or duct; sometimes ductus deferens (vas deferens)

*In some words, *pen/o* means punishment (e.g., penology is the study of punishment).

WRITE IT! EXERCISE 19

Write combining forms for the following.

1. genitals or reproduction _____
2. penis _____
3. prostate _____
4. scrotum _____

5. semen _____
6. sperm _____
7. testes _____
8. vas deferens _____

The testes produce an important male hormone, **testosterone**, that induces and maintains male secondary sex characteristics. In addition, the testes are responsible for **spermato+genesis**, the formation of mature functional sperm. Human sperm are produced in vast numbers after puberty. Each sperm has a head with a nucleus, a neck, and a tail that provides propulsion (Fig. 11.30). The formation of sperm is also influenced by hormones produced by the brain and the pituitary gland.

spermat/o = sperm
-genesis = formation

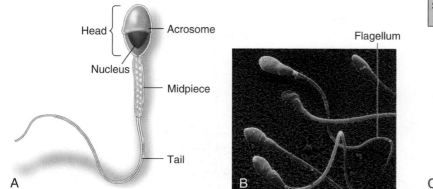

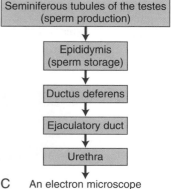

Fig. 11.30 The Human Spermatozoon and Passageway of Sperm. **A,** A sperm in cross section. The nucleus contains the chromosomes and is located in the head. The tip of the head is covered by an acrosome, which contains enzymes that help the sperm penetrate the ovum. The midpiece contains mitochondria that provide energy, and the tail is a typical flagellum for movement. **B,** Five spermatozoa are seen with an electron microscope. **C,** The pathway of sperm from where they are produced in the testes to ejaculation in semen.

VESIC/O MEANS BLADDER, CYST, OR SAC

The term *vesicle*, however, means a small sac containing fluid or a small, blisterlike elevation on the skin containing serous fluid. Seminal vesicles refer to small sacs that store semen, whereas vesicular rash refers to an eruption of blisters on the skin.

Semen, also called seminal fluid, is a mixture of sperm cells and secretions. Both the number of sperm and their motility (movement) can be observed with a light microscope. Although millions of sperm are ejaculated in semen, only one sperm fertilizes an ovum. The production of sperm outside the body cavity is necessary for viability of the sperm. The testes develop in the abdominal cavity of the fetus and normally descend through the inguinal canal into the scrotum shortly before birth (sometimes shortly after birth).

semin/o = semen

Sperm leave the male's body in semen, the fluid that is discharged from the penis at the height of sexual excitement. **Seminal vesicles** serve as a reservoir for semen until it is discharged. The seminal vesicles, the **prostate**, and other glands produce fluids necessary for survival of the sperm. The prostate is also called the prostate gland.

WORD ORIGIN

semen (L.), seed

Spermatozoa are mature male sex cells. **Spermato+cidal** or **spermicidal** refers to the killing of sperm. Contraceptive foams and creams are spermicidal, and as such are designed to prevent pregnancy.

-cidal = killing

FIND IT!
EXERCISE 20

Write the meaning of the combining forms in these new terms.

Term	Meaning of Combining Form	Term	Meaning of Combining Form
1. **penile**	_____	4. **seminal**	_____
2. **prostatic**	_____	5. **testicular**	_____
3. **scrotal**	_____		

 Diseases, Disorders, and Diagnostic Terms

anorchidism Congenital absence of one or both testicles; same as **anorchism**.

aspermia or aspermatogenesis Absence of sperm in semen.

benign prostatic hyperplasia (BPH) (hyper-, increase + -plasia, formation) Nonmalignant, noninflammatory enlargement of the prostate, most common among men older than 50 (Fig. 11.31).

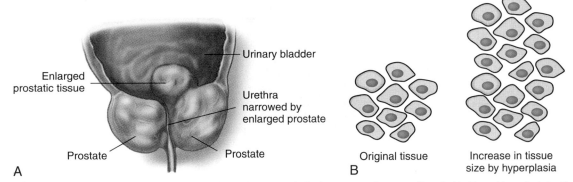

Fig. 11.31 Benign Prostatic Hyperplasia. **A,** Prostate (shown in cross section) enlarges, extending upward into the bladder and inward, obstructing the outflow of urine. **B,** Representation of tissue enlargement by hyperplasia. **prostat/o** = prostate; **urin/o** = urine

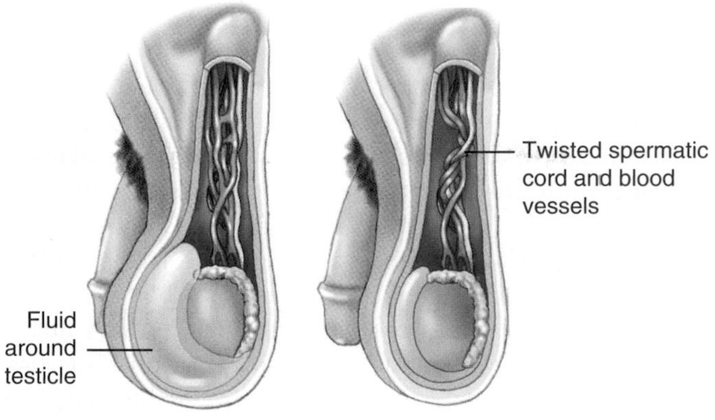

Fig. 11.32 Hydrocele and Testicular Torsion. **hydr/o** = water; **-cele** = hernia

cryptorchidism (crypt/o, hidden + orchid/o, testis + -ism, condition) Undescended testicles; failure of the testicles to descend into the scrotum before birth.

hydrocele (hydr/o, water + -cele, hernia) Accumulation of fluid in a saclike cavity, especially serous tumors of the testes or associated parts. Serous (ser/o, serum + -ous, pertaining to) means resembling serum or producing or containing serum (Fig. 11.32).

intersexuality A rare chromosomal abnormality in which both testicular and ovarian elements exist in the same person and may result in abnormal genitalia; hermaphrodism. The affected individual is referred to as intersex.

(In Greek mythology, Hermaphroditus was the child of the goddess Aphrodite and the god Hermes. Hermaphroditus was bisexual, and his name is the basis for the term *hermaphrodite*.)

orchiditis or orchitis (orchid/o or orchi/o, testis + -itis, inflammation) Inflammation of a testis. (Notice the spelling of orchitis. In joining orchi/o + -itis, one *i* is dropped to avoid double *i*.)

prostatic carcinoma Slowly progressing cancer of the prostate; typically detected by a prostate-specific antigen (PSA) test and rectal examination. The treatment is surgery, radiation therapy, or hormones.

prostatitis Inflammation of the prostate.

testicular cancer Malignant neoplastic disease of the testes, occurring most frequently in men between 15 and 35 years of age.

testicular torsion (testicul/o, testicle) Axial rotation of the spermatic cord, which cuts off the blood supply to the testicle (see Fig. 11.32).

WRITE IT! **EXERCISE 21**

Write a term in the blanks to complete each sentence.

1. A term for undescended testicles is _____.
2. A nonmalignant, noninflammatory enlargement of the prostate is benign prostatic _____.
3. The term that means inflammation of the prostate is _____.
4. A synonym for orchiditis is _____.
5. Accumulation of fluid in the testicle is called a(n) _____.
6. Congenital absence of one or both testicles is anorchidism, also called _____.
7. Accumulation of fluid in a testicle is a _____.
8. A rare chromosomal abnormality in which both testicular and ovarian elements exist in the same person is _____.
9. Malignant neoplastic disease of the testes is _____ cancer.
10. Axial rotation of the spermatic cord is testicular _____.

Surgical and Therapeutic Interventions

Learn the following terms.

circumcision Surgical removal of the end of the foreskin that covers the head of the penis. This is usually performed shortly after birth for hygienic or religious reasons.

orchidectomy (orchid/o, testes, + -ectomy, excision) Surgical removal of a testicle (often done to treat malignancy of a testicle). Excision of both testes is **castration**. **Orchiectomy** is a synonym for orchidectomy.

orchidoplasty (-plasty, surgical repair) Plastic surgery of the testis, particularly the surgery performed to correct a testicle that has not descended properly into the scrotum.

orchiopexy (-pexy, surgical fixation) Surgical fixation of an undescended testicle in the scrotum. Also called **orchidopexy**.

orchiotomy (-tomy, incision) Incision and drainage of a testis.

prostatectomy (prostat/o, prostate) Removal of all or part of the prostate.

transurethral microwave thermotherapy (TUMT) (trans-, across + urethr/o, urethra; therm/o, heat) Treatment of BPH performed through the urethra using microwave energy to raise the temperature selectively and destroy prostatic tissue.

transurethral needle ablation (TUNA) Treatment of BPH performed through the urethra using low-level radio frequency energy. *Ablation* is a general term for excision or removal of a growth or any part of the body.

transurethral prostatectomy Partial or complete removal of prostatic tissue by means of a cystoscope passed through the urethra. It is also called **transurethral resection** of the prostate (TURP). *Resection* is a term that means excision of all or part of a structure.

vasectomy (vas/o, vas deferens) Removal of all or a segment of the vas deferens, usually done bilaterally to produce sterility (Fig. 11.33).

vasovasostomy (-stomy, new opening) Surgically reconnecting the ends of the severed ductus deferens, done to correct an obstruction or as a form of vasectomy reversal.

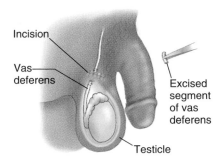

Incision
Vas deferens
Excised segment of vas deferens
Testicle

vas/o = vas deferens
-ectomy = excision
contra- = against
-plasty = surgical repair

Fig. 11.33 Vasectomy. This surgical procedure is performed as a permanent method of contraception, although it sometimes can be surgically reversed by vasoplasty (vasovasostomy). In a vasectomy, a small incision is made in the scrotum, and a piece of the vas deferens is removed.

WRITE IT! EXERCISE 22

Write a term in each blank to complete these sentences.

1. The term for surgical fixation of an undescended testicle is _____.
2. Surgical removal of the end of the foreskin that covers the head of the penis is _____.
3. Surgical removal of a segment of the ductus deferens is a _____.
4. Surgical removal of a testicle is _____.
5. Surgical removal of all or part of the prostate is called a _____.
6. A general term for excision or removal of a growth or any part of the body is _____.

Sexually Transmitted Diseases or Infections

An infection acquired through sexual contact is a sexually transmitted infection (STI) or a sexually transmitted disease (STD), sometimes called venereal disease (venereal was named for Venus, goddess of love). In general, STDs cause one of these problems: male **urethr+itis**, female lower genitourinary tract infection, and **vagin+itis**. The term **genito+urin+ary** (GU) pertains to the genitals and the urinary organs.

urethr/o	= urethra
vagin/o	= vagina
genit/o	= genitals
-ur/o	= urinary tract

Study Table 11.2 to learn the names and characteristics of several STDs. You may want to refer to the table to complete Exercises 23 and 24.

TABLE 11.2   SEXUALLY TRANSMITTED DISEASES (STDS) AND THEIR CAUSES

Disease of the Genitals*	Causative Agent	Characteristics
Bacterial		
Gonorrhea	*Neisseria gonorrhoeae*, commonly called **gonococcus** (GC)	Males: Urethral discharge (presence of gonorocci in smears and/or culture [Fig. 11.34]), dysuria Females: Often asymptomatic
Syphilis	*Treponema pallidum* (a **spirochete**)	Primary stage: Painless **chancre** (Fig. 11.35) Secondary stage: Rash Late stage: Only about one third of untreated cases progress to syphilitic involvement of the viscera, cardiovascular system, and central nervous system.
Chlamydial infection	*Chlamydia trachomatis*	Males: Urethritis, dysuria, frequent urination Females: Mild symptoms to none; one of the most common STDs in North America; frequent cause of pelvic inflammatory disease (PID) and sterility
Chancroid (nonsyphilitic venereal ulcer)	*Haemophilus ducreyi*	Painful ulceration of the genitals
Nonspecific genital infection	Various organisms, not all of which are bacteria	Males: Nongonococcal urethritis Females: PID, cervicitis

Continued

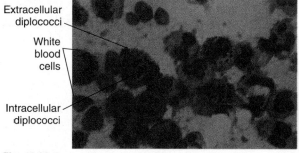

Fig. 11.34 Gram-Negative Intracellular Diplococci. The presence of gram-negative intracellular diplococci in a urethral smear is usually indicative of gonorrhea in males. The same finding in females is considered presumptive and is generally followed by culture to confirm the diagnosis. Note also the presence of many extracellular diplococci. **intra-** = within; **cellul/o** = cell; **-ar** = pertaining to; **dipl/o** = double; **gon/o** = reproduction or genital; **extra-** = outside

Labels: Extracellular diplococci; White blood cells; Intracellular diplococci

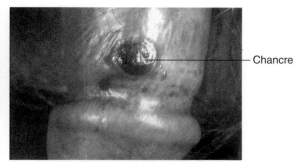

Fig. 11.35 Syphilitic Chancre. The lesion of primary syphilis generally develops about 2 weeks after exposure. Scrapings from the ulcer show spirochetes, the causative organism of syphilis, when examined microscopically using special illumination.

Label: Chancre

TABLE 11.2	SEXUALLY TRANSMITTED DISEASES (STDS) AND THEIR CAUSES—cont'd	
Disease of the Genitals*	**Causative Agent**	**Characteristics**
Viral		
Acquired immunodeficiency syndrome (AIDS)	Human immunodeficiency virus (HIV)	A fatal late stage of HIV infection that involves profound immunosuppression. To be diagnosed as having AIDS, one must be infected with HIV and have a clinical disease that indicates cellular immunodeficiency, or have a specified level of markers in the blood, including certain T lymphocytes. AIDS is characterized by opportunistic infections and malignant neoplasms that rarely affect healthy individuals, especially **Kaposi sarcoma** (Fig. 11.36). HIV is transmitted by infected body fluids (sexual contact, blood and blood products, breast milk).
Herpes genitalis (genital herpes)	Herpes simplex type 2 (HSV-2)	Blisters and ulceration of the genitalia, fever, and dysuria (Fig. 11.37)
Condyloma acuminatum (genital warts)	Human **papillomavirus** (HPV)	Cauliflower-like genital and anal warts (Fig. 11.38); infection puts females at high risk for cervical cancer. A vaccine is available that prevents infection with the two types of HPV responsible for most cervical cancer cases.
Hepatitis B, C, and D	Hepatitis B, C, and D viruses (HBV, HCV, and HDV)	These inflammatory conditions of the liver are separate diseases acquired by sexual contact, contaminated blood, or use of contaminated needles or equipment. Diseases vary from mild symptoms to serious complications. Hepatitis B vaccine is available for those at high risk; hepatitis B immune globulin provides postexposure passive immunity.
Protozoal		
Trichomoniasis	*Trichomonas vaginalis* (Fig. 11.38)	Females: Frothy discharge of varying severity Males: Often asymptomatic
Fungal		
Candidiasis	*Candida albicans* (Fig. 11.39)	Vulvovaginitis: white patches, cheeselike discharge
Parasitic		
Pubic lice	*Phthirus pubis*	Severe itching, redness, and inflammation of the skin and mucous membranes

*Although diseases of the genitals are given emphasis here, many of the organisms can infect other organs.

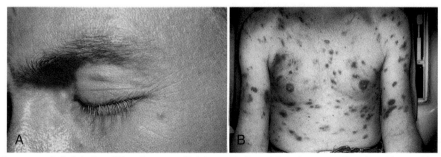

Fig. 11.36 Kaposi Sarcoma. **A,** Early lesion of Kaposi sarcoma. **B,** Advanced lesions of Kaposi sarcoma. Note the widespread hemorrhagic plaques and nodules.

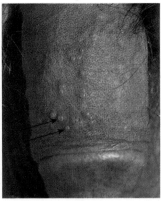

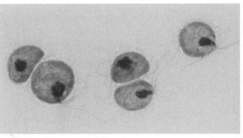

Fig. 11.39 *Trichomonas* in a Stained Smear. *Trichomonas* is a sexually transmitted protozoon that is pathogenic to humans. Five protozoa are shown. Perhaps the origin of their name is their hair-like flagella. **trich/o** = hair

Fig. 11.37 Genital Herpes. These unruptured vesicles (arrows) of herpes simplex virus type 2 (HSV-2) appear on the penis.
genit/o = genitals

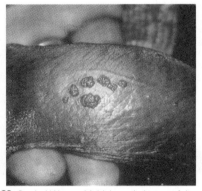

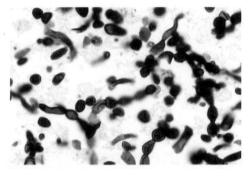

Fig. 11.40 *Candida albicans*, a Fungal Organism. Stained appearance of the microscopic fungi, showing the way in which the fungi multiply by budding.

Fig. 11.38 Genital Warts. Multiple genital warts of the penis.

MATCH IT!
EXERCISE 23

Choose the category of causative agent in the right column to classify these STDs.

_____ 1. AIDS
_____ 2. candidiasis
_____ 3. chlamydial infection
_____ 4. genital herpes
_____ 5. genital warts
_____ 6. gonorrhea
_____ 7. hepatitis B, C, or D
_____ 8. syphilis
_____ 9. trichomoniasis

A. bacteria
B. fungi
C. protozoa
D. virus

WRITE IT!

EXERCISE 24

Write a term in each blank to complete these sentences.

1. An STD caused by a gonococcus is _____.
2. Where are intracellular diplococci of gonorrhea located relative to the cell, within or outside?

   _____

3. A lesion that is characteristic of the primary stage of syphilis is called a _____.
4. A disease that may be asymptomatic in females but is one of the most common STDs in North America is a _____ infection.
5. A late-stage infection with HIV is called acquired _____ syndrome.
6. A malignant lesion of AIDS that is rarely seen in healthy individuals is _____ sarcoma.
7. A viral infection that causes blisters and ulceration of the genitalia is _____ genitalis.
8. Cauliflower-like genital and anal warts are characteristic of the infection commonly called genital

   _____.

9. HBV, HCV, or HDV causes an inflammatory condition of the liver called _____.
10. The STD caused by *Trichomonas vaginalis* is _____.
11. Inflammation of the vulva and vagina accompanied by a cheeselike discharge is characteristic of

    _____.

12. A parasitic STD that causes severe itching, redness, and inflammation of the skin and mucous membranes is pubic _____.

⚠ **Be Careful With These!**

cervic/o can refer to the uterine cervix or the neck.

cyst/o means bladder, cyst, or sac.

metr/o can mean uterine tissue, but sometimes means measure.

vas/o means vessel or duct, but sometimes specifically means the ductus deferens.

colposcopy vs. laparoscopy vs. hysteroscopy

amenorrhea vs. dysmenorrhea

menorrhagia vs. metrorrhagia

anorchism vs cryptorchidism

Chlamydia vs *Condyloma* vs. candidiasis

A Career as an Ultrasonographer

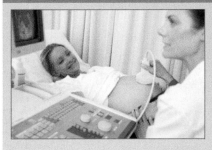

Chelsey Jones is really proud of her decision to study sonography. She had always wanted a career helping people directly. She works mostly with obstetric patients and truly feels that her talents are being used for an important purpose. Chelsey almost studied architecture because she knew she had a talent for visualizing objects in three dimensions, but that talent also applies to sonography. A bachelor's degree is not always required for ultrasonographers, but most employers prefer individuals registered through the American Registry for Diagnostic Medical Sonography or the American Registry of Radiologic Technologists. For more information, visit www.sdms.org, and click on the resources tab or www.arrt.org.

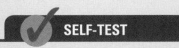

SELF-TEST

Work the following exercises to test your understanding of the material in Chapter 11. It is best to do all the exercises before checking your answers against the answers in Appendix III. Pay particular attention to spelling.

A. LABELING!   *Label the diagram with the following combining forms that correspond to numbered lines 1 through 5 (the first one is done as an example): cervic/o, colp/o, hyster/o, oophor/o, salping/o.*

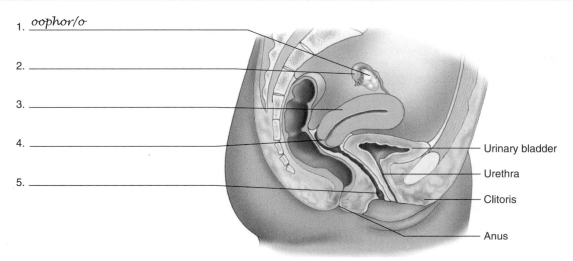

1. *oophor/o*
2.
3.
4.
5.

Urinary bladder
Urethra
Clitoris
Anus

Label the diagram with the following combining forms that correspond to numbered lines 6 through 11 (the first one is done as an example): orchi/o, pen/o, prostat/o, scrot/o, urethr/o, vas/o.

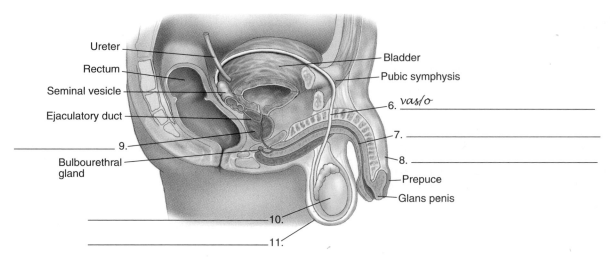

Ureter
Rectum
Seminal vesicle
Ejaculatory duct
9.
Bulbourethral gland
10.
11.

Bladder
Pubic symphysis
6. *vas/o*
7.
8.
Prepuce
Glans penis

B. MATCHING!   *Match the terms on the left with the descriptions in the right column.*

_____ 1. ovary
_____ 2. placenta
_____ 3. progesterone
_____ 4. testis
_____ 5. uterus
_____ 6. vagina

A. afterbirth
B. important hormone of pregnancy
C. normal site of implantation
D. site of production of ova
E. site of production of sperm
F. where sperm are received during intercourse

C. IDENTIFYING!   *Label these illustrations using of the following: antepartum, hysteroscopy, leiomyoma, oophorohysterogram, orchidoplasty, unipara, vasectomy*

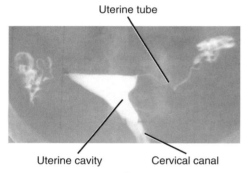

1. X-ray image of the uterus and ovarian tubes

_____

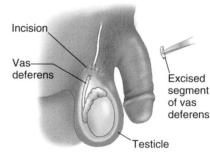

2. Excision of a portion of the vas deferens

_____

D. CHOOSING!   *Circle the one correct answer (A, B, C, or D) for each question.*

1. Which term refers to the lining of the uterus?
    (A) cervix uteri   **(B)** endometrium   **(C)** myometrium   **(D)** perimetrium

2. Which of the following is the hormone tested for in a pregnancy test?
    (A) BPH   **(B)** EDD   **(C)** HCG   **(D)** LMP

3. Which of the following is a genetic disorder in which the fetus has an extra chromosome?
    (A) Down syndrome   **(B)** endometriosis   **(C)** erythroblastosis fetalis   **(D)** hemolytic anemia

4. Which of the following is abnormal placement of the placenta in the uterus?
    (A) abruptio placentae   **(B)** cesarean section   **(C)** ectopic pregnancy   **(D)** placenta previa

5. Which term refers to the normal presentation of the fetus during labor?
    (A) breech   **(B)** cephalic   **(C)** shoulder   **(D)** transverse

6. Which of the following is a lighted instrument that allows direct visualization of the abdominal contents?
    (A) colposcope   **(B)** dilation and curettage   **(C)** fetal monitoring   **(D)** laparoscope

7. Which branch of medicine specializes in the care of women during pregnancy and childbirth?
    (A) gynecology   **(B)** internal medicine   **(C)** obstetrics   **(D)** pediatrics

8. Which hormone has the primary responsibility of induction and maintenance of male sexual characteristics?
   (A) amnion   (B) estrogen   (C) testosterone   (D) uterine

9. Which term means a woman who has never given birth to a viable offspring?
   (A) nullipara   (B) secundipara   (C) tripara   (D) unipara

10. What are reproductive organs called?
    (A) genitalia   (B) gonadotropin   (C) uteri   (D) vulva

11. What is the name of the transparent sac that encloses the fetus in utero?
    (A) amniocentesis sac   (B) amniotic sac   (C) congenital membrane   (D) trisomic membrane

12. Which term is the same as pregnancy?
    (A) climacteric   (B) dysmenorrheal   (C) fistula   (D) gestation

13. Which term means an abnormal tubelike passage?
    (A) adhesion   (B) colposcopy   (C) fistula   (D) polyp

14. Which of the following means childbirth?
    (A) gestation   (B) neonatality   (C) obstetrics   (D) parturition

15. What is the term for a tumor found on a mucous membrane?
    (A) curettage   (B) Pap   (C) polyp   (D) ovum

16. A chancre is characteristic of the primary stage of which disease?
    (A) chancroid   (B) chlamydial infection   (C) syphilis   (D) trichomoniasis

17. Which of the following is characterized by cauliflower-like genital and anal warts?
    (A) candidiasis   (B) condyloma acuminatum   (C) gonorrhea   (D) nonspecific genital infection

18. Which of the following is a parasitic STD that causes severe itching, redness, and inflammation?
    (A) chancroid   (B) papillomavirus   (C) pubic lice   (D) syphilis

19. Which of the following means direct visual inspection of the cervical canal and uterine cavity?
    (A) colposcopy   (B) hysteroscopy   (C) laparoscopy   (D) mammography

20. Which of the following means destruction of a thin layer of the uterus?
    (A) chorionic villus sampling   (B) endometrial ablation   (C) hysterectomy   (D) transurethral resection

E. WRITING!   *Write one word for each of the following.*

1. a newborn   _____
2. attachment of a fertilized ovum to the endometrium   _____
3. deliberate rupture of the fetal membranes to induce labor   _____
4. incision made to enlarge the vaginal opening for delivery   _____
5. menopause   _____
6. painful menstruation   _____
7. pertaining to the cervix uteri   _____
8. prolapse of the uterus   _____
9. surgical puncture of the amnion   _____
10. release of an ovum from the ovary   _____

F. SPELLING AND PRONUNCIATION! *Circle all incorrectly spelled terms and write their correct spelling. Then pronounce all the terms.*

cervicokolpitis   epididymis   korionic   sistocele   sifilis

_____

G. QUICK CHALLENGE! *Find an incorrect term in each sentence and write the correct term.*

1. Mastalgia or mastodynia means pain in the pelvis. _____
2. Metrorrhagia is excessive flow during menstruation. _____
3. Vasectomy reversal is called vasotomy. _____
4. A female who is pregnant for the first time is a secundipara. _____
5. Inflammation of an ovary and its uterine tube is endometriosis. _____

H. READING HEALTH CARE REPORTS *Read the laboratory report and answer the questions that follow the report.*

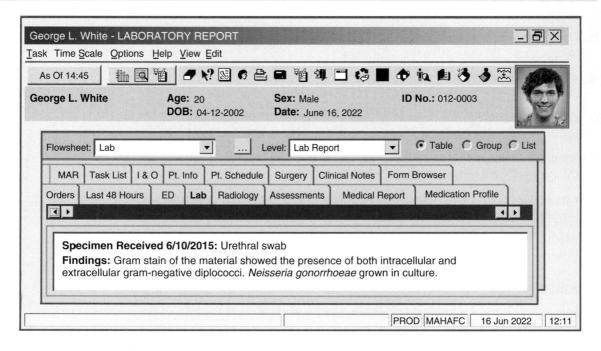

George L. White - LABORATORY REPORT

Task Time Scale Options Help View Edit

As Of 14:45

George L. White   **Age:** 20   **Sex:** Male   **ID No.:** 012-0003
DOB: 04-12-2002   **Date:** June 16, 2022

Flowsheet: Lab   …   Level: Lab Report   ⦿ Table ○ Group ○ List

MAR | Task List | I & O | Pt. Info | Pt. Schedule | Surgery | Clinical Notes | Form Browser

Orders | Last 48 Hours | ED | **Lab** | Radiology | Assessments | Medical Report | Medication Profile

Specimen Received 6/10/2015: Urethral swab
Findings: Gram stain of the material showed the presence of both intracellular and extracellular gram-negative diplococci. *Neisseria gonorrhoeae* grown in culture.

PROD | MAHAFC | 16 Jun 2022 | 12:11

1. What is meant by intracellular and extracellular diplococci? _____
   _____

2. What is the name of the sexually transmitted disease that is implied? _____

3. What is the common name of the organism that causes this disease? _____

I.   *Read the following office visit note, then circle one answer for each of the questions that follow the report.*

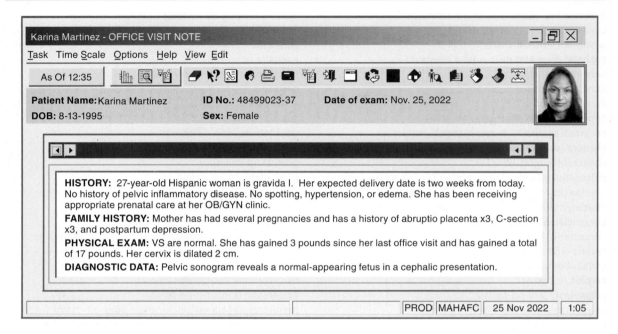

Karina Martinez - OFFICE VISIT NOTE

Task Time Scale Options Help View Edit

As Of 12:35

Patient Name: Karina Martinez   **ID No.:** 48499023-37   **Date of exam:** Nov. 25, 2022
DOB: 8-13-1995   **Sex:** Female

HISTORY: 27-year-old Hispanic woman is gravida I. Her expected delivery date is two weeks from today. No history of pelvic inflammatory disease. No spotting, hypertension, or edema. She has been receiving appropriate prenatal care at her OB/GYN clinic.
FAMILY HISTORY: Mother has had several pregnancies and has a history of abruptio placenta x3, C-section x3, and postpartum depression.
PHYSICAL EXAM: VS are normal. She has gained 3 pounds since her last office visit and has gained a total of 17 pounds. Her cervix is dilated 2 cm.
DIAGNOSTIC DATA: Pelvic sonogram reveals a normal-appearing fetus in a cephalic presentation.

PROD | MAHAFC | 25 Nov 2022 | 1:05

1. Abruptio placentae means premature detachment of which of the following? (fetus, ovary, placenta, uterus)
2. Pelvic inflammatory disease is infection of the upper genital organs beyond the (cervix, ovary, uterus, vagina).
3. When did the patient' mother suffer depression? (after birth, before birth, during birth)
4. What does the abbreviation "C" in C-section refer to? (cesarean, chancre, circumcision, conization)
5. What is an alternative term for prenatal? (antenatal, antepartum, neonatal, postnatal)

*Use Appendix III to check your answers.

QUICK & EASY (Q&E) LIST

Use the Evolve website (http://evolve.elsevier.com/Leonard/quick) to review the terms presented in Chapter 11. Look closely at the spelling of each term as it is pronounced.

abruptio placentae *(ab-**rup**-shē-ō pluh-**sen**-tē)*
acquired immunodeficiency syndrome *(uh-**kwīrd** im-ū-nō-duh-**fish**-un-sē **sin**-drōm)*
amenorrhea *(uh-men-ō-**rē**-uh)*
amniocentesis *(am-nē-ō-sen-**tē**-sis)*
amnion *(**am**-nē-on)*
amniotic *(am-nē-**ot**-ik)*
amniotomy *(am-nē-**ot**-uh-mē)*

anorchidism *(an-**or**-ki-diz-um)*
anorchism *(an-**or**-kiz-um)*
antepartum *(an-tē-**pahr**-tum)*
areola *(uh-**rē**-ō-luh)*
aspermatogenesis *(ā-spur-muh-tō-**jen**-uh-sis)*
aspermia *(uh-**spur**-mē-uh)*
benign prostatic hyperplasia *(buh-**nīn** pros-**tat**-ik hī-pur-**plā**-zhuh)*

QUICK & EASY (Q&E) LIST—cont'd

breech presentation *(brēch **prē**-zun-**tā**-shun)*
bulbourethral gland *(bul-bō-ū-**rē**-thrul gland)*
candidiasis *(kan-di-**dī**-uh-sis)*
castration *(kas-**trā**-shun)*
cephalic presentation (suh-**fal**-ik prē-zun-**tā**-shun)
cervical *(**sur**-vi-kul)*
cervical polyp *(**sur**-vi-kul **pol**-ip)*
cervicocolpitis
cervix uteri *(**sur**-viks **ū**-tur-ī)*
cesarean section *(suh-**zar**-ē-un **sek**-shun)*
chancre *(**shang**-kur)*
chancroid *(**shang**-kroid)*
chlamydial infection *(kluh-**mid**-ē-ul in-**fek**-shun)*
chorion *(**kor**-ē-on)*
chorionic villus sampling *(kor-ē-**on**-ik **vil**-us **sam**-pling)*
circumcision *(sur-kum-**sizh**-un)*
climacteric *(klī-**mak**-tur-ik)*
clitoris *(**klit**-uh-ris)*
coitus *(**kō**-i-tus)*
colpitis *(kol-**pī**-tis)*
colpoplasty *(**kol**-pō-plas-tē)*
colporrhaphy *(kol-**por**-uh-fē)*
colposcope *(**kol**-pō-skōp)*
colposcopy *(kol-**pos**-kuh-pē)*
condyloma acuminatum *(kon-duh-**lō**-muh uh-kū-mi-**nāt**-um)*
conization of the cervix *(kon-i-**zā**-shun ov thuh **sur**-viks)*
contraception *(kon-truh-**sep**-shun)*
contraceptive *(kon-truh-**sep**-tiv)*
cryptorchidism *(krip-**tor**-ki-diz-um)*
curettage *(kū-ruh-**tahzh**)*
cystocele *(**sis**-tō-sēl)*
cytology *(sī-**tol**-uh-jē)*
dilation and curettage *(dī-**lā**-shun and kū-ruh-**tahzh**)*
Down syndrome *(doun **sin**-drōm)*
ductus deferens *(**duk**-tus **def**-ur-enz)*
dysmenorrhea *(dis-men-uh-**rē**-uh)*
dysplasia *(dis-**plā**-zhuh)*
ectopic *(ek-**top**-ik)*
endometrial ablation *(en-dō-**mē**-trē-ul ab-**lā**-shun)*
endometriosis *(en-dō-mē-trē-**ō**-sis)*
endometritis *(en-dō-mē-**trī**-tis)*
endometrium *(en-dō-**mē**-trē-um)*
epididymis *(ep-i-**did**-uh-mis)*
episiotomy *(uh-piz-ē-**ot**-uh-mē)*
erythroblastosis fetalis *(uh-rith-rō-blas-**tō**-sis fi-**ta**-lus)*
estrogen *(**es**-truh-jen)*
extrauterine *(eks-truh-**ū**-tur-in)*
fallopian *(fuh-**lō**-pē-un)*
fertilization *(fur-ti-li-**zā**-shun)*

fetal *(**fē**-tul)*
fetal monitoring *(**fē**-tul **mon**-i-tur-ing)*
fetus *(**fē**-tus)*
fistula *(**fis**-tū-luh)*
genitalia *(jen-i-**tā**-lē-uh)*
genitourinary *(jen-i-tō-**ū**-ri-nar-ē)*
gestation *(jes-**tā**-shun)*
glans penis (glanz **pē**-nis)
gonads *(**gō**-nads)*
gonococcus *(gon-ō-**kok**-us)*
gonorrhea *(gon-ō-**rē**-uh)*
gravida *(**grav**-i-duh)*
gynecologist *(gī-nuh-**kol**-uh-jist)*
gynecology *(gī-nuh-**kol**-uh-jē)*
hepatitis *(hep-uh-**tī**-tis)*
herpes genitalis *(**hur**-pēz jen-i-**tal**-is)*
human chorionic gonadotropin *(**hū**-mun kor-ē-**on**-ik gō-nuh-dō-**trō**-pin)*
hydrocele (**hī**-drō-sēl)
hysterectomy *(his-tur-**ek**-tuh-mē)*
hysteroptosis *(his-tur-op-**tō**-sis)*
hysterosalpingogram *(his-tur-ō-sal-**ping**-gō-gram)*
hysterosalpingography *(his-tur-ō-sal-ping-**gog**-ruh-fē)*
hysteroscope *(**his**-tur-ō-skōp)*
hysteroscopy *(his-tur-**os**-kuh-pē)*
implantation *(im-plan-**tā**-shun)*
intersexuality *(in-tur-sek-shōō-**al**-i-tē)*
intrauterine *(in-truh-**ū**-tur-in)*
in utero *(in **ū**-tur-ō)*
in vitro fertilization *(in **vē**-trō fur-ti-li-**zā**-shun)*
Kaposi sarcoma *(**kah**-pō-sē sahr-**kō**-muh)*
labia majora *(**lā**-bē-uh muh-**jor**-uh)*
labia minora *(**lā**-bē-uh muh-**nor**-uh)*
lactation *(lak-**tā**-shun)*
lactiferous *(lak-**tif**-ur-us)*
laparohysterectomy *(lap-uh-rō-his-tuh-**rek**-tuh-mē)*
laparoscope *(**lap**-uh-rō-skōp)*
laparoscopy *(lap-uh-**ros**-kuh-pē)*
leiomyoma *(lī-ō-mī-**ō**-muh)*
lobule *(**lob**-ūl)*
lumpectomy *(lum-**pek**-tuh-mē)*
mammalgia *(muh-**mal**-juh)*
mammary *(**mam**-ur-ē)*
mammogram *(**mam**-uh-gram)*
mammography *(muh-**mog**-ruh-fē)*
mammoplasty *(**mam**-ō-plas-tē)*
mastalgia *(mas-**tal**-juh)*
mastectomy *(mas-**tek**-tuh-mē)*
mastitis *(mas-**tī**-tis)*
mastodynia *(mas-tō-**din**-ē-uh)*

QUICK & EASY (Q&E) LIST—cont'd

mastopexy (*mas*-tō-pek-sē)
mastoptosis (mas-tō-*tō*-sis)
menopause (*men*-ō-pawz)
menorrhagia (men-uh-*rā*-juh)
menses (*men*-sēz)
menstruation (men-strōō-*ā*-shun)
metrorrhagia (mē-trō-*rā*-juh)
mons pubis (monz *pū*-bis)
myoma (mī-*ō*-muh)
myometrium (mī-ō-*mē*-trē-um)
neonatal (nē-ō-*nā*-tul)
neonate (*nē*-ō-nāt)
nonspecific genital infection (non-spuh-*sif*-ik *jen*-i-tul in-*fek*-shun)
nullipara (nuh-*lip*-uh-ruh)
obstetrician (ob-stuh-*tri*-shun)
obstetrics (ob-*stet*-riks)
oophorectomy (ō-of-uh-*rek*-tuh-mē)
oophoritis (ō-of-uh-*rī*-tis)
oophorosalpingitis (ō-of-uh-rō-sal-pin-*jī*-tis)
orchidectomy (or-ki-*dek*-tuh-mē)
orchiditis (or-ki-*dī*-tis)
orchidopexy (*or*-ki-dō-pek-sē)
orchidoplasty (*or*-ki-dō-plas-tē)
orchiectomy (or-kē-*ek*-tuh-mē)
orchiopexy (*or*-kē-ō-pek-sē)
orchiotomy (or-kē-*ot*-uh-mē)
orchitis (or-*kī*-tis)
ovarian (ō-*var*-ē-un)
ovarian carcinoma (ō-*var*-ē-un kahr-si-*nō*-muh)
ovarian cyst (ō-*var*-ē-un sist)
ovaries (*ō*-vuh-rēz)
ovulation (ov-ū-*lā*-shun)
ovum (*ō*-vum)
Pap smear (pap smēr)
papillomavirus (pap-i-*lō*-muh-vī-rus)
parturition (pahr-tū-*ri*-shun)
pelvic inflammatory disease (*pel*-vik in-*flam*-uh-tor-ē di-zēz)
penile (*pē*-nīl)
penis (*pē*-nis)
perimetrium (per-i-*mē*-trē-um)
placenta (pluh-*sen*-tuh)
placenta previa (pluh-*sen*-tuh *prē*-vē-uh)
postnatal (pōst-*nā*-tul)
postpartum (pōst-*pahr*-tum)
premenstrual syndrome (prē-*men*-strōō-ul *sin*-drōm)
prenatal (prē-*nā*-tul)
prepuce (*prē*-pūs)
primigravida (prī-mi-*grav*-i-duh)

progesterone (prō-*jes*-tuh-rōn)
prostate (*pros*-tāt)
prostatectomy (pros-tuh-*tek*-tuh-mē)
prostatic (pro-*stat*-ik)
prostatic carcinoma (pro-*stat*-ik kahr-si-*nō*-muh)
prostatitis (pros-tuh-*tī*-tis)
pubic lice (*pū*-bik līs)
radical hysterectomy (*rad*-i-kul his-tur-*ek*-tuh-mē)
rectovaginal (rek-tō-*vaj*-i-nul)
salpingectomy (sal-pin-*jek*-tuh-mē)
salpingitis (sal-pin-*jī*-tis)
salpingocele (sal-*ping*-gō-sēl)
salpingo-oophorectomy (sal-ping-gō-ō-of-uh-*rek*-tuh-mē)
salpingorrhaphy (sal-ping-*gor*-uh-fē)
scrotal (*skrōt*-ul)
scrotum (*skrō*-tum)
secundipara (sē-kun-*dip*-uh-ruh)
semen (*sē*-mun)
seminal (*sem*-i-nul)
seminal vesicles (*sem*-i-nul *ves*-i-kuls)
shoulder presentation (*shōl*-dur prē-zun-*tā*-shun)
speculum (*spek*-ū-lum)
spermatocidal (spur-muh-tō-*sī*-dul)
spermatogenesis (spur-muh-tō-*jen*-uh-sis)
spermatozoa (spur-muh-tō-*zō*-uh)
spermatozoon (spur-muh-tō-*zō*-on)
spermicidal (spur-mi-*sī*-dul)
spermicide (*spur*-mi-sīd)
spirochete (*spī*-rō-kēt)
sterilization (ster-i-li-*zā*-shun)
syphilis (*sif*-i-lis)
testes (*tes*-tēz)
testicle (*tes*-ti-kul)
testicular (tes-*tik*-ū-lur)
testicular cancer (tes-*tik*-ū-lur *kan*-sur)
testicular torsion (tes-*tik*-ū-lur *tor*-shun)
testis (*tes*-tis)
testosterone (tes-*tos*-tuh-rōn)
transabdominal (trans-ab-*dom*-i-nul)
transurethral microwave thermotherapy (trans-ū-*rē*-thrul *mī*-krō-wāv thur-mō-*ther*-uh-pē)
transurethral needle ablation (trans-ū-*rē*-thrul *nē*-dul ab-*lā*-shun)
transurethral prostatectomy (trans-ū-*rē*-thrul pros-tuh-*tek*-tuh-mē)
transurethral resection (trans-ū-*rē*-thrul rē-*sek*-shun)
trichomoniasis (trik-ō-mō-*nī*-uh-sis)
trimester (trī-*mes*-tur)
tripara (*trip*-uh-ruh)
tubal ligation (*tōō*-bul lī-*gā*-shun)

QUICK & EASY (Q&E) LIST—cont'd

unipara (ū-*nip*-uh-ruh)	**vasectomy** (vuh-*sek*-tuh-mē)
urethritis (ū-ruh-*thrī*-tis)	**vasovasostomy** (vā-zō-vā-*zos*-tuh-mē)
uterine cancer (ū-tur-in *kan*-sur)	**vesicovaginal** (ves-i-kō-*vaj*-i-nul)
uterine fibroid (ū-tur-in *fī*-broid)	**vulva** (*vul*-vuh)
uterus (ū-tur-us)	**vulval** (*vul*-vul)
vagina (vuh-*jī*-nuh)	**vulvar** (*vul*-vur)
vaginal (*vaj*-i-nul)	**vulvectomy** (vul-*vek*-tuh-mē)
vaginitis (vaj-i-*nī*-tis)	**vulvitis** (vul-*vī*-tis)
vas deferens (vas *def*-ur-ens)	**zygote** (*zī*-gōt)

Don't forget the games and other activities available at http://evolve.elsevier.com/Leonard/quick.

QUICK CONNECT

Review all lists of word parts and their meanings for this chapter using the flashcards you prepared or the flashcards on the Evolve site.

The function of the reproductive system is to produce offspring. Genitalia are reproductive organs, whether male or female, particularly those external to the body.

Gonads: testes (singular: spermatozoon) and ovaries (singular ovum) production of sperm and ova. Ducts transport and receive ovum or sperm and important fluids. Also secrete important hormones.

FEMALE REPRODUCTIVE SYSTEM:

Gynecology: study of diseases of the female reproductive organs.

External genitalia are called vulva, which include: mons pubis, labia majora, labia minora, clitoris, openings for glands.

Internal structures: left and right ovaries and associated uterine (fallopian) tubes, uterus, vagina, special glands. Know their functions.

Human embryo is the period time from fertilization until the end of the eighth week. A fetus is the latter stages of a developing offspring (in humans, that time in utero after the first 8 weeks).

Remember the location of the three layers of uterus: endometrium, myometrium, and perimetrium.

Know the meaning of these terms: puberty, menstruation, climacteric, menses, vulval/vulvar, coitus.

DISEASES AND OTHER DIAGNOSTIC TERMS: What is the function of a speculum, Pap smear, dysplasia, and cytology? How is an examination with a speculum different from colposcopy, laparoscopy, hysteroscopy, and hysterosalpingography? Be able to differentiate these terms: amenorrhea, dysmenorrhea, menorrhagia, and metrorrhagia. Know these additional terms: cervical polyp, cervicocolpitis, colpitis, cystocele, endometriosis, endometritis, fistula, hysteroptosis, myoma. Can you differentiate these terms pertaining to the ovaries (oophoritis, oophorsalpingitis, carcinoma, cyst)? Recognize the difference in salpingitis vs. salpingocele. Differentiate pelvic inflammatory disease, premenstrual syndrome, uterine cancer, uterine fibroid, and vulvitis. Describe the difference in colpoplasty and colporrhaphy, as well as these terms: oophorectomy, salpingectomy, salpingo-oophorectomy, salpingorrhaphy, and vulvectomy.

DIFFERENTIATE CONTRACEPTIVES. Recognize the meaning of each and how it works. Recognize the effectiveness.

Recognize these surgical and therapeutic terms: in vitro fertilization, sterilization, tubal ligation. What does dilation and curettage mean and how does it differ from endometrial ablation? What is the difference in hysterectomy, laparohysterectomy, and radical hysterectomy?

PREGNANCY AND CHILDBIRTH: Know the meaning of these terms: fertilization, implantation, zygote, human embryo vs. human fetus, and human chorionic gonadotropin. Know these obstetrical terms: amnion, parous, gestation, parturition, antepartum vs. postpartum. Know the difference in nullipara, primipara, unipara, secundipara, and tripara. Name three types of fetal presentations. Also know the meaning of abruptio placenta, amniotic sac, amniocentesis vs. chorionic villus sampling. Differentiate amniotomy, episiotomy, placenta previa, and cesarean section. Describe the difference in Down syndrome and erythroblastosis fetalis?

FEMALE BREASTS (mammary glands): Know these structures: lobules, areola, lactiferous ducts. Diagnostic terms: mammography/mammogram, mammalgia, mastoptosis. Surgical terms: lumpectomy, mastectomy, mammoplasty.

MALE REPRODUCTIVE SYSTEMS:

Structures to remember: testes, penis, prepuce, glans penis, epididymis, scrotum, ductus/vas deferens, bulbourethral glands, and prostate. Testes produce testosterone and are responsible for spermatogenesis. Seminal vesicles are a reservoir for semen until it is discharged; in addition, they as well as the prostate and other glands produce essential fluids for survival of sperm. Know these terms: spermatozoa, and spermatocidal/spermicidal.

Diseases, disorders and diagnostic terms: anorchidism/anorchism, aspermia/aspermatogenesis, benign prostatic hyperplasia, cryptorchidism, hydrocele, intersexuality, orchiditis/orchitis, prostatic carcinoma, prostatitis, testicular cancer, and testicular torsion.

Know the meaning of these surgical and therapeutic terms: circumcision, transurethral needle ablation, transurethral prostatectomy, vasectomy, and vasovasostomy. Differentiate these terms that relate to the testes: orchidectomy, orchidoplasty, orchiopexy, and orchiotomy.

STDS:

Know its meaning and the difference in gonorrhea (caused by gonococcus), syphilis (caused by a spirochete and produces a chancre in first stage), chlamydial infection, chancroid, nonspecific genital infection. AIDS (caused by HIV), genital herpes (know its cause), genital warts (know its cause), hepatitis, trichomoniasis, candidiasis, and pubic lice.

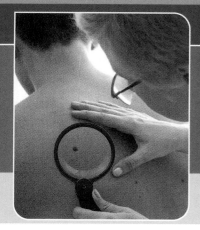

CHAPTER 12

Integumentary System

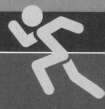

Dermatology is the study of the skin, including its pathologic characteristics and the diagnosis and treatment of skin disorders. A dermatologist is shown examining the patient for skin cancer.

OBJECTIVES

After completing Chapter 12, you will be able to:

1. Recognize or write the functions of the integumentary system.
2. Recognize or write the meanings of Chapter 12 word parts and use them to build and analyze terms.
3. Write terms for select structures of the integumentary system, or match them with their descriptions.
4. Write the names of the diagnostic terms and pathologies related to the integumentary system when given their descriptions, or match terms with their meanings.
5. Match surgical and therapeutic interventions for the integumentary system or write the names of the interventions when given their descriptions.
6. Spell terms for the integumentary system correctly.

Function First

QUICK TIP

When you see *sebaceous*, think of sebum, the oily secretion of the skin.

WORD ORIGIN

integument (L.), a covering

The integumentary system is the skin and its appendages, hair, nails, sweat glands (which help eliminate waste salt and control body temperature by excreting water), and sebaceous glands. The skin is the **integument**, or external covering of the body. We are more familiar with the skin than many other organs because it is external. Skin has many important functions, and the mnemonic DERMA will help you remember them:

- **D** vitamin synthesis
- **E**limination of wastes through perspiration
- **R**egulation of body temperature through perspiration
- **M**akes information about the environment available to the brain
- **A**cts as a barrier to moisture loss, harmful light rays, and invasion of microbes

WRITE IT!
EXERCISE 1

Write an answer in each blank to complete these sentences.

1. The skin is the external covering and is called the _____.
2. The skin protects the underlying tissues from drying out, harmful light rays, and invasion of _____.
3. The skin makes information about the environment available to the _____.
4. The sweat glands help control body temperature and excrete water and _____.

Structures of the Integumentary System

Layers of the Skin

The skin covers the surface of the body and consists of two main parts: the **epi+dermis** and the **dermis**. Remembering that epi- means above, it is easy to remember that the epidermis is located above the dermis. Label Fig. 12.1 as you read the following information. The epidermis *(1)* is the thin outer layer of the skin that is **avascular** (without blood vessels). The dermis *(2)* is the thick layer under the epidermis. A layer of **sub+cutane+ous adipose tissue** *(3)* is located under the dermis. **Cutaneous** means pertaining to the skin, and subcutaneous means beneath the skin. **Adipose** means fatty because adip/o means fat. The subcutaneous adipose tissue is composed of fat that serves as insulation and a cushion against shock.

When it is intact, the skin serves as protection from microorganisms. The outermost part of the epidermis contains scalelike, nonliving cells that are constantly being shed and replaced. The primary component of these nonliving cells is **keratin**, a **sclero+protein**, which is insoluble in most solvents. The dermis contains numerous blood vessels, nerves, and glands. Hair follicles are also embedded in this layer. The upper region of the dermis has many fingerlike projections that result in ridges on the outermost layer of the skin. The ridge patterns on the fingertips and thumbs (fingerprints) are unique to each person.

Modified skin continues into various parts of the body, for example, the mucous membrane that lines the mouth, the nose, the intestines, and other cavities or canals that open to the outside. The mucous membrane, also called mucosa, protects the underlying structure.

WORD ORIGIN

derma (G.), skin
cutis (L.), skin

---

epi- = above
sub- = below
cutane/o = skin
-ous = pertaining to
adip/o = fat

---

scler/o = hard

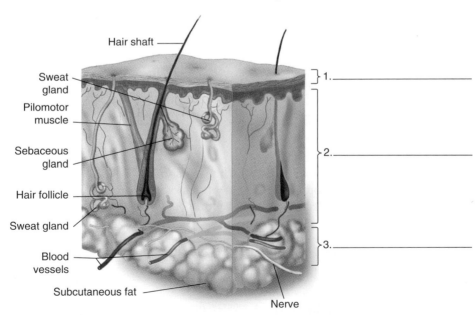

epi- = above or upon
cutane/o, derm/a = skin
seb/o = sebum
sub- = under
adip/o = fat
pil/o = hair

Hair shaft

Sweat gland

Pilomotor muscle

Sebaceous gland

Hair follicle

Sweat gland

Blood vessels

Subcutaneous fat

Nerve

1.
2.
3.

Fig. 12.1 Layers and Structures of the Skin. The epidermis *(1)*, the thin outer layer, is composed of four to five layers. Underneath the epidermis is the thicker dermis *(2)*, which is composed of connective tissue containing lymphatics, nerves, blood vessels, hair follicles, sebaceous glands, and sweat glands. Beneath the dermis is a layer of subcutaneous adipose tissue *(3)*.

MATCH IT!* **EXERCISE 2**

Match the terms in the left column with their descriptions.

_____ 1. dermis
_____ 2. epidermis
_____ 3. subcutaneous adipose tissue

A. composed of fat
B. thicker layer of skin
C. thin outer layer of skin

*Use Appendix III, Answers, to check your answers to all the exercises in Chapter 12.

Commit to memory the word parts in the following table.

WORD PARTS: INTEGUMENTARY SYSTEM

Combining Forms	Meaning	Suffixes	Meaning
adip/o, lip/o	fat	-cidal	killing
axill/o	axilla (armpit)	-derm	skin or a germ layer
bacter/i, bacteri/o	bacteria	-static	keeping stationary
cutane/o, derm/a, derm/o, dermat/o	skin		
erythemat/o	erythema or redness		
follicul/o	follicle		
ichthy/o	fish		
kerat/o*	horny tissue (tissue containing keratin)		
onych/o, ungu/o	nail		
pil/o, trich/o	hair		
seb/o	sebum		
seps/o	infection		
sept/o	infection or septum		
xer/o	dry		

Use the electronic flashcards on the Evolve site or make your own set of flashcards using the above list. Select the word parts just presented, and study them until you know their meanings. Do this each time a set of word parts is presented.

*Sometimes kerat/o means cornea (eye structure).

The skin is derived from a tissue layer called ectoderm that forms during embryonic development. Sense receptors of the skin and other parts of the nervous system are also derived from ectoderm.

THE SUFFIX -DERM CAN MEAN EITHER SKIN OR AN EMBRYONIC LAYER

Soon after fertilization, the fertilized egg undergoes cell division, producing a ball of cells that eventually differentiates into three distinct layers: **endoderm**, **mesoderm**, and **ectoderm** (innermost, middle, and outermost layers, respectively). In endoderm, mesoderm, and ectoderm, -derm is used to refer to an embryonic layer, a primary layer of cells of the developing embryo from which various organ systems develop. The suffix can also mean skin.

The term **dermatome** has three different meanings.
- In embryology, dermatome refers to a layer in early human development that gives rise to the dermal layers of the skin.
- In surgery, a dermatome is an instrument used to cut thin slices of skin for grafting.
- In anatomy and physiology, a dermatome refers to the skin surface area innervated (supplied) by a spinal nerve. A dermatome is named according to the nerve's source from the spinal cord. Dermatomes C, T, L, and S designate cervical, thoracic, lumbar, and sacral spinal nerves, respectively (Fig. 12.2).

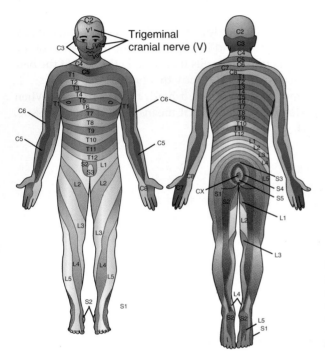

Fig. 12.2 Dermatome Distribution of Spinal Nerves. The dermatomes are named C, T, L, and S (cervical, thoracic, lumbar, and sacral), which correspond to a single spinal nerve that innervates each of them. Trigeminal, as used here, pertains to the three branches of the fifth cranial nerve. Persons with shingles develop painful skin eruptions that follow the underlying route of cranial or spinal nerves inflamed by the latent *varicella zoster* virus, which caused chickenpox when they were younger.

WRITE IT!

EXERCISE 3

Write combining forms for these meanings.

1. dry _____
2. erythema or redness _____
3. fat _____ or _____
4. fish _____
5. follicle _____
6. hair _____ or _____
7. horny tissue _____
8. infection _____ or _____
9. nail _____ or _____
10. sebum _____

pil/o = hair
motor = mover, pertaining to motion

Accessory Skin Structures

The accessory skin structures include the hair, nails, sebaceous glands, and sweat glands. Locate these structures in Fig. 12.1. **Pilomotor muscles** cause erection of the hairs of the skin in response to a chilly environment, emotional stimulus, or skin irritation.

Hair protects the scalp from injury. Hair in the nostrils and external ear canal protects these structures from dust and insects. Eyebrows and lashes protect the eyes. **Axilla** means armpit. Hair develops in the **axillary** region at puberty.

Sweat glands are also called **sudoriferous glands**. Certain sweat glands produce perspiration when they are stimulated by increased temperature or emotional stress. Although elimination of waste in the form of **perspiration** is a function of the sweat glands, their principal function is to help regulate body temperature.

> **QUICK TIP**
>
> *kerat/o* also refers to the cornea, the transparent structure at the front of the eye.

Sebaceous glands generally arise from the hair follicles and produce **sebum**, the oily substance that inhibits the growth of bacteria and is responsible for lubrication of the skin. The hair **follicles** are tiny tubes of epidermal cells that contain the root of the hair shaft. Sebaceous glands are found in all areas of the body that have hair.

kerat/o = horny tissue
ungu/o = nail

Fingernails and toenails are composed of keratin, a hard, fibrous protein. When kerat/o is used in discussions pertaining to the skin, it means hard or horny tissue. **Ungual** means pertaining to the nail.

WRITE IT!
EXERCISE 4

Write an answer in each blank to complete these sentences.

1. Hair, nails, sebaceous glands, and sweat glands are the _____ skin structures.
2. A term that means pertaining to the armpit is _____.
3. Sweat glands are _____ glands.
4. Another term for sweat is _____.
5. Glands that produce sebum are called _____ glands.
6. A term that means pertaining to the nail is _____.

🚑 Diseases, Disorders, and Diagnostic Terms

The skin is a reflection of the general health of a person, and it can communicate information to the trained observer. Normal skin has an even tone that is free of lesions, bruises, or signs of inflammation. Skin changes may be related to specific skin diseases, but also may reflect an underlying systemic disorder.

A skin test is one that is performed to determine the reaction of the body to a substance by observing the results of either injecting the substance or applying it to the skin. When it is done to determine whether an allergy to a particular substance exists, it is called an *allergy test* or a *patch test*.

kerat/o = horny tissue
-rrhea = flow or discharge
seb/o = sebum

Skin Lesions

A skin **lesion** is any visible, localized abnormality of the skin, such as a wound, rash, or sore. This includes spots that appear on the skin, in addition to swellings and changes of shape, such as an underlying tumor. Perhaps you are familiar with the benign skin lesions of **seborrheic keratosis** that are often seen in older persons. Some lesions of this type are deeply pigmented (Fig. 12.3). A lesion that is **circumscribed** is well defined, giving the appearance of being able to draw a circle around it.

WORD ORIGIN

circum- (L.), around
scribere (L.), to draw

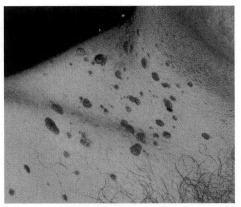

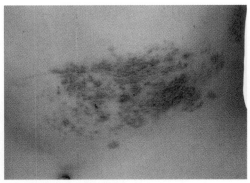

Fig. 12.4 Shingles. These painful skin eruptions follow the underlying route of cranial or spinal nerves that are inflamed by the virus.

Fig. 12.3 Seborrheic Keratoses, Benign Skin Lesions. Numerous seborrheic keratoses are present, some of which are deeply pigmented with melanin. The large lesions show the characteristic stuck-on appearance.

Skin infections are caused by specific types of bacteria, viruses, and fungi. A **verruca** is a benign warty skin lesion (wart) with a rough surface caused by a common contagious virus.

Herpes simplex virus (HSV) infection is the most common viral infection of adult skin. Herpes simplex virus type 1 (HSV-1) causes the classic fever blisters. Another type of herpes virus, herpes zoster, causes shingles and occurs with reactivation of the herpes virus in individuals who have previously had chickenpox (Fig. 12.4). Vaccination to prevent shingles is available.

The skin lesions just discussed are examples of *primary* lesions, initial reactions to an underlying problem that alters one of the structural components of the skin. Both a cyst and a **nodule** cause a raised area of the overlying skin, but the **cyst** is filled with fluid or a semisolid material (Fig. 12.5).

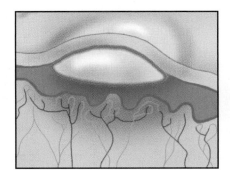

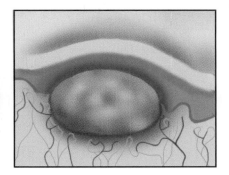

A **cyst** is a sac filled with fluid or semisolid material.

A **nodule** is a marble-like, solid lesion more than 1 cm wide and deep.

Fig. 12.5 Differentiation of a Cyst vs. a Nodule (seen here in cross section).

See other primary lesions of the skin in Fig. 12.6 and read the characteristics of each type. **Macules** (e.g., freckles) are small and nonraised, unlike **papules** (e.g., moles). A **plaque** (e.g., dandruff) is elevated and appears as a large patch. Blisters or fluid-filled lesions include **vesicles**, **bullae**, and pustules. Vesicles are smaller than bullae, and **pustules** are filled with cloudy fluid or pus.

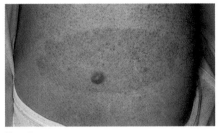

Macules
Nonraised, discolored spots less than 1 cm in diameter

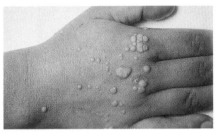

Papules
Elevated lesion less than 1 cm in diameter

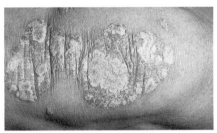

Plaques
Elevated and circumscribed patches more than 1 cm in diameter

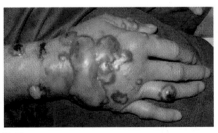

Bullae
Blisters greater than 1 cm and filled with clear fluid

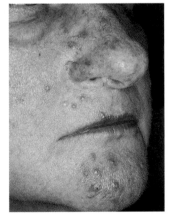

Pustules
Vesicles filled with cloudy fluid or pus

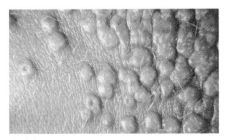

Vesicles
Blisters less than 1 cm and filled with clear fluid

Fig. 12.6 Primary Lesions of the Skin. These are initial reactions to an underlying problem that alters one of the structural components of the skin.

Wheals (Fig. 12.7), often seen in an allergic skin eruption, are irregularly shaped, slightly raised lesions that usually itch and can be caused by food, insect stings, and certain medications.

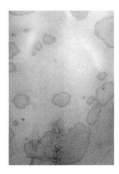

Fig. 12.7 Wheals. This irregularly shaped, slightly raised lesion is seen in urticaria (hives), an allergic skin eruption. Note the irregular shapes of the lesions.

MATCH IT! EXERCISE 5

Match the skin lesions in the left column with their descriptions.

_____ 1. bulla
_____ 2. macule
_____ 3. papule
_____ 4. pustule
_____ 5. vesicle

A. blister larger than 1 cm
B. blister less than 1 cm, filled with clear fluid
C. discolored spot, not elevated
D. small elevated lesion
E. fluid-filled sac containing pus

Secondary lesions of the skin are changes in the appearance of the primary lesion and can occur with normal progression of a disease. Atrophy of the skin, ulcers, and fissures are secondary lesions (Fig. 12.8). **Atrophy** of the skin (e.g., stretch marks) is characterized by thinning with the loss of skin markings. **Ulcers** are deep, irregular erosions that extend into the dermis. Athlete's foot produces linear cracks in the epidermis and is an example of a **fissure**. **Scales** (not shown in the illustration) are dried fragments of sloughed epidermis that are whitish and irregular in size and shape.

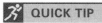

QUICK TIP

Secondary lesions:
atrophy
ulcer
fissure
scales

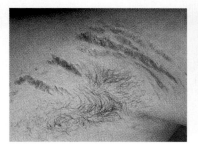

Atrophy
Wasting of the epidermis; skin appears thin and transparent

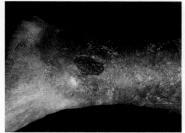

Ulcer
Irregularly shaped erosions that extend into the dermis

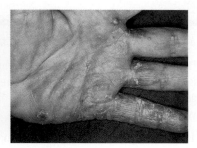

Fissures
Deep linear splits through the epidermis into the dermis

Fig. 12.8 Secondary Lesions of the Skin. Atrophy of the skin, ulcers, and fissures results from changes in the initial skin lesion.

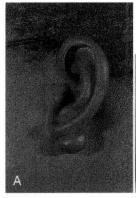

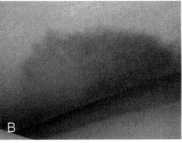

Fig. 12.9 Examples of Injuries to the Skin. **A,** Keloids resulting from overgrowth of scar tissue after a skin injury. **B,** A large contusion caused by a blow to the body and characterized by swelling, discoloration, and pain.

Injuries to the Skin

> **QUICK TIP**
>
> Examples of wounds:
>   laceration
>   incision
>   puncture
>   abrasion
>   contusion
>   burn

> **a-** = without
> **sept/o** = infection
> **-ic** = pertaining to

A wound is a physical injury involving a break in the skin, usually caused by an act or accident rather than a disease. The trauma (injury) to the skin and underlying tissues requires healing to repair the defect. If damage to the skin is severe, a scar remains after healing of a wound. A **keloid** is excessive overgrowth of scar tissue at the sight of a skin injury, particularly wounds or surgical incisions (Fig. 12.9, *A*). A **laceration** is a torn, jagged wound, whereas an **incision** is a smooth-edged wound produced by a sharp instrument. Surgical incisions generally heal faster than other wounds because they are performed under a+sept+ic conditions, and because minimal damage is done by the sharp instruments used. **Aseptic** means free of pathogenic organisms. A puncture is a wound made by piercing. An **abrasion** results when skin is scraped or rubbed away by friction. A **contusion** (bruise) is caused by an injury to the body that does not break the skin and is characterized by swelling and discoloration (Fig. 12.9, *B*).

WRITE IT! EXERCISE 6

Match the injuries to the skin in the left column with their descriptions.

_____ 1. abrasion   A. a bruise
_____ 2. contusion   B. skin is scraped or rubbed away by friction
_____ 3. incision   C. smooth-edged wound produced by a sharp instrument
_____ 4. laceration   D. torn, jagged wound
_____ 5. puncture   E. wound made by piercing

QUICK CASE STUDY | EXERCISE 7

Match terms from the report with descriptions 1 through 5.

Dermatologist Amy Sadighi examined three patients and made the following diagnoses: Follow-up visit with Adam Burns, keloid resulting from laceration requiring stitches 1 month ago; 17-year-old Noah Dearing, acne vulgaris with several cysts, abscesses, and scarring; 45-year-old Ardith Castillo has developed severe urticaria with various-sized wheals post antibiotic.

1. sacs under the skin filled with fluid or semisolid material _____
2. elevated and irregularly shaped lesions _____
3. excessive overgrowth of unsightly scar tissue _____
4. skin eruption that is also known as hives _____
5. torn, jagged wound _____

Burns are tissue injuries resulting from excessive exposure to heat, electricity, chemicals, radiation, or gases. The extent of the injury is determined by the amount of exposure and the nature of the agent that caused the burn.

The American Burn Association recommends categorizing a burn injury,

---

THE "RULE OF NINES" CALCULATES THE SIZE OF A BURN INJURY

The rule of nines is a formula for estimating the percentage of adult body surface covered by burns (Fig. 12.10). The formula can be used for adults whose weight is proportional to their height, but it is modified for infants and children because of their proportionately larger head size. The rule of nines assigns 9% to the head and each arm, 18% to each leg and the anterior and posterior of the trunk, and 1% to the perineum.

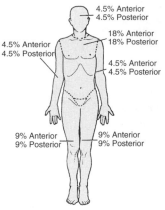

4.5% Anterior
4.5% Posterior
18% Anterior
18% Posterior
4.5% Anterior
4.5% Posterior
4.5% Anterior
4.5% Posterior
9% Anterior
9% Posterior
9% Anterior
9% Posterior

Fig. 12.10 Rule of Nines.

according to the depth of tissue destruction, as a superficial burn, a deep partial-thickness burn, a full-thickness burn, or a deep full-thickness burn (Fig. 12.11). These were formerly called first-degree, second-degree, third-degree, and fourth-degree burns. In addition to the burn depth, burn severity includes factors such as the size and location of the burn, mechanism of the injury, duration and intensity of the burn, and the age and health of the patient. TBSA refers to the total body surface area that is burned. Very young and older persons are most at risk. Severe burns usually require skin grafting, usually from the patient's own body. In a **skin graft**, skin is implanted to cover areas where skin has been lost.

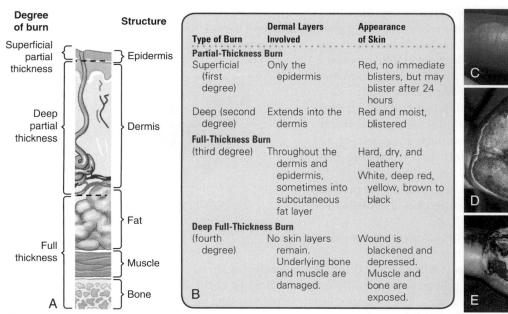

Type of Burn	Dermal Layers Involved	Appearance of Skin
Partial-Thickness Burn		
Superficial (first degree)	Only the epidermis	Red, no immediate blisters, but may blister after 24 hours
Deep (second degree)	Extends into the dermis	Red and moist, blistered
Full-Thickness Burn		
(third degree)	Throughout the dermis and epidermis, sometimes into subcutaneous fat layer	Hard, dry, and leathery White, deep red, yellow, brown to black
Deep Full-Thickness Burn		
(fourth degree)	No skin layers remain. Underlying bone and muscle are damaged.	Wound is blackened and depressed. Muscle and bone are exposed.

Fig. 12.11 Burn Classifications. **A,** Cross section of skin indicating the degree of burn and the structures involved. **B,** Descriptions of burns. **C,** Partial-thickness burn. **D,** Deep-partial thickness burn. **E,** Deep full-thickness burn.

Write a word to complete each of these sentences.

1. Only the epidermis is damaged in a _____ partial-thickness burn.
2. In a deep partial-thickness burn, damage does not extend beyond the layer of skin called the _____.
3. Underlying bone and muscle are damaged in a _____ full-thickness burn.

Skin Disorders

abscess Cavity that contains pus caused by an infectious microorganism and surrounded by inflamed tissue (Fig. 12.12).

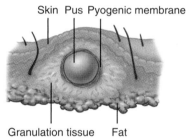

Skin Pus Pyogenic membrane

Granulation tissue   Fat

Fig. 12.12 Abscess. Note the collection of pus.

albinism (albin/o, white + -ism, condition) Absence of normal pigmentation, present at birth, caused by a defect in **melanin** precursors. The person affected with albinism is an **albino** (see Fig. 3.12).

cellulitis Acute infection of the skin and subcutaneous tissue characterized most often by local heat, redness, pain, and swelling (see Fig. 6.21).

contact dermatitis Skin rash resulting from exposure to an irritant or to a sensitizing agent that initiates an allergic response, such as poison ivy and allergic reaction to nickel in jewelry (see Fig. 2.20).

cyanosis (cyan/o, blue + -osis, condition) Bluish discoloration of the skin and mucous membranes caused by lack of oxygenated blood to tissues (see Fig. 3.13).

dermatitis (dermat/o, skin + -itis, inflammation) Inflammatory condition of the skin.

discoid lupus erythematosus (DLE) Chronic disorder, primarily of the skin, characterized by lesions that are covered with scales. The disorder was so named because of the reddish facial rash that appears in some patients (Fig. 12.13), giving them

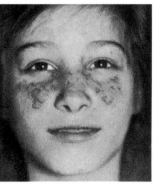

Fig. 12.13 Characteristic "Butterfly" Rash of Lupus Erythematosus. *Lupus* is the Latin term for wolf; the name perhaps originated from the rash over the nose and cheeks.

a wolflike appearance. Erythemat/o means **erythema**, a redness or inflammation of the skin or mucous membranes. Also called cutaneous lupus erythematosus.

frostbite Damage to skin, tissues, and blood vessels as a result of prolonged exposure to cold (Fig. 12.14).

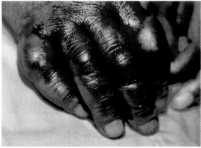

Fig. 12.14 Frostbite. Second-degree frostbite of the fingers, including vesicles and swelling.

furuncle Localized skin infection originating in a gland or hair follicle and characterized by pain, redness, and swelling. Also called a boil.

hypopigmentation Decreased tissue pigmentation, but not complete absence of skin color as in albinism.

ichthyosis (ichthy/o, fish) Any of several generalized skin disorders marked by skin that is dry and scaly, resembling fish skin (Fig. 12.15).

Fig. 12.15 Ichthyosis. The type shown here is hereditary and is characterized by large, dry, dark scales.

lipoma (lip/o, fat + -oma, tumor) Benign tumor consisting of mature fat cells (see Fig. 2.7, *A*).

Lyme disease Infection transmitted by the bite of an infected tick. A red macule or papule appears at the bite site and is accompanied by flulike symptoms (Fig. 12.16). Other symptoms appear weeks or months later.

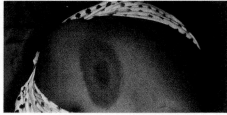

Fig. 12.16 Lyme Disease. Note the targetlike appearance of the bite.

malignant melanoma (melan/o, black + -oma, tumor) Any of a group of malignant tumors that originate in the skin and that are composed of **melanocytes** (see Fig. 2.6, *B*). Excessive sun exposure increases the risk of melanoma.

mycodermatitis (myc/o, fungus) Inflammation of the skin caused by a fungus.

necrosis Death of areas of damaged or diseased tissue or bone surrounded by healthy tissue (Fig. 12.17).

pediculosis Infestation by lice and named for a genus of sucking lice, *Pediculus*. There are head lice, body lice, and pubic lice.

petechiae Tiny purple or red spots appearing on the skin as a result of tiny hemorrhages within dermal or submucosal layers (Fig. 12.18).

psoriasis Common chronic skin disorder characterized by circumscribed red patches covered by thick, dry, silvery scales (Fig. 12.19).

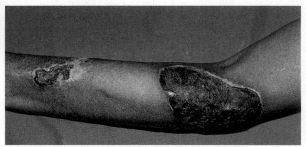

Fig. 12.17 Skin Necrosis. This skin eruption began as red, painful plaques that became necrotic.

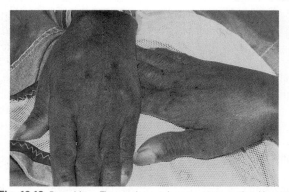

Fig. 12.18 Petechiae. Tiny purple or red spots appear on the skin as a result of tiny hemorrhages beneath the surface.

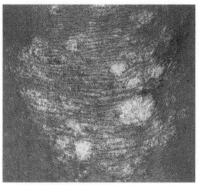

Fig. 12.19 Psoriasis. This skin disorder is characterized by circumscribed red patches covered by thick, dry, silvery scales.

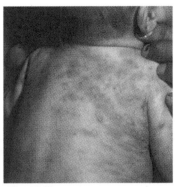

Fig. 12.20 Scabies rash in an infant.

scabies Contagious dermatitis caused by the itch mite that is transmitted by close contact (Fig. 12.20).

scleroderma (scler/o, hard + -derma, skin) Chronic hardening and thickening of the skin.

skin cancer Any of several neoplasms of the skin; the most common and most curable malignancies. Skin cancers are caused by ionizing radiation, certain genetic defects, chemical carcinogens, and overexposure to the sun or other sources of ultraviolet radiation.

urticaria Skin eruption characterized by wheals of varying shapes and sizes with well-defined margins and pale centers. Its causes include drugs, foods, and insect bites. Also called **hives** (see Fig. 12.7).

xerosis (xer/o, dry) Minor irritation of the skin characterized by excessive dryness, which can lead to scaling, thinning, and injury.

Disorders of Accessory Skin Structures

acne vulgaris Skin disease characterized by blackheads (the result of blocked hair follicles becoming infected with bacteria), whiteheads, and pus-filled lesions; common where sebaceous glands are numerous (faces, upper back, and chest); acne.

folliculitis Inflammation of a hair follicle.

hidradenitis (hidr/o, sweat + aden/o, gland + -itis, inflammation) Inflammation of a sweat gland caused by occlusion (closing off) of the pores with subsequent bacterial infection of the gland.

onychomycosis Fungal condition of the nails (Fig. 12.21).

onychopathy Any disease of the nails.

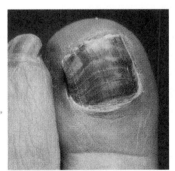

Fig. 12.21 Onychomycosis. This is a fungal condition of the nails. Note the discoloration of the nail and the redness around the nail, indicating inflammation.

seborrhea (seb/o, sebum + -rrhea, discharge) Excessive production of sebum.

seborrheic dermatitis Inflammatory condition of the skin that begins with the scalp but may involve other areas, particularly the eyebrows; commonly called dandruff.

trichosis (trich/o, hair + -osis, condition) Any abnormal condition of hair growth, including baldness or excessive hair growth in an unusual place (Fig. 12.22).

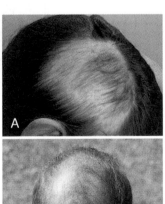

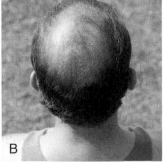

Fig. 12.22 Trichosis. **A,** Abnormal hair pattern, in this case associated with an irresistible urge to pull out one's hair. **B,** Alopecia prematura. This man is in his early thirties and is experiencing premature baldness.

MATCH IT!
EXERCISE 9

Match the skin disorders in the left column with their descriptions.

_____ 1. abscess
_____ 2. albinism
_____ 3. cyanosis
_____ 4. furuncle
_____ 5. ichthyosis
_____ 6. lipoma
_____ 7. mycodermatitis
_____ 8. onychomycosis
_____ 9. petechiae
_____ 10. xerosis

A. a boil
B. benign tumor composed of fat cells
C. bluish discoloration of the skin
D. cavity that contains pus
E. congenital absence of normal pigment
F. dry and scaly skin, resembling fish skin
G. excessive dryness of the skin
H. fungal infection of the nails
I. inflammation of the skin caused by a fungus
J. tiny purple or red spots on the skin

Surgical and Therapeutic Interventions

Superficial wounds often heal without suturing. Deep wounds or those located where movement opens the cut edges are stapled or sutured. Adhesive sprays are sometimes used if wounds are not deep.

Wound irrigation is the flushing of an open wound using a medicated solution, water, sterile saline (balanced salt solution), or an antimicrobial liquid preparation. This is done to cleanse and remove debris or excessive drainage. Superficial wounds often heal without suturing. Deep wounds that are located where movements open the wound edges are often stapled or sutured.

Lipo+**suction**, also called suction-assisted lipectomy, removes adipose tissue with a suction pump device and is used primarily as cosmetic surgery to remove or reduce localized areas of fat, particularly in the neck, arms, legs, and belly (Fig. 12.23).

adip/o, lip/o = fat

Collagen injections use an insoluble protein, collagen, to enhance the lips or fatten sunken facial skin. The injections are a nonsurgical means of smoothing out facial lines and wrinkles but require ongoing treatments to maintain the improvements achieved. Ongoing cosmetic treatments are also necessary for injections of minute doses of the *Clostridium botulinum* toxin (e.g., Botox) administered by a physician (Fig. 12.24). The injections reduce contractions of the muscles that cause persistent frown lines,

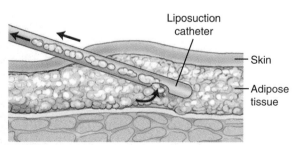

Fig. 12.23 Liposuction. This procedure, also called suction lipectomy, removes adipose tissue with a suction pump device.
adip/o, lip/o = fat; **-ectomy** = excision

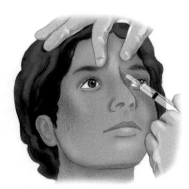

Fig. 12.24 Injections to Reduce Facial Lines. Botulinum toxin (Botox) is injected between the brows to reduce frown lines. The injection must be repeated every 3 months.

especially those between the brows. The toxin was used to treat several spastic muscle disorders long before it was used for cosmetic effects.

top/o = place
bacteri/o, bacter/i = bacteria
-cidal = killing
-static = keeping stationary

Topical medications are drugs placed directly on the skin. Topical antimicrobial agents and dressings are often applied to prevent infection when the skin has been broken. **Bacterio+static** means inhibiting the growth of bacteria, whereas **bactericidal** means killing bacteria. **Asepsis** means the absence of germs (its literal translation is the absence of infection), such as in the description of a wound that is not infected. The opposite of asepsis is **sepsis**, which means infection or contamination. An infected wound is described as **septic**.

trans- = across or through
derm/o = skin

Transdermal drug delivery is a method of applying a drug to unbroken skin (see Fig. 3.8). The drug is absorbed through the skin and then enters the circulatory system. Transdermal delivery is used particularly for estrogen and nicotine and to deliver drugs to prevent motion sickness. Unfortunately, not all medications can be administered transdermally.

Treatment of acne vulgaris includes the use of topical and oral antibiotics, special skin washes, and other products (e.g., Retin-A) that produce a mild, superficial peel of the epidermis. The latter products also improve the appearance of aged or sun-damaged skin. Superficial scars, wrinkles, blemishes, and sun-damaged areas of the outermost layers of the skin can be reduced or removed by laser, chemical peels, or physical sanding of the skin. The top layers peel away, and new, smoother skin layers replace the old ones. One technique, dermabrasion, is included in the following list of additional surgical or therapeutic terms pertaining to the skin.

derm/a = skin

Most surgical procedures involving the skin are performed to repair or treat damaged skin, remove lesions, or penetrate the skin to allow diagnostic or other procedures. Review additional interventions below.

antimicrobial Medicine applied to broken skin to prevent infection.

antiperspirants Compounds that act against or inhibit perspiration.

aspiration Withdrawal of fluid from a cyst with a syringe.

biopsy Removal of a small piece of tissue for microscopic examination to confirm or establish a diagnosis; abbreviated Bx or bx. In a **punch biopsy**, an instrument called a punch is used to remove a small amount of material (at least to the level of the dermis) for microscopic study (Fig. 12.25). A skin biopsy may involve removal of part of a tumor (**incisional biopsy**) to establish a diagnosis, or removal of the entire tumor (**excisional biopsy**) (Fig. 12.26).

cryosurgery Use of subfreezing temperature to destroy tissue.

curettage Scraping of material from a surface to remove abnormal tissue).

debridement Removal of foreign material and dead or damaged tissue, especially from a wound.

dermabrasion Treatment for the removal of superficial scars on the skin by the use of revolving wire brushes or sandpaper.

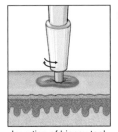
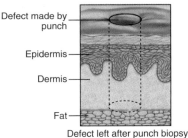

Insertion of biopsy tool   Defect left after punch biopsy

Fig. 12.25 Punch Biopsy. With the use of a punch, living tissue is removed for examination.

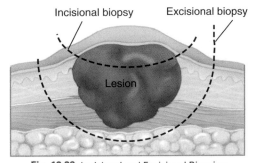

Fig. 12.26 Incisional and Excisional Biopsies.

electrolysis (electr/o, electricity + -lysis, destruction) Destruction of a substance by passing electrical current through it. Laser treatments are sometimes used to destroy the hair follicles when hair is growing in an undesirable place.

electrosurgery Surgery performed with electrical instruments that operate on high-frequency electric current and are often used to destroy skin lesions.

Mohs surgery Tissue-sparing surgery, especially for the face; layers are removed and examined until the specimen is clear of malignancy (Fig. 12.27).

tattoo removal Multiple treatments, either dermabrasion or laser removal. The age, density, type, and color of ink, as well as depth of pigment insertion, determine the number of treatments.

MATCH IT!
EXERCISE 10

Match the terms in the left column with their descriptions.

_____ 1. cryosurgery
_____ 2. curettage
_____ 3. dermabrasion
_____ 4. liposuction

A. physical sanding of the skin
B. removal of localized areas of fat
C. scraping a surface to remove abnormal tissue
D. use of subfreezing temperatures to destroy tissue

 Be Careful With These!

macule (nonraised, discolored spot) versus *papule* (elevated lesion <1 cm in diameter)
vesicles (blisters <1 cm) versus *bullae* (blisters >1 cm)
cyst (sac filled with fluid or semisolid material) versus *nodule* (solid lesion >1 cm wide and deep)

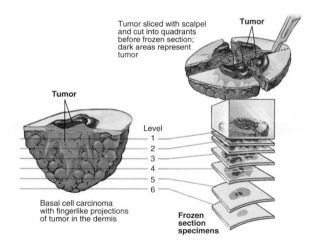

Tumor sliced with scalpel and cut into quadrants before frozen section; dark areas represent tumor

Tumor

Tumor

Level
1
2
3
4
5
6

Basal cell carcinoma with fingerlike projections of tumor in the dermis

Frozen section specimens

Fig. 12.27 Mohs Surgery. Dark areas represent the tumor. Layers are removed until the specimen is clear of malignancy.

A Career as a Licensed Practical Nurse

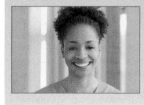

Jeanne had always wanted to work in nursing, and she discovered that becoming a licensed practical nurse (LPN) has its advantages. LPNs provide care under the supervision of a registered nurse, physician, or dentist, but their formal training only takes approximately 1 or 2 years, depending on the state. Jeanne's compassion and decision-making skills, plus the study skills she used to pass the licensure examination, have given her a great career. For more information, visit this website: www.nflpn.org.

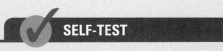

SELF-TEST

Work the following exercises to test your understanding of the material in Chapter 12. It is best to do all the exercises before checking your answers against the answers in Appendix III. Pay particular attention to spelling.

A. WRITING! *List five functions of the skin.*

1. _____ 3. _____ 5. _____

2. _____ 4. _____

B. WRITING! *Write the names of the three skin layers.*

1. _____ 2. _____ 3. _____

C. SPELLING AND PRONUNCIATION! *Circle all incorrectly spelled terms, and write the correct spellings. Then pronounce the terms.*

anteperspiratant   axilary   follikle   integumant   petechie

D. READING HEALTH CARE REPORTS *Find the correct terms in the medical report to match the descriptions that follow.*

Michael Turner - MEDICAL REPORT   _ 🗗 ✕

Task Time Scale Options Help View Edit

Turner, Michael   **Age:** 38   **Sex:** Male   **Loc:**
                        DOB: 07-07-1984 **MRN:** 523892   **FIN:**

Flowsheet: Clinical Notes ▾ ... Level: Consultation ▾   ⦿ Table ○ Group ○ List

MAR | Task List | I & O | Pt. Info | Pt. Schedule | Surgery | **Clinical Notes** | Form Browser

Orders | Last 48 Hours | ED | Lab | Radiology | Assessments | Medical Report | Medication Profile

Reason for Plastic Surgery Consultation: Hypertrophic scarring and keloid formation, left upper extremity and neck.
History of Present Illness: 38-year-old black male who suffered 25% TBSA full- and partial-thickness flame burns to bilateral upper extremities and neck after tripping and falling into a camp fire four months ago. Patient was treated with Silvadene dressing changes and split-thickness skin grafts to the bilateral upper extremities and neck, with right and left thighs as donor sites. Donor sites were treated with a single layer of petrolatum gauze and have healed well. Right upper extremity graft site has healed without sepsis or excessive scarring. Left upper extremity and neck show hypertrophic scarring and keloid formation despite wearing of elastic pressure bandage.
Medical History: Unremarkable except for onychomycosis of the toenails.

1. an overgrowth of collagenous scar tissue at the site of a wound   _____
2. areas of skin removed from one site and transplanted to another site   _____
3. infection   _____
4. the classification of the type of burn   _____
5. fungal condition of the nails   _____

E. CHART NOTE   *Write terms from the report to match the descriptions.*

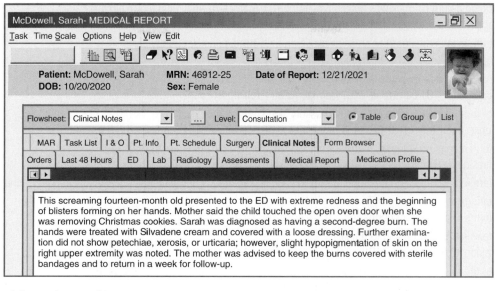

McDowell, Sarah- MEDICAL REPORT   — ⊡ ☒

Task Time Scale Options Help View Edit

Patient: McDowell, Sarah   **MRN:** 46912-25   **Date of Report:** 12/21/2021
DOB: 10/20/2020   **Sex:** Female

Flowsheet: Clinical Notes ▼   ...   Level: Consultation ▼   ⦿ Table ○ Group ○ List

| MAR | Task List | I & O | Pt. Info | Pt. Schedule | Surgery | **Clinical Notes** | Form Browser |

| Orders | Last 48 Hours | ED | Lab | Radiology | Assessments | Medical Report | Medication Profile |

This screaming fourteen-month old presented to the ED with extreme redness and the beginning of blisters forming on her hands. Mother said the child touched the open oven door when she was removing Christmas cookies. Sarah was diagnosed as having a second-degree burn. The hands were treated with Silvadene cream and covered with a loose dressing. Further examination did not show petechiae, xerosis, or urticaria; however, slight hypopigmentation of skin on the right upper extremity was noted. The mother was advised to keep the burns covered with sterile bandages and to return in a week for follow-up.

1. decreased tissue pigmentation   _____
2. descriptive of burn extension into the dermis   _____
3. excessive dryness of the skin   _____
4. skin eruption characterized by wheals   _____
5. tiny hemorrhages in dermal skin layer   _____

F. IDENTIFYING!   *Label these illustrations using one of the following: abrasion, atrophy, bullae, ichthyosis, onychomycosis.*

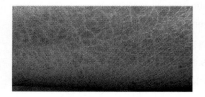

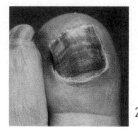

1. Scaly, fishlike skin condition

_____

2. Fungal condition of the nails

_____

G. MATCHING!   *Match the skin lesions in the left column with their descriptions.*

_____ 1. bulla   **A.** blister, larger than 1 cm
_____ 2. cyst   **B.** blister, smaller than 1 cm
_____ 3. fissure   **C.** cracklike lesion of the skin
_____ 4. macule   **D.** discolored spot, not elevated
_____ 5. papule   **E.** fluid-filled sac containing pus
_____ 6. pustule   **F.** sac filled with clear fluid
_____ 7. vesicle   **G.** solid elevation, less than 0.5 cm in diameter

H. CHOOSING!   *Circle the one correct answer (A, B, C, or D) for each question.*

1. In describing a burn by thickness, which type of burn is characterized by immediate blisters?
   (A) deep partial-thickness   **(B)** deep full-thickness   **(C)** full-thickness   **(D)** superficial partial-thickness

2. Which term means the death of areas of tissue or bone surrounded by healthy parts?
   (A) atrophy   **(B)** erosion   **(C)** fissure   **(D)** necrosis

3. Which procedure destroys tissue by using very cold temperatures?
   (A) cryosurgery   **(B)** curettage   **(C)** dermabrasion   **(D)** liposuction

4. Which of the following terms is not an accessory skin structure?
   (A) adipose   **(B)** hair   **(C)** nails   **(D)** sebaceous glands

5. Which term means scraping of material from a surface to remove abnormal tissue?
   (A) aspiration   **(B)** curettage   **(C)** electrosurgery   **(D)** fissure

6. Which term means an acute infection of the skin and subcutaneous tissue characterized by local heat, redness, pain, and swelling?
   (A) cellulitis   **(B)** contact dermatitis   **(C)** ichthyosis   **(D)** lipoma

7. Which term means pertaining to the skin?
   (A) abrasion   **(B)** abscess   **(C)** cutaneous   **(D)** dermatitis

8. Which of the following is a general term for any visible, localized abnormality of the skin?
   (A) abrasion   **(B)** abscess   **(C)** lesion   **(D)** wound

9. Which of the following is a skin eruption characterized by wheals?
   (A) lupus erythematosus   **(B)** malignant melanoma   **(C)** pediculosis   **(D)** urticaria

10. Which of the following is a primary component of epidermis?
   (A) adipose   **(B)** keratin   **(C)** plaque   **(D)** sebum

I. WRITING!   *Write one-word terms for each of these meanings.*

1. a boil   _____
2. torn, jagged wound   _____
3. lack of skin pigment   _____
4. another name for a bruise   _____
5. any disease of the nails   _____

6. benign, fatty tumor   _____
7. chronic skin hardening   _____
8. excessive dryness of the skin   _____
9. inflammation of a sweat gland   _____
10. pertaining to the nails   _____

J. QUICK CHALLENGE!   *Find an incorrect term in each sentence and write the correct term.*

1. Small blisters less than 1 cm are called bullae.
   _____

2. Psoriatic muscles cause erection of the hairs of the skin.
   _____

3. Necrotic means well-defined, with definite borders.
   _____

4. Damage as a result of prolonged exposure to cold is called pediculosis.
   _____

5. Drugs placed directly on the skin are called antimicrobial medications.
   _____

*Use Appendix III to check your answers.

QUICK & EASY (Q&E) LIST

Use the Evolve website (http://evolve.elsevier.com/Leonard/quick) to review the terms presented in Chapter 12. Look closely at the spelling of each term as it is pronounced.

abrasion *(uh-**brā**-zhun)*
abscess *(**ab**-ses)*
acne vulgaris *(**ak**-nē vul-**gar**-is)*
adipose *(**ad**-i-pōs)*
albinism *(**al**-bi-niz-um)*
albino *(al-**bī**-nō)*
antimicrobial *(an-tē-mī-**krō**-bē-ul)*
antiperspirant *(an-tē-**pur**-spur-unt)*
asepsis *(ā-**sep**-sis)*
aseptic *(ā-**sep**-tik)*
aspiration *(as-pi-**rā**-shun)*
atrophy *(**at**-ruh-fē)*
avascular *(ā-**vas**-kū-lur)*
axilla *(ak-**sil**-uh)*
axillary *(**ak**-si-lar-ē)*
bactericidal *(bak-tēr-i-**sī**-dul)*
bacteriostatic *(bak-tēr-ē-ō-**stat**-ik)*
biopsy *(**bī**-op-sē)*
bullae *(**bul**-ē)*
cellulitis *(sel-ū-**lī**-tis)*
circumscribed *(**sur**-kum-skrībd)*
contact dermatitis *(**kon**-takt dur-muh-**tī**-tis)*
contusion *(kun-**tōō**-zhun)*
cryosurgery *(krī-ō-**sur**-jur-ē)*
curettage *(kū-ruh-**tahzh**)*
cutaneous *(kū-**tā**-nē-us)*
cyanosis *(sī-uh-**nō**-sis)*
cyst *(sist)*
debridement *(dā-brēd-**maw**)*
dermabrasion *(dur-muh-**brā**-zhun)*
dermatitis *(dur-muh-**tī**-tis)*
dermatome *(**dur**-muh-tōm)*
dermis *(**dur**-mis)*
discoid lupus erythematosus *(**dis**-koid **lōō**-pus er-uh-them-uh-**tō**-sis)*
ectoderm *(**ek**-tō-durm)*
electrolysis *(ē-lek-**trol**-uh-sis)*
electrosurgery *(ē-lek-trō-**sur**-jur-ē)*
endoderm *(**en**-dō-durm)*
epidermis *(ep-i-**dur**-mis)*
erythema *(er-uh-**thē**-muh)*
excisional biopsy *(ek-**sizh**-shu-nul **bī**-op-sē)*
fissure *(**fish**-ur)*
follicle *(**fol**-i-kul)*
folliculitis *(fuh-lik-ū-**lī**-tis)*

frostbite *(**frost**-bīt)*
furuncle *(**fū**-rung-kul)*
hidradenitis *(hī-drad-uh-**nī**-tis)*
hives *(hīvz)*
hypopigmentation *(hī-pō-pig-mun-**tā**-shun)*
ichthyosis *(ik-thē-**ō**-sis)*
incision *(in-**sizh**-un)*
incisional biopsy *(in-**sizh**-un-ul **bī-op-sē**)*
integument *(in-**teg**-ū-ment)*
keloid *(**kē**-loid)*
keratin *(**ker**-uh-tin)*
laceration *(las-ur-**ā**-shun)*
lesion *(**lē**-zhun)*
lipoma *(lip-**ō**-muh)*
liposuction *(**lip**-ō-suk-shun)*
Lyme disease *(līm di-**zēz**)*
macule *(**mak**-ūl)*
malignant melanoma *(muh-**lig**-nunt mel-uh-**nō**-muh)*
melanin *(**mel**-uh-nin)*
melanocyte *(**mel**-uh-nō-sīt, muh-**lan**-ō-sīt)*
mesoderm *(**mez**-ō-durm)*
mycodermatitis *(mī-kō-dur-muh-**tī**-tis)*
necrosis *(nuh-**krō**-sis)*
nodule *(**nod**-ūl)*
onychomycosis *(on-i-kō-mī-**kō**-sis)*
onychopathy *(on-i-**kop**-uh-thē)*
papule *(**pap**-ūl)*
pediculosis *(puh-dik-ū-**lō**-sis)*
perspiration *(pur-spi-**rā**-shun)*
petechiae *(puh-**tē**-kē-ē)*
pilomotor muscle *(pī-lō-**mō**-tur **mus**-ul)*
plaque *(plak)*
psoriasis *(suh-**rī**-uh-sis)*
punch biopsy *(punch **bī**-op-sē)*
pustule *(**pus**-tūl)*
scabies *(**skā**-bēz)*
scales *(skālz)*
scleroderma *(sklēr-ō-**dur**-muh)*
scleroprotein *(sklēr-ō-**prō**-tēn)*
sebaceous gland *(suh-**bā**-shus gland)*
seborrhea *(seb-ō-**rē**-uh)*
seborrheic dermatitis *(seb-ō-**rē**-ik dur-muh-**tī**-tis)*
seborrheic keratosis *(seb-ō-**rē**-ik ker-uh-**tō**-sis)*
sebum *(**sē**-bum)*
sepsis *(**sep**-sis)*

QUICK & EASY (Q&E) LIST—cont'd

septic (**sep**-tik)

skin cancer (skin **kan**-sur)

skin graft (skin graft)

subcutaneous adipose tissue (sub-kū-**tā**-nē-us **ad**-i-pōs **tish**-o͞o)

sudoriferous gland (s͞o͞o -dō-**rif**-ur-us gland)

tattoo removal (ta-**to͞o** ri-**mo͞o** -vul)

topical medication (**top**-i-kul med-i-**kā**-shun)

transdermal (trans-**dur**-mul)

trichosis (tri-**kō**-sis)

ulcer (**ul**-sur)

ungual (**ung**-gwul)

urticaria (ur-ti-**kar**-ē-uh)

verruca (vuh-**ro͞o** -kuh)

vesicle (**ves**-i-kul)

wheals (hwēlz, wēlz)

xerosis (zēr-**ō**-sis)

Don't forget the games and other activities available at http://evolve.elsevier.com/Leonard/quick.

 QUICK CONNECT

Review all lists of word parts and their meanings for this chapter using the flashcards you prepared or the flashcards on the Evolve site.

The skin is the integument. Cutaneous means pertaining to the skin and subcutaneous means beneath the skin. The suffix -derm can mean either skin or an embryonic layer (fertilized egg differentiates into endoderm, mesoderm, and ectoderm).

Functions of the integumentary system:

D vitamin synthesis

Elimination of wastes through perspiration

Regulation of body temperature through perspiration

Makes information about the environment available to the brain

Acts as a barrier to moisture loss, harmful light rays, and invasion of microbes

Layers of the skin (outer to innermost):

- epidermis (avascular): contains scalelike, nonliving cells (composed primarily of keratin, a scleroprotein, which is insoluble in most solvents)
- dermis (contains blood vessels, nerves, and glands)
- subcutaneous adipose tissue (composed of fat that serves as insulation and cushions against shock)

Accessory skin structures include hair, nails, sebaceous glands, and sweat glands. Pilomotor muscles cause erection of the hairs of the skin. Hair protects the nose and eyes, skin, and scalp. Sudoriferous (sweat) glands produce sebum, oily substance that lubricates the skin and inhibits bacterial growth. Secondary sex characteristics occur at puberty, including hair development in the axillary and genital regions. Ungual means pertaining to the nail (composed of keratin, protein that is the primary component of epidermis, hair, nails, and tooth enamel that is insoluble in most solvents).

Skin lesions: A lesion is any visible, localized abnormality of the skin. A circumscribed lesion has defined edges, such as those of seborrheic keratosis (benign skin lesions often seen in older persons). A verruca is a benign warty skin lesion caused by a contagious virus.

Herpes simplex virus infection is the most common viral infection of adults. HSV-1 causes the classic fever blister. Herpes zoster causes shingles, reactivation of latent chicken pox virus, generally preventable or reduced by vaccination.

Primary lesions are initial reactions to an underlying problem that alters the structural components of the skin. Secondary lesions (changes that occur with normal progression of a disease; examples are atrophy, ulcers, fissures or scales) alter the structural components of the skin.

Primary lesions: Both cysts (sacs filled with fluid or semisolid material) and nodules (marble-like solid lesions more than 1 cm wide and deep) cause raised areas of the overlying skin. Be able to recognize the characteristics of other primary lesions (macules, papules, plaques, bullae, vesicles, and pustules). Wheals, often seen in an allergic skin eruption, are irregularly shaped, slightly raised lesions that usually itch.

Injuries to the skin: Wound (physical break in the skin). If skin damage is severe, a scar remains after healing. Excessive overgrowth of unsightly scar tissue after skin injury is a keloid. Differentiate these terms: abrasion and a laceration and an incision; abrasion and contusion. Know the meaning of aseptic.

Burns are tissue injuries resulting from excessive injury to heat, electricity, chemicals, radiation, or gases (extent of injury is determined by amount of exposure and nature of the agent that caused the burn). Differentiate the three categories of destruction by the depth of tissue destruction.

Know the meanings of these skin disorders: abscess, cellulitis, discoid lupus erythematosus, frostbite, furuncle, ichthyosis, lipoma, Lyme disease, malignant melanoma, myodermatitis, necrosis, pediculosis, petechiae, psoriasis, scleroderma, urticarial, xerosis. Differentiate albinism, hypopigmentation and cyanosis. Recognize that Lyme disease and scabies are transmitted by insects. What distinguishes contact dermatitis from the term "dermatitis" in general?

Know the meanings of the terms associated with the accessory skin structures. Distinguish these terms associated with the nails: onychomycosis and onychopathy. Know the meanings of these terms: acne vulgaris, folliculitis, hidradenitis, seborrhea, seborrheic dermatitis, trichosis.

Surgical and Therapeutic Interventions: Wound irrigation is the flushing of an open wound to cleanse and remove debris or excessive drainage. Liposuction removes or reduces localized areas of fat. Collagen injections enhance the lips or fatten sunken facial skin. Botox injections reduce contractions of the muscles that cause frown lines as well as prevention of certain spastic muscle disorders, such as blepharospasm. Topical medications: Know the difference in bacteriostatic vs. bactericidal; asepsis vs. sepsis. Know the meaning of transdermal drug delivery.

Differentiate these terms: antimicrobial vs. antiperspirants; aspiration vs. biopsy; curettage vs. debridement vs. dermabrasion; electrolysis vs. electrosurgery.

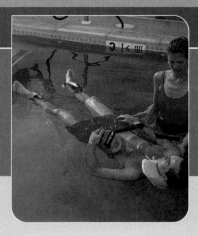

CHAPTER 13

Nervous System and Psychologic Disorders

Aquatic physical therapy (aqua therapy) or pool therapy uses the benefits of heat and the buoyancy of water to reduce the stress on joints and assist in healing and strengthening of muscles in stroke survivors, persons with osteoarthritis, and those recovering from shoulder, hip, or knee replacement.

OBJECTIVES

After completing Chapter 13, you will be able to:

1. Recognize or write the functions of the nervous system.
2. Recognize or write the meanings of Chapter 13 word parts and use them to build and analyze terms.
3. Write terms for select structures of the nervous system, or match them with their descriptions.
4. Write the names of the diagnostic terms and pathologies related to the central nervous system when given their descriptions, or match terms with their meanings.
5. Match the names of psychologic disorders with their descriptions.
6. Match surgical and therapeutic interventions for the central nervous system or write the names of the interventions when given their descriptions.
7. Spell terms for the nervous system and psychologic disorders correctly.

 Function First

Each of the body systems has specific functions, yet all are interrelated and work together to sustain life. It has been said that the human body is more complex than the greatest computer. The nervous system keeps us in touch with both our internal and external environments. Serving as the control center and communications network, the nervous system stores and processes information, stimulates movement, and detects change. In addition, working with the endocrine system, the nervous system helps maintain homeostasis, a dynamic equilibrium of the internal environment of the body.

The nervous system affects both psychologic and physiologic (pertaining to physical and chemical processes) functions. The study of behavior and the function and processes of the mind is called psychology. The nervous system influences other body systems; for example, damage to certain nerves may result in respiratory arrest.

home/o = sameness
-stasis = controlling

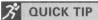 **QUICK TIP**

Physiologic pertains to function; *psychologic* pertains to the mind.

physi/o = nature

Sensory, or **afferent**, receptors detect changes that occur inside and outside the body and convey them to the brain. Some receptors monitor changes in the outside environment, such as in room temperature, and other receptors monitor changes within the body, such as in body temperature. Integrative functions create sensations, produce thoughts and memory, and make decisions based on what is received from the sensory receptors. The nervous system responds by sending motor, or **efferent**, signals from the brain to muscles and glands to cause an effect. The interrelation of these activities is more easily understood when shown in a diagram (Fig. 13.1). The part of the nervous system under conscious or voluntary control is called the **somatic** nervous system. The part of the nervous system that relates to involuntary or automatic body functions is called the **autonomic nervous system**.

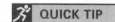

QUICK TIP

Somatic usually pertains to the body, as distinguished from the mind.

aut/o = self

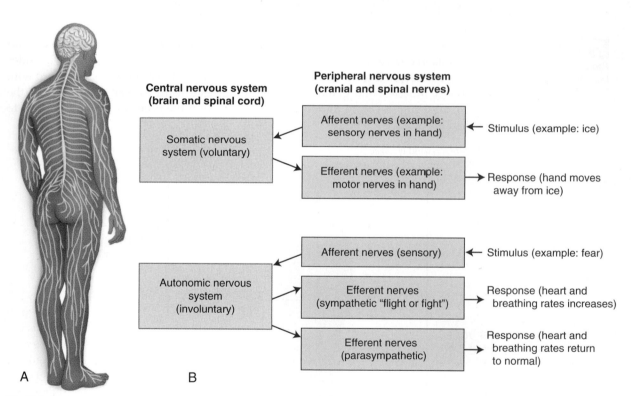

Fig. 13.1 Divisions of the Nervous System. **A,** The central nervous system *(yellow)* includes the brain and spinal cord. The peripheral nervous system *(blue)* is made up of nerves that take impulses away from and toward the central nervous system (CNS) to receptors, muscles, and glands. **B,** Schematic drawing of the interrelationship of the central and peripheral nervous systems.

WRITE IT!*

EXERCISE 1

Write a word in each blank to complete these sentences.

As the control center and communication network, the nervous system has several functions:

- stores and processes (1) _____;
- stimulates (2) _____;
- detects (3) _____ in both the internal and external environment;
- works with the endocrine system to maintain (4) _____ (internal equilibrium).

Receptors that detect internal or external changes are called sensory or (5) _____ receptors. Motor or (6) _____ signals to muscles and glands bring about an effect. The part of the nervous system under voluntary control is the (7) _____ nervous system, and the part that relates to involuntary body functions is the (8) _____ nervous system.

*Use Appendix III, Answers, to check your answers to all the exercises in Chapter 13.

Structures of the Nervous System

Organization of the Nervous System

QUICK TIP

Peripheral means away from the center.

Two major divisions of the nervous system are the **central nervous system** (CNS) and the **peripheral nervous system** (PNS) (Fig. 13.2). The CNS, the control center, includes the brain and spinal cord. The second division connects the brain and spinal cord with receptors, muscles, and glands (carrying impulses toward as well as away from the CNS), allowing the brain to detect sensations within the body, as well as respond to sensations outside the body.

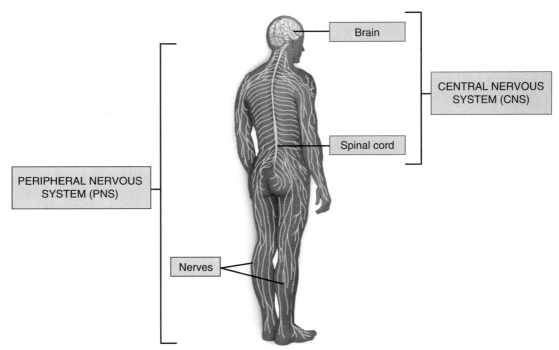

Fig. 13.2 Simplified View of the Divisions of the Nervous System.

HEALTH CARE CONNECTION

The full meaning of *peripheral* is pertaining to the outside, surface, or surrounding area of an organ, structure, or field of vision. *Periphery* means parts or areas near or outside the perimeter or boundary. These terms are used in other body systems as well as the nervous system.

WRITE IT! EXERCISE 2

Write the names of the two major divisions of the nervous system.

1. _____

2. _____

The nervous system is composed of two types of cells: **neurons** and glial (neuroglial) cells. The two types of cells have different functions.

WORD ORIGIN
glia (G.), glue

- Neurons conduct impulses either to or from the nervous system (Fig. 13.3, *A*). Note the **cytoplasmic** projections: a single axon and several dendrites that project from the cell body. **Dendrites** transmit impulses to the cell body and the **axon** carries impulses away from the cell body. Many axons are surrounded by a white fatty covering called a **myelin sheath** (Fig. 13.3, *B*). These fibers conduct nerve impulses faster than axons that lack the myelin sheath. The outermost layer of the axon is called the **neurilemma** (or neurolemma).

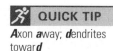 **QUICK TIP**
Axon **a**way; **d**endrites towar**d**

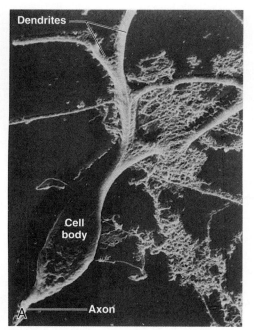

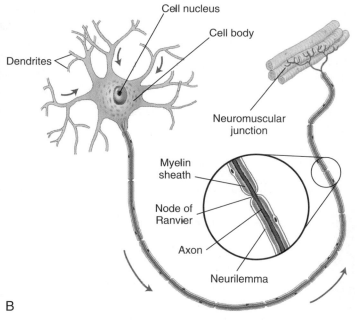

Fig. 13.3 Structure of a Typical Neuron. **A,** Micrograph of a neuron with labeled nerve processes: dendrites and an axon. **B,** The basic parts of a neuron are the cell body, a single axon, and several dendrites. Arrows indicate the direction that an impulse travels to or from the cell body. Some axons are surrounded by a segmented myelin sheath. The myelinated regions provide much faster conduction of the nerve impulse than parts of the axon that are not myelinated. **neur/o** = nerve; **muscul/o** = muscle

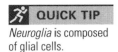

QUICK TIP

Neuroglia is composed of glial cells.

• **Neuroglia**, or **glia**, are the supporting tissue cells of the nervous system. Neuroglial cells provide special support and protection. If glial cells are destroyed, they can replace themselves; however, if an axon is destroyed, it cannot be replaced.

QUICK REVIEW!

Two types of cells: 1. neurons (conduct impulses);   2. neuroglia (provide support)

WRITE IT!
EXERCISE 3

Write a term in each blank to complete these sentences.

1. The _____ nervous system includes the brain and spinal cord.
2. The _____ nervous system consists of nerves that carry impulses toward, as well as away from, the brain and spinal cord.
3. A nerve cell that has dendrites and an axon is called a _____.
4. The supporting structure of nervous tissue is composed of _____ cells.

Commit to memory the word parts in the following table.

WORD PARTS: NERVOUS SYSTEM AND PSYCHOLOGIC DISORDERS

Combining Forms	Meaning	Combining Forms	Meaning
aut/o	self	mening/o	meninges
cerebell/o	cerebellum	ment/o, psych/o	mind
cerebr/o,* encephal/o	brain	myel/o	bone marrow or spinal cord
cervic/o	neck (sometimes cervix uteri)	nerv/o, neur/o	nerve
coccyg/o	coccyx (tailbone)	phren/o	mind or diaphragm
crani/o	cranium (skull)	physi/o	nature
dendr/o	tree	sacr/o	sacrum
dur/o	dura mater	spin/o	spine
gli/o	neuroglia or a sticky substance	thorac/o	thorax (chest)
lumb/o	lower back	ventricul/o	ventricle

Use the electronic flashcards on the Evolve site or make your own set of flashcards using the above list. Select the word parts just presented, and study them until you know their meaning. Do this each time a set of word parts is presented.

*Sometimes *cerebr/o* means cerebrum.

MATCH IT!
EXERCISE 4

Match the terms in the left column with their descriptions.

_____ 1. aut/o
_____ 2. cerebr/o
_____ 3. cervic/o
_____ 4. crani/o
_____ 5. dendr/o
_____ 6. lumb/o
_____ 7. myel/o
_____ 8. phren/o

A. brain
B. lower back
C. mind
D. neck
E. self
F. skull
G. spinal cord
H. tree

WRITE IT!
EXERCISE 5

Write the meanings of these word parts.

1. cerebell/o _____
2. coccyg/o _____
3. dur/o _____
4. encephal/o _____

5. gli/o _____
6. ment/o _____
7. physi/o _____
8. spin/o _____

Central Nervous System

The central nervous system consists of the brain and spinal cord, both encased in bone—the skull (or **cranium**) and the spinal column, respectively. Additional protection for the brain and spinal cord is provided by **cerebrospinal fluid** (CSF), produced by the ventricles, and three membranes (dura mater, arachnoid, and pia mater) that are collectively called the **meninges** (Fig. 13.4). Ventricles of the brain are cavities filled with CSF produced by special cells within them.

cerebr/o = brain
spin/o = spine

HEALTH CARE CONNECTION

The brain has an anatomic feature, the blood-brain barrier, which prevents or slows the passage of chemical compounds, toxins, pathogens, microorganisms, and some drugs. For example, penicillin can be used to treat infections in other parts of the body but cannot cross the blood-brain barrier.

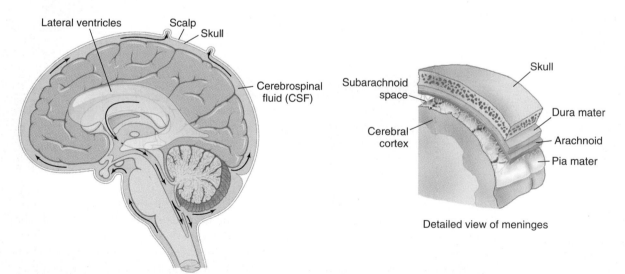

Fig. 13.4 The Brain and Its Protective Membranes, the Meninges.   The tough outer membrane, the dura mater, lies just inside the skull. The threadlike strands of the middle layer, the arachnoid, resemble a cobweb. The pia mater is the innermost meningeal layer and is so tightly bound to the brain that it cannot be removed from the brain without damaging the surface.

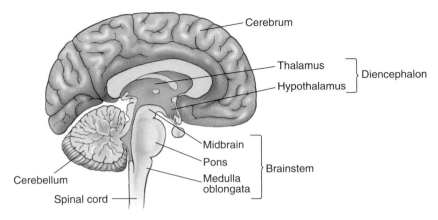

Fig. **13.5** Principal Structures of the Brain (Midsagittal View). The brainstem consists of the midbrain, the pons, and the medulla. Its lower end is a continuation of the spinal cord. The diencephalon is above the brainstem and consists of the thalamus and the hypothalamus. The cerebrum is about ⅞ of the total weight of the brain and spreads over the diencephalon. The cerebellum is inferior to the cerebrum.

The principal structures of the brain are shown in Fig. 13.5. Major structures are the **cerebrum**, the **diencephalon**, the **cerebellum**, and the brainstem. The **hypothalamus** (located beneath the **thalamus**) communicates directly with the pituitary gland, which is discussed in Chapter 15. The brainstem (midbrain, **pons**, and **medulla oblongata**) connects the cerebrum with the spinal cord.

A longitudinal fissure almost completely divides the cerebrum into two **cerebral hemispheres** (hemi- means half). The surface of each hemisphere (right and left) is covered with a convoluted layer of grey matter called the **cerebral cortex**. Division of the cortex into lobes provides useful reference points. Different lobes of the brain are identified with speech, vision, movement of the body, and so forth (Fig. 13.6).

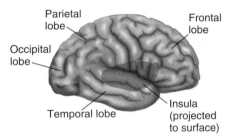

Fig. **13.6** Lateral View of the Cerebrum. The surface of the cerebrum is marked by convolutions. The pia mater closely follows the convolutions and goes deep into the grooves (sulci). Each cerebral hemisphere is divided into five lobes: the frontal lobe, the occipital lobe, the temporal lobe, the parietal lobe, and an insula that is covered by parts of the other lobes.

HEALTH CARE CONNECTION

Note that different lobes are associated with different functions. The frontal lobes are associated with personality, behavior, emotion, and intellectual functions. The temporal lobes are associated with hearing and smell, the occipital lobes are associated with vision, and the parietal lobes are associated with language and general function of sensation.

Peripheral Nervous System

The peripheral nervous system is the part of the nervous system that is outside the central nervous system. The PNS consists of both sensory nervous tissue and motor nervous tissue. Thirty-one pairs of nerves emerge from the spinal cord and are named and numbered according to the region and level of the spinal cord from which they emerge: **cervical**, **thoracic**, **lumbar**, **sacral**, and **coccygeal** nerves (Fig. 13.7). Special sense organs—the eyes, the ears, the skin, the mouth, and the nose—have receptors that detect sensations, and the information is then transmitted to the brain (see Chapter 14).

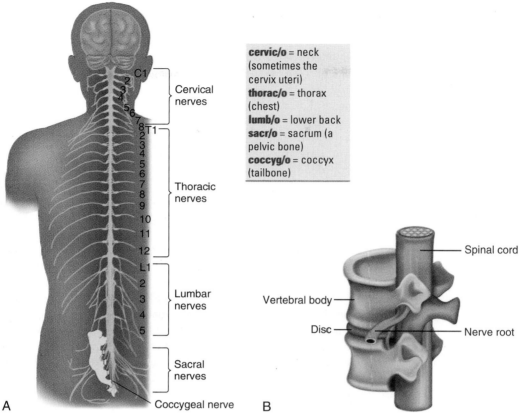

cervic/o = neck
(sometimes the
cervix uteri)
thorac/o = thorax
(chest)
lumb/o = lower back
sacr/o = sacrum (a
pelvic bone)
coccyg/o = coccyx
(tailbone)

Fig. 13.7 Spinal Cord and Nerves Emerging from It. **A,** The spinal cord, about 44 cm (16 to 18 inches) long, extends from the medulla to the second lumbar vertebra. It ends at the cauda equina (meaning horse's tail), a group of nerves that arise from the lower portion of the cord and hang like wisps of coarse hair. There are 31 pairs of spinal nerves: 8 cervical, 12 thoracic, 5 lumbar, 5 sacral, and 1 coccygeal. **B,** Protection of the spinal cord by the vertebrae, the 33 bones of the spinal column.

A simple example shows how light is transmitted to the brain:

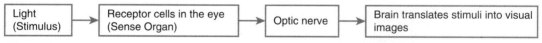

The **spinal cord** is a cylindric structure located in the canal of the vertebral column. It extends from the base of the skull to the first or second lumbar vertebra. The **sciatic nerve** is actually two nerves bound together; it is often considered the largest nerve in the body. Neuralgia along the course of this nerve is called sciatica.

Write a term to complete these sentences.

1. Another name for the skull is _____

2. Collectively, the dura mater, arachnoid, and pia mater are called _____.

3. The structure that represents most of the brain's weight is the _____.

4. A longitudinal fissure almost completely divides the cerebrum into two cerebral _____.

5. The gray matter is the cerebral _____.

6. The structure located in the canal of the vertebral column is the _____ cord.

🚑 Diseases, Disorders, and Diagnostic Terms

Certain illnesses involving the nervous system may require chemical analysis and microscopic examination of the cerebrospinal fluid, obtained by spinal puncture (usually a lumbar puncture; see Fig. 6.29). A large number of leukocytes in CSF may indicate infection, and bacterial and fungal cultures are done if indicated.

A change in the level of consciousness may be the first indication of a decline in CNS function. Memory is another means of assessing neurologic function. Nerve cells that are lost as a person ages do not regenerate. This explains why balance, reflex, and coordinated movement generally deteriorate with advancing age. Vision, hearing, taste, and smell also typically decline.

electr/o = electric
encephal/o = brain
-graphy = recording

Electro+encephalo+graphy (EEG) is the recording and analysis of the electrical activity of the brain (see Fig. 3.16). The record obtained is an **electroencephalogram**. The diagnosis of brain death may require electroencephalography to demonstrate that electrical activity of the brain is absent.

epi- = on, upon
dur/o = dura mater
sub- = under
intra- = within

Magnetic resonance imaging (MRI), computed tomography (CT), and scans using radioisotopes are used to assess structural changes of the brain and spinal cord. CT is especially helpful in diagnosing head injuries (see Fig. 4.10). Three types of hematomas associated with head injuries are subdural, epidural, and intracerebral hematomas (Fig. 13.8). In an **epidural hematoma**, blood accumulates in the epidural space, the space outside the dura mater (the outermost and toughest of the three meninges surrounding the brain and spinal cord). Accumulation of blood beneath the dura mater is called a **subdural hematoma**, and bleeding occurs within the brain in an **intracerebral hematoma**. All hematomas within the skull are serious and can result in compression of the brain, so they are treated promptly and may require removal.

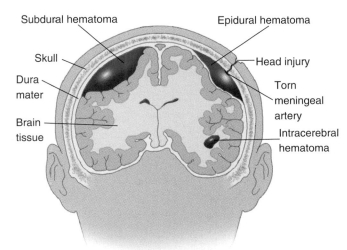

Subdural hematoma
Skull
Dura mater
Brain tissue
Epidural hematoma
Head injury
Torn meningeal artery
Intracerebral hematoma

cerebr/o = brain
dur/o = dura mater
hemat/o = blood
-oma = tumor
mening/o = meninges

Fig. 13.8 Hematomas. Three types associated with head injuries: subdural hematoma, epidural hematoma, and intracerebral hematoma.

🏃 QUICK TIP

Cerebrovascular accident is CVA, stroke, stroke syndrome, or a "brain attack."

In a **cerebro+vascul+ar accident** (CVA), normal blood supply to the brain is disrupted. CVA results in insufficient oxygen to brain tissue and is caused by hemorrhage, occlusion (closing), or constriction of the blood vessels that normally supply oxygen to the brain. Paralysis, weakness, speech defect, and other complications, as well as death, may occur. Some types of strokes are often preceded by warning signs, such as a **transient ischemic attack** (TIA), which is caused by a brief interruption in cerebral blood flow. Ischemic refers to deficient blood circulation. TIA symptoms often include disturbance of normal vision, dizziness, weakness, and numbness. They usually last only a few minutes and do not cause permanent disabilities.

Disorders that interfere with CSF flow, such as brain tumors, can cause **hydrocephalus**, or accumulation of fluid in the skull. The fluid accumulation usually causes increased intracranial pressure. When this happens in an infant, before the cranial bones fuse, the skull enlarges (see Fig. 5.25). In an older child or adult, the pressure damages the soft brain tissue.

A cerebral aneurysm (localized dilation of the wall of a cerebral artery) may require cerebral angiography for diagnosis (Fig. 13.9). Cerebral aneurysms pose a danger of rupture, intracranial hemorrhage, and hemorrhagic stroke.

> **QUICK TIP**
> *Transient* means temporary.

hydr/o = water
cephal/o = head

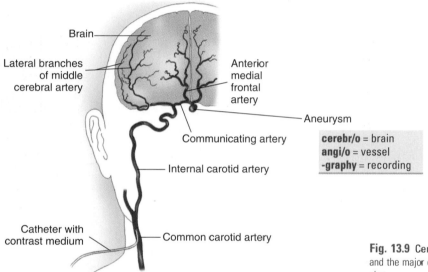

cerebr/o = brain
angi/o = vessel
-graphy = recording

Fig. 13.9 Cerebral Aneurysm. Diagram of an aneurysm and the major cerebral arteries visible in cerebral angiography.

WRITE IT! **EXERCISE 7**

Write a one-word term for each of these descriptions.

1. common name for a cerebrovascular accident _____
2. fluid accumulation in the skull _____
3. the recording of the electrical activity of the brain _____
4. type of hematoma in which blood accumulates beneath the dura mater _____
5. type of hematoma in which blood accumulates outside the dura mater _____
6. type of hematoma in which bleeding occurs within the brain _____

Fractures as well as excessive bending or extension of the spine can result in spinal cord injuries. These spinal injuries include excessive hyperflexion (beyond normal bending), hyperextension (beyond normal maximum extension), and vertical compression (Fig. 13.10).

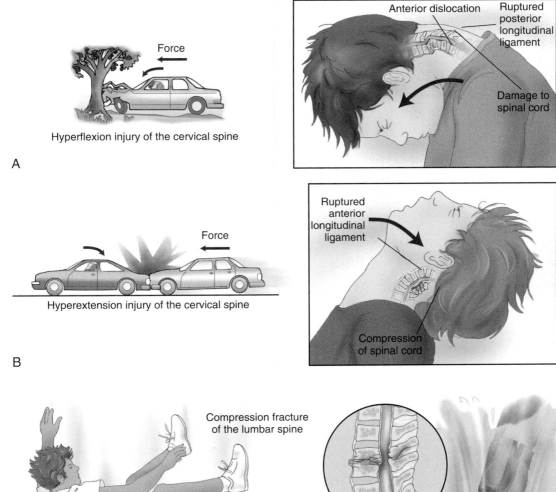

Fig. 13.10 Closed Spinal Cord Injuries. Fractures and dislocations of the vertebral column can result in injury to the spinal cord. These types of vertebral injuries occur most often at points where a relatively mobile portion of the spine meets a relatively fixed segment. **A,** Hyperflexion of the cervical vertebrae. **B,** Hyperextension of the cervical vertebrae. **C,** Vertical compression of the lumbar spine and the cervical spine.

The following list provides information on additional disorders and diagnostic terms related to the nervous system.

akinesia (a-, no + kinesi/o, movement + -ia, condition) Complete or partial loss of muscle movement.

anesthesia (an-, no + esthesi/o, feeling) Partial or complete loss of sensation with or without loss of consciousness; results from disease, injury, or administration of an anesthetic.

aphagia (a-, no + -phagia, eating) Inability or refusal to swallow; characterized by abstention from eating because swallowing is painful.

aphasia (-phasia, speech) An abnormal neurologic condition in which there is absence or impairment of the ability to communicate through speech, writing, or signs.

bradykinesia (brady-, slow + -kinesia, movement) Abnormal slowness of movement or sluggishness of mental and physical processes.

brain tumor A neoplasm of the intracranial portion of the CNS; may be primary or secondary (metastasized from another area) (Fig. 13.11).

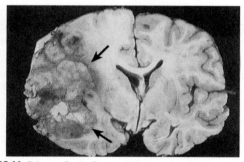

Fig. 13.11 Primary Brain Tumor. This autopsy specimen of the brain shows a large tumor *(arrows)*. The patient had multiple distant metastases in the lung and spine. Compare the size of the two hemispheres.

cephalalgia (cephal/o, head + -algia, pain) Headache; **cephalgia**.

cerebral concussion (cerebr/o, brain + -al, pertaining to) Loss of consciousness, either temporary or prolonged, as a result of a blow to the head.

cerebral contusion Bruising of brain tissue as a result of head injury.

cerebral hemorrhage (hem/o, blood + -rrhage, excessive bleeding) Result of the rupture of a sclerosed, diseased, or injured blood vessel in the brain.

cerebral palsy Brain disorder characterized by paralysis and lack of muscle coordination; it results from developmental defects in the brain or trauma at birth.

coma State of unconsciousness from which the patient cannot be aroused, even by powerful stimulation.

diplegia (di-, two + -plegia, paralysis) Paralysis affecting like parts on both sides of the body.

dyslexia (dys-, difficult + -lexia, words) Inability to read, spell, and write words despite the ability to see and recognize letters.

dysphagia (-phagia, eating, swallowing) Difficulty in swallowing, usually associated with obstruction or other disorder of the esophagus.

dysphasia (-phasia, speech) Speech impairment caused by a lesion in the brain; characterized by lack of coordination and failure to arrange words properly.

electromyography (my/o, muscle) Preparation, study, and interpretation of an electromyogram, a graphic record of the contraction of a muscle as a result of electrical stimulation.

encephalitis (encephal/o, brain + -itis, inflammation) Inflammation of the brain.

encephalocele Hernial protrusion of brain substance through a congenital or traumatic opening of the skull; craniocele.

encephalomalacia (-malacia, softening) Softening of the brain.

encephalomeningitis (mening/o, meninges) Inflammation of the brain and meninges.

encephalopathy (-pathy, disease) Any disease of the brain.

epilepsy (-lepsy, seizure) A group of neurologic disorders characterized by recurrent episodes of convulsive seizures, sensory disturbances, loss of consciousness, or all of these. An uncontrolled electrical discharge from the nerve cells of the cerebral cortex is common to all types of epilepsy. Epilepsy is diagnosed in persons of all ages by electroencephalography, the process of measuring the electrical impulses of the brain (Fig. 13.12).

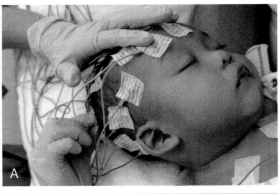

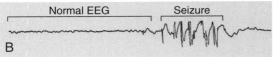

Fig. 13.12 Electroencephalography. **A,** Baby undergoing EEG. This procedure is painless, but the patient must be quiet during the procedure. **B,** Electroencephalogram comparison of the normal part of an EEG, followed by seizure activity.

hemiplegia (hemi-, half) Paralysis of one side of the body. Compare hemiplegia with **paraplegia** (para-, near or beside), paralysis of the legs and lower part of the body, and **quadriplegia** (quadri-, four), paralysis of all four extremities; also called **tetraplegia** (Fig. 13.13).

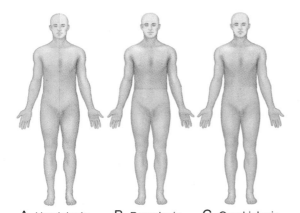

A. Hemiplegia   B. Paraplegia   C. Quadriplegia

Fig. 13.13 Comparison of Affected Areas in Three Types of Paralysis. **A,** Hemiplegia. **B,** Paraplegia. **C,** Quadriplegia.

hyperkinesia (hyper-, excessive + -kinesia, movement) Abnormally increased activity or motor function.

meningitis (mening/o, meninges) Inflammation of the meninges, usually by either a bacterium or a virus.

meningocele Herniation of the meninges through a defect in the skull (cranial meningocele) or vertebral column (spinal meningocele) (Fig. 13.14).

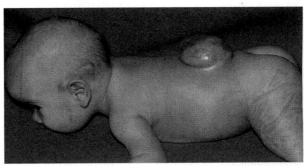

Fig. 13.14 Meningocele. The spinal meninges have formed a hernial cyst that is filled with cerebrospinal fluid and is protruding through a defect in the vertebral column. **-cele** = herniation;   **mening/o** = meninges

multiple sclerosis (scler/o, hard + -osis, condition) Chronic CNS disease with progressive destruction of the myelin sheaths of the neurons. The resulting scar tissue interferes with the normal transmission of nerve impulses (Fig. 13.15). It begins slowly, usually in young adulthood, and continues throughout life.

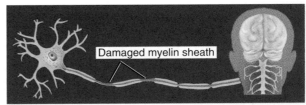

Damaged myelin sheath

Fig. 13.15 Nerve Damage to the Spinal Cord and Brain in Multiple Sclerosis. This results in multiple areas of destruction and scarring of the myelin sheath. Depending on where the damage occurs, symptoms may include problems with muscular control, balance, or vision.
multi- = many;   **scler/o** = hard;   **-osis** = condition

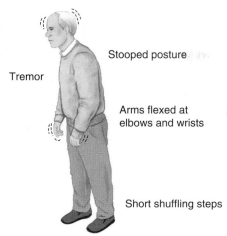

Fig. 13.16 Later Stage of Parkinson Disease. Characteristics of this degenerative neurologic disorder include resting tremor, pill rolling of the fingers, muscle rigidity and weakness, a shuffling gait, a masklike and immobile facial expression, and forward flexion of the trunk. Some of the latter signs are evident in this patient.

myasthenia gravis (my/o, muscle + -asthenia, weakness) Disease characterized by muscle weakness and abnormal fatigue.

myelitis (myel/o, bone marrow or spinal cord) Inflammation of the bone marrow or spinal cord.

myelography Radiographic examination of the spinal cord by injection of a radiopaque medium.

narcolepsy (narc/o, sleep) Chronic ailment involving sudden attacks of sleep that occur at intervals, usually beginning in adolescence or early adulthood.

neuralgia (neur/o, nerve) Pain along the course of a nerve.

neuritis Inflammation of a nerve.

neuropathy Any disease of the nerves, especially disease or degeneration of the peripheral nerves.

Parkinson disease Chronic nervous disease characterized by a fine, slowly spreading tremor, muscular weakness, rigidity, and often a peculiar gait (Fig. 13.16).

peripheral neuropathy Any functional or organic disorder of the PNS.

shingles (herpes zoster) Acute, infectious eruption of vesicles, usually on the trunk of the body along a peripheral nerve caused by reactivation of the latent chickenpox virus. (See Fig. 12.4).

MATCH IT!

EXERCISE 8

Match the terms in the left column with the meanings in the right column.

1. akinesia
2. aphagia
3. bradykinesia
4. cephalgia
5. dysphasia
6. encephalocele
7. myelitis
8. meningocele
9. narcolepsy
10. paraplegia

A. headache
B. herniation of the brain through the skull
C. herniation of the meninges
D. inability or refusal to swallow
E. iinflammation of the bone marrow
F. loss of muscle movement
G. paralysis of the legs and lower part of the body
H. slowness of movement
I. speech impairment
J. sudden attacks of sleep

Psychologic Disorders

Psychologic disorders are unlike most diseases or disorders that confront health professionals because there often is no change in the body structure, and sometimes not even detectable changes in chemistry, thus making the abnormalities difficult to demonstrate and treat in the usual sense. **Psycho+somat+ic** means expression of an emotional conflict through physical symptoms.

psych/o = mind
somat/o = body

WORD PARTS: NERVOUS SYSTEM AND PSYCHOLOGIC DISORDERS

Combining Forms	Meaning	Prefix/Suffix	Meaning
arachn/o	spider	agora-	open marketplace
claustr/o	closed space	-asthenia	weakness
pseud/o	false	-esthesia	sensation, perception
zo/o	animal	-lexia	words, phrases
		-orexia	appetite

Use the electronic flashcards on the Evolve site or make your own set of flashcards using the above list. Select the word parts just presented, and study them until you know their meaning. Do this each time a set of word parts is presented.

WRITE IT!
EXERCISE 9

Write the combining form (CF), prefix (P), or suffix (S) as indicated in the following blanks.

1. animal (CF) _____
2. appetite (S) _____
3. closed space (CF) _____
4. false (CF) _____
5. open marketplace (P) _____

6. sensation or perception (S) _____
7. spider (CF) _____
8. weakness (S) _____
9. words or phrases (S) _____

QUICK TIP

Atrophy of the cerebral cortex occurs in Alzheimer disease.

aut/o = self
-ism = condition

Only a few psychologic disorders have observable pathologic conditions of the brain. Examples of observable pathologic conditions are some neurodevelopmental disorders, dementia, and Alzheimer disease.

Neurodevelopmental disorders are impairments of the growth and development of the brain or CNS. An **intellectual disability** is below-average cognitive functioning that causes delays and impairments in multiple areas, including social participation and education. **Dementia** is a progressive mental disorder characterized by chronic personality disintegration, confusion, disorientation, and deterioration of intellectual capacity and function. **Alzheimer disease** is characterized by progressive mental deterioration, often with confusion, disorientation, restlessness, speech disturbances, and inability to carry out purposeful movement. Three stages of disease progression are recognized: first stage, slight changes in changes in behavior and memory, may not be recognized; second stage shows mild changes in memory and thinking; third stage, dementia.

Signs of psychologic disorders can appear in a very young child. Such is the case with autism and attention deficit disorder. **Autism** is characterized by withdrawal and impaired development in social interaction and communication. **Attention deficit disorder** and **attention deficit hyperactivity disorder** are abbreviated ADD and ADHD, respectively. These are characterized by several patterns of behavior, such as short attention span, poor concentration, and, in ADHD, hyperactivity. Hyperactivity is also called **hyperkinesia**. Translated literally, hyperkinesia, or **hyperkinesis**, is above normal movement.

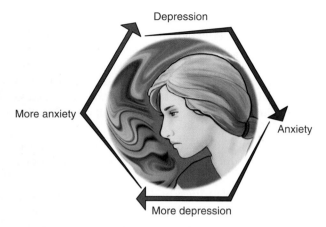

Depression

More anxiety

Anxiety

More depression

Fig. 13.17 Schematic of the Anxiety Cycle. When the natural stress response causes more stress, a cycle becomes established. A permanent state of nervousness, worry, and apprehension can lead to depression.

Anxiety disorders are characterized by anticipation of impending danger and dread, the source of which is largely unknown or unrecognized (Fig. 13.17). An anxiety attack is an acute, psychobiologic reaction that usually includes several of the following: restlessness, tension, tachycardia, and breathing difficulty. A **psychobiological response** involves both the mind and physical body.

Posttraumatic stress disorder is characterized by an acute emotional response after a traumatic event or situation involving severe environmental stress, such as physical assault or military combat.

A panic disorder or **panic attack** is an episode of acute anxiety that occurs unpredictably with feelings of intense apprehension or terror, accompanied by dyspnea (difficult breathing), dizziness, sweating, trembling, and chest pain.

Emotional conflicts are so repressed in a **dissociative disorder** that a separation or split in the personality occurs, resulting in an altered state of consciousness or a confusion of identity. Symptoms may include amnesia, and in this case the loss of memory is generally caused by severe emotional trauma.

An **obsessive-compulsive disorder** (OCD) is an anxiety disorder characterized by recurrent and persistent thoughts, ideas, feelings, or compulsions sufficiently severe to cause distress, consume considerable time, or interfere with the person's occupational, social, or interpersonal functioning. An **obsession** is a persistent thought or idea that occupies the mind and cannot be erased by logic or reasoning. A **compulsion** is an irresistible, repetitive impulse to act contrary to one's ordinary standards.

Phobias are obsessive, irrational, and intense fears of an object, an activity, or a physical situation. Phobias range from abnormal fear of public places, **agoraphobia**, to abnormal fear of animals, **zoophobia**, and even include an abnormal fear of acquiring a phobia, **phobophobia**. **Arachnophobia** is a morbid fear of spiders. **Acrophobia** (acr/o = extremity [heights]) is an irrational fear of heights. **Claustrophobia** is a morbid fear of closed spaces. An abnormal fear of fire is **pyrophobia**.

WORD ORIGIN

obsession *obsidere* (L.), to haunt

WORD ORIGIN

agoraphobia *agora* (G.), marketplace *phobos* (G.), fear
Ancient Greek marketplaces were large, open spaces.

WORD ORIGIN

claustrophobia *clausdere* (L.), to shut

HEALTH CARE CONNECTION

The bite of some spiders is dangerous to humans, including the black widow, the brown recluse, and species of jumping spiders and tarantulas. Spider venom may contain enzymatic proteins that affect neuromuscular transmission or cardiovascular function.

Anorexia nervosa is an eating disorder primarily seen in adolescent girls and usually associated with emotional stress or conflict, such as anxiety, irritation, anger, and fear. It is characterized by prolonged refusal to eat, resulting in wasting, emotional disturbance concerning body image, and fear of becoming obese. **Bulimia nervosa** occurs predominantly in females with usual onset in adolescence or late childhood, and is characterized by episodes of binge eating followed by behavior designed to rid the body of the excess calories (most commonly purging behaviors such as self-induced vomiting or laxative abuse, but sometimes other methods, i.e., excessive exercise or fasting).

A **mood disorder** is a variety of conditions characterized by a disturbance in mood as the main feature. Examples of mood disorders include depression, mania, and bipolar disorder.

Most persons experience occasional feelings of sadness or discouragement resulting from personal loss or tragedy; however, **clinical depression** is an abnormal emotional state characterized by exaggerated feelings of sadness, despair, discouragement, emptiness, and hopelessness.

A **mania** is an unstable emotional state that includes excessive excitement, elation, ideas, and psychomotor activities. In an extreme manic episode a delusion of grandeur may occur. The suffix -mania is used to write terms pertaining to excessive preoccupation. **Megalo+mania** is an abnormal mental state in which one believes oneself to be a person of great importance, power, fame, or wealth.

> **WORD ORIGIN**
>
> megalomania *megas* (G.), greater, large
> *mania* (G.), madness

DICTATORS AND OTHER "BIG EGO" PERSONS ARE SOMETIMES CALLED MEGALOMANIACS

During his final years, Alexander the Great is said to have exhibited signs of megalomania. His extraordinary achievements, coupled with his own sense of destiny, and the flattery of his companions may have contributed to the effect.

A **bipolar disorder** is a major mental disorder characterized by the occurrence of manic episodes, major depressive episodes, or mixed moods. The term *bipolar* in the name indicates that the disorder has two distinct aspects. Megalomania may occur in an extreme manic episode of bipolar disorder.

Pyro+mania is excessive preoccupation with fire. A **pyro+maniac** has an obsessive preoccupation with fires, either to set or watch them.

Klepto+mania is characterized by an abnormal, uncontrollable, and recurrent urge to steal.

Sexual disorders are those caused at least in part by psychologic factors. Such a disorder, characterized by a decrease or disturbance in sexual desire that is not the result of a general medical condition, is called a sexual dysfunction. Sexual perversion or deviation, in which the sexual instinct is expressed in ways that are biologically undesirable, socially prohibited, or socially unacceptable, is termed **paraphilia**.

Somatoform disorders are any of a group of disorders characterized by symptoms suggesting physical illness or disease, for which there are no demonstrable organic causes or physiologic dysfunctions. Somato+form is derived from somat/o, meaning body, and -form, which is a suffix for shape.

What was formerly called **hypochondriasis** or hypochondria has been replaced by two diagnoses: somatic symptom disorder and illness anxiety disorder (IAD). To meet the criteria for somatic symptom disorder, patients must have one or more chronic somatic symptoms about which they are excessively preoccupied or fearful. Patients

> **bi-** = two
>
> **pyr/o** = fire
> **-mania** = excessive preoccupation

> **WORD ORIGIN**
>
> kleptomania *kleptien* (G.), to steal

> **somat/o** = body

> **WORD ORIGIN**
>
> hypochondriasis *chondros* (G.), cartilage
> *hypo* (G.) under

with IAD may or may not have a medical condition, but have heightened bodily sensations, are anxious about the possibility of an undiagnosed illness, and devote excessive time and energy to health concerns.

Neur+asthenia (neur/o, nerve; -asthenia, weakness) is a nervous disorder characterized by weakness and sometimes nervous exhaustion. It is often associated with a depressed state and is believed by some to be psychosomatic. **Psychosomatic disorders** are emotional states that influence the physical body's functioning.

Pseudo+mania is a false or pretended mental disorder. **Pseudo+plegia** is hysterical paralysis. There is loss of muscle power without real paralysis.

A psychotic disorder, or **psychosis**, is any major mental disorder characterized by a gross impairment in reality testing in which the individual incorrectly evaluates the accuracy of thoughts or perceptions and makes incorrect inferences, even in the face of contrary evidence.

Schizophrenia is any of a large group of psychotic disorders. **Schizo+phrenia** is characterized by gross distortion of reality, hallucinations, disturbances of language and communication, and disorganized or catatonic behavior (psychologically induced immobility with muscular rigidity that is interrupted by agitation).

> **schiz/o** = split
> **phren/o** = mind

Translated literally, schizophrenia means "split mind" and relates to the splitting off of a part of the psyche, which may dominate the psychic life of the patient even though it may express behavior contrary to the original personality. The concept of multiple personalities, two or more distinct subpersonalities, is not necessarily a characteristic of schizophrenia.

A number of personality disorders exist with which you may already be familiar. These include antisocial behavior, paranoia, and others. **Anti+social behavior** is acting against the rights of others. **Paranoia** is characterized by persistent delusions of persecution, mistrust, and combativeness.

Additional information about psychologic disorders can be found in the *Diagnostic and Statistical Manual of Mental Disorders* (DSM-5), published by the American Psychiatric Association. It relates to the International Classification of Diseases and uses diagnostic codes, which are fundamental to medical record keeping, greatly facilitating data record keeping and retrieving.

MATCH IT!
EXERCISE 10

Match the psychologic terms in the left column with their descriptions.

_____ 1. acrophobia
_____ 2. Alzheimer disease
_____ 3. anorexia nervosa
_____ 4. claustrophobia
_____ 5. hypochondriasis
_____ 6. kleptomania
_____ 7. neurasthenia
_____ 8. paranoia
_____ 9. pseudomania
_____ 10. pyromania

A. abnormal uncontrollable and recurring urge to steal
B. chronic abnormal concern about one's health
C. chronic weakness and fatigue, often following depression
D. eating disorder that results in wasting of the body
E. false or pretended mental disorder
F. irrational fear of heights
G. morbid fear of closed spaces
H. persistent mistrust and delusions of persecution
I. progressive mental deterioration
J. uncontrollable urge to set fires

QUICK CASE STUDY | EXERCISE 11

Select terms from the report to match the descriptions.

George Goodwin was referred to neurologist Dr. Thomas Smith for severe cephalgia of 2 months' duration. Tests results were negative, and there was no indication of dyskinesia, dysphasia, or dyslexia. Family history indicated a father who suffered frequent narcolepsy. George was admitted to the hospital. Hydrocodon-APAP 5-325 four times a day was effective in treating the pain, and he was sent home after 3 days with a Rx for this medication. The son notified us 4 months later that Mr. Goodwin had died. Autopsy showed an inoperable brain tumor.

1. difficulty in swallowing   _____

2. headache   _____

3. impairment of voluntary movement   _____

4. inability to read, spell, and write words   _____

5. recurrent, uncontrollable brief episodes of sleep   _____

 Surgical and Therapeutic Interventions

 PROGRAMMED LEARNING

Remember to cover the answers (left column) with folded paper or the bookmark. Write an answer in each blank, and then check your answer before proceeding to the next frame.

1. **Neuroplasty** is plastic surgery to repair a nerve or nerves. **Neuro+rrhaphy** is _____ of a cut nerve. **Neuro+lysis** has several meanings: release of a nerve sheath by cutting it longitudinally; surgery to break up adhesions surrounding a nerve; relief of tension on a nerve; and disintegration of nerve tissue.

2. Nerve blocks are used to reduce pain by temporarily blocking transmission of nerve impulses. Pain management may be for a short time (e.g., after surgery) or longer, as in chronic pain. **Analgesics** are agents that relieve _____ without causing loss of consciousness. **Hypnotics** are drugs often used as sedatives to produce a calming effect.

3. In addition to analgesics and anesthetics, many drugs act on the central nervous system. **Antidepressants** treat depression and other mental disorders; **antimigraine** drugs treat migraine headaches; **antiparkinsonian** agents relieve symptoms of Parkinson disease. **Antianxiety drugs** induce relaxation to relieve anxiety. **Anticonvulsants** relieve or prevent _____. Antipyretics are used to reduce fever. There are numerous treatments for depression and psychologic disorders that are beyond the scope of this book. Check the pharmacology section for Chapter 13 at: http://evolve.elsevier.com /Leonard/quick/

craniotomy	4. Cranial surgery may be needed for vascular abnormalities, brain tumors, trauma, or removal of pus and necrotic products of infection. Any surgical opening into the skull is a _____.
removal (or excision)	5. Craniotomies are performed to gain access to the brain, relieve intracranial pressure, or control bleeding inside the skull. **Craniectomy** (see Fig. 6.28) is surgical _____ of a portion of the skull to perform surgery on the brain. This type of surgery may be necessary to repair the brain or its vessels, remove a brain tumor, or repair an aneurysm (a localized dilation of the wall of a blood vessel).
cranioplasty	6. Surgical repair of the skull after surgery or injury to the skull is called _____. **Shunts** (passages or bypasses between two vessels) are used to redirect cerebrospinal fluid from one area to another using a tube or an implanted device, as in a **ventriculoperitoneal shunt** (Fig. 13.18).
electrical	7. Trans+cutane+ous electrical nerve stimulation (TENS) is a method of pain control by the application of _____ impulses to the nerve endings (Fig. 13.19).
	8. **Stereotactic radiosurgery** involves closed-skull destruction of a target (e.g., tumor) using ionizing radiation. The patient's head is held in a frame. In a gamma knife

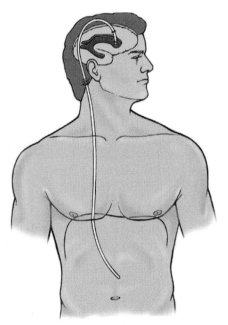

Fig. 13.18 Ventriculoperitoneal Shunt. This type of shunt consists of plastic tubing between a cerebral ventricle and the peritoneum, to drain excess cerebrospinal fluid from the brain in hydrocephalus.
ventricul/o = ventricle; **periton/o** = peritoneum;
-eal = pertaining to

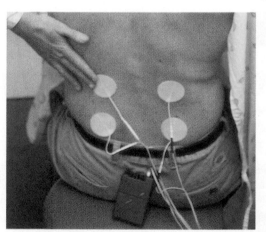

Fig. 13.19 Transcutaneous Electrical Nerve Stimulation (TENS). The TENS unit is being used in this example to control low back pain. Electrodes are placed on the skin and attached to a stimulator by flexible wires. The electrical impulses block transmission of pain signals to the brain. TENS is nonaddictive and has no known side effects, but it is contraindicated in patients with artificial cardiac pacemakers.
trans- = across; **cutane/o** = skin; **-ous** = pertaining to

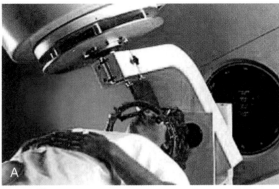
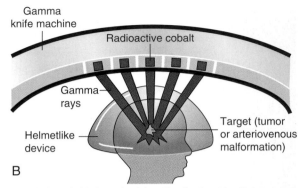

Fig. 13.20 Gamma "Knife" Treatment Assisted by Stereotaxis. **A,** The stereotactic frame holds the patient's head in a fixed position. **B,** In a gamma knife treatment, beams are intense only at the targeted area.

knife	**procedure,** a high dose of radiation is delivered to precisely targeted tumor tissue (Fig. 13.20). This is called gamma _____ procedure because controlled radiation replaces a surgical knife.

MATCH IT! EXERCISE 12

Match the surgical terms in the left column with their descriptions.

_____ 1. analgesics

_____ 2. cranioplasty

_____ 3. craniotomy

_____ 4. hypnotics

_____ 5. neurolysis

_____ 6. neuroplasty

_____ 7. neurorrhaphy

A. agents that are often used as sedatives

B. agents that relieve pain

C. incision of the skull

D. surgical relief of tension on a nerve

E. surgical repair of a nerve

F. surgical repair of the skull

G. suturing of a cut nerve

Be Careful With These!

aphagia versus *dysphagia*

cerebell/o (cerebellum) versus *cerebr/o* (brain)

-asthenia (weakness) versus *-esthesia* (sensation, perception)

-lexia (words, phrases) versus *-orexia* (appetite)

A Career as an EEG Technologist

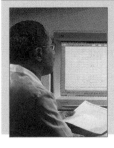

Gregory is an electroencephalography (EEG) and polysomnography technologist. He enjoys his work at a center that studies sleep disorders. He knows that the test results help physicians determine treatment and that improving patients' sleep is one of the best aids to better health. Gregory studied electroneurodiagnostic technology, earned his associate's degree, and passed the national board examination. There are also programs that specifically focus on polysomnographic technology. For more information, visit this website: www.aset.org

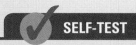

SELF-TEST

Work the following exercises to test your understanding of the material in Chapter 13. It is best to do all the exercises before checking your answers against the answers in Appendix III. Pay particular attention to spelling.

A. WRITING!   *Write a word in each blank to complete these sentences.*

1. The brain and spinal cord are part of the _____ nervous system.
2. The various nerves that connect the brain and the spinal cord with receptors, muscles, and glands make up the _____ nervous system.
3. The _____ nervous system is the control center of the body.
4. The main type of nerve cell is called a _____.
5. Nerve cells that provide special support and protection are called _____ cells.
6. Protective membranes called _____ cover the brain and spinal cord.
7. Disorders that are characterized by anticipation of impending danger and dread are _____ disorders.
8. Agents that relieve pain without causing loss of consciousness are called _____.

B. WRITING!   *Write one-word terms for these meanings.*

1. abnormal preoccupation with fire   _____
2. incision of the skull   _____
3. any disease of the brain   _____
4. destruction of nerve tissue   _____
5. uncontrollable urge to steal   _____
6. abnormal fear of spiders   _____
7. persistent, irrational fear or dread _____
8. inability to read and write words   _____
9. surgical repair of the skull   _____
10. suturing of a cut nerve   _____

C. CHOOSING!   *Circle the one correct answer (A, B, C, or D) for each question.*

1. What is the term for protrusion of the brain through a defect in the skull?
   (A) cranioplasty   **(B)** encephalitis   **(C)** encephalocele   **(D)** encephalomyeloma

2. In which type of hematoma is blood found within the brain tissue itself?
   (A) epidural   **(B)** intracerebral   **(C)** subdural   **(D)** vascular

3. Which of the following diseases or disorders is characterized by sudden attacks of sleep?
   (A) astigmatism   **(B)** diplegia   **(C)** encephalomalacia   **(D)** narcolepsy

4. Which of the following is an infectious eruption that usually occurs on the trunk of the body?
   (A) Alzheimer disease   **(B)** multiple sclerosis   **(C)** myelitis   **(D)** shingles

5. Which of the following means recording of the electrical activity of the brain?
   (A) akinesia   **(B)** electroencephalography   **(C)** encephalopathy   **(D)** narcolepsy

6. Which term means inflammation of the brain?   **(A)** adrenitis   **(B)** encephalitis   **(C)** meningitis   **(D)** myelitis

7. Which term means a headache?   **(A)** cephalalgia   **(B)** cephalotomy   **(C)** dyslexia   **(D)** dysphagia

8. Which of the following is an abnormal emotional state characterized by exaggerated feelings of sadness and hopelessness?   **(A)** clinical depression   **(B)** myopia   **(C)** psychosis   **(D)** psychosomatic disorder

9. Which of the following is an irrational fear of open spaces, characterized by marked fear of venturing out alone?   **(A)** agoraphobia   **(B)** anorexia nervosa   **(C)** attention deficit disorder   **(D)** autism

10. Which term means complete loss of muscle movement?   **(A)** akinesia   **(B)** aphasia   **(C)** aphonia   **(D)** dyskinesia

D. IDENTIFYING!   *Label these illustrations using one of the following: hemiplegia, hypothalamus, paraplegia, quadriplegia, meningocele.*

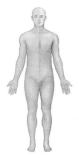
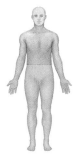
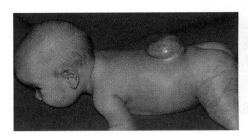

1. paralysis of one side of the body   2. paralysis of the legs and lower part of the body   3. herniation of the meninges

_____   _____   _____

E. READING HEALTH CARE REPORTS   *Read the report and select one answer for questions 1 through 5.*

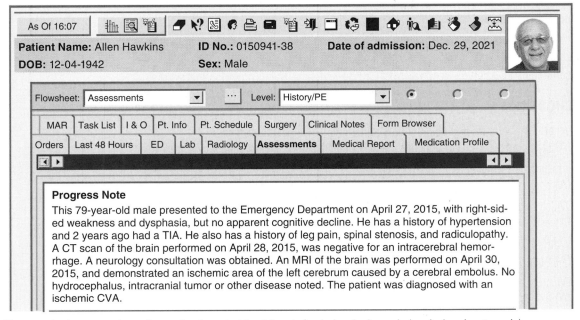

As Of 16:07				

Patient Name: Allen Hawkins   **ID No.:** 0150941-38   **Date of admission:** Dec. 29, 2021
DOB: 12-04-1942   **Sex:** Male

Flowsheet: Assessments   Level: History/PE

MAR | Task List | I & O | Pt. Info | Pt. Schedule | Surgery | Clinical Notes | Form Browser
Orders | Last 48 Hours | ED | Lab | Radiology | **Assessments** | Medical Report | Medication Profile

Progress Note
This 79-year-old male presented to the Emergency Department on April 27, 2015, with right-sided weakness and dysphasia, but no apparent cognitive decline. He has a history of hypertension and 2 years ago had a TIA. He also has a history of leg pain, spinal stenosis, and radiculopathy. A CT scan of the brain performed on April 28, 2015, was negative for an intracerebral hemorrhage. A neurology consultation was obtained. An MRI of the brain was performed on April 30, 2015, and demonstrated an ischemic area of the left cerebrum caused by a cerebral embolus. No hydrocephalus, intracranial tumor or other disease noted. The patient was diagnosed with an ischemic CVA.

1. The term in the report that refers to inadequate blood flow is (embolus, hydrocephalus, ischemic, stenosis).

2. The "T" in the abbreviation TIA stands for (temporal, transient, transcutaneous, tumor).

3. Dysphasia is a condition that refers to a patient's (attention span, cognition, movement, speech).

4. The abbreviation that indicates a stroke is (CVA, CT, MRI, TIA).

5. A term in the report that means an accumulation of fluid in the skull is
   (dysphasia, hypertension, hydrocephalus, radiculopathy).

F. READING HEALTH CARE REPORTS   *Read the health care report, then write terms from the report that match the descriptions.*

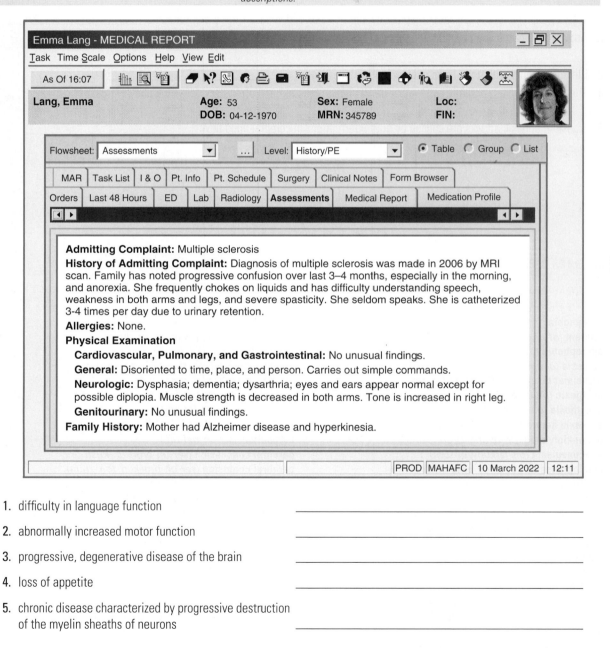

Emma Lang - MEDICAL REPORT

Task Time Scale Options Help View Edit

As Of 16:07

Lang, Emma   **Age:** 53   **Sex:** Female   **Loc:**
                        DOB: 04-12-1970   **MRN:** 345789   **FIN:**

Flowsheet: Assessments   ...   Level: History/PE   • Table ○ Group ○ List

| MAR | Task List | I & O | Pt. Info | Pt. Schedule | Surgery | Clinical Notes | Form Browser |

| Orders | Last 48 Hours | ED | Lab | Radiology | **Assessments** | Medical Report | Medication Profile |

Admitting Complaint: Multiple sclerosis
History of Admitting Complaint: Diagnosis of multiple sclerosis was made in 2006 by MRI scan. Family has noted progressive confusion over last 3–4 months, especially in the morning, and anorexia. She frequently chokes on liquids and has difficulty understanding speech, weakness in both arms and legs, and severe spasticity. She seldom speaks. She is catheterized 3-4 times per day due to urinary retention.
Allergies: None.
Physical Examination
   Cardiovascular, Pulmonary, and Gastrointestinal: No unusual findings.
   General: Disoriented to time, place, and person. Carries out simple commands.
   Neurologic: Dysphasia; dementia; dysarthria; eyes and ears appear normal except for possible diplopia. Muscle strength is decreased in both arms. Tone is increased in right leg.
   Genitourinary: No unusual findings.
Family History: Mother had Alzheimer disease and hyperkinesia.

PROD MAHAFC 10 March 2022 12:11

1. difficulty in language function   _____

2. abnormally increased motor function   _____

3. progressive, degenerative disease of the brain   _____

4. loss of appetite   _____

5. chronic disease characterized by progressive destruction
   of the myelin sheaths of neurons   _____

G. SPELLING AND PRONUNCIATION!   *Circle all incorrectly spelled terms, and write the correct spelling. Then pronounce all the terms.*

akrophobia   periferal   sudoplegia   subdural   thalmus

_____

H. QUICK CHALLENGE!   *Find an incorrect term in each sentence and write the correct term.*

1. A coccygeal shunt redirects cerebrospinal fluid from a cerebral ventricle to the peritoneum. _____

2. An adjective for having physical symptoms of emotional disorder is pseudoplegia.

   _____

3. Bleeding occurs within the brain in an epidural hematoma. _____

4. The cervical nerve is actually two lumbar nerves bound together and often considered the body's largest nerve.

   _____

5. Transient aphasic attacks are caused by brief interruptions in cerebral flood flow. _____

*Use Appendix III to check your answers.

QUICK & EASY (Q&E) LIST

Use the Evolve website (http://evolve.elsevier.com/Leonard/quick) to review the terms presented in Chapter 13. Look closely at the spelling of each term as it is pronounced.

acrophobia *(ak-rō-**fō**-bē-uh)*
afferent *(**af**-ur-unt)*
agoraphobia *(ag-uh-ruh-**fō**-bē-uh)*
akinesia *(ā-ki-**nē**-zhuh)*
Alzheimer disease *(**awltz**-hī-mur di-**zēz**)*
analgesic *(an-ul-**jē**-zik)*
anesthesia *(an-es-**thē**-zhuh)*
anorexia nervosa *(an-ō-**rek**-sē-uh nur-**vō**-suh)*
antianxiety drug *(an-tē-ang-**zī**-uh-tē drug)*
anticonvulsant *(an-tē-kun-**vul**-sunt)*
antidepressants *(an-tē-dē-**pres**-unts)*
antimigraine *(an-tē-**mī**-grān)*
antiparkinsonian *(an-tē-pahr-kin-**sō**-nē-un)*
antisocial behavior *(an-tē-**sō**-shul bē-**hāv**-yur)*
anxiety disorders *(ang-**zī**-uh-tē dis-**or**-durz)*
aphagia *(uh-**fā**-juh)*
aphasia *(uh-**fā**-zhuh)*
arachnophobia *(uh-rak-nō-**fō**-bē-uh)*
attention deficit disorder *(uh-**ten**-shun **def**-i-sit dis-**or**-dur)*
attention deficit hyperactivity disorder *(uh-**ten**-shun **def**-i-sit hī-pur-ak-**tiv**-i-tē dis-**or**-dur)*
autism *(**aw**-tiz-um)*
autonomic nervous system *(aw-tuh-**nom**-ik **nur**-vus **sis**-tum)*

axon *(**ak**-son)*
bipolar disorder *(bī-**pō**-lur dis-**or**-dur)*
brain tumor *(brān **too**-mur)*
bulimia nervosa *(boo-**lē**-mē-uh nur-**vō**-suh)*
bradykinesia *(brad-ē-ki-**nē**-zhuh)*
central nervous system *(**sen**-trul **nur**-vus **sis**-tum)*
cephalalgia *(sef-uh-**lal**-juh)*
cephalgia *(suh-**fal**-juh)*
cerebellum *(ser-uh-**bel**-um)*
cerebral concussion *(**ser**-uh-brul kun-**kush**-un)*
cerebral contusion *(**ser**-uh-brul kun-**too**-zhun)*
cerebral cortex *(**ser**-uh-brul **kor**-teks)*
cerebral hemispheres *(**ser**-uh-brul **hem**-i-sfērz)*
cerebral hemorrhage *(**ser**-uh-brul **hem**-uh-ruj)*
cerebral palsy *(**ser**-uh-brul **pawl**-zē)*
cerebrospinal fluid *(ser-uh-brō-**spī**-nul **floo**-id)*
cerebrovascular accident *(ser-uh-brō-**vas**-kū-lur **ak**-si-dunt)*
cerebrum *(**ser**-uh-brum, suh-**rē**-brum)*
cervical *(**sur**-vi-kul)*
claustrophobia *(klaws-trō-**fō**-bē-uh)*
clinical depression *(**klin**-i-kul di-**presh**-un)*
coccygeal *(kok-**sij**-ē-ul)*

QUICK & EASY (Q&E) LIST—cont'd

coma *(kō-muh)*
compulsion *(kum-**pul**-shun)*
craniectomy *(krā-nē-**ek**-tuh-mē)*
cranioplasty *(**krā**-nē-ō-plas-tē)*
craniotomy *(krā-nē-**ot**-uh-mē)*
cranium *(**krā**-nē-um)*
cytoplasmic *(sī-tō-**plaz**-mik)*
dementia *(duh-**men**-shuh)*
dendrite *(**den**-drīt)*
diencephalon *(dī-un-**sef**-uh-lon)*
diplegia *(dī-**plē**-jē-uh)*
dissociative disorder *(dis-**ō**-shē-āt-iv dis-**or**-dur)*
dyslexia *(dis-**lek**-sē-uh)*
dysphagia *(dis-**fā**-jē-uh)*
dysphasia *(dis-**fā**-zhuh)*
efferent *(**ef**-ur-unt)*
electroencephalogram *(ē-lek-trō-en-**sef**-uh-lō-gram)*
electroencephalography *(ē-lek-trō-un-sef-uh-**log**-ruh-fē)*
electromyography *(ē-lek-trō-mī-**og**-ruh-fē)*
encephalitis *(en-sef-uh-**lī**-tis)*
encephalocele *(en-**sef**-uh-lō-sēl)*
encephalomalacia *(en-sef-uh-lō-muh-**lā**-shuh)*
encephalomeningitis *(en-sef-uh-lō-men-in-**jī**-tis)*
encephalopathy *(en-sef-uh-**lop**-uh-thē)*
epidural hematoma *(ep-i-**doo**-rul hē-muh-**tō**-muh)*
epilepsy *(**ep**-i-lep-sē)*
glia *(**glī**-uh)*
hemiplegia *(hem-ē-**plē**-juh)*
hydrocephalus *(hi-drō-**sef**-uh-lus)*
hyperkinesia *(hī-pur-ki-**nē**-zhuh)*
hyperkinesis *(hī-pur-ki-**nē**-sis)*
hypnotic *(hip-**not**-ik)*
hypochondriasis *(hī-pō-kon-**drī**-uh-sis)*
hypothalamus *(hī-pō-**thal**-uh-mus)*
intracerebral hematoma *(in-truh-**ser**-uh-brul hē-muh-**tō**-muh)*
kleptomania *(klep-tō-**mā**-nē-uh)*
lumbar *(**lum**-bur, **lum**-bahr)*
mania *(**mā**-nē-uh)*
medulla oblongata *(muh-**dul**-uh ob-long-**gah**-tuh)*
megalomania *(meg-uh-lō-**mā**-nē-uh)*
meninges *(muh-**nin**-jēz)*
meningitis *(men-in-**jī**-tis)*
meningocele *(muh-**ning**-gō-sēl)*
mood disorder *(mo͞od dis-**or**-dur)*
multiple sclerosis *(**mul**-ti-pul skluh-**rō**-sis)*
myasthenia gravis *(mī-us-**thē**-nē-uh **gra**-vis)*
myelin sheath *(**mī**-uh-lin shēth)*
myelitis *(mī-uh-**lī**-tis)*

myelography *(mī-uh-**log**-ruh-fē)*
narcolepsy *(**nahr**-kō-lep-sē)*
neuralgia *(noo-**ral**-juh)*
neurasthenia *(noor-us-**thē**-nē-uh)*
neurilemma *(noor-i-**lem**-uh)*
neuritis *(noo-**rī**-tis)*
neurodevelopmental disorders *(noor-ō-dē-vel-op-**men**-tul dis-**or**-durz)*
neuroglia *(noo-**rog**-lē-uh)*
neurolysis *(noo-**rol**-i-sis)*
neuron *(**noor**-on)*
neuropathy *(noo-**rop**-uh-thē)*
neuroplasty *(**noor**-ō-plas-tē)*
neurorrhaphy *(noo-**ror**-uh-fē)*
obsession *(ob-**sesh**-un)*
obsessive-compulsive disorder *(ub-**ses**-iv kum-**pul**-siv dis-**or**-dur)*
panic attack *(**pan**-ik uh-**tak**)*
paranoia *(par-uh-**noi**-uh)*
paraphilia *(par-uh-**fil**-ē-uh)*
paraplegia *(par-uh-**plē**-juh)*
Parkinson disease *(**pahr**-kin-sun di-**zēz**)*
peripheral nervous system *(puh-**rif**-ur-ul **nur**-vus **sis**-tum)*
peripheral neuropathy *(puh-**rif**-ur-ul noo-**rop**-uh-thē)*
phobias *(**fō**-bē-uhz)*
phobophobia *(fō-bō-**fō**-bē-uh)*
pons *(ponz)*
posttraumatic stress disorder *(pōst-traw-**mat**-ik stres dis-**or**-dur)*
pseudomania *(so͞o-dō-**mā**-nē-uh)*
pseudoplegia *(so͞o-dō-**plē**-juh)*
psychobiological response *(sī-kō-bī-ō-**loj**-i-kul rē-**spons**)*
psychosis *(sī-**kō**-sis)*
psychosomatic *(sī-kō-sō-**mat**-ik)*
psychosomatic disorders *(sī-kō-sō-**mat**-ik dis-**or**-durz)*
pyromania *(pī-rō-**mā**-nē-uh)*
pyromaniac *(pī-rō-**mā**-nē-ak)*
pyrophobia *(pī-rō-**fō**-bē-uh)*
quadriplegia *(kwod-ri-**plē**-juh)*
sacral *(**sā**-krul)*
schizophrenia *(skit-sō-**frē**-nē-uh)*
sciatic nerve *(sī-**at**-ik nurv)*
sexual disorders *(**sek**-sho͞o-ul dis-**or**-durz)*
shingles *(**shing**-gulz)*
shunt *(shunt)*
somatic *(sō-**mat**-ik)*
somatoform disorders *(sō-**mat**-ō-form dis-**or**-durz)*
spinal cord *(**spī**-nul kord)*
stereotactic radiosurgery *(ster-ē-ō-**tak**-tik rā-dē-ō-**sur**-jur-ē)*

QUICK & EASY (Q&E) LIST—cont'd

subdural hematoma *(sub-**doo**-rul hē-muh-**tō**-muh)*
tetraplegia *(tet-ruh-**plē**-juh)*
thalamus *(**thal**-uh-mus)*
thoracic *(thuh-**ras**-ik)*

transient ischemic attack *(**tran**-shent, **tran**-sē-unt is-**kē**-mik uh-**tak**)*
ventriculoperitoneal shunt *(ven-trik-ū-lō-per-i-tō-**nē**-ul shunt)*
zoophobia *(zō-ō-**fō**-be-uh)*

Don't forget the games and other activities available at *http://evolve.elsevier.com/Leonard/quick.*

  QUICK CONNECT

Review all lists of word parts and their meanings for this chapter using the flashcards you prepared or the flashcards on the Evolve site.

The nervous system, the body's control center and communication network, stores and processes information, stimulates movement, and detects environmental changes (internal and external). It activates and coordinates all the functions of the body. Its organization:

Central nervous system (CNS, brain and spinal cord) is voluntary.

Peripheral nervous system (PNS, cranial and spinal nerves): communication network between the CNS and the rest of the body: afferent (sensory) or efferent (parasympathetic) is involuntary.

The CNS is composed of two types of cells:

• Neurons (conduct impulses to or from the CNS) have an axon (carries impulses away from the neuron) and dendrites (carries impulses to the neuron). Myelin sheaths covering many axons conduct nerve impulses faster. Neurotransmitters (acetylcholine, epinephrine, dopamine, endorphins, serotonin) inhibit or enhance a nervous response. Neurons *cannot* replace themselves.

Brain and spinal cord are encased in bone: cranium and spinal column, respectively. Additional protection is provided by CSF and three membranes (dura mater, arachnoid, and pia mater).

Principal structures of the brain: cerebrum, diencephalon, cerebellum and the brainstem (midbrain, pons, and medulla oblongata). Each cerebral hemisphere is covered with grey matter. Lobes of the brain are occipital, parietal, frontal, temporal, and insula.

• Neuroglia provide support and protection. These *can* replace themselves.

The PNS: afferent (sensory, sympathetic) or efferent (parasympathetic) nerves

Cervical, thoracic, lumbar, sacral and coccygeal nerves emerge from the spinal cord. Sense organs (eyes, ears, skin, mouth, and nose) have receptors that detect sensations, and the information is then transmitted to the brain. The sciatic nerve is often considered the body's largest nerve.

DISEASE AND DIAGNOSTIC TERMS:

Testing: Includes changes in level of consciousness, memory, balance, reflex, and coordinated movement, chemical and microscopic analysis of the CSF; electroencephalography, MRI, electromyography, myelography

Diseases/disorders: cerebrovascular accident, TIA, hydrocephalus, cerebral aneurysm, spinal fractures as well as excessive hyperflexion, hyperextension, and vertical compression. Know the meaning of other terms related to disorders or diagnostic terms: akinesia, anesthesia, aphagia vs. aphasia, bradykinesia, cephalgia, cerebral concussion vs. cerebral contusion vs. cerebral hemorrhage, cerebral palsy, coma, diplegia, dyslexia vs. dysphagia vs. dysphasia, encephalitis vs. encephalocele vs. encephalomalacia vs. encephalomeningitis vs. encephalopathy, epilepsy, four types of paralysis (hemiplegia, paraplegia, quadriplegia [tetraplegia]), hyperkinesia, meningitis, meningocele, multiple sclerosis, myasthenia gravis, myelitis, narcolepsy, neuralgia vs. neuralgia vs. neuropathy, Parkinson disease, peripheral neuropathy, shingles.

Differentiate three types of hematomas associated with head injuries: hematomas (epidural, subdural, and intracerebral); cerebrovascular

Psychologic disorders: Know the meaning of these terms: psychosomatic, neurodevelopmental disorders, dementia, Alzheimer disease, autism, ADD vs. ADHD, hyperkinesia (hyperkinesis), anxiety disorders, posttraumatic stress disorder, panic disorder/attack; dissociative disorder, obsessive-compulsive disorder, phobias (including agoraphobia, zoophobia, phobophobia, arachnophobia, claustrophobia, pyrophobia), eating disorders include anorexia nervosa and bulimia, mood disorder, clinical depression, mania (includes megalomania, pyromania), kleptomania, bipolar disorder, pyromania, hypochondriasis, sexual and somatoform disorders, neurasthenia, psychosomatic disorders, pseudoplegia, pseudomania, psychosis, schizophrenia, paranoia, and antisocial behavior

Surgical interventions: neuroplasty, craniectomy, shunts, stereotactic radiosurgery

Therapeutic interventions: analgesics, hypnotics, antidepressants, antiparkinsonian agents, anticonvulsants, and antianxiety drugs

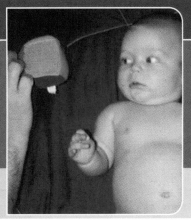

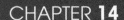

CHAPTER 14

Special Sense Organs of the Peripheral Nervous System

Pregnant females report that fetuses kick after sudden loud noises. At birth, an infant may turn toward a parent who is whispering. Here an audiologist demonstrates how a 3-month-old infant responds to interesting sounds by looking in the direction of the sound.

OBJECTIVES

After completing Chapter 14, you will be able to:

1. Recognize or write the function of the peripheral nervous system.
2. Recognize or write the meaning of receptors in the peripheral nervous system.
3. List or recognize the names of the special sense organs.
4. Write or recognize the brain's interpretation(s) of the special sense organs.
5. Recognize or write the meanings of Chapter 14 word parts and use them to build or analyze terms.

6. Write terms for selected structures of the sense organs or match terms with their descriptions.
7. Write the names of the diagnostic terms and pathologies related to the special sense organs.
8. Match surgical and therapeutic interventions in Chapter 14 or write the names of the interventions when given their descriptions.
9. Correctly spell terms pertaining to the special senses.

 Function First

The peripheral nervous system (PNS) forms the communication network between the central nervous system and the rest of the body. The PNS consists of the nerves that branch out from the brain and spinal cord, which communicate with the rest of the receptors, muscles, and glands (see Chapter 13).

    Receptors are sensory nerve endings that respond to various kinds of stimulation. The awareness that results is what we know as sensation. Special **sense organs**—the eyes, ears, skin, mouth, and nose—have receptors that detect sensations, and then sensory neurons transmit the information to the central nervous system, where it is interpreted as sight, hearing, touch, taste, or smell, for example.

QUICK TIP

Sensory nerve endings are also called sensory receptors.

THERE ARE OTHER TYPES OF RECEPTORS

This chapter concentrates on five sense organs; however, remember that there are other types of receptors, such as those that tell us when we're full and those found in muscles.

Write a word in each blank to complete these sentences.

1. Communication between the central nervous system and the rest of the body is accomplished by the _____ nervous system.
2. Sensory nerve endings that respond to various stimuli are called _____.
3. List the names of the five special sense organs: _____.

*Use Appendix III, Answers, to check your answers to all the exercises in Chapter 14.

Eyes

The eyes are paired organs of sight. Eyelids open and close the eye and keep foreign objects from entering most of the time. Each of our eyes is encased in a protective, bony socket. Our binocular vision sends two slightly different images to the brain, which the brain uses to determine depth of vision. Eye dominance is an unconscious preference to use one eye rather than the other for certain purposes, such as looking through a telescope or a mononuclear microscope.

Label the structures in Fig. 14.1 as you read the next paragraphs.

Light rays enter the **pupil** *(1)*, the small, dark, circular structure in the center of the eye, which is surrounded by the colored portion of the eye that we regularly see, the **iris** *(2)*. Muscles of the iris constrict the pupil in bright light and dilate the pupil in dim light, thereby regulating the amount of light entering the eye. The tough outer layer of the eye is the **sclera** *(3)*, the white opaque membrane covering most of the eyeball.

Associated with the eye are certain accessory organs: muscle, fascia, eyebrow, eyelid, conjunctiva, and the lacrimal glands. The **conjunctiva** is the mucous membrane lining the inner surface of the eyelid that acts as a protective covering for the exposed surface of the eye. You learned in Chapter 5 that dacry/o and lacrim/o mean tear, tearing, or crying. The **lacrimal glands** *(4)* produce and store tears (**lacrimal fluid**) that keep the eyeballs moist. Tears produced by the lacrimal gland wash over the eyeball and are drained through small openings in the inner corner of the eye. Tears pass through these openings into small **lacrimal ducts** *(5)* that drain into the large **nasolacrimal sac** *(6)*. From here the tears pass into the large **nasolacrimal duct** *(7)* that ends in the nasal cavity. If more lacrimal fluid is produced than can be removed, we say the person is crying. This is also called **tearing**.

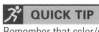

QUICK TIP

Remember that scler/o means hard.

WORD ORIGIN

conjunctivus (L.), connecting
iris (G.), rainbow, halo

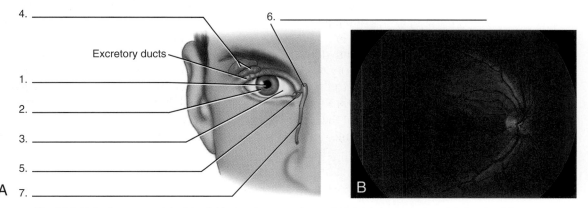

4. _____   6. _____

Excretory ducts

1. _____
2. _____
3. _____
5. _____
A 7. _____

B

Fig. 14.1 Major Structures of the Eye. A, Numbered structures (see text). **B,** Ophthalmoscopic view of the interior of the eye.

Observe and label Fig. 14.2 as indicated in the following discussion. The eyeball is composed of three layers:

- **sclera,** the tough outer layer that covers most of the eye and that you labeled in Fig. 14.1; locate it in Fig. 14.2.
- **cornea** (8), the transparent structure at the front of the eyeball that bends or refracts light rays so they are focused properly on the sensitive receptor cells in the posterior region of the eye.
- **choroid** (9) a dark brown membrane inside the sclera that is continuous with the iris and the **ciliary body** (10) on the anterior surface of the eye.

> ### HEALTH CARE CONNECTION
>
> Corneas are easily transplanted for people with scarred or opaque corneas. Transplants are generally successful because antibodies responsible for rejection of foreign tissue usually do not reach the avascular, transplanted cornea.

The ciliary body surrounds the outside of the **lens** (11) in a circular fashion, allowing change in the shape and thickness of the lens. These changes cause **refraction** of light rays in the posterior region of the eye, causing flattening of the lens (for distant vision) or thickening and rounding of the lens (for close vision). This refractory adjustment for close vision is called **accommodation**.

The ciliary body also secretes a fluid called aqueous humor, which is found in the **anterior chamber** (12). Another cavity of the eye is the **vitreous chamber** (13), which is filled with a soft, jellylike material, the **vitreous humor**. Escape of this fluid due to trauma may result in significant damage to the eye.

The **retina** (14) is the delicate nervous tissue membrane of the eye, which is continuous with the **optic nerve** (15) and enables vision. The **optic disc** (16) is the region of the eye where the optic nerve meets the retina. There are no light receptors in the optic disc; therefore, it is known as the blind spot of the eye.

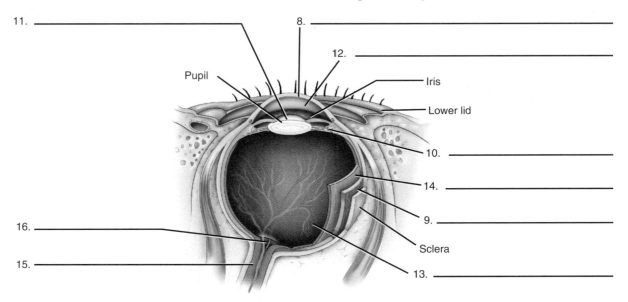

Fig. 14.2 Structures of the Eyeball, Transverse Section.

TABLE 14.1   FUNCTIONS OF THE MAJOR COMPONENTS OF THE EYE

Structure	Function
cornea	refraction of light
choroid	blood supply
ciliary body	secretion of vitreous fluid, helps change the shape of lens
external ocular muscles	movement of the eyeball
eyelid	protection for the eye
iris	contracts or relaxes to control the amount of light entering the eye through the pupil
lacrimal glands	secretion of tears
lens	light refraction
optic nerve	transmission of visual information to the brain
retina	transforms optic signals into nerve impulses
rods	distinguish light from dark, perceive shape and movement
cones	color vision
sclera	external protection

Light waves travel through the eye so they are focused on sensitive receptor cells of the retina called the **rods and cones** (Fig. 14.3). Rods are responsible for peripheral vision, night vision, and detection of motion. Three types of cones function in bright light and are responsible for color and central vision. Read about the two forms of color blindness, **daltonism** and **achromatic vision** in Health Care Connection below. Table 14.1 presents a summary of the eye structures and their functions.

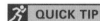

> ### QUICK TIP
> There are about 3 million cones and 100 million rods in the retina. Rods are also called retinal rods.

HEALTH CARE CONNECTION

Most cases of color blindness affect either the green or red receptor cones, so that the two colors cannot be distinguished from each other. This is called *daltonism*, and in most cases it is not a blindness but a weakness in perceiving colors distinctly. It is an inherited, sex-linked disorder. Normal color vision sees various shades of color in a color blindness chart (Fig. 14.4). Total color blindness, or achromatic vision, is characterized by an inability to see any color at all. It may be the result of a defect or absence of the cones.

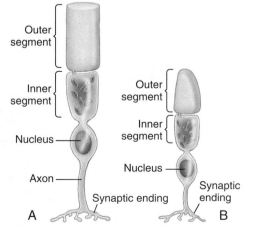

Fig. 14.3 Drawings of Rod and Cone Photoreceptor Cells of the Eye. **A,** Retinal rod. **B,** Retinal cone.

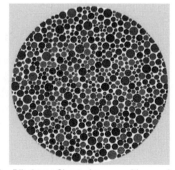

Fig. 14.4 Color Blindness Chart. A person with normal color vision sees different shades of green (representing the number 74), red, and orange. A person with daltonism sees different shades but does not see different colors distinctly.

MATCH IT!

EXERCISE 2

Match the anatomical terms in the left column with correct responses in the right column.

_____ 1. ciliary body
_____ 2. conjunctiva
_____ 3. cornea
_____ 4. iris
_____ 5. lacrimal gland
_____ 6. nasolacrimal duct
_____ 7. optic disc
_____ 8. pupil
_____ 9. retina
_____ 10. sclera

A. also known as the blind spot
B. channel that carries tears from the nasolacrimal sac to the nose
C. colored portion of the eye
D. delicate, nervous tissue of the eye
E. lines the inner surface of the eyelid
F. produces and stores tears
G. small, dark, circular structure located in the center of the eye
H. surrounds the outside of the lens and causes flattening or thickening of it
I. transparent structure at the front of the eye that refracts light rays
J. white, opaque membrane covering most of the eyeball

Learn the following word parts.

WORD PARTS: EYE

Combining Form	Meaning	Combining Form	Meaning
choroid/o	choroid	ocul/o, ophthalm/o	eye
chrom/o	color	opt/o, optic/o	vision
conjunctiv/o	conjunctiva	presby/o	old or old age
corne/o, kerat/o*	cornea	pupill/o	pupil
dacry/o, lacrim/o	tear	retin/o	retina
ir/o, irid/o	iris	ton/o	tone or tension

*kerat/o sometimes means hard or horny.

WRITE IT!

EXERCISE 3

Write the meanings of these combining forms.

1. conjunctiv/o _____
2. dacry/o _____
3. corne/o _____
4. irid/o _____
5. kerat/o _____
6. lacrim/o _____
7. ocul/o _____
8. retin/o _____

Diseases, Disorders, and Diagnostic Terms

Diseases of the eye are common, and minor visual problems are not even considered to be true diseases. For example, eyeglasses and eye drops can be bought without a prescription. Optometrists treat eye problems such as nearsightedness or farsightedness; ophthalmologists are medical doctors who treat other pathologies of the eye. Clearness or sharpness of vision is tested with a common **Snellen chart**; normal vision is described as 20/20; the top number is the number of feet the patient is standing from the chart, and the bottom number is the number of feet a person with normal vision would be from the chart and still be able to read the smallest number.

You learned in an earlier chapter that ophthalmoscopy is visual examination of the eyes using an ophthalmoscope. An **ophthalmometer** is an instrument used to measure the eye, specifically the cornea.

FIND IT!

EXERCISE 4

Write the combining forms and their meanings for these new terms.

1. **conjunctival**
   pertaining to the conjunctiva
   conjunctiv/o, conjunctiva

2. **choroidal**
   pertaining to the choroid
   _____

3. **corneal**
   pertaining to the cornea
   _____

4. **iridic**
   pertaining to the iris
   _____

5. **lacrimal**
   pertaining to the tears
   _____

6. **ocular, optic** (also **ophthalmic**)
   of, pertaining to, or affecting the eye
   _____

7. **pupillary**
   pertaining to the pupil
   _____

8. **retinal**
   pertaining to the retina
   _____

Three common irregularities in vision are refractive disorders (the lens is unable to focus an image accurately on the retina).

- **Myopia** is nearsightedness; parallel rays entering the eye are focused in front of the retina.
- **Hyperopia** is farsightedness, or inability of the eyes to focus on nearby objects; rays of light entering the eye are brought to focus behind the retina.
- **Astigmatism** is uneven focusing of the image, resulting from distortion of the curvature of the lens or cornea.

Compare these three irregularities, which are illustrated in Fig. 14.5.

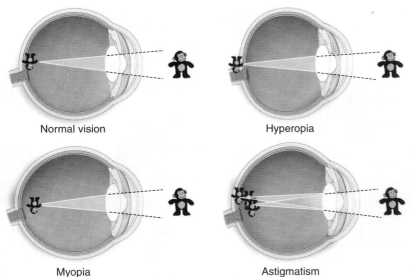

Normal vision

Hyperopia

Myopia

Astigmatism

Fig. 14.5 Refraction of the Eye. Normal versus three common irregularities.

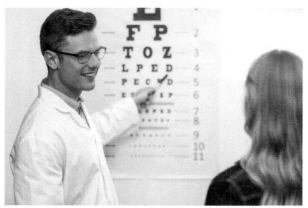

Fig. 14.6 Snellen Chart. Charts are used to test visual acuity as patients distinguish letters and numbers ordinarily seen at different distances.

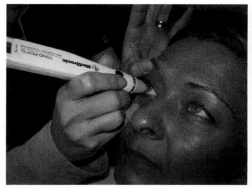

Fig. 14.7 Tono-Pen Tonometry. Several types of tonometers are used. The Tono-Pen method measures and records the resistance of the eyeball to indentation after exerting a tiny pressure.

Visual acuity is a measure of the ability to distinguish letters and numbers at a given distance. A **Snellen chart** (Fig. 14.6) is one of several charts that test visual acuity. An individual who can read at 20 feet what the average person can read at this distance has 20/20 vision, whereas an individual who can read at 20 feet what the average person can read at 30 feet has 20/30 vision.

Tonometry is measurement of the intraocular pressure using a tonometer (Fig. 14.7), usually after numbing the eye with an anesthetic. Everyone who has had an eye exam has probably experienced tonometry, in addition to **assessment of visual fields** (determines the physical space visible to an individual in a fixed position) (Fig. 14.8). Ophthalmologists also commonly perform a slit-lamp examination (Fig. 14.9), which examines the various layers of the eye with a bright light, usually after the pupils have been dilated using a **mydriatic** (agent that dilates the pupil), often an anesthetic, and sometimes a dye.

Presbyopia is hyperopia and impairment of vision caused by advancing years or old age.

Accommodation reflex is the ability of the eye to adjust to variations in distance. The **fluorescein angiography** procedure uses fluorescein (a bright green fluorescent dye) to examine movement of blood through blood vessels in the eye.

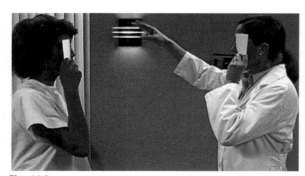

Fig. 14.8 Assessment of Visual Fields. A normal test is 65 degrees upward, 75 degrees downward, 60 degrees inward, and 90 degrees outward. Defects in the vision that remain constant are usually caused by damage to the retina or visual pathways.

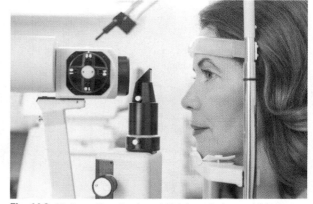

Fig. 14.9 Slit-Lamp Examination. A high-intensity beam of light is projected through a narrow slit, and a cross section of the illuminated part of the eye is examined through a magnifying lens.

Match the terms on the left with their meanings in the right column.

_____ 1. hyperopia
_____ 2. myopia
_____ 3. mydriatic
_____ 4. presbyopia
_____ 5. tonometry
_____ 6. visual fields

A. agent that dilates the eye
B. farsightedness
C. impairment of vision caused by advancing age
D. measurement of intraocular pressure
E. nearsightedness
F. physical space visible when head is held still

Additional irregularities or abnormal conditions of the eye are included in the following list.

amblyopia, strabismus (Fig. 14.10) Reduced vision in one eye, not correctable by glasses but by wearing eye patch.

blepharitis Inflammation of the eyelid (Fig. 14.11).

cataract An abnormal progressive condition of the lens, characterized by loss of transparency (Fig. 14.12). Cataract comes from the Latin word *cataracta*, meaning waterfall.

color vision deficiencies
  achromatic vision (see p. 391).
  achromatopsia Profound inability to see color
  daltonism (see p. 391).

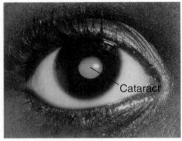

Fig. 14.12 Cataract. The lens appears cloudy due to the cataract.

conjunctivitis Inflammation of the conjunctiva; also called red eyes or pink eye.

glaucoma An abnormal condition of increased pressure within the eye. Prolonged pressure can damage the retina and optic nerve.

hordeolum Sty, or stye, resulting from an infected sebaceous gland of an eyelash (see Fig. 14.11).

macular degeneration A progressive deterioration of the retina associated with new vessel formation that can progress to blindness (Fig. 14.13).

nyctalopia Poor vision at night or in dim light.

photophobia Excessive sensitivity of the eyes to light.

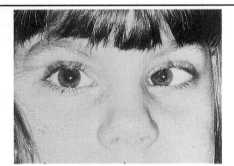

Fig. 14.10 Amblyopia. Lazy eye.

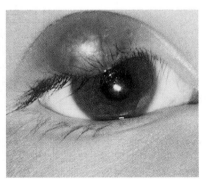

Fig. 14.11 Blepharitis Caused by a Sty. This infection of a gland of the eye shows a great deal of redness and swelling.

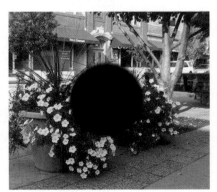

Fig. 14.13 Macular Degeneration. The blind spot in the center shows the loss of central vision.

ptosis Drooping of the upper eyelids; blepharoptosis.

retinal detachment Separation of the retina from the choroid, usually resulting from a hole or tear in the retina (Fig. 14.14). If detachment is not halted, total blindness of the eye results.

retinopathy Any disease of the retina. Diabetic retinopathy is an abnormality of the retina caused by diabetes mellitus (Fig. 14.15).

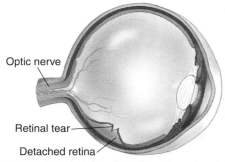

Optic nerve

Retinal tear

Detached retina

Fig. 14.14 Retinal Detachment. The onset of separation of the retina from the back of the eye is usually sudden and painless. The person may experience bright flashes of light or floating dark spots in the affected eye. Sometimes there is loss of visual field, as though a curtain is being pulled over part of the visual field.

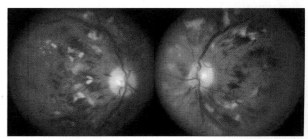

Fig. 14.15 Ophthalmoscopic View in Diabetic Retinopathy. Note retinal hemorrhages and abnormal pigmentation in both eyes.

HEALTH CARE CONNECTION

Legal blindness is defined in most states as best corrected visual acuity less than 20/200 in the better eye or marked constriction of the visual fields.

WRITE IT! EXERCISE 6

Write terms in the blanks to complete these sentences.

1. any disease of the retina _____
2. drooping of the upper eyelids _____
3. poor vision at night or in dim light _____
4. red eyes or pink eye _____
5. condition of increased pressure within the eye _____
6. inflammation of the eyelid _____
7. also called strabismus _____
8. excessive sensitivity of the eyes _____
9. sty _____
10. profound inability to see color _____

 Surgical and Therapeutic Interventions

Covering an eye in childhood is one example of a therapeutic intervention for amblyopia. Glaucoma is often treated with eye drops and laser; in extreme cases, **iridectomy** (surgical removal of part of the iris) is performed to restore proper drainage. Ophthalmic creams, ointments, or liquid drops are prescribed to relieve pressure within the eye, to provide moisture, or as anesthetic or antibiotic preparations for the eye.

PROGRAMMED LEARNING

Remember to cover the answers (left column) with folded paper or the bookmark. Write an answer in each blank, and then check your answer before proceeding to the next frame.

eyelid	1. **Blepharoplasty** is surgical repair of the _____ to repair ptosis.
corneal	2. A **corneal transplant** is transplantation of _____ tissue from a donor or the patient's own cornea.
cold	3. **Ophthalmic cryosurgery** is a general term for the use of extreme _____ to remove a cataract or to cause the edges of a detached retina to heal. **Cryo+extraction** is removal of a cataract using an extremely cold probe.
cornea	4. As a therapeutic measure, **corneal abrasion** means scraping away of the outer layers of the _____, perhaps to smooth one that is abnormally buckled.
lens	5. **Extraction of the lens** means removal of the lens to treat a cataract. **Intraocular lens transplant** is replacing the _____ with an artificial lens. This surgery may also be used for patients with extreme myopia, diplopia, and certain other abnormalities.
retina	6. **Laser retinal photocoagulation** uses laser to make pinpoint scars to stabilize a detached _____.
myopia	7. **LASIK** (laser-assisted in situ keratomileusis) is corneal surgery in which the excimer laser and a microkeratome (instrument used to create a thin hinged flap on the surface of the cornea) are combined to correct nearsightedness, also called _____.

MATCH IT! EXERCISE 7

Match the word parts in the left column with their meanings (a choice may be used more than once).

_____ 1. blepharoplasty
_____ 2. cryoextraction
_____ 3. intraocular lens transplant
_____ 4. laser retinal photocoagulation
_____ 5. LASIK

A. corneal surgery using laser and a microkeratome
B. removal of a cataract
C. replacing the lens with an artificial lens
D. stabilizing a detached retina with the use of laser
E. surgical repair of the eyelids
F. use of extreme cold for cataract removal or retinal reattachment

QUICK CASE STUDY | EXERCISE 8

Select terms from the report to match the descriptions.

Rachel Harlow, 80 years of age, was examined by Dr. Chein in the Ophthalmology Clinic for blurry vision and nyctalopia. Accommodation reflex and visual field are normal. Tono-Pen tonometry shows increased pressure in the right eye, likely glaucoma.

1. ability of the eye to adjust to variations in distance _____
2. increased pressure within the eye _____
3. measuring of intraocular pressure _____
4. physical space visible to an individual in a fixed position _____
5. poor vision at night or in dim light _____

Ears

WORD ORIGIN

cera (L.), wax

The ears have receptors that detect touch, pain, heat and cold, but we usually think of the ears as enabling us to hear. We depend on our ears not only for hearing but also for the sense of equilibrium (commonly called balance). Several glands secrete a yellowish brown, waxy substance called **cerumen**, which lubricates and protects the ear.

Refer to Fig. 14.16. Anatomically, the ear is divided into the external ear, middle ear, and inner ear:

- external ear: the visible part of the ear; ends at the **tympanic membrane** (eardrum)
- middle ear: air-filled cavity containing three tiny bones
- inner ear: contains the cochlea and semicircular canals

The external ear functions in collecting sound waves and directing them into the ear canal, where they strike the tympanic membrane. As the eardrum vibrates, it moves three small bones (ossicles) in the middle ear (the **malleus, incus,** and **stapes**) that conduct the sound waves through the middle ear. Locate these bones in Fig. 14.16. As the stapes moves, it touches a membrane called the **oval window**, which separates the middle ear from the inner ear. The inner ear is a complex inner structure that contains receptors for the sense of balance (semicircular canals) and hearing (cochlea). The **cochlea** is a spiral tunnel resembling a snail shell. The **semicircular canals** are fluid-filled canals that open into the cochlea. A simplified version of the pathway of sound is:

Sound →	Auditory canal →	Eardrum →	Ossicles →	Cochlea →	Auditory nerve fibers →	Auditory region of the brain

The **auditory tube** or **eustachian tube** leads from the middle ear to the pharynx (throat). This tube can prevent damage to the eardrum by equalizing pressure in the middle ear with the atmospheric pressure.

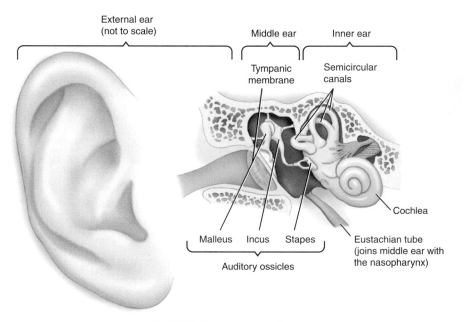

Fig. 14.16 Structures of the Ear.

HEALTH CARE CONNECTION

Normally the pressure of air in the middle ear is equal to that of the environment; however, if you ascend to high altitudes (flying or climbing a high mountain), the atmospheric pressure in the middle ear is greater than that in the outer ear, causing the eardrum to bulge outward. Swallowing opens the eustachian tube so that air can leave the middle ear until the pressures are balanced. The eardrum relaxes and avoids the danger of bursting by equalizing the pressure in the middle ear to atmospheric pressure.

QUICK REVIEW: EAR STRUCTURES

Outer ear ends at the tympanic membrane.
Middle ear has three auditory ossicles (malleus, incus, and stapes).
Inner ear contains the cochlea and semicircular canals.
Eustachian (auditory) tube leads from the middle ear to the pharynx.

Learn the following word parts.

WORD PARTS

Combining Form	Meaning	Suffix	Meaning
acoust/o, audi/o	hearing	-ory	pertaining to
adenoid/o	adenoids		
aur/o, auricul/o, ot/o	ear		
cerumin/o	ear wax		
cochle/o	cochlea		
myring/o, tympan/o	eardrum*		
salping/o	eustachian tube		

*The eardrum is also called the tympanic membrane.

FIND IT!
EXERCISE 9

Find the combining form in these new terms and write its meaning. A short definition is provided for each term.

Term	Combining Form	Meaning of Combining Form
1. **acoustic** pertaining to sound or hearing	_____	_____
2. **audible** capable of being heard	_____	_____
3. **auditory** pertaining to the sense of hearing and the organs involved	_____	_____
4. **aural, auricular, otic** pertaining to the external ear	_____	_____
5. **cochlear** pertaining to the cochlea	_____	_____

Diseases, Disorders, and Diagnostic Terms

Ear trauma can occur from a blow by a blunt object. The eardrum can be damaged by extended exposure to loud noises, penetrating injury, rupture, or perforation by shock-waves from an explosion, deep sea diving, trauma, or acute middle ear infections. A perforated eardrum can be seen during an otoscopic examination (Fig. 14.17). An **otoscopic examination**, also called **otoscopy**, is examination of the ear using an **otoscope**.

Various **tuning fork tests** screen for both function of the auditory nerve and ability of ear structures to conduct sound waves to the inner ear. **Audiometry** is the measurement of hearing (Fig. 11.18)

An **audiologist** detects and evaluates hearing loss and determines how a patient can best make use of remaining hearing. An **audiometer** is an electronic device for measuring hearing. The record produced is an **audiogram**. Hearing is tested by using tones from very low to very high frequencies at various decibels (dB) of intensity. The lowest intensity at which a young, normal ear can detect sound (about 51% of the time) is 0 dB. Conversational speech is around 60 dB, and sounds at that decibel intensity are not harmful. Exposure to loud noises, even for a short time, can damage the cochlear hair cells and result in hearing loss. Looking at Table 14.2, note that only 3 minutes is considered a safe exposure time if you are sitting in the front row at a rock concert. **Deafness** is inability to hear. Having some degree of hearing impairment is termed "hearing impaired."

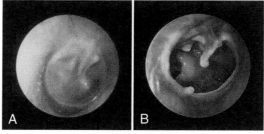

Fig. 14.17 Comparison of the Appearance of a Normal Eardrum and a Perforated Eardrum. **A,** Otoscopic view of a normal, intact eardrum. **B,** Otoscopic view of a perforated eardrum.

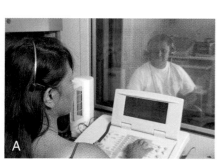
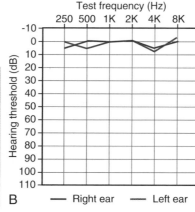
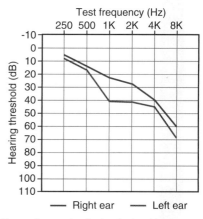

Fig. 14.18 Audiometry. **A,** Audiologist is shown using an audiometer. **B,** Normal audiogram pattern (left) vs audiogram showing hearing loss (right).

TABLE 14.2   DECIBEL INTENSITY AND SAFE EXPOSURE TIME FOR COMMON SOUNDS

Sound	Decibel Intensity (dB)	Safe Exposure Time*	Sound	Decibel Intensity (dB)	Safe Exposure Time*
Threshold of hearing	0		Motorcycle	90	8 hr
Whispering	20		Chain saw	100	2 hr
Average residence or office	40		Rock concert, front row	120	3 min
Conversational speech	60		Jet engine	140	Immediate danger
Car traffic	70	>8 hr	Rocket launching pad	180	Immediate danger

*For every 5-dB increase in intensity, the safe exposure time is cut in half.
From Ignatavicius DD, Workman ML: *Medical-surgical nursing: critical thinking for collaborative care,* ed 5, St Louis, 2006, Saunders.

Otitis means inflammation of the ear. A discharge from the ear, **otorrhea**, may accompany otitis. Otorrhea may contain blood, pus, or even spinal fluid. Ear infections are just one cause of otorrhea. Otitis may produce **otalgia**, pain in the ear, which is also called an earache.

Otitis media is inflammation of the middle ear. The middle ear is separated from the external ear by the eardrum. **Myringitis** is inflammation of the tympanic membrane. **Mastoiditis** is an infection of one of the mastoid bones of the skull, usually an extension of a middle ear infection. It is difficult to treat and can result in hearing loss. Antibiotic therapy is aimed at treating middle ear infections before they progress to mastoiditis.

Otitis externa means an external ear infection, often caused by fungus, also called **otomycosis** (commonly called swimmer's ear). **Otitis interna** is inner ear infection, inflammation of the inner ear, and can affect both hearing and equilibrium.

Otosclerosis is hardening of the ear. This condition is caused by formation of spongy bone around structures of the middle and inner ear. It is hereditary and leads to hearing impairment that is usually first noticed in young or middle-aged persons.

Tinnitus, noise in the ears, is one of the most common complaints of persons with ear or hearing disorders. The noise includes ringing, buzzing, roaring, or clicking. It may be a sign of something as simple as accumulation of earwax or cerumen or as serious as **Meniere disease**. The latter is a chronic disease of the inner ear with recurring episodes of hearing loss, tinnitus, and vertigo. **Vertigo** is also called dizziness.

WORD ORIGIN
medius (L.), middle

WORD ORIGIN
tinnire (L.), to tinkle

MATCH IT!   EXERCISE 10

Match the terms in the left column with their descriptions in the right column.

_____ 1. cerumen
_____ 2. otalgia
_____ 3. otorrhea
_____ 4. otosclerosis
_____ 5. tinnitus
_____ 6. vertigo

A. abnormal hardening of the bones in the middle ear
B. earwax
C. discharge or draining from the ear
D. dizziness
E. earache
F. ringing or other noise in one or both ears

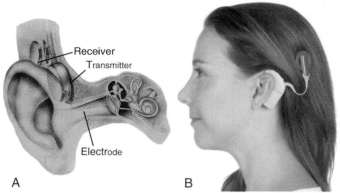

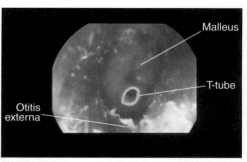

Fig. 14.20 Pressure-Equalizing Tube in Place in the Eardrum. An incision is made in the eardrum, and a tube is positioned to relieve pressure and release pus or fluid from the middle ear. The tube is left in place for a time to allow the ear to drain.

Fig. 14.19 Cochlear Implant. **A,** Drawing of an electronic device that is surgically implanted into the cochlea of a deaf person. **B,** Young girl with a cochlear implant.

 ## Surgical and Therapeutic Interventions

A hearing aid is an electronic device that amplifies sound. In complete hearing loss, a **cochlear implant** is an implanted device that assists hearing by electrically stimulating the cochlea (Fig. 14.19). A hearing aid consists of a microphone, a battery power supply, an amplifier, and a receiver. Since the microphone receives sound waves directed *toward* the person, wearers hear best when you are in front of them. Programmable hearing aids are customized on the basis of the individual's hearing loss.

Otoplasty is surgical repair or reconstruction of the external ear.

Tympanostomy is surgical creation of an opening through the eardrum to promote drainage and/or allow the introduction of artificial tubes (pressure-equalizing tubes) to maintain the opening (Fig. 14.20).

Antibiotics are used to treat bacterial ear infections. **Ceruminolytics** are medications that are used to soften and break down earwax.

WRITE IT! **EXERCISE 11**

Complete the following by writing a word in each sentence.

1. A term for surgical creation of an opening through the eardrum is _____.
2. Surgical repair or reconstruction of the ear is _____.
3. Ceruminolytics are medications that soften and break down _____.
4. A _____ implant assists hearing by electrically stimulating the _____.

 ## The Skin

The skin is equipped with sensory nerve endings that respond to various kinds of stimulation. In addition, modified skin structures continue into various body parts, such as the mucous membrane in the lining of the nose, the mouth, and the eyes.

Learn the following word parts.

WORD PARTS: TYPES OF RECEPTORS			
Combining Form	**Meaning**	**Combining Form**	**Meaning**
chem/o	chemical	phot/o	light
mechan/o	mechanical	therm/o	heat
noc/i	cause harm, injury, or pain		

Mechano+receptors that are sensitive to mechanical changes in touch or pressure are widely distributed in the skin. Mechanoreceptors for hearing are located within the ear.

The eyes contain **photoreceptors** that detect light.

Thermoreceptors are located immediately under the skin and are widely distributed throughout the body. Thermo+receptors detect changes in temperature, sensing both cool and heat, as the name implies.

The sense of pain is initiated by special receptors, **nociceptors**, that are widely distributed throughout the skin and internal organs.

WRITE IT!
EXERCISE 12

Complete the following by writing a word in each sentence.

1. Nerve endings that detect light are called _____.
2. Nerve endings that detect changes in temperature are called _____.
3. Nerve endings that detect pain are called _____.
4. Receptors that are sensitive to mechanical changes in touch or pressure are called _____.

Mouth and Nose

Chemoreceptors are nerve endings in the nose and tongue that are adapted for excitation by chemicals that enable taste. With openings on the surface of the nose and mouth, **taste buds** are taste organs which have chemoreceptors for sweet, sour, bitter, and salty tastes (Fig. 14.21).

WORD ORIGIN
chemeia (G.), chemical

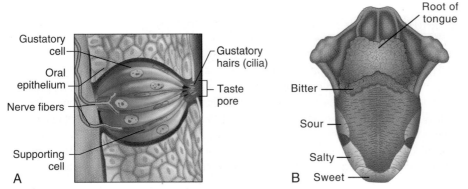

Fig. 14.21 Taste Buds and Taste Regions of the Tongue. A, Drawing of an individual taste bud. Each taste bud rests in a pocket. Many taste buds containing gustatory (L. *gustare*, to taste) cells are distributed over the tongue and the roof of the mouth. **B,** Taste regions of the tongue. In addition to the four basic taste sensations (sweet, sour, bitter, and salty), there are combined perceptions plus the input from olfactory receptors.

Learn the following word part.

Suffix	Meaning
-osmia	sense of smell

WORD ORIGIN

olfacere (L.), to smell

The nose is also responsible for the sense of smell, and this sense is intricately linked with chemoreceptors that enable us to experience different tastes of food and other substances. The term **olfaction** means the sense of smell, and **olfactory** means pertaining to the sense of smell. **Anosmia** is loss or impairment of the sense of smell, which can occur as a temporary condition when one has a respiratory infection or a permanent anosmia when the olfactory nerve is destroyed. **Hyperosmia** is an abnormally increased sensitivity to odors.

MATCH IT!
EXERCISE 13

Match the terms in the left column with their descriptions in the right column.

_____ 1. anosmia
_____ 2. chemoreceptors
_____ 3. hyperosmia
_____ 4. olfactory

A. increased sensitivity to odors
B. loss or impairment of the sense of smell
C. nerve endings that are adapted for detecting chemicals
D. pertaining to the sense of smell

 Be Careful With These!

accommodation vs. refraction   daltonism vs. achromatic vision
anosmia vs. hyperosmia   myopia vs. hyperopia
cornea vs. choroid   retinal rods vs. cones

A Career as an Ophthalmic Assistant

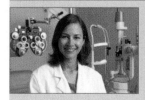

Danielle is a certified ophthalmic assistant (COA). She completed an independent study course and passed the COA exam. Danielle enjoys the patient contact in her career and knowing that she is helping patients maintain the amazing sense of sight. She is considering getting additional training to become a certified ophthalmic technician (COT), as that would allow her to perform additional duties and be more valuable as an employee. Visit the Joint Commission on Allied Health Personnel in Ophthalmology website (www.jcahpo.org) for information on becoming a certified ophthalmic assistant, and the American Speech-Language-Hearing Association (www.asha.org) for information on becoming an audiologist's assistant.

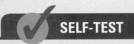

SELF-TEST

Work the following exercises to test your understanding of the material in Chapter 14. It is best to do all the exercises before checking your answers against the answers in Appendix III. Pay particular attention to spelling.

A. MATCHING!   *Match the terms on the left with the descriptions on the right.*

_____ 1. chemoreceptor	A. a vascular layer inside the sclera
_____ 2. cornea	B. filled with a soft, jelly-like material
_____ 3. choroid	C. produces and stores tears
_____ 4. lacrimal gland	D. sensory nerve ending that responds to various chemical stimuli
_____ 5. pupil	E. small, dark, circular structure located in the center of the eye
_____ 6. vitreous chamber	F. transparent structure that bends or refracts light rays

B. IDENTIFYING!   *Label these illustrations using one of the following: astigmatism, cochlear, hyperopia, malleus, myopia, stapes*

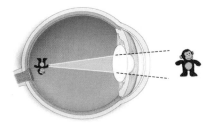

1. nearsightedness

    _____

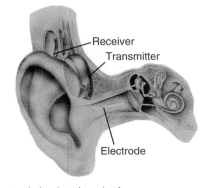

Receiver
Transmitter
Electrode

2. electronic implant in a deaf person

    _____ implant

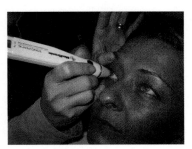

3. Measurement of the eye's intraocular pressure

    _____

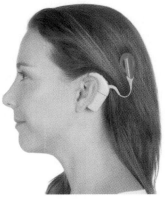

4. Implanted device to assist complete hearing loss

    _____

C. CHOOSING!   *Choose the one correct answer (A, B, C, or D) for each question.*

1. Kallie is a 72-year-old female who tells the optometrist that her eyes do not adjust as quickly when she goes into a dark theater as they used to. Muscles of which eye structure regulate the amount of light entering the eye?
   (A) conjunctiva   **(B)** choroid   **(C)** cornea   **(D)** iris

2. The ophthalmologist explains to Seth that he has total color blindness. Which of the following is Seth's condition?
   (A) achromatic vision   **(B)** day vision   **(C)** double vision   **(D)** night vision

3. What is tested when Dr. Johnson uses a Tono-Pen tonometer during an ophthalmic examination?
   (A) assessment of visual field   **(B)** intraocular pressure   **(C)** refractory adjustment   **(D)** sensory nerve response

4. Manuel is told he needs blepharoplasty to correct droopy eyelids. What problem does blepharoplasty correct?
   (A) amblyopia   **(B)** ptosis   **(C)** nyctalopia   **(D)** retinopathy

5. The flight attendant told Carrie to swallow when she experienced painful pressure in the middle ear while flying, and the pressure was relieved. How did swallowing help equalize the pressure in her ears?   **(A)** opening of the eustachian tube   **(B)** response of the oval window   **(C)** vibration of the bones in the middle ear   **(D)** vibration of the eardrum

6. Which part of the ear is responsible for the sense of balance?
   (A) cochlea   **(B)** semicircular canals   **(C)** stapes   **(D)** tympanic membrane

7. Tina is 65 years old and her vision is deteriorating. What is the name of the vision impairment caused by advancing years?
   (A) abrasion   **(B)** astigmatism   **(C)** photophobia   **(D)** presbyopia

8. What is the term for the agent that the optical assistant drops in Tina's eyes to dilate the pupils?
   (A) mydriatic   **(B)** nyctalopia   **(C)** photocoagulation   **(D)** tinnitus

D. WRITING!   *Write one word for the following.*

1. earwax   _____
2. farsightedness   _____
3. loss or impairment of the sense of smell   _____
4. pertaining to the sense of smell   _____
5. receptor that detects pain   _____
6. receptor that is sensitive to mechanical change   _____
7. removal of a cataract using an extremely cold probe   _____
8. surgical creation of an opening through the eardrum   _____
9. synonym for ptosis   _____
10. three bones in the middle ear: incus, stapes, and ?   _____

E. READING HEALTH REPORTS

Read the following emergency department report and find the correct terms to match the descriptions that follow the report.

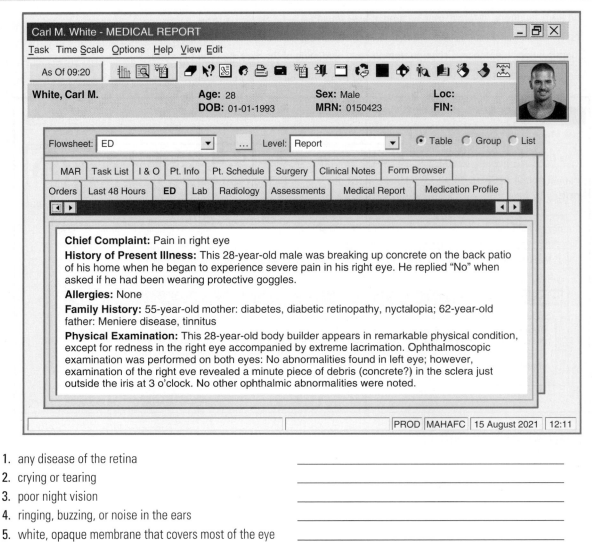

Carl M. White - MEDICAL REPORT	− 🗗 ✕

Task Time Scale Options Help View Edit

| As Of 09:20 | 📊 🔍 📑 | ✎ ⚲ ? 🖼 🔗 🖨 💾 📋 🔌 🖵 ♻ ■ ◆ 👥 📒 ✋ 👇 📊 | |

White, Carl M.   **Age:** 28   **Sex:** Male   **Loc:**
DOB: 01-01-1993   **MRN:** 0150423   **FIN:**

Flowsheet: ED   ▼   …   Level: Report   ▼   ⦿ Table ○ Group ○ List

| MAR | Task List | I & O | Pt. Info | Pt. Schedule | Surgery | Clinical Notes | Form Browser |

| Orders | Last 48 Hours | ED | Lab | Radiology | Assessments | Medical Report | Medication Profile |

Chief Complaint: Pain in right eye

History of Present Illness: This 28-year-old male was breaking up concrete on the back patio of his home when he began to experience severe pain in his right eye. He replied "No" when asked if he had been wearing protective goggles.

Allergies: None

Family History: 55-year-old mother: diabetes, diabetic retinopathy, nyctalopia; 62-year-old father: Meniere disease, tinnitus

Physical Examination: This 28-year-old body builder appears in remarkable physical condition, except for redness in the right eye accompanied by extreme lacrimation. Ophthalmoscopic examination was performed on both eyes: No abnormalities found in left eye; however, examination of the right eye revealed a minute piece of debris (concrete?) in the sclera just outside the iris at 3 o'clock. No other ophthalmic abnormalities were noted.

| | | PROD | MAHAFC | 15 August 2021 | 12:11 |

1. any disease of the retina   _____
2. crying or tearing   _____
3. poor night vision   _____
4. ringing, buzzing, or noise in the ears   _____
5. white, opaque membrane that covers most of the eye   _____

F. READING HEALTH REPORTS   *Read the health report and circle the correct answer in sentences 1 through 5.*

1. The term "otalgia" means (earwax, ear infection, ear pain, hearing loss).
2. The term "auditory" refers to (ear, hearing, noise, sound).
3. The tympanic membrane is also referred to as the (cochlea, eardrum, Eustachian tube, stapes).
4. Tinnitus means (deafness, discharge from the ear, hardening of the ears, noise in the ears).
5. Vertigo is characterized by (buzzing, clicking, dizziness, ringing).

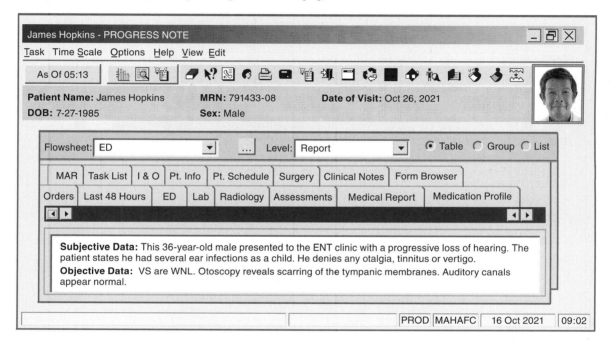

James Hopkins - PROGRESS NOTE

Task Time Scale Options Help View Edit

As Of 05:13

Patient Name: James Hopkins   **MRN:** 791433-08   **Date of Visit:** Oct 26, 2021
DOB: 7-27-1985   **Sex:** Male

Flowsheet: ED   ...   Level: Report   ⦿ Table ○ Group ○ List

| MAR | Task List | I & O | Pt. Info | Pt. Schedule | Surgery | Clinical Notes | Form Browser |

| Orders | Last 48 Hours | ED | Lab | Radiology | Assessments | Medical Report | Medication Profile |

Subjective Data: This 36-year-old male presented to the ENT clinic with a progressive loss of hearing. The patient states he had several ear infections as a child. He denies any otalgia, tinnitus or vertigo.
Objective Data: VS are WNL. Otoscopy reveals scarring of the tympanic membranes. Auditory canals appear normal.

PROD MAHAFC   16 Oct 2021   09:02

G. SPELLING AND PRONUNCIATION!   *Circle all incorrectly spelled terms, and write the correct spellings.*

catarack   eustakian   okular   olfactory   serumenolytics

H. WRITING!   *Write a word to complete each sentence.*

1. The sense organs that are continuous with the optic nerve and enable vision are the _____.
2. Total color blindness is the same as _____.
3. Use of a tonometer to measure intraocular pressure is called _____.
4. The ear structure that contains receptors for hearing is the _____.
5. The auditory or _____ tube leads from the middle ear to the pharynx.
6. An _____ is one who is trained to detect and evaluate hearing.
7. Otitis _____ means inflammation of the middle ear.
8. Surgical creation of an opening through the eardrum is called a _____.
9. The organ or modifications of it that is associated with mechanoreceptors, nociceptors, and thermoreceptors is the _____.
10. The nose and _____ have nerve endings that enable taste.

I. QUICK CHALLENGE!   *Find an incorrect term in each sentence and write the correct term.*

1. A chronic disease characterized by ringing, buzzing, or other noise in the ears is tinnitus disease. _____ _____
2. A term for pink eye is amblyopia. _____
3. Loss or impairment of the sense of smell is called olfaction. _____
4. Pertaining to sound or hearing is the adjective, aural. _____
5. Uneven focusing of light rays on the retina is called presbyopia. _____

*Use Appendix III to check your answers.

🔊 QUICK & EASY (Q&E) LIST

Use the Evolve website (http://evolve.elsevier.com/Leonard/quick) to review the terms presented in Chapter 14. Look closely at the spelling of each term as it is pronounced.

accommodation *(uh-kom-uh-**dā**-shun)*
accommodation reflex *(uh-kom-uh-**dā**-shun **rē**-fleks)*
achromatic vision *(ak-rō-**mat**-ik **vizh**-un)*
achromatopsia *(uh-krō-muh-**top**-sē-uh)*
acoustic *(uh-**kōōs**-tik)*
amblyopia *(am-blē-**ō**-pē-uh)*
anosmia *(an-**oz**-mē-uh)*
anterior chamber *(an-**tēr**-ē-ur **chām**-bur)*
assessment of visual fields *(uh-**ses**-munt uv **vizh**-o͞o-ul fēldz)*
astigmatism *(uh-**stig**-muh-tiz-um)*
audible *(**aw**-duh-bul)*
audiogram *(**aw**-dē-ō-gram)*
audiologist *(aw-dē-**ol**-uh-jist)*

audiometer *(aw-dē-**om**-uh-tur)*
auditory *(**aw**-di-tor-ē)*
auditory tube *(**aw**-di-tor-ē to͞ob)*
aural *(**aw**-rul)*
auricular *(aw-**rik**-ū-lur)*
blepharitis *(blef-uh-**rī**-tis)*
blepharoplasty *(**blef**-uh-rō-plas-tē)*
cataract *(**kat**-uh-rakt)*
cerumen *(suh-**ro͞o**-mun)*
ceruminolytics *(suh-ro͞o-mi-nō-**lit**-iks)*
chemoreceptors *(kē-mō-rē-**sep**-turz)*
choroid *(**kor**-oid)*
choroidal *(kor-**oid**-ul)*
ciliary body *(**sil**-ē-ar-ē **bod**-ē)*

QUICK & EASY (Q&E) LIST—cont'd

cochlea (*kok*-lē-uh)
cochlear (*kok*-lē-ur)
cochlear implant (*kok*-lē-ur *im*-plant)
color vision deficiencies (*kul*-ur *vizh*-un dē-*fish*-un-sēz)
conjunctiva (kun-*junk*-ti-vuh)
conjunctival (kun-*junk*-ti-vul)
conjunctivitis (kun-junk-ti-*vī*-tis)
cornea (*kor*-nē-uh)
corneal (*kor*-nē-ul)
corneal abrasion (*kor*-nē-ul uh-*brā*-zhun)
corneal transplant (*kor*-nē-ul *trans*-plant)
cryoextraction (krī-ō-ek-*strak*-shun)
daltonism (*dawl*-tun-iz-um)
deafness (*def*-nis)
eustachian tube (ū-*stā*-kē-un to͞ob)
extraction of the lens (ek-*strak*-shun uv thuh lenz)
fluorescein angiography (floo-*res*-ēn an-jē-*og*-ruh-fē)
glaucoma (glaw-*kō*-muh)
hordeolum (hor-*dē*-ō-lum)
hyperopia (hī-pur-*ō*-pē-uh)
hyperosmia (hī-pur-*oz*-mē-uh)
incus (*ing*-kus)
intraocular lens transplant (in-truh-*ok*-ū-lur lenz *trans*-plant)
iridectomy (ir-i-*dek*-tuh-mē)
iridic (ī-*rid*-ik)
iris (*ī*-ris)
lacrimal (*lak*-ri-mul)
lacrimal ducts (*lak*-ri-mul dukts)
lacrimal fluid (*lak*-ri-mul flo͞o-id)
lacrimal glands (*lak*-ri-mul glandz)
laser retinal photocoagulation (*lā*-zur *ret*-i-nul fō-tō-kō-ag-ū-*lā*-shun)
LASIK (*lā*-sik)
lens (lenz)
macular degeneration (*mak*-ū-lur dē-jen-ur-*ā*-shun)
malleus (*mal*-ē-us)
mastoiditis (mas-toid-*ī*-tis)
mechanoreceptors (mek-uh-nō-rē-*sep*-turz)
Meniere disease (me-*nyār* di-*zēz*)
mydriatic (mid-rē-*at*-ik)
myopia (mī-*ō*-pē-uh)
myringitis (mir-in-*jī*-tis)
nasolacrimal duct (na-zō-*lak*-ri-mul dukt)
nasolacrimal sac (na-zō-*lak*-ri-mul sak)
nociceptors (nō-si-*sep*-turz)
nyctalopia (nik-tuh-*lō*-pē-uh)
ocular (*ok*-ū-lur)
olfaction (ol-*fak*-shun)
olfactory (ol-*fak*-tuh-rē)
ophthalmic (of-*thal*-mik)

ophthalmic cryosurgery (of-*thal*-mik krī-ō-*sur*-jur-ē)
ophthalmometer (of-thul-*mom*-uh-tur)
optic (*op*-tik)
optic disc (*op*-tik disk)
optic nerve (*op*-tik nurv)
otalgia (ō-*tal*-juh)
otic (*ō*-tik)
otitis (ō-*tī*-tis)
otitis externa (ō-*tī*-tis eks-*tur*-nuh)
otitis interna (ō-*tī*-tis in-*tur*-nuh)
otitis media (ō-*tī*-tis *mē*-dē-uh)
otomycosis (ō-tō-mī-*kō*-sis)
otoplasty (*ō*-tō-plas-tē)
otorrhea (ō-tō-*rē*-uh)
otosclerosis (ō-tō-skluh-*rō*-sis)
otoscope (*ō*-tō-skōp)
otoscopic examination (ō-tō-*skop*-ik eg-zam-i-*nā*-shun)
otoscopy (ō-*tos*-kuh-pē)
oval window (*ō*-vul *win*-dō)
photophobia (fō-tō-*fō*-bē-uh)
photoreceptors (fō-tō-rē-*sep*-turz)
presbyopia (pres-bē-*ō*-pē-uh)
ptosis (*tō*-sis)
pupil (*pū*-pil)
pupillary (*pū*-pi-lar-ē)
receptors (rē-*sep*-turz)
refraction (rē-*frak*-shun)
retina (*ret*-i-nuh)
retinal (*ret*-i-nul)
retinal detachment (*ret*-i-nul dē-*tach*-munt)
retinopathy (ret-i-*nop*-uh-thē)
rods and cones (rodz and kōnz)
sclera (*sklēr*-uh)
semicircular canals (sem-ē-*sur*-kyuh-lur kuh-*nalz*)
sense organs (sens *or*-gun)
Snellen chart (*snel*-un chahrt)
stapes (*stā*-pēz)
strabismus (struh-*biz*-mus)
taste buds (tāst budz)
tearing (*tēr*-ing)
thermoreceptors (thur-mō-rē-*sep*-turz)
tinnitus (*tin*-i-tus, ti-*nī*-tus)
tonometry (tō-*nom*-uh-trē)
tuning fork tests (*to͞on*-ing fork tests)
tympanic membrane (tim-*pan*-ik *mem*-brān)
tympanostomy (tim-puh-*nos*-tuh-mē)
vertigo (*vur*-ti-gō)
visual acuity (*vizh*-o͞o-ul uh-*kū*-i-tē)
vitreous chamber (vit-rē-us *chām*-bur)
vitreous humor (*vit*-rē-us *hū*-mur)

Don't forget the games and other activities available at *http://evolve.elsevier.com/Leonard/quick*.

QUICK CONNECT

Review all lists of word parts and their meanings for this chapter using the flashcards you prepared or the flashcards on the Evolve site.

The peripheral nervous system forms the communication network between the central nervous system and the rest of the body. This system consists of the nerves that branch out from the brain and spinal cord to communicate with receptors, muscles, and glands. Special sense organs (eyes, ears, skin, mouth, and nose) have receptors that detect sensations, then sensory neurons transmit the information to the CNS where it is interpreted as sight, hearing, touch, taste, and smell.

THE EYES: *Recognize the terms and functions of main structures of the eye.* Light rays enter the pupil, which is surrounded by the iris. Muscles of the iris regulate the amount of light entering the eye by constricting or dilating the pupil. The sclera is the tough white membrane covering most of the eyeball. Accessory organs of the eye: The conjunctiva is the membrane lining the inner surface of the eyelid. The lacrimal glands produce and store lacrimal fluid (tears). Excess tears are drained into lacrimal ducts that drain into the large lacrimal sac, then into the nasal cavity via nasolacrimal ducts. The three layers of the eyeball are: sclera, cornea, choroid. The ciliary body surrounds the outside of the lens, allowing it to change shape and thickness to accommodate distant or near vision. The retina is the delicate nervous tissue membrane of the eye that is continuous with the optic nerve and enables vision. Retinal rods and cones are responsible for peripheral vision, night vision, and detection of motion.

Ophthalmometry is used to measure the eye (especially the cornea). Optometrists treat eye problems such as nearsightedness or farsightedness with corrective lens. Common tests include visual acuity (i.e., using a Snellen chart), tonometry (intraocular pressure measurement), assessment of visual fields, and a slit-lamp examination after use of a mydriatic to dilate the pupils. Accommodation reflex is the ability of the eye to adjust to variations in distance. Fluorescein angiography is used to measure movement of blood through blood vessels in the eye. Three common irregularities in vision: myopia (nearsightedness), hyperopia (farsightedness) and astigmatism (uneven focusing of the image). Presbyopia is hyperopia common in older persons.

Ophthalmologists are physicians who specialize in diagnosis and treatment of disorders of the eye. Differentiate these irregularities or abnormal conditions of the eye: amblyopia, blepharitis, cataract, color vision deficiencies (achromatic vision, achromatopsia, Daltonism), conjunctivitis, glaucoma, hordeolum, macular degeneration, nyctalopia, photophobia, ptosis, retinal detachment, retinopathy.

Surgical and therapeutic interventions: Conservative methods include ophthalmic creams or drops. Surgical procedures: iridectomy, blepharoplasty, corneal transplant, cryosurgery, corneal abrasion, lens extraction, intraocular lens transplant, laser retinal photocoagulation, and LASIK.

THE EARS: The ears are important not only for hearing but also equilibrium. Cerumen lubricates and protects the ears. Important anatomic features: External ear collects sound waves and directs them into the ear canal, where they strike the tympanic membrane. Important structures of the middle ear: tympanic membrane, malleus, incus, and stapes. Inner ear contains semicircular canals and cochlea. Eustachian tube joins middle ear with the nasopharynx. Know these terms: acoustic, audible, auditory, aural (auricular, otic), and cochlear.

Diagnostic tests: otoscopy, audiometry, tuning fork tests. Disorders: otitis externa, otitis interna, otorrhea, otalgia, otitis media, myringitis, mastoiditis, otomycosis, tinnitus, Meniere disease.

Therapeutic terms: hearing aid, ceruminolytics, antibiotics

Surgical terms: cochlear implant, otoplasty, tympanostomy

THE SKIN: Four types of modified skin structures. Recognize the stimuli that stimulate these sensory nerve endings: mechanoreceptors, photoreceptors, thermoreceptors, and nociceptors.

MOUTH & NOSE: Chemoreceptors (nerve endings that are adapted for excitation) in the nose and mouth enable taste. Nose is also responsible for smell (olfaction). Anosmia is loss or impairment of smell. Hyperosmia is abnormally increased sensitivity to odors.

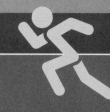

CHAPTER 15

Endocrine System and Cancer Treatments

A sonographer scans the patient's thyroid using the ultrasound probe, and images are captured and projected on the screen. Permanent records are made for study to determine if a mass is present, and cysts are differentiated from solid masses/tumors.

OBJECTIVES

After completing Chapter 15, you will be able to:

1. Recognize or write the functions of the endocrine system.
2. Recognize or write the meanings of Chapter 15 word parts; use them to build and analyze terms.
3. Write terms for selected structures of the endocrine system and their associated hormones and functions or match them with descriptions.
4. Write the names of the diagnostic terms and pathologies for the endocrine system when

given descriptions or match terms with their meanings.
5. Match surgical and therapeutic interventions for the endocrine system or write the names of the interventions when given their descriptions.
6. Match cancer treatments with their descriptions or write the treatments when given the descriptions.
7. Spell terms for the endocrine system and cancer treatments correctly.

ENDOCRINE SYSTEM

Function First

The endo+crine system coordinates with the nervous system to regulate body activities. This is accomplished by endocrine hormones that affect various processes throughout the body, such as growth, metabolism, and secretions from other organs. Dysfunctional hormone production may involve either a deficiency (**hyposecretion**) or an excess (**hypersecretion**).

dys- = bad, impaired

WRITE IT! EXERCISE 1

Write answers to these questions.

1. What is the function of the endocrine system? _____
2. What is the meaning of hyposecretion? _____
3. What is the meaning of hypersecretion? _____

*Use Appendix III, Answers, to check your answers to all the exercises in Chapter 15.

Structures of the Endocrine System

The endocrine system, also called the "hormonal system," is composed of glands that have the ability to manufacture or release chemical substances (**hormones**) that are discharged into the bloodstream and used in other parts of the body.

endo- = inside
-crine = secrete

GLANDS ARE CLASSIFIED BASED ON THE PRESENCE OR ABSENCE OF DUCTS

Endocrine glands are ductless and secrete their hormones into the bloodstream. **Exocrine glands** open onto a body surface and discharge their secretions through ducts (e.g., sweat glands) (Fig. 15.1). Exocrine glands are not part of the endocrine system.

exo- = outside

Major Endocrine Glands

Endocrine glands release hormones directly into the circulatory system. The organ or structure toward which the effects of a hormone are primarily directed is called the **target organ**. The target cell concept (Fig. 15.2) explains how only certain tissue responds to a specific hormone. Endocrine glands release hormones in one of two ways:
1. Hormones are released in response to the nervous system.
2. The pituitary produces stimulating (or tropic) hormones that act on endocrine glands, which then produce hormones.

Thus the pituitary gland is nicknamed the "master gland." Another way to understand pituitary function follows:

Pituitary produces stimulating hormones → Other endocrine glands → Other hormones

An example of the master gland acting on another gland involves gonado+tropic hormones (also called gonadotropins), which are produced by the pituitary gland and act on the gonads (ovaries or testicles).

 QUICK TIP

Gonadotropins act on the ovaries or testicles, the target organs.

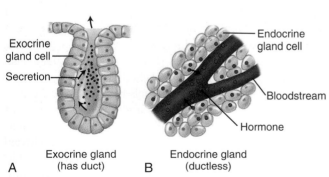

Fig. 15.1 Comparison of the Structures of an Exocrine Gland and an Endocrine Gland. **A,** Exocrine glands, such as sweat glands, are simple glands that have a duct that enables them to empty secretions onto a body surface. **B,** Endocrine glands are ductless and produce and secrete hormones into the blood or lymph nodes.
exo- = outside; **endo-** = inside; **-crine** = secrete

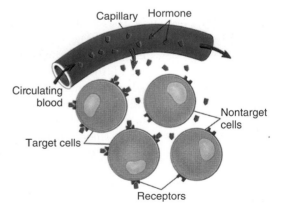

Fig. 15.2 Target Cell Concept. The hormone recognizes the target tissue through receptors (the site that interacts with the hormone), so the hormones act only on cells that have receptors specific for that hormone. The shape of the receptor determines which hormone can react with it.

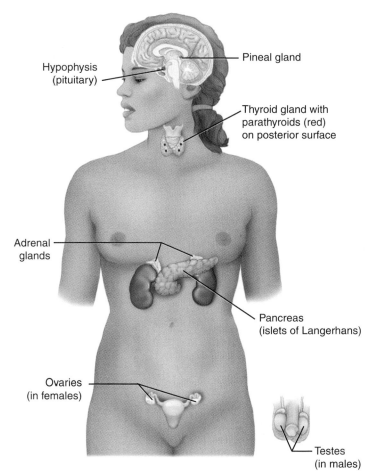

Hypophysis (pituitary)

Pineal gland

Thyroid gland with parathyroids (red) on posterior surface

Adrenal glands

Pancreas (islets of Langerhans)

Ovaries (in females)

Testes (in males)

Fig. 15.3 Location of Major Glands of the Endocrine System. **hypo-** = below normal;   **-physis** = growth

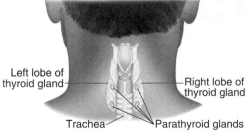

Larynx

Thyroid gland

Pyramidal lobe

Lateral lobe

Isthmus of thyroid gland

Trachea

Fig. 15.4 Thyroid gland. Located at the front of the neck. Its hormones are essential to normal body growth in infancy and childhood.

Left lobe of thyroid gland

Right lobe of thyroid gland

Trachea

Parathyroid glands

Fig. 15.5 Parathyroid Glands. Each parathyroid gland, embedded in the posterior surface of the thyroid, is about the size of a grain of rice.   **para-** = near or beside

hypo- = below
-physis = growth

The locations of the major glands of the endocrine system, including the pituitary, are shown in Fig. 15.3. The **pituitary** gland is also called the **hypophysis**, so named because it is attached by a stalk at the base of the brain. Other endocrine glands include the pineal gland, the thyroid and parathyroid glands, islets of Langerhans within the **pancreas**, adrenal glands, the ovaries in females, and the testes in males. The **pineal gland**, also called the pineal body, is shaped like a pinecone and is attached to the posterior part of the brain. It uses information regarding changing light levels to adjust its output of the hormone melatonin, helping control circadian rhythms and also the function of females' ovaries. The **thyroid** gland, located at the front of the neck, consists of bilateral lobes that are connected by a narrow strip of thyroid tissue (Fig. 15.4). **Parathyroid** glands are located near the thyroid, as the name implies, and are actually embedded in the posterior surface of the thyroid (Fig. 15.5). The pancreas is an elongated structure that has digestive functions and endocrine functions (Fig. 15.6). The **islets of Langerhans** are **pancreatic** cells that perform an endocrine function. An **adrenal** gland lies above each of the two kidneys. The ovaries and testes are endocrine glands as well as organs that produce ova or sperm, respectively.

🏃 **QUICK TIP**

Islets of Langerhans is an eponym because they are named for their discoverer, Dr. Paul Langerhans.

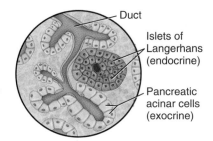

Duct
Islets of Langerhans (endocrine)
Pancreatic acinar cells (exocrine)

Fig. 15.6 Cells of the Pancreas. More than 98% of the pancreas consists of exocrine tissue (ducts and acinar cells), the main source of digestive enzymes. The endocrine cells secrete important hormones, including insulin and glucagon.
exo- = outside; **endo-** = inside

WRITE IT! EXERCISE 2

Write answers to these questions.

1. What is the general name for the structures that compose the endocrine system?
   _____

2. What is the term that means the chemical substances that are secreted by endocrine glands?
   _____

3. Describe the difference between endocrine and exocrine glands. _____
   _____

4. Which type of gland functions as part of the endocrine system? _____

5. What is the general term for the organ or structure toward which the effects of a hormone are directed?
   _____

6. Describe two ways in which endocrine glands are stimulated to release hormones.
   _____
   _____

7. Write the name of the master gland: _____

8. In no particular order, list the names of seven endocrine glands, not including the master gland (*hint:* two are the male and female sex glands): (a) _____, (b) _____,
   (c) _____, (d) _____, (e) _____,
   (f) _____, and (g) _____.

Commit to memory the word parts in the following table.

WORD PARTS: ENDOCRINE SYSTEM

Combining Forms	Meaning	Combining Forms	Meaning
aden/o	gland	pituitar/o, hypophys/o	pituitary gland
adren/o, adrenal/o	adrenal glands	ren/o, nephr/o	kidney
andr/o	male or masculine	thyr/o, thyroid/o	thyroid gland
gigant/o	giant	toxic/o	poison
gonad/o	gonad	**Suffixes**	
insulin/o	insulin	-gen	beginning, origin
iod/o	iodine	-physis	growth
myx/o	mucus	-tropic	stimulate
pancreat/o	pancreas	-tropin	that which stimulates
parathyroid/o	parathyroids	-uria	urine, urination

Use the electronic flashcards on the Evolve site or make your own set of flashcards using the above list. Select the word parts just presented, and study them until you know their meanings. Do this each time a set of word parts is presented.

Match terms in numbers 1-8 with the combining forms.

_____ 1. adrenal gland   _____ 5. kidney   A. aden/o   E. iod/o

_____ 2. giant   _____ 6. male or masculine   B. adren/o   F. myx/o

_____ 3. gland   _____ 7. mucus   C. andr/o   G. ren/o

_____ 4. iodine   _____ 8. poison   D. gigant/o   H. toxic/o

Select Hormones

Some of the most discussed hormones include cortisone and steroids that are banned by most major sports organizations. Growth hormone injections are included in the list of athletic performance-enhancing drugs (Fig. 15.7).

You may also be familiar with cortisone injections to relieve pain and inflammation, or the use of cortisone in topical creams and ointments to relieve skin inflammation. Female sex hormones are used in several birth control methods, including oral contraceptives (pills, patches, and subdermal implants).

The body's insufficient secretion or improper use of the hormone insulin leads to diabetes mellitus. Important hormones are summarized in Table 15.1.

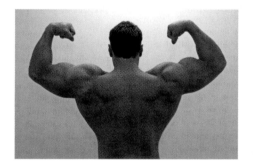

Fig. 15.7 Steroid Use. Body builders sometimes take steroid hormones to achieve muscular definition, which can lead to endocrine disorders. Physicians can order tests of steroids when they see overdevelopment of muscles in a patient and suspect abuse.

TABLE 15-1   SELECT HORMONES AND CORRESPONDING ENDOCRINE GLANDS

Hormone	Endocrine Gland	Major Function(s)
adrenaline (also known as epinephrine)	adrenals	Potent stimulator of the "fight or flight" response, increasing blood pressure and cardiac output
androgen (major androgen is testosterone)	testicles	Development and maintenance of masculinizing characteristics
antidiuretic hormone (ADH)	pituitary*	Suppression of urine formation
cortisone	adrenals	Important in regulation of body metabolism
estrogens (female sex hormones; includes estradiol and estrone)	ovaries (primarily)	During menstrual cycle, act on the female genitalia to produce a suitable site for fertilization, implantation, and nutrition of the early embryo
growth hormone	pituitary	Stimulation of body growth and maintenance of size once growth has been obtained
insulin	pancreas	Regulation of blood glucose by coordinating with other hormones
thyroxine (iodine-containing hormone)	thyroid	Cell metabolism

*ADH is synthesized by the hypothalamus (a structure of the brain), which also controls its secretion by the pituitary.

WRITE IT!   **EXERCISE 4**

Write suffixes for these meanings.

1. beginning _____
2. growth _____
3. origin _____

4. stimulate _____
5. that which stimulates _____
6. urination _____

MATCH IT!   **EXERCISE 5**

Match the endocrine glands in the left column with the hormone they secrete.

_____ 1. adrenals
_____ 2. ovaries
_____ 3. pancreas
_____ 4. pituitary
_____ 5. testicles

A. androgen
B. antidiuretic hormone
C. epinephrine
D. estrogen
E. insulin

Diseases, Disorders, and Diagnostic Terms

Most endocrine glands are not accessible for examination in a routine physical examination; however, the testicles and thyroid gland are exceptions. The testicles are examined for masses or a difference in size. The thyroid gland can be observed and palpated for any unusual bulging over the thyroid area (Fig. 15.8, *A*). Both enlargement and masses are abnormal findings and indicate that additional testing is necessary. **Hyperthyroidism** is abnormally increased activity of the thyroid. A classic finding associated with hyperthyroidism is **ex+ophthalmos**, that is, protrusion of the eyeballs, but further tests are required with this condition because hyperthyroidism is not always the cause. The patient in Fig. 15.8, *B*, has both exophthalmos and a **goiter**, an enlarged thyroid gland that is usually evident as a pronounced swelling in the neck.

A person who is described as **eu+thyroid** has normal thyroid function.

hyper- = above normal
ex- = outward
ophthalm/o = eye
eu- = normal

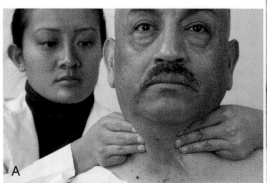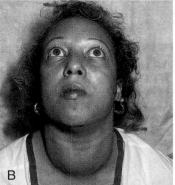

Fig. 15.8 Physical Examination of the Thyroid Gland. A, Using the hands to feel for thyroid enlargement or masses. **B,** Observing the patient for thyroid enlargement and exophthalmos, protrusion of the eyeballs. This patient shows both exophthalmos and a goiter, which is an enlarged thyroid gland, evidenced by the swelling in the neck.
ex- = outward;   **ophthalm/o** = eye

hypo- = below normal

Hypo+thyroid+ism is decreased activity of the thyroid. Several blood tests and radiologic studies are used to determine thyroid function. Thyroid scans consist of administering a radioactive substance, allowing time for the thyroid gland to absorb the radiation, scanning the thyroid, and imaging the radiation distribution.

Physical indications of endocrine disorders also include unusually tall or short stature, coarsening of facial features, edema (accumulation of fluid in the interstitial tissues), hair loss, or excessive facial hair in women. Laboratory testing includes blood tests and urine tests, depending on the symptoms. Magnetic resonance imaging (MRI) is useful in identifying tumors involving the pituitary.

Diabetes insipidus is a disorder associated with a deficiency of antidiuretic hormone (ADH) produced by the pituitary gland, or inability of the kidneys to respond to ADH. Do not confuse diabetes insipidus with **diabetes mellitus** (DM), the well-known type of diabetes that produces hyperglycemia and is associated with insufficient or improper use of insulin. Type 1 diabetes mellitus is characterized by abrupt onset of symptoms and a dependence on insulin injections to sustain life. Type 2 diabetes mellitus is usually characterized by a gradual onset; dietary control, sometimes combined with oral hypoglycemic medications, may be effective in regulating the disorder. "Diabetics" are persons who have diabetes mellitus. Diabetes insipidus has some of the characteristics of diabetes mellitus: **poly+uria** and **poly+dipsia**. The two terms mean "frequent urination" and "increased thirst," respectively. However, diabetes insipidus is not associated with insulin deficiency, **hyper+glyc+emia** (increased level of glucose in the blood), or **glycos+uria** (sugar in the urine). Table 15.2 compares the characteristics of these two types of diabetes.

> ### 🏃 QUICK TIP
> *Diuretic* means promoting urine excretion. *Antidiuretic* has the opposite meaning.

poly- = many
-uria = urination
-dipsia = thirst
hyper- = increased
glyc/o = sugar
-emia = blood

TABLE 15.2   COMPARISON OF DIABETES INSIPIDUS AND DIABETES MELLITUS

Characteristic	Diabetes Insipidus	Diabetes Mellitus
Antidiuretic hormone (ADH) deficiency	Yes	No
Polyuria	Yes	Yes
Polydipsia	Yes	Yes
Insufficient or improper use of insulin	No	Yes*
Hyperglycemia	No	Yes
Glycosuria	No	Yes

*Diabetes mellitus is classified as type 1 or type 2.

WRITE IT!

EXERCISE 6

Write terms for these descriptions.

1. disorder associated with a deficiency of ADH _____
2. disorder associated with insufficient or improper use of insulin _____
3. decreased activity of the thyroid _____
4. frequent urination _____
5. increased level of blood glucose _____
6. increased thirst _____
7. protrusion of the eyeballs _____
8. sugar in the urine _____

The following list provides information about other disorders of the endocrine system.

acromegaly (acr/o, extremity + -megaly, enlarged) Disorder in which there is abnormal enlargement of the extremities of the skeleton—nose, jaws, fingers, and toes—caused by hypersecretion of growth hormone after maturity (Fig. 15.9).

adenoma (-oma, tumor) Tumor of a gland.

cretinism Condition caused by congenital deficiency of thyroid secretion and marked by arrested physical and mental development (Fig. 15.10).

dwarfism Disease caused by hyposecretion of growth hormone during childhood; it causes a person to be much smaller than normal size (Fig. 15.11).

gigantism (gigant/o, large + -ism, condition) Condition in which a person reaches an abnormal stature; it results from hypersecretion of growth hormone during childhood. Compare dwarfism and gigantism (Fig. 15.12).

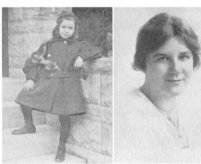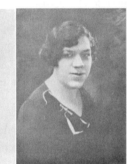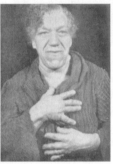

**acr/o =
extremities
-megaly =
enlargement**

Fig. 15.9 Progression of Acromegaly. The patient is shown at age 9 years, age 16, age 33 (with well-established acromegaly), and age 52 in the late stage of acromegaly.

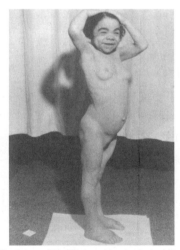

Fig. 15.10 Cretinism. This 33-year-old untreated adult with cretinism exhibits characteristic features. She is only 44 inches tall, has underdeveloped breasts, a protruding abdomen, an umbilical hernia, widened facial features, and scant axillary and pubic hair.
umbilic/o = umbilicus (navel); **faci/o** = facial;
axill/o = axilla; **pub/o** = pubis

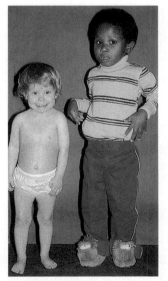

Fig. 15.11 Growth Hormone Deficiency. A normal 3-year-old boy and a short 3-year-old girl who exhibits the characteristic "Kewpie doll" appearance, suggesting a diagnosis of growth hormone deficiency. This deficiency leads to dwarfism unless identified early and treated.

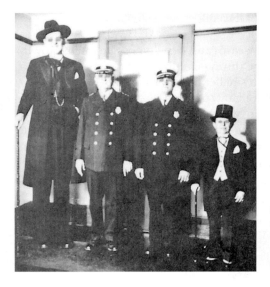

Fig. 15.12 Gigantism and Dwarfism Resulting From Abnormal Secretions of Growth Hormone (GH). Hypersecretion of GH during the early years results in gigantism (person on the far left). The person usually has normal body proportions and normal sexual development. The same hypersecretion in an adult causes acromegaly. Hyposecretion of GH during the early years produces a dwarf (person on the far right) unless the child is treated with GH injections. **gigant/o** = large; **-ism** = condition; **hyper-** = more than normal; **hypo-** = less than normal

hyperinsulinism Excessive secretion of insulin by the pancreas, which causes hypoglycemia.

hyperparathyroidism Increased activity of the parathyroid glands.

hypoglycemia (hypo-, decreased) Abnormally low blood sugar.

hypoparathyroidism Decreased activity of the parathyroid glands.

hypopituitarism Diminished activity of the pituitary gland.

myxedema (myx/o, mucus + -edema, swelling) Condition resulting from hypofunction of the thyroid gland, characterized by a dry, waxy swelling of the skin.

thyrotoxicosis (thyr/o, thyroid + toxic/o, poison + -osis, condition) Morbid condition caused by excessive thyroid secretion; also known as thyroid storm.

MATCH IT! EXERCISE 7

Match the diagnostic terms in the left column with their descriptions.

_____ 1. acromegaly

_____ 2. cretinism

_____ 3. diabetes insipidus

_____ 4. diabetes mellitus

_____ 5. exophthalmos

_____ 6. gigantism

_____ 7. goiter

A. abnormal enlargement of the extremities

B. abnormally tall stature

C. condition caused by congenital deficiency of thyroid secretion

D. disorder associated with insufficient or improper use of insulin

E. disorder caused by insufficient ADH or inability of kidneys to respond to ADH

F. enlarged thyroid gland that results in swelling of the neck

G. outward protrusion of the eyeballs

WRITE IT! EXERCISE 8

Write terms for these descriptions.

1. abnormally low blood sugar _____

2. an iodine-containing thyroid hormone _____

3. excessive secretion of insulin _____

4. normal thyroid function _____

5. tumor of a gland _____

QUICK CASE STUDY | EXERCISE 9

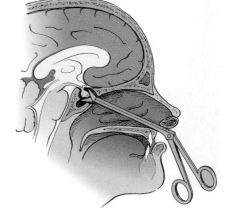

Select terms from the report to match the descriptions.

Humberto Cordova suddenly began experiencing polyuria, polydipsia, and polyphagia. Laboratory findings showed a normal level of antidiuretic hormone but hyperglycemia, glycosuria, and ketonuria. Further testing indicated diabetes mellitus.

1. a greater than normal amount of glucose in the blood   _____
2. excessive, uncontrolled eating   _____
3. increased urination   _____
4. pertaining to the suppression of urine excretion   _____
5. presence of sugar, especially glucose, in the urine   _____

 Surgical and Therapeutic Interventions

 PROGRAMMED LEARNING

Remember to cover the answers (left column) with folded paper or the bookmark. Write an answer in each blank, and then check your answer before proceeding to the next frame.

hypophysis (pituitary)	1. Because the most common cause of hypopituitarism is a pituitary tumor, treatment consists of surgery or radiation to remove the tumor, followed by administration of the deficient hormones. Certain types of pituitary tumors can cause overproduction of growth hormone (GH), and the treatment of choice is surgery to remove the tumor. Irradiation of the tumor and drugs may also be indicated. **Hypophysectomy** is surgical removal or destruction of the _____ (Fig. 15.13).
target	2. Increased production of a single tropic hormone by the pituitary gland usually causes oversecretion by the _____ organ. Drug therapy may be useful in suppressing the hormone production.

Fig. 15.13 Hypophysectomy. Surgical removal of the pituitary gland may be performed to excise a pituitary tumor or to slow the growth and spread of endocrine-dependent malignant tumors. Hypophysectomy is done only if other treatments fail to destroy all of the pituitary tumor. **hypophys/o** = pituitary

excision

3. The treatment of hyperthyroidism is destruction of large amounts of the thyroid tissue by surgery or radioactive materials or the use of **antithyroid drugs** to block the production of thyroid hormones. **Thyroidectomy** is _____ of the thyroid.

parathyroids

4. **Parathyroidectomy** is excision of one or more _____.

adrenalectomy

5. It may be necessary to surgically remove adrenal tumors that cause the adrenals to produce excess corticoids. Using adrenal/o, write a word that means excision of an adrenal gland: _____

adenectomy

6. Write a term that means removal of a gland, but not a specific one:

    _____

insulin

7. The goal of treatment of DM is to maintain a balance of the body's insulin and glucose. Type 1 diabetes is controlled by administration of insulin, proper diet, and exercise. Insulin is administered by injection on a regular basis, either subcutaneous injection or via an insulin pump. An **insulin pump** is a portable, battery-operated instrument that delivers a measured amount of insulin through the abdominal wall. It can be programmed to deliver doses of insulin according to the body's needs (Fig. 15.14). The individual with type 1 diabetes requires an outside source of _____ to sustain life.

    Insulin is a **glucose-lowering agent**. Type 2 diabetes is controlled by diet, **exercise,** oral agents, and sometimes insulin. Oral agents are another means of **lowering** blood glucose.

excessive

8. Treatment of hypoglycemia may consist of a glucose paste placed inside the cheek, administration of glucose (dextrose) such as that found in orange juice, or intravenously if the person is unconscious. Strict attention to diet is important for patients with hypoglycemia caused by _____ secretion of insulin.

    Glands may become overactive or sometimes cancerous. Read the next section about various cancer treatments.

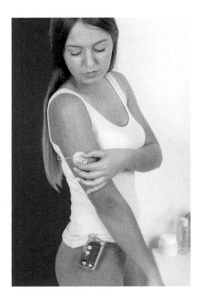

Fig. 15.14 External Insulin Pump. This insulin pump is about the size of a small cell phone and is worn externally. It delivers precise doses of rapid-acting insulin to closely match your body's needs. Additional insulin can be delivered "on demand" before an unusually large meal or to correct a high blood sugar.

Write a one-word term in each blank to complete these sentences.

1. A term for surgical removal or destruction of the pituitary gland is _____.
2. Type 1 diabetes is controlled by administration of _____, proper diet, and exercise.
3. Type 2 diabetes is generally controlled by diet, exercise, and _____-lowering agents, if needed.
4. The term for removal of a gland is _____.
5. The term for removal of the thyroid gland is _____.
6. Excision of one or more parathyroids is called _____.

CANCER TREATMENTS

9. Certain vaccinations can reduce the risk of developing cancer associated with specific chronic infections, including hepatitis B vaccine and human papilloma virus (HPV) vaccine. Three major methods of treating cancer are: surgical excision, radiation therapy, and systemic or biological therapy (chemotherapy, bone marrow transplant, and immunotherapy).

    Surgical excision is the primary treatment for cancer; however, the cancer must be small and present in only that organ. Surgical removal of the following may be successful at stopping cancer if it has not spread: skin, stomach, colon, lung, breast, and uterus. Therefore, when possible, the primary way to remove cancer is surgical _____.

    Resection is excision of a significant part of an organ plus surrounding tissue that contains lymph nodes, whereas **exenteration** is extensive surgical removal of the tumor, its origin, and all surrounding tissue. Exenteration is more extensive than resection.

excision

10. The extent and location of metastases determines the therapeutic strategy in breast cancer. For breast cancer with distant metastases, nonsurgical treatment (chemotherapy, hormone therapy, and sometimes radiation) may be prescribed. For women with breast cancer at a stage for which surgery is recommended, follow-up after the surgery with chemotherapy, radiation, hormone therapy, or targeted therapy may be prescribed.

    Excision of the lump with removal of varying amounts of tissue is often the treatment of choice in breast cancer. The amount of extra tissue removed ranges from a small amount of surrounding healthy tissue to the entire breast. A lumpectomy is surgical excision of a tumor that is known to be or suspected of being cancer. Mast/ectomy is removal of the _____. Only breast tissue is removed in a simple mastectomy, whereas axillary lymph nodes and muscles of the chest are removed in a radical mastectomy (Fig. 15.15).

breast

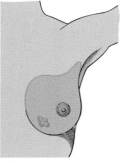

A — Total or simple mastectomy

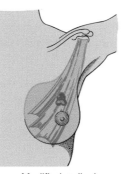

B — Modified radical mastectomy

Fig. 15.15 Simple vs. Radical Mastectomy. These are most commonly performed to remove a malignant tumor. **A,** In a simple mastectomy, only breast tissue is removed. **B,** In a radical mastectomy, axillary lymph nodes and some of the muscles of the chest are removed with the breast.

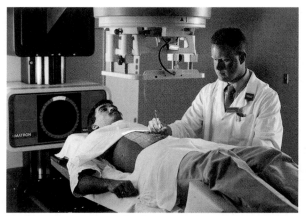

Fig. 15.16 Male Patient Being Prepared to Receive Radiation Therapy. The external beam of radiation is generated by the equipment.

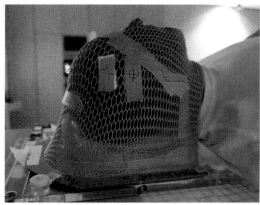

Fig. 15.17 Patient Receiving Radiotherapy Treatments for Brain Cancer. A custom-made mask gently holds the head in the correct position for treatment.

11. Radiation therapy is the treatment of neoplastic disease by using x-rays or gamma rays to destroy malignant cells (Figs. 15.16 and 15.17). Some cancers are treated solely with radiation, but radiation is sometimes done before surgical removal to shrink the tumor or after excision of the tumor.

    The goal of radiotherapy is to deliver a maximum dose of radiation to the tumor tissue and a minimal dose to the surrounding normal tissue. Cancerous tumors that are destroyed by radiation are said to be **radiosensitive**, whereas those that are not affected are **radioresistant**. Radiotherapy is another term for _____ therapy.

12. When **fractionation** is used in radiology, radiation is administered in smaller units over time to minimize tissue damage compared with a single large dose. Write this term that is used when radiation is administered several times in smaller units: _____.

13. A **linear accelerator** (LINAC) is an apparatus used in radiology that accelerates charged subatomic particles to deliver supervoltage x-rays for radiotherapy (see Fig. 4.17). Write this new term that is abbreviated LINAC: linear _____.

14. **Brachy/therapy,** internal radiotherapy, is implantation of radiation seeds or beads of radioactive material directly into the tumor or a cavity of the tumor, and these may be temporary or permanent. Write the name of this type of cancer therapy that uses radioactive beads or seeds: _____.

15. **Stereotactic radiosurgery** (gamma knife stereotactic surgery) delivers a large dose of radiation from several different angles to treat small intracranial tumors or to destroy a vascular abnormality (arteriovenous malformation in the brain). Write this term for gamma knife surgery: _____ radiosurgery (see Fig. 13.20).

16. **Chemotherapy** is the use of _____ to treat cancer. Ideally, the cytotoxic drug selectively kills large numbers of tumor cells without harming healthy cells. Chemotherapy may be used alone or in combination with radiation and/or surgery. Many agents used in chemotherapy can be injected intravenously; in addition, various types of catheters may be used.

    A PET scan provides information about the metabolism, size, and shape of an internal structure (Fig. 15.18). After invasive cancer has been detected, full-body PET scans can detect areas of metastases, called "hot spots" (Fig. 15.19)

(answer column, left margin)

radiation

fractionation

accelerator

brachytherapy

stereotactic

chemicals

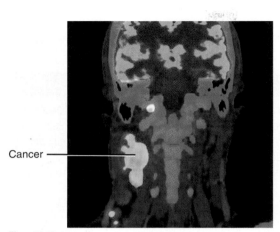

Fig. 15.18 High-Resolution PET Scan. Providing information about the metabolism of an internal structure, this PET scan shows neck cancer (arrow).

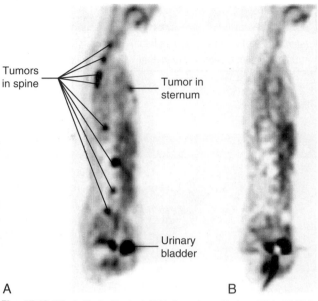

Fig. 15.19 Whole-Body Sagittal PET Scan in a Patient With Multiple Breast Cancer Metastases, Before and After Treatment. **A,** Numerous tumors (dark spots) are seen. **B,** Image obtained after chemotherapy.

transplant

17. Biological therapy includes bone marrow transplant and immunotherapy, both using the body's own defenses to fight cancer. A **bone marrow transplant** (BMT) may be previously harvested or may use bone marrow from a matching donor to stimulate normal blood cell growth in specific types of leukemia. Bone marrow is ideally harvested from the donor on the day it is infused into the patient. BMT means bone marrow _____.

transplantation

18. **Immunotherapy** is the use of immunostimulants and immunosuppressants to prevent and treat disease. This includes the transfer of immunocompetent cells from one person to another. **Stem cell transplantation** is collection of stem cells from a compatible donor and administration to a recipient. Patients with certain malignancies are candidates for this procedure. Both patient and recipient undergo conditioning processes before donation or receiving the stem cells. In autologous stem cell transplantion, the patient's own stem cells are collected, then reinfused after chemotherapy. Collection of stem cells, then administration to a recipient, is called stem cell _____.

WRITE IT!   EXERCISE 11

Write a one-word term in each blank to complete these sentences.

1. Extensive surgical removal of a tumor, its origin, and surrounding tissue is _____.
2. In describing cancerous tumors, the opposite of radiosensitive is _____.
3. Radiation administered several times in smaller units is called _____.
4. An apparatus that accelerates charged subatomic particles in radiotherapy is a _____ accelerator.
5. Another name for internal radiotherapy is _____.
6. The use of immunostimulants and immunosuppressants to prevent and treat disease is _____.

Be Careful With These!

aden/o (gland) versus adren/o (adrenal gland) versus andr/o (male)
-tropic (stimulate) versus -tropin (that which stimulates)

A Career as a Medical Technologist

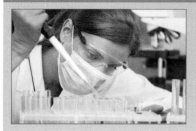

Bethany Euclid is a medical technologist. She completed a bachelor's degree to prepare for the certification exam and is employed in a small hospital lab. She mainly runs tests on body fluids (e.g., blood, sputum, urine) and uses equipment to run many of the analyses. Bethany knows she is an integral part of the diagnostic medical process. For more information, visit *ascp.org* or *www.ameri canmedtech.org*.

 SELF-TEST

Work the following exercises to test your understanding of the material in Chapter 15. It is best to do all the exercises before checking your answers against the answers in Appendix III. Pay particular attention to spelling.

A. WRITING!   *List the names of seven endocrine glands, not including the master gland:*

_____

_____

B. WRITING!   *Write answers to these questions.*

1. What is the function of the endocrine system? _____

2. What is the difference between a gland and a hormone? _____

3. Which gland is the "master gland"? _____

4. What is a target organ? _____

5. What are two general types of dysfunctions in hormone production? _____

C. CHOOSING!   *Circle the one correct answer (A, B, C, or D) for each question.*

1. What is the general term for chemical substances that are discharged into the bloodstream and used in some other part of the body?   **(A)** cortisones   **(B)** estrogens   **(C)** excretions   **(D)** hormones

2. Which of the following is characterized by an abnormal enlargement of the extremities?
   (A) acromegaly   **(B)** hyperparathyroidism   **(C)** hypoglycemia   **(D)** thyrotoxicosis

3. Which term means increased activity of the thyroid gland?
   (A) euthyroid   **(B)** hyperthyroidism   **(C)** hypothyroidism   **(D)** thyroxine

4. The presence or absence of what determines whether a gland is classified as an endocrine gland or an exocrine gland?
   (A) blood vessels   **(B)** ducts   **(C)** fluids   **(D)** islets

5. Which term means an enlargement of the thyroid gland resulting in swelling at the front of the neck?
   (A) goiter   **(B)** hyperparathyroidism   **(C)** hyperthyroidism   **(D)** hypothyroidism

6. Which of the following is associated with insufficient production or improper use of insulin?
   (A) diabetes insipidus   **(B)** diabetes mellitus   **(C)** myxedema   **(D)** thyrotoxicosis

7. Which of the following is a disease caused by insufficient secretion of growth hormone during childhood?
   (A) acromegaly   **(B)** cretinism   **(C)** dwarfism   **(D)** gigantism

8. Which term means excessive secretion of insulin?
   (A) diabetes   **(B)** hyperinsulinism   **(C)** hypoinsulinism   **(D)** polydipsia

9. Which gland is responsible for the production of insulin?
   (A) adrenal   **(B)** pancreas   **(C)** parathyroid   **(D)** thyroid

10. Which of the following disorders results from hypofunction of the thyroid gland?
    (A) acromegaly   **(B)** exophthalmos   **(C)** hypoparathyroidism   **(D)** myxedema

11. Extensive surgical removal of a tumor, its origin, and surrounding tissue is called
    (A) biopsy   **(B)** exenteration   **(C)** fractionation   **(D)** resection

12. Cancerous tumors that are destroyed by radiation are said to be
    (A) immune   **(B)** neoplastic   **(C)** radioresistant   **(D)** radiosensitive

13. Another name for internal radiotherapy
    (A) brachytherapy   **(B)** excision   **(C)** lumpectomy   **(D)** parathyroidectomy

14. Use of immunostimulants and immunosuppressants to prevent and treat disease is
    (A) chemotherapy   **(B)** excision   **(C)** immunotherapy   **(D)** radiotherapy

D. WRITING!   *Write a one-word term for each meaning.*

1. abnormally large stature   _____
2. abnormally low blood sugar   _____
3. decreased activity of the parathyroid gland   _____
4. removal of the pituitary   _____
5. increased thirst   _____
6. frequent urination   _____
7. tumor of a gland   _____
8. removal of a gland   _____
9. removal of the thyroid gland   _____
10. toxic condition of the thyroid _____

E. READING HEALTH CARE REPORTS   *Write the meanings of underlined terms in the following medical report.*

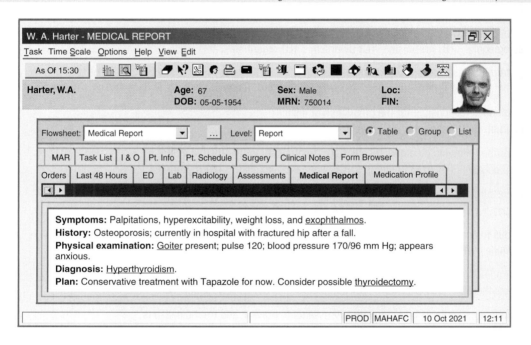

Symptoms: Palpitations, hyperexcitability, weight loss, and <u>exophthalmos</u>.
History: Osteoporosis; currently in hospital with fractured hip after a fall.
Physical examination: <u>Goiter</u> present; pulse 120; blood pressure 170/96 mm Hg; appears anxious.
Diagnosis: <u>Hyperthyroidism</u>.
Plan: Conservative treatment with Tapazole for now. Consider possible <u>thyroidectomy</u>.

1. exophthalmos   _____
2. goiter   _____
3. hyperthyroidism _____
4. thyroidectomy   _____

F.   *Read the sentences that follow the report and write "T" for true or "F" for false.*

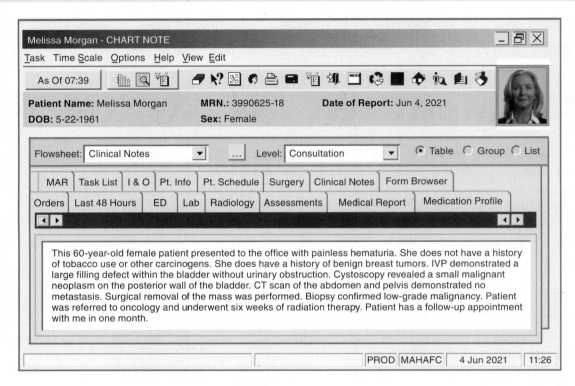

Melissa Morgan - CHART NOTE

Task Time Scale Options Help View Edit

As Of 07:39

Patient Name: Melissa Morgan   **MRN.:** 3990625-18   **Date of Report:** Jun 4, 2021
DOB: 5-22-1961   **Sex:** Female

Flowsheet: Clinical Notes   ...   Level: Consultation   ⦿ Table ○ Group ○ List

MAR | Task List | I & O | Pt. Info | Pt. Schedule | Surgery | Clinical Notes | Form Browser

Orders | Last 48 Hours | ED | Lab | Radiology | Assessments | Medical Report | Medication Profile

This 60-year-old female patient presented to the office with painless hematuria. She does not have a history of tobacco use or other carcinogens. She does have a history of benign breast tumors. IVP demonstrated a large filling defect within the bladder without urinary obstruction. Cystoscopy revealed a small malignant neoplasm on the posterior wall of the bladder. CT scan of the abdomen and pelvis demonstrated no metastasis. Surgical removal of the mass was performed. Biopsy confirmed low-grade malignancy. Patient was referred to oncology and underwent six weeks of radiation therapy. Patient has a follow-up appointment with me in one month.

PROD | MAHAFC | 4 Jun 2021 | 11:26

1. Oncology deals with all new growths, even nonmalignancies. _____
2. Malignant cancers can also be termed benign. _____
3. Radiotherapy is an alternative term for radiation therapy. _____
4. Tobacco use is not a carcinogen. _____
5. Radiology is the study of tumors. _____

G. IDENTIFYING!   *Label these illustrations using one of the following: brachytherapy, exenteration, goiter, hypophysectomy, parathyroidectomy, thyroidectomy.*

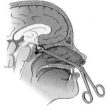

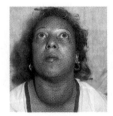

1. Surgical removal of the pituitary gland

_____

2. Enlargement of the thyroid gland

_____

H. SPELLING AND PRONUNCIATION!   *Circle all incorrectly spelled terms, and write the correct spelling. Then pronounce the terms.*

adrenalene   cretenism   goiture   hypersekretion   mixedema

I. QUICK CHALLENGE!   *Find an incorrect term in each sentence and write the correct term.*

1. A congenital deficiency of thyroid secretion can lead to thyrotoxicosis. _____

2. An adrenal pump delivers a measured amount of insulin through the abdominal wall. _____

3. Exophthalmos, protrusion of the extremities, is a classic finding associated with hyperthyroidism.

   _____

4. The adrenal gland is attached to the posterior part of the brain. _____

5. Two parathyroid glands are embedded in the posterior surface of the thyroid. _____

*Use Appendix III to check your answers.

QUICK & EASY (Q&E) LIST

Use the Evolve website (http://evolve.elsevier.com/Leonard/quick) to review the terms presented in Chapter 15. Look closely at the spelling of each term as it is pronounced.

acromegaly (ak-rō-**meg**-uh-lē)
adenectomy (ad-uh-**nek**-tuh-mē)
adenoma (ad-uh-**nō**-muh)
adrenal (uh-**drē**-nul)
adrenalectomy (uh-drē-nul-**ek**-tuh-mē)
adrenaline (uh-**dren**-uh-lin)
androgen (**an**-drō-jun)
antidiuretic hormone (an-tē-dī-ū-**ret**-ik **hor**-mōn)
antithyroid drugs (an-tē-**thī**-roid drugz)
bone marrow transplant (bōn **mar**-ō **trans**-plant)
brachytherapy (brak-ē-**ther**-uh-pē)
chemotherapy (kē-mō-**ther**-uh-pē)
cortisone (**kor**-ti-sōn)
cretinism (**krē**-tin-iz-um)
diabetes insipidus (dī-uh-**bē**-tēz in-**sip**-i-dus)
diabetes mellitus (dī-uh-**bē**-tēz **mel**-luh-tus, muh-**lī**-tis)
dwarfism (**dworf**-iz-um)
endocrine glands (**en**-dō-krin glandz)
estrogen (**es**-truh-jun)
euthyroid (ū-**thī**-roid)
exenteration (ek-sen-tur-**ā**-shun)
exocrine glands (ek-**sō**-krin glandz)
exophthalmos (ek-sof-**thal**-mos)
fractionation (frak-shun-**ā**-shun)
gigantism (jī-**gan**-tiz-um)

glucose-lowering agent (**glū**-kōs lō-wur-ing **ā**-junt)
glycosuria (glī-kō-**sū**-rē-uh)
goiter (**goi**-tur)
growth hormone (grōth **hor**-mōn)
hormone (**hor**-mōn)
hyperglycemia (hī-pur-glī-**sē**-mē-uh)
hyperinsulinism (hī-pur-**in**-suh-lin-iz-um)
hyperparathyroidism (hī-pur-par-uh-**thī**-roid-iz-um)
hypersecretion (hī-pur-sē-**krē**-shun)
hyperthyroidism (hī-pur-**thī**-roid-iz-um)
hypoglycemia (hī-pō-glī-**sē**-mē-uh)
hypoparathyroidism (hī-pō-par-uh-**thī**-roid-iz-um)
hypophysectomy (hī-pof-uh-**sek**-tuh-mē)
hypophysis (hī-**pof**-uh-sis)
hypopituitarism (hī-pō-pi-**too**-i-tuh-riz-um)
hyposecretion (hī-pō-suh-**krē**-shun)
hypothyroidism (hī-pō-**thī**-roid-iz-um)
immunotherapy (im-ū-nō-**ther**-uh-pē)
insulin (**in**-suh-lin)
insulin pump (**in**-suh-lin pump)
islets of Langerhans (ī-lets ov **lahng**-uhr-hahnz)
linear accelerator (**lin**-ē-ur ak-**sel**-ur-ā-tur)
myxedema (mik-suh-**dē**-muh)
pancreas (**pan**-krē-us)
pancreatic (pan-krē-**at**-ik)

QUICK & EASY (Q&E) LIST—cont'd

parathyroid *(par-uh-**thī**-roid)*
parathyoidectomy *(par-uh-thī-roid-**ek**-tuh-mē)*
pineal gland *(**pin**-ē-ul gland)*
pituitary *(pi-**too**-i-tar-ē)*
polydipsia *(pol-ē-**dip**-sē-uh)*
polyuria *(pol-ē-**ū**-rē-uh)*
radioresistant *(rā-dē-ō-rē-**zis**-tunt)*
radiosensitive *(rā-dē-ō-**sen**-si-tiv)*

resection *(rē-**sek**-shun)*
stem cell transplantation *(stem sel trans-plan-**tā**-shun)*
stereotactic radiosurgery *(ster-ē-ō-**tak**-tik rā-dē-ō-**sur**-jur-ē)*
target organ *(**tahr**-gut **or**-gun)*
thyroid *(**thī**-roid)*
thyroidectomy *(thī-roid-**ek**-tuh-mē)*
thyrotoxicosis *(thī-rō-tok-si-**kō**-sis)*
thyroxine *(thī-**rok**-sin)*

Don't forget the games and other activities available at *http://evolve.elsevier.com/Leonard/quick.*

 QUICK CONNECT

Review all lists of word parts and their meanings for this chapter using the flashcards you prepared or the flashcards on the Evolve site.

The endocrine system, composed of glands and also called the hormonal system, uses hormones to coordinate with the nervous system to regulate body activities. Dysfunction includes a deficiency (hyposecretion) or an excess (hypersecretion).

Endocrine glands are ductless and secrete their hormones into the bloodstream. Exocrine glands discharge their secretions through ducts and are not part of the endocrine system.

ENDOCRINE SYSTEM:

Major Endocrine Glands And Their Target Organs (organ or structure toward which the effects of the hormone are primarily directed):

Endocrine glands release hormones in one of two ways:

1. In response to the nervous system, or
2. The pituitary gland (master gland) produces stimulating (or tropic) hormones that act on endocrine glands, which then release hormones.

MAJOR GLANDS OF THE ENDOCRINE SYSTEM: pituitary (hypophysis), pineal gland, thyroid, parathyroid, pancreas (islets of Langerhans) adrenal, ovaries, and testes.

Select endocrine glands and hormones they secrete:

adrenals: adrenaline (epinephrine) and cortisone

testicles: androgen (testosterone is major one)

pituitary: antidiuretic hormone

ovaries: estrogens

pituitary: growth hormone

pancreas: insulin

thyroid: thyroxine (iodine-containing hormone for cell metabolism)

Increased production of a tropic hormone by the pituitary usually causes oversecretion by the target organ. Drug therapy may suppress the hormone production.

Remember the meaning of these diagnostic terms:

- Changes in physical appearance may be associated with hormonal dysfunctions: unusually short or tall stature, coarsening of facial features, edema, hair loss, or excessive facial hair in women, exophthalmos, and enlarged thyroid
- Blood and urine tests for hormone levels; radiologic studies (i.e., thyroid scans, MRI)
- Differentiate these diseases/disorders: hyperthyroidism (associated with exophthalmos, goiter, and thyrotoxicosis) vs. hypothyroidism; diabetes mellitus vs. diabetes insipidus; hypoparathyroidism, hypopituitarism, myxedema, acromegaly, adenoma, cretinism, dwarfism vs. gigantism, hypoparathyroidism, and hypoglycemia vs. hypoparathyroidism vs. hypopituitarism.
- Would hyperinsulinism bring about hypoglycemia or hyperglycemia?
- How are hyperglycemia, polyuria, glycosuria, and polydipsia related to diabetes mellitus?

Differentiate these surgical terms: hypophysectomy, thyroidectomy, parathyroidectomy, adrenalectomy, and adrenectomy.

Therapeutic terms: insulin pump, glucose-lowering agents, insulin, glucose paste and glucose for hypoglycemia, steroids

CANCER TREATMENTS:

Three major methods of treating cancer are:

(1) Surgical excision is the primary method, but cancer must be small and present in only one organ. Resection (excision of a significant part of an organ plus surrounding tissue that contains lymph nodes) vs. exenteration (excision of a significant part of an organ plus surrounding tissue that contains lymph nodes). Breast (lumpectomy vs. simple mastectomy vs. radical mastectomy)

(2) Radiation (radiosensitive vs. radioresistant); fractionation, LINAC, brachytherapy, stereotactic radiosurgery or gamma knife stereotactic surgery

(3) Systemic (chemotherapy) or biological therapy (bone marrow transplant and immunotherapy, stem cell transplant)

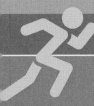

Medical Abbreviations

A. Abbreviations and Their Meanings

PART ONE

Chapter 2

CA	cancer, carcinoma
ED	emergency department
ENT	ear, nose, and throat
ER	emergency room
GP	general practitioner
GYN, Gyn, gyn	gynecology
ICU	intensive care unit
OB	obstetrics

Chapter 3

ECG, EKG	electrocardiogram
EEG	electroencephalogram
UV	ultraviolet

Chapter 4

AMA	American Medical Association
BP	blood pressure
CPT	Current Procedural Terminology
CT, CAT	computed tomography, computerized (computed) axial tomography
Dx	diagnosis
ICD	International Classification of Diseases
mm Hg	millimeters of mercury
MRI	magnetic resonance imaging
OD	overdose (also right eye)
OTC	over-the-counter (drug)
P	pulse
PET	positron emission tomography

R	respirations
Sx	symptoms
T	temperature
WHO	World Health Organization
WNL	within normal limits

Chapter 5

AIDS	acquired immunodeficiency syndrome
AP	anteroposterior
CBC, cbc	complete blood count
CDC	Centers for Disease Control and Prevention
CSF	cerebrospinal fluid
DNA	deoxyribonucleic acid
FEMA	Federal Emergency Management Agency
HIV	human immunodeficiency virus
HPF	high-power field
IV	intravenous
LLQ	left lower quadrant
LPF	low-power field
LUQ	left upper quadrant
PA	physician assistant; posteroanterior
RBC	red blood cell, red blood cell count
RLQ	right lower quadrant
RUQ	right upper quadrant
SOB	shortness of breath
STD	sexually transmitted disease
STI	sexually transmitted infection
WBC	white blood cell, white blood cell count
WMD	weapons of mass destruction

PART TWO

Chapter 6

BMT	bone marrow transplant
C1 … C7	first cervical vertebra … seventh cervical vertebra
COX-2	cyclooxygenase inhibitors
DJD	degenerative joint disease
DMARD	disease-modifying antirheumatic drug
fx	fracture
L1 … L5	first lumbar vertebra … fifth lumbar vertebra
LE	lupus erythematosus
NSAID	nonsteroidal antiinflammatory drug
RA	rheumatoid arthritis; right atrium
ROM	range of motion
T1 … T12	first thoracic vertebra … twelfth thoracic vertebra
WBC	white blood cell, white blood cell count

Chapter 7

ASD	atrial septal defect
AV, A-V	atrioventricular (also arteriovenous)
CABG	coronary artery bypass graft
CAD	coronary artery disease
CHD	coronary heart disease
CHF	congestive heart failure
CPR	cardiopulmonary resuscitation
CVA	cerebrovascular accident
echo	echocardiography
ICD	implantable cardioverter defibrillation
MI, AMI	myocardial infarction (acute MI)
SA	sinoatrial
T&A	tonsillectomy and adenoidectomy
VSD	ventricular septal defect

Chapter 8

ARDS	adult respiratory distress syndrome; acute respiratory distress syndrome
CAL	chronic airflow limitation
COLD	chronic obstructive lung disease
COPD	chronic obstructive pulmonary disease
LRT	lower respiratory tract
SARS	severe acute respiratory syndrome
SIDS	sudden infant death syndrome
SOB	shortness of breath
TB	tuberculosis
URT	upper respiratory tract
VC	vital capacity

Chapter 9

DM	diabetes mellitus
ERCP	endoscopic retrograde cholangiopancreatography
GERD	gastroesophageal reflux disease
GI	gastrointestinal
IBS	inflammatory bowel syndrome

LGI	lower gastrointestinal tract
UGI	upper gastrointestinal tract

Chapter 10

ADH	antidiuretic hormone
ARF	acute renal failure
BUN	blood urea nitrogen
ESWL	extracorporeal shock wave lithotripsy
IVP	intravenous pyelogram
IVU	intravenous urography
pH	hydrogen ion concentration, "potential" hydrogen
TUR	transurethral resection
TURP	transurethral resection of the prostate
U/A, UA	urinalysis
UTI	urinary tract infection

Chapter 11

AIDS	acquired immunodeficiency syndrome
BPH	benign prostatic hyperplasia
C-section	cesarean section
D&C	dilation and curettage
EDD	expected delivery date
FDA	U.S. Food and Drug Administration
GC	gonococcus
GU	genitourinary
HBV	hepatitis B virus
HCV	hepatitis C virus
HCG, hCG	human chorionic gonadotropin
HDV	hepatitis D virus
HIV	human immunodeficiency virus
HPV	human papillomavirus
HRT	hormone replacement therapy
HSV-2	herpes simplex virus type 2 (genital herpes)
IUD	intrauterine device
IVF	in vitro fertilization
LMP	last menstrual period
OCs	oral contraceptives
Pap	Papanicolaou smear, stain, or test
PID	pelvic inflammatory disease
PMS	premenstrual syndrome
PSA	prostate-specific antigen
STD	sexually transmitted disease
STI	sexually transmitted infection
TUMT	transurethral microwave thermotherapy
TUNA	transurethral needle ablation
TURP	transurethral resection of the prostate

Chapter 12

Bx, bx	biopsy
DLE	discoid lupus erythematosus
HSV	herpes simplex virus
TBSA	total body surface area

Chapter 13

ADD	attention deficit disorder
ADHD	attention deficit–hyperactivity disorder
CNS	central nervous system
CSF	cerebrospinal fluid
CVA	cerebrovascular accident; costovertebral angle
DSM	Diagnostic and Statistical Manual of Mental Disorders
IAD	illness anxiety disorder
OCD	obsessive-compulsive disorder
PNS	peripheral nervous system
TENS	transcutaneous electrical nerve stimulation
TIA	transient ischemic attack

Chapter 14

dB	decibel
LASIK	laser-assisted in situ keratomileusis
PNS	peripheral nervous system

Chapter 15

ADH	antidiuretic hormone
BMT	bone marrow transplant
DM	diabetes mellitus
GH	growth hormone
HPV	human papillomavirus
LINAC	linear accelerator

B. Finding Medical Abbreviations

acquired immunodeficiency syndrome	AIDS	decibel	dB
acute myocardial infarction	AMI	degenerative joint disease	DJD
acute renal failure	ARF	deoxyribonucleic acid	DNA
adult respiratory distress syndrome	ARDS	diabetes mellitus	DM
anteroposterior	AP	diagnosis	Dx
antidiuretic hormone	ADH	Diagnostic and Statistical Manual of Mental Disorders	DSM
atrial septal defect	ASD		
atrioventricular	AV, A-V	dilation and curettage	D&C
attention deficit disorder	ADD	discoid lupus erythematosus	DLE
attention deficit-hyperactivity disorder	ADHD	disease-modifying antirheumatic drug	DMARD
benign prostatic hyperplasia	BPH	ear, nose, and throat	ENT
biopsy	Bx, bx	echocardiography	ECHO, echo
blood pressure	BP		
blood urea nitrogen	BUN	electrocardiogram	ECG, EKG
bone marrow transplant	BMT	electroencephalogram	EEG
cancer	CA	emergency department	ED
carcinoma	CA	emergency room	ER
cardiopulmonary resuscitation	CPR	endoscopic retrograde cholangiopancreatography	ERCP
Centers for Disease Control and Prevention	CDC		
		expected delivery date	EDD
central nervous system	CNS	extracorporeal shock wave lithotripsy	ESWL
cerebrospinal fluid	CSF	Federal Emergency Management Agency	FEMA
cerebrovascular accident	CVA	fracture	fx
cervical vertebrae	C1-C7	gastroesophageal reflux disease	GERD
cesarean section	C-section	gastrointestinal	GI
chronic airflow limitation	CAL	general practitioner	GP
chronic obstructive lung disease	COLD	genitourinary	GU
chronic obstructive pulmonary disease	COPD	gonococcus	GC
complete blood count	CBC, cbc	growth hormone	GH
computed tomography, computerized (computed) axial tomography	CT, CAT	gynecology	Gyn
		hepatitis B virus	HBV
congestive heart failure	CHF	hepatitis C virus	HCV
coronary artery bypass graft	CABG	hepatitis D virus	HDV
coronary artery disease	CAD	herpes simplex virus	HSV
coronary heart disease	CHD	herpes simplex virus type 2 (genital herpes)	HSV-2
costovertebral angle	CVA	high-power field	HPF
cyclooxygenase inhibitors	COX-2	hormone replacement therapy	HRT

human chorionic gonadotropin	HCG, hCG	prostate-specific antigen	PSA
human immunodeficiency virus	HIV	pulse	P
human papillomavirus	HPV	range of motion	ROM
illness anxiety disorder	IAD	red blood cell, red blood cell count	RBC
in vitro fertilization	IVF	respiration	R
inflammatory bowel syndrome	IBS	rheumatoid arthritis	RA
intensive care unit	ICU	right atrium	RA
intrauterine device	IUD	right lower quadrant	RLQ
intravenous	IV	right upper quadrant	RUQ
intravenous pyelogram	IVP	severe acute respiratory syndrome	SARS
intravenous urography	IVU	sexually transmitted disease	STD
laser-assisted in situ keratomileusis	LASIK	sexually transmitted infection	STI
last menstrual period	LMP	shortness of breath	SOB
left atrium	LA	sinoatrial	SA
left lower quadrant	LLQ	sudden infant death syndrome	SIDS
left upper quadrant	LUQ	symptoms	Sx
linear accelerator	LINAC	temperature	T
low-power field	LPF	thoracic vertebrae	T1-T12
lower gastrointestinal tract	LGI	tonsillectomy and adenoidectomy	T&A
lower respiratory tract	LRT	total body surface area	TBSA
lumbar vertebrae	L1-L5	transcutaneous electrical nerve stimulation	TENS
lupus erythematosus	LE	transient ischemic attack	TIA
magnetic resonance imaging	MRI	transurethral microwave thermotherapy	TUMT
millimeters of mercury	mm Hg	transurethral needle ablation	TUNA
myocardial infarction	MI	transurethral resection	TUR
nonsteroidal antiinflammatory drug	NSAID	transurethral resection of the prostate	TURP
obsessive-compulsive disorder	OCD	tuberculosis	TB
obstetrics	OB	ultraviolet	UV
overdose	OD	upper gastrointestinal tract	UGI
oral contraceptives	OCs	upper respiratory tract	URT
over the counter (drug)	OTC	urinalysis	UA, U/A
Papanicolaou smear, stain, or test	Pap	urinary tract infection	UTI
pelvic inflammatory disease	PID	U.S. Food and Drug Administration	FDA
peripheral nervous system	PNS	ventricular septal defect	VSD
positron emission tomography	PET	vital capacity	VC
posteroanterior; physician assistant	PA	weapons of mass destruction	WMD
"potential" hydrogen, hydrogen ion concentration	pH	white blood cell, white blood cell count	WBC
		within normal limits	WNL
premenstrual syndrome	PMS	World Health Organization	WHO

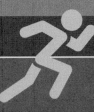

Word Parts

A. Alphabetized Word Parts and Meanings

Word Parts	Meaning	Word Parts	Meaning
a-	no, not, without	-ation	action or process
ab-	away from	audi/o	hearing
abdomin/o	abdomen	auro, auricul/o, o/to	ear
-able, -ible	capable of, able to	aut/o	self
-ac, -al, -an, -ar, -ary	pertaining to	axill/o	axilla (armpit)
acoust/o	hearing	bacter/i, bacteri/o	bacteria
acr/o	extremities (arms and legs)	bi-	two
ad-	toward	bil/i	bile
aden/o	gland	bi/o	life or living
adenoid/o	adenoids	blast/o	embryonic form
adip/o	fat	blephar/o	eyelid
adren/o	adrenal glands	brady-	slow
aer/o	air	bronch/o, bronchi/o	bronchi
agora-	open marketplace	bronchiol/o	bronchiole
alb/o, albin/o	white	burs/o	bursa
albumin/o	albumin	calcane/o	calcaneus (heel bone)
algesi/o	sensitivity to pain	calc/i	calcium
-algia	pain	cancer/o, carcin/o	cancer
alveol/o	alveolus	cardi/o	heart
amni/o	amnion	carp/o	carpus (wrist)
amyl/o	starch	caud/o	tail, in a posterior direction
an-	no, not, without	cec/o	cecum
ana-	upward, excessive, or again	-cele	hernia
an/o	anus	cellul/o	little cell or compartment
andr/o	male, masculine	-centesis	surgical puncture
angi/o, vascul/o	vessel	centi-	one hundred or one-hundredth
ankyl/o	stiff	cephal/o	head, toward the head
ante-	before	cerebell/o	cerebellum
anter/o	anterior, toward the front	cerebr/o	brain, cerebrum
anti-	against	cerumin/o	cerumen
aort/o	aorta	cervic/o	neck, uterine cervix
append/o, appendic/o	appendix	cheil/o	lips
arachn/o	spider	chem/o	chemical
arter/o, arteri/o	artery	chir/o	hand
arteriol/o	articulation, joint	chlor/o	green
arthr/o	joint	chol/e	bile
-ase	enzyme	cholecyst/o	gallbladder
-asthenia	weakness	choledoch/o	common bile duct
atel/o	imperfect	chondr/o	cartilage
ather/o	yellow fatty plaque	choroid/o	choroid

Word Parts	Meaning	Word Parts	Meaning
chrom/o	color	encephal/o	brain
-cidal	killing	end-, endo-	inside
circum-	around	enter/o	intestines, small intestine
cirrh/o	orange-yellow	epi-	above or upon (on)
claustr/o	barrier, closed space	epiglott/o	epiglottis
clavicul/o	clavicle (collarbone)	-er	one who
coccyg/o	coccyx	erythemat/o	erythema or redness
cochle/o	cochlea	erythr/o	red
col/o, colon/o	colon or large intestine	-esis	action, process, or result of
colp/o	vagina	esophag/o	esophagus
coni/o	dust	-esthesia	sensation, perception
conjunctiv/o	conjunctiva	esthesi/o	feeling
contra-	against	eu-	normal, good
corne/o	cornea	-eum, -ium	membrane
corpor/o	body	ex-, exo-	outside, without, away from
cost/o	rib	extern/o	external, outside
crani/o	cranium, skull	extra-	outside
crin/o, -crine	secrete	faci/o	face
cry/o	cold	femor/o	femur (thigh bone)
crypt/o	hidden	fet/o	fetus
cutane/o	skin	fibr/o	fiber
cyan/o	blue	fibul/o	fibula
cyst/o	cyst, bladder, sac	fluor/o	emitting or reflecting light
cyt/o, -cyte	cell	follicul/o	follicle
dacry/o	tear, tearing, crying	gastr/o	stomach
dactyl/o	digit (toe, finger, or both)	gen/o, -gen	beginning, origin
de-	down, from, removing, reversing	-genesis	producing, forming
dendr/o	tree	-genic	produced by or in
dent/i, dent/o	teeth	genit/o	genitals
-derm	skin or a germ layer	ger/a, ger/o, geront/o	aged, elderly
derm/a, dermat/o, derm/o, -derm	skin	gigant/o	giant
		gingiv/o	gums
di-	two	gli/o	neuroglia or sticky substance
dia-	through	glomerul/o	glomerulus
diplo-	double	gloss/o	tongue
dips/o	thirst	glyc/o, glycos/o	sugar
dist/o	far or distant from the origin or point of attachment	gon/o	genitals, reproduction
		gonad/o	gonad
dors/o	directed toward or situated on the back side	gram/o	to record
		-gram	a record
duoden/o	duodenum	-graph	recording instrument
dur/o	dura mater	-graphy	process of recording
-dynia	pain	gynec/o	female
dys-	"bad," difficult	hem/a, hem/o, hemat/o	blood
-eal	pertaining to	hemi-	half, partly
ech/o	sound	hepat/o	liver
-ectasia, -ectasis	dilation, stretching	herni/o	hernia
ecto-	outside, without, away from	hidr/o	perspiration
-ectomy	excision	hist/o	tissue
-edema	swelling	home/o	sameness
electr/o	electricity	humer/o	humerus
embol/o	embolus	hydr/o	water
-emesis	vomiting	hyper-	excessive, more than normal
-emia	blood	hypo-	beneath or below normal
en-	inside	hypophys/o	pituitary (hypophysis)

Word Parts	Meaning	Word Parts	Meaning
hyster/o	uterus	macro-	large
-ia, -iasis	condition	mal-	"bad," poor, abnormal
-iac	one who suffers	malac/o	soft, softening
-iatrician	practitioner	-malacia	softening
-iatrics, -iatric, -iatry	medicine	mamm/o, mast/o	breast
-ic	pertaining to	-mania	excessive preoccupation
ichthy/o	fish	mechan/o	mechanical
ile/o	ileum	medio-	middle or nearer the middle
ili/o	ilium	megal/o, mega-	enlargement
immun/o	immune	-megaly	large, enlarged
in-	not, inside, in	melan/o	black
infer/o	lowermost, below	men/o	month
infra-	below	mening/o	meninges
insulin/o	insulin	ment/o	mind, chin
inter-	between	meso-	middle
intern/o	internal	meta-	change or next in a series
intestin/o	intestines	metacarp/o	metacarpals
intra-	within	metatars/o	metatarsals
iod/o	iodine	-meter	instrument used to measure
ir/o, irid/o	iris	metr/i	uterine tissue
ischi/o	ischium	metr/o	measure, uterine tissue
-ism	condition, theory	-metry	process of measuring
-ist	one who	micro-	small
-itis	inflammation	mid-	middle
-ium	membrane	milli-	one thousand or one-thousandth
-ive	pertaining to	mono-	one or single
jejun/o	jejunum	muc/o	mucus
kerat/o	hard or horny tissue, cornea	multi-	many
kinesi/o, -kinesia, -kinesis	movement, motion	muscul/o	muscle
lacrim/o	tear, tearing, crying	my/o	muscle
lact/o	milk	myc/o	fungus
lapar/o	abdominal wall	myel/o	bone marrow, spinal cord
laryng/o	larynx	myring/o	eardrum
later/o	toward the side, farther from the midline of the body or a structure	myx/o	mucus
		narc/o	stupor
		nas/o	nose
leps/o, -lepsy	seizure	nat/i, nat/o	birth
leuc/o, leuk/o	white	ne/o	new
-lexia	words, phrases	necr/o	dead, death
lingu/o	tongue	nephr/o	kidney
lip/o	fat, lipid	nerv/o, neur/o	nerve
lith/o, -lith	stone, calculus	noc/i	cause harm, injury, or pain
lob/o	lobe	non-	not
log/o	knowledge, words	nulli-	none
-logic, -logical	pertaining to the science or study of	obstetr/o	midwife
		ocul/o	eye
-logist	one who studies, specialist	odont/o	teeth
-logy	study or science of	-oid	resembling
lumb/o	lower back	-ole	little
lymph/o	lymph, lymphatics	olig/o	few
lymphat/o	lymphatics	-oma	tumor (occasionally, swelling)
lys/o	destruction, dissolving	omphal/o	umbilicus (navel)
-lysin	that which destroys	-on	body
-lysis	dissolving, destruction, freeing	onc/o	tumor
-lytic	capable of destroying	onych/o	nail

Word Parts	Meaning	Word Parts	Meaning
oophor/o	ovary	pleur/o	pleura
ophthalm/o	eye	-poiesis	production
-opia	vision	-poietin	substance that causes production
optic/o, opt/o	vision	poly-	many
or/o	mouth	post-	after, behind
orchi/o, orchid/o	testes	poster/o	posterior toward the back, situated behind
-orexia	appetite		
orth/o	straight	-pnea	breathing
-ory	pertaining to	pneum/o	lung, air
-ose	sugar	pneumon/o	lung
-osis	condition	pre-	before
-osmia	sense of smell	presby/o	old or old age
oste/o	bone	primi-	first
ot/o	ear	pro-	before
-ous	pertaining to, characterized by	proct/o	anus, rectum
ovar/o	ovary	prostat/o	prostate
ox/o	oxygen	prote/o, protein/o	protein
pan-	all	proxim/o	nearer the origin or point of attachment
pancreat/o	pancreas		
par/o	to bear offspring	pseud/o	false
para-	near, beside, abnormal	psych/o	mind
-para	female who has given birth	-ptosis	sagging, prolapse
parathyroid/o	parathyroids	pub/o	pubis
patell/o	patella (kneecap)	pulm/o, pulmon/o	lung
path/o	disease	pupill/o	pupil
-pathy	disease	py/o	pus
ped/o	child, foot	pyel/o	renal pelvis
pelv/i	pelvis	pyr/o	fire
pen/o	penis (occasionally, punishment)	quad-, quadri-	four
-penia	deficiency	rach/i, rachi/o	spine
-pepsia	digestion	radi/o	radius, radiant energy
per-	through, by	rect/o	rectum
peri-	around	ren/o	kidney
periton/o	peritoneum	retin/o	retina
-pexy	surgical fixation	retro-	behind, backward
phag/o, -phagia, -phagic, -phagy	eating, swallowing, ingesting	rheumat/o	rheumatism
		rhin/o	nose
phalang/o	phalanges (bones of fingers or toes)	roentgen/o	x-ray
		-rrhage	excessive bleeding
pharmac/o, pharmaceut/i	drugs, medicine	-rrhagia	hemorrhage
pharyng/o	pharynx	-rrhaphy	suture
phas/o, -phasia	speech	-rrhea	flow, discharge
phleb/o	vein	-rrhexis	rupture
-phobia	abnormal fear	sacr/o	sacrum
phon/o	voice	salping/o	uterine tube or eustachian tube
phot/o	light	-sarcoma	malignant tumor arising from connective tissue
phren/o	mind, diaphragm		
physi/o	nature	scapul/o	scapula (shoulder blade)
-physis	growth	schis/o, schiz/o, schist/o, -schisis	split, cleft
pil/o	hair		
pituitar/o	pituitary	scler/o, -sclerosis	hard, hardening
-plasia	development or formation of tissue	scop/o	to examine, to view
plast/o	repair	-scope	instrument used for viewing
-plasty	surgical repair	-scopy	process of visually examining
pleg/o, -plegia	paralysis	scrot/o	scrotum

Word Parts	Meaning	Word Parts	Meaning
seb/o	sebum	-tome	instrument used for cutting
semi-	half, partly	-tomy	incision
semin/o	semen	ton/o	tone or tension
seps/o	infection	tonsill/o	tonsil
sept/o	infection or septum	top/o	place, position
ser/o	serum	tox/o, toxic/o	poison
sial/o	saliva, salivary gland	trache/o	trachea (windpipe)
sigmoid/o	sigmoid colon	trans-	across, through
silic/o	silica	tri-	three
som/a, somat/o	body	trich/o	hair
son/o	sound	-tripsy	surgical crushing
-spasm	twitching, cramp	troph/o, -trophic, -trophy	nutrition
spermat/o	sperm	-tropic	stimulate
spin/o	spine	-tropin	that which stimulates
spir/o	spiral, to breathe	tympan/o	eardrum
splen/o	spleen	uln/o	ulna
spondyl/o	vertebra	ultra-	beyond, excess
-stasis	stopping, controlling	ungu/o	nail
-static	keeping stationary	uni-	one, single
stern/o	sternum (breastbone)	ur/o	urine, urinary tract
stomat/o	mouth	ureter/o	ureter
-stomy	formation of an opening	urethr/o	urethra
sub-	under	-uria	urine, urination
super-	excessive or above	urin/o	urine or urination
supra-	above, beyond	uter/o	uterus
super/o	uppermost, above	vag/o	vagus nerve
sym-, syn-	joined, together	vagin/o	vagina
tachy-	fast	vas/o	vessel, ductus deferens
tars/o	tarsals (ankle bones)	vascul/o	vessel
ten/o, tend/o, tendin/o	tendon	ven/o	vein
test/o, testicul/o	testicle, testis	ventr/o	ventral or belly side
tetra-	four	venul/o	venule
therapeut/o, -therapy	treatment	vertebr/o	vertebra
therm/o	heat	vesic/o	bladder or vesicle
thorac/o	thorax, chest	viscer/o	viscera
thromb/o	thrombus, clot	vulv/o	vulva
thyr/o, thyroid/o	thyroid gland	xanth/o	yellow
tibi/o	tibia	xer/o	dry
-tic	pertaining to	-y	state, condition
tom/o	to cut	zo/o	animal

B. English Terms and Corresponding Word Parts

English Term(s)	Word Parts	English Term(s)	Word Parts
abdomen	abdomin/o	again	ana-
abdominal wall	lapar/o	against	anti-, contra-
abnormal	mal-, para-	aged	ger/a, ger/o, geront/o
above	epi-, super-, supra-	air	aer/o, pneum/o
across	trans-	air sac	alveol/o
action	-ation, -esis	all	pan-
adenoids	adenoid/o	alveolus	alveol/o
adrenal glands	adren/o	amnion	amni/o
after	post-	animal	zo/o

English Term(s)	Word Parts	English Term(s)	Word Parts
ankle bone	tars/o	cerebellum	cerebell/o
anus	an/o	cerebrum	cerebr/o
anus and rectum	proct/o	cerumen	cerumin/o
aorta	aort/o	cervix uteri	cervic/o
appendix	append/o, appendic/o	chemical	chem/o
armpit	axill/o	chest	thorac/o
arms and legs	acr/o	child	ped/o
around	circum-, peri-	chin	ment/o
arteriole	arteriol/o	choroid	choroid/o
artery	arter/o, arteri/o	clavicle	clavicul/o
articulation	arthr/o	closed space, barrier	claustr/o
away from	ab-, ex-	clot (thrombus)	thromb/o
back	dors/o	coccyx	coccyg/o
backward	retr/o	cochlea	cochle/o
bacteria	bacter/i, bacteri/o	cold	cry/o
"bad" (difficult, poor)	dys-, mal-	collarbone	clavicul/o
before	ante-, pre-, pro-	colon	col/o, colon/o
beginning	gen/o, -gen, -genic, -genesis, -genous	color	chrom/o
		common bile duct	choledoch/o
behind	poster/o, post-, retro-	condition	-ia, -iasis, -osis, -y
belly side	ventr/o	conjunctiva	conjunctiv/o
below or beneath	hypo-, sub-, infra-	constant	home/o
below normal	hypo-	controlling	-stasis
beside	par-, para-	cornea	kerat/o, corne/o
between	inter-	cramp	-spasm
beyond	supra-	cranium	crani/o
bile	bil/i, chol/e	cut (to cut)	tom/o
birth	nat/i, nat/o	incision or cutting	-tomy
birth (give birth)	par/o	instrument used to cut	-tome
woman who has given birth	para-	cyst	cyst/o
		death	necr/o
black	melan/o	decreased or deficient	-penia
bladder	cyst/o	destruction	lys/o
blood	hem/a, hem/o, hemat/o, -emia	that which destroys	-lysin
blue	cyan/o	process of destroying	-lysis
body	corpor/o, som/a, somat/o	capable of destroying	-lytic
bone	oste/o	development	-plasia
bone marrow	myel/o	diaphragm	phren/o
brain	cerebr/o, encephal/o	difficult	dys-
breast	mamm/o, mast/o	digestion	-pepsia
breastbone	stern/o	digit	dactyl/o
breathing	-pnea	dilation	-ectasia, -ectasis
bronchi	bronch/o, bronchi/o	discharge	-rrhea
bronchiole	bronchiol/o	disease	path/o, -osis, -pathy
bursa	burs/o	dissolving	lys/o
calcaneus	calcane/o	distant	dist/o
calcium	calc/i	double	diplo-
calculus	lith/o, -lith	down	de-
cancer	cancer/o, carcin/o	drooping	-ptosis
carpus	carp/o	drugs	pharmac/o, pharmaceut/i
cartilage	chondr/o	dry	xer/o
cause harm, injury, or pain	noc/i	duct	vas/o
cecum	cec/o	ductus deferens	vas/o
cell	cyt/o, -cyte	duodenum	duoden/o
compartment or little cell	cellul/o	dura mater	dur/o

English Term(s)	Word Parts
dust	coni/o
ear	ot/o, aur/o, auricul/o
eardrum	myring/o, tympan/o
eat	phag/o
elderly	ger/a, ger/o, geront/o
electricity	electr/o
embolus	embol/o
embryonic form	-blast, blast/o
emitting or reflecting light	fluor/o
enzyme	-ase
epiglottis	epiglott/o
esophagus	esophag/o
eustachian tube	salping/o
examine	scop/o
instrument used	-scope
process of examining	-scopy
excessive	hyper-, super-, ana-
excision	-ectomy
extremities	acr/o
eye	ophthalm/o, ocul/o
eyelid	blephar/o
face	faci/o
false	pseud/o
far	dist/o
fast	tachy-
fat	adip/o, lip/o
fear (abnormal)	-phobia
feeling	esthesi/o
female	gynec/o
femur	femor/o
fetus	fet/o
few	olig/o
fiber, fibrous	fibr/o
fibula	fibul/o
fingers or toes	dactyl/o
fire	pyr/o
first	primi-
fish	ichthy/o
flow	-rrhea
follicle	follicul/o
for	pro-
formation of an opening	-stomy
formation of tissue	-plasia
four	quadri-, tetra-
from	de-
front	anter/o
fungus	myc/o
gall	chol/e
gallbladder	cholecyst/o
giant	gigant/o
gland	aden/o
glomerulus	glomerul/o
gonad	gonad/o
good	eu-
green	chlor/o

English Term(s)	Word Parts
growth	-physis
gums	gingiv/o
hair	pil/o, trich/o
half	hemi-, semi
hand	chir/o
hard, hardening	scler/o, kerat/o
head	cephal/o
hearing	audi/o, acoust/o
heart	cardi/o
heat	therm/o
hemorrhage	-rrhagia
hernia	-cele, herni/o
hidden	crypt/o
horny tissue	kerat/o
humerus	humer/o
ileum	ile/o
ilium	ili/o
immune	immun/o
incision	tom/o, -tomy
instrument used	-tome
increase	-osis
infection	seps/o, sept/o
inferior	infer/o
inflammation	-itis
ingest	phag/o, -phagia, -phagic, -phagy
inside	in-, en-, end-, endo-
insulin	insulin/o
intestine	enter/o, intestin/o
iodine	iod/o
iris	ir/o, irid/o
ischium	ischi/o
jejunum	jejun/o
joined or together	sym-, syn-
joint	arthr/o
keeping stationary	-static
kidney	nephr/o, ren/o
killing	-cidal
kneecap	patell/o
large	gigant/o, macro-, megalo-, -megaly
large intestine	col/o
larynx	laryng/o
life or living	bi/o
light	phot/o
lip	cheil/o
liver	hepat/o
location	top/o
lower back	lumb/o
lung	pneum/o, pneumon/o, pulm/o, pulmon/o
lymph	lymph/o
lymphatics	lymph/o, lymphat/o
male, masculine	andr/o
malignant tumor	-sarcoma
many	multi-, poly-

English Term(s)	Word Parts
marketplace	agora-
measure	metr/o
instrument used	-meter
process	-metry
mechanical	mechan/o
medicine	-iatrics, -iatric, -iatry, pharmac/o
membrane	-eum, -ium
meninges	mening/o
middle	medi/o, meso-, mid-
midwife	obstetr/o
milk	lact/o
mind	ment/o, phren/o, psych/o
month	men/o
more than normal	hyper-
mouth	or/o, stomat/o
movement	kinesi/o
mucus	muc/o, myx/o
muscle	muscul/o, my/o
nail	onych/o, ungu/o
narrowing	-stenosis
nature	physi/o
near	par-, para-, proxim/o
neck	cervic/o
nerve	nerv/o, neur/o
neuroglia	gli/o
new	ne/o
new opening	-stomy
no	a-, an-
none	nulli-
normal	norm/o, eu-
nose	nas/o, rhin/o
not	a-, an-, in-, non-
nutrition	troph/o, -trophy
obsessive preoccupation	-mania
old, elderly	ger/o, geront/o
old or old age	presby/o
one	uni-, mono-
one hundred, one-hundredth	centi-
one-thousandth	milli-
one who	-er, -ist
one who studies	-logist
orange-yellow	cirrh/o
organs of reproduction	genit/o, gon/o
origin	gen/o, -gen, -genic, -genesis
outside	ecto-, ex-, exo-, extra-
ovary	oophor/o
oxygen	ox/o
pain	-algia, -dynia
painful	dys-
pancreas	pancreat/o
paralysis	pleg/o, -plegia
parathyroids	parathyroid/o
patella (kneecap)	patell/o
pelvis	pelv/i
perception	-esthesi/o, -esthesia

English Term(s)	Word Parts
peritoneum	periton/o
perspiration	hidr/o
pertaining to	-ac, -al, -an, -ar, -ary, -eal, -ic, -ive, -ory, -ous, -tic
pertaining to the science or study of	-logic, -logical
phalanges	phalang/o
pharynx	pharyng/o
phrases	-lexia
pituitary	pituitar/o, hypophys/o
place (position)	top/o
pleura	pleur/o
poison	tox/o, toxic/o
practitioner	-iatrician
preoccupation (excessive)	-mania
process	-ation, -esis
production	-poiesis
prolapse	-ptosis
prostate gland	prostat/o
protein	prote/o, protein/o
pubis	pub/o
pupil	pupil/o
pus	py/o
radiant energy	radi/o
radius	radi/o
record (to record)	gram/o
process of recording	-graphy
the record	-gram
recording instrument	-graph
rectum	rect/o
red	erythr/o
redness	erythemat/o
removal	-ectomy
renal pelvis	pyel/o
repair	plast/o
reproduction	gon/o
resembling	-oid
result of	-esis
retina	retin/o
reversing	de-
rheumatism	rheumat/o
ribs	cost/o
rupture	-rrhexis
sac	cyst/o
sacrum	sacr/o
sag	-ptosis
saliva, salivary glands	sial/o
sameness	home/o
scapula (shoulder blade)	scapul/o
sebum	seb/o
secrete	crin/o, -crine
seizure	-lepsy
self	aut/o
semen	semin/o
sensation	esthesi/o, -esthesia
sense of smell	-osmia

English Term(s)	Word Parts
sensitivity to pain	algesi/o
septum	sept/o
shoulder blade	scapul/o
side	later/o
sigmoid colon	sigmoid/o
single	mono-
situated above	super/o, super-, supra-
situated below	infer/o, infra-
skin	cutane/o, derm/a, dermat/o, derm/o, -derm
skull	crani/o
slow	brady-
small	micro-, -ole
small intestine	enter/o
smell	-osmia
soft, softening	malac/o, -malacia
sound	ech/o, son/o
specialist	-ist
speech	phas/o
sperm, spermatozoa	spermat/o
spider	arachn/o
spinal cord	myel/o
spine	rach/i, rachi/o, spin/o, spondyl/o
spleen	splen/o
split	schis/o, schiz/o, -schisis, schist/o
starch	amyl/o
sternum (breastbone)	stern/o
sticky substance	gli/o
stimulate	-tropic
stomach	gastr/o
stone	lith/o, -lith
stopping	-stasis
straight	orth/o
stretching	-ectasia, -ectasis
study or science of	-logy
stupor	narc/o
substance that causes production	-poietin
sugar	glyc/o, glycos/o, -ose
surgical crushing	-tripsy
surgical fixation	pex/o, -pexy
surgical puncture	-centesis
surgical repair	-plasty
suture	-rrhaphy
sweat	hidr/o
swelling	-edema
tail	caud/o
tailbone	coccyg/o
tarsals (ankle bones)	tars/o
tear (crying)	dacry/o, lacrim/o
teeth	dent/i, dent/o, odont/o
tendon	ten/o, tend/o
testis, testicle	orchi/o, orchid/o, test/o, testicul/o
that which stimulates	-tropin
thirst	dips/o
thorax	thorac/o

English Term(s)	Word Parts
three	tri-
throat	pharyng/o
thrombus	thromb/o
through	dia-, trans-
thyroid gland	thyr/o, thyroid/o
tibia	tibi/o
tissue	hist/o
to cut	tom/o
tone or tension	ton/o
tongue	gloss/o, lingu/o
tonsil	tonsill/o
toward	ad-
trachea	trache/o
treatment	therapeut/o, -therapy
tree	dendr/o
tumor	onc/o, -oma
twice	di-
twitching	-spasm
two	bi-, di-
ulna	uln/o
umbilicus	omphal/o
under	sub-
upon (on)	epi-
uppermost	super/o
upward	ana-
ureter	ureter/o
urethra	urethr/o
urinary tract	ur/o
urination	urin/o
urine	ur/o, urin/o
uterine tissue	metr/o
uterine tube	salping/o
uterus	hyster/o, uter/o
vagina	colp/o, vagin/o
vagus nerve	vag/o
vein	phleb/o, ven/o
ventral	ventr/o
venule	venul/o
vertebra	spondyl/o, vertebr/o
vessel	angi/o, vas/o, vascul/o
viscera	viscer/o
vision	opt/o, optic/o, -opia, ocul/o
voice	phon/o
vomiting	-emesis
vulva	vulv/o
water	hydr/o
weakness	-asthenia
white	alb/o, albin/o, leuk/o
windpipe	trache/o
within	intra-
without	a-, an-, ex-
words	-lexia
wrist bone	carp/o
x-ray	roentgen/o
yellow	xanth/o
yellow fatty plaque	ather/o

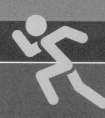

Answers

PART ONE

Chapter 1

Exercises

1.
1. CF
2. CF
3. CF
4. WR
5. CF
6. WR

2.
1. P
2. S
3. P
4. S
5. CF
6. S
7. P
8. CF
9. S

3.
1. P
2. S
3. S
4. S
5. P
6. S
7. P
8. P
9. P

4.
1. trich/o, pil/o
2. ocul/o, ophthalm/o
3. nas/o, rhin/o
4. or/o, stomat/o
5. thorac/o

5.
1. otic
2. otitis
3. otology
4. otoplasty
5. otorrhea
6. ototomy

6.
1. dyspnea
2. enteric
3. eupepsia
4. tonsillitis

5. uremia
6. antianxiety
7. leukocyte
8. appendicitis
9. hyperemia
10. endocardial

7.
1. Alzheimer disease
2. Beckman thermometer
3. cesarean section
4. Foley catheter
5. Holter monitor
6. Alzheimer disease
7. Heimlich maneuver
8. Lyme disease
9. Parkinson syndrome
10. Wilms' tumor

8.
1. A
2. A
3. B
4. A
5. B

9.
1. alveoli
2. appendices
3. atria
4. bacilli
5. carcinomas
6. diagnoses
7. larynges
8. prognoses
9. protozoa
10. varices

10.
1. prefix
2. suffix
3. Holter monitor
4. ED, OP

11.
1. three
2. ek
3. kos
4. six
5. net

Self-Test

A.
1. C
2. C
3. B
4. C
5. B
6. C
7. A
8. A
9. B
10. C
11. B
12. C
13. B
14. C
15. B
16. C
17. C
18. C
19. B
20. A

B.
1. C
2. B
3. A
4. B
5. A

C.
1. A
2. A
3. B
4. B
5. A
6. A
7. B
8. A

D.
1. hypodermic
2. leukemia
3. melanoid
4. myocardial
5. thrombosis
6. dyspnea
7. antiserum

8. hyperemia
9. hyperpnea
10. psychosis

E.
1. appendixes or appendices
2. bronchi
3. ilea
4. pharynges
5. prognoses
6. alveoli
7. bacteria
8. psychoses
9. vertebrae
10. varices

F.
1. alveolus
2. appendix
3. atrium
4. bacillus
5. cortex
6. diagnosis
7. phalanx
8. protozoon
9. septum
10. vertebra

G.
1. Prognosis should be prognoses.
2. Bacterium should be bacteria.
3. The last "atrium" should be atria.
4. The second "spermatozoa" should be spermatozoon.
5. The second "phalanx" should be phalanges.
6. Phalanx should be phalanges.
7. The 2nd patella should be patellae.

8. Vertebra should be vertebrae.
9. Eponyms should be eponym.

10. Petechia should be petechiae.
H. (Listening exercise)
I. 1. (acronym) eponym

2. (atrium) atria
3. (bacillus) bacilli
4. (diagnosis) diagnoses

5. (carcinomata) carcinoma

Chapter 2
Exercises

1. 1. E
   2. B
   3. D
   4. A
   5. E
   6. B
   7. C
   8. F

2. 1. cardi/o; heart
   2. dermat/o; skin
   3. gynec/o; female
   4. immun/o; immune
   5. neur/o; nerve
   6. onc/o; tumor
   7. ophthalm/o; eye
   8. path/o; disease
   9. psych/o; mind
   10. radi/o; radiation
   11. rhin/o; nose
   12. ur/o; urinary tract

3. 1. to secrete
   2. intestines or small intestine
   3. feeling or sensation
   4. stomach
   5. elderly
   6. larynx
   7. birth
   8. new
   9. midwife
   10. straight
   11. ear
   12. child or foot

4. 1. neonatology
   2. otolaryngology
   3. rheumatologist
   4. endocrine
   5. oncologist
   6. gastroenterologist

5. 1. cardi/ac: cardi, heart; -ac, pertaining to
   2. derm/al: derm, skin; -al, pertaining to
   3. dermato/logic, dermato/logical: dermat/o, skin; -logic and -logical,

pertaining to the study of
4. gastr/ic: gastr, stomach; -ic, pertaining to
5. gyneco/logic, gyneco/logical: gynec/o, female; -logic and -logical, pertaining to the study of
6. neuro/logic, neuro/logical: neur/o, nerve; -logic and -logical, pertaining to the study of
7. obstetr/ic, obstetr/ical: obstetr/o, midwife; -ic and -ical, pertaining to
8. ophthalm/ic, ophthalmo/logic, ophthalmo/logical: ophthalm/o, eye; -ic, pertaining to; -logic and -logical, pertaining to the study of
9. ot/ic: ot, ear; -ic, pertaining to
10. pediatr/ic: ped, child; -iatrics, medical profession or treatment. The "s" is deleted to form the adjective.
11. radio/logic, radio/logical: radi/o, radiation; -logic and -logical, pertaining to the study of
12. uro/logic, uro/logical, urin/ary: ur/o, urinary tract or urine; -logic and -logical, pertaining to the study of; urin/o, urine; -ary, pertaining to

6. 1. D
   2. I

3. H
4. E
5. G
6. F
7. J
8. C
9. B
10. A

7. 1. cardiology
   2. radiology
   3. immunology
   4. endocrinology
   5. rhinology
   6. obstetrics
   7. gastroenterology
   8. urology
   9. orthopedics
   10. rheumatology

8. 1. J
   2. G
   3. B
   4. I
   5. K
   6. C
   7. L
   8. D
   9. A
   10. E
   11. F
   12. H

9. 1. angi/o
   2. oste/o
   3. encephal/o
   4. mast/o
   5. derm/a

10. 1. -pexy, surgical fixation
    2. -ectomy, excision
    3. -stomy, formation of an opening
    4. -scopy, visual examination
    5. -logist, specialist
    6. -ectomy, excision
    7. -pexy, surgical fixation
    8. -ectomy, excision
    9. -lysis, loosening, freeing, or destroying

10. -plasty, surgical repair

11. 1. H
    2. D
    3. J
    4. G
    5. B
    6. I

12. 1. puncture of the amniotic sac to remove fluid
    2. drug that produces loss of feeling
    3. physician specializing in females, in general
    4. physician specializing in pregnant females

13. 1. angioplasty
    2. mammoplasty
    3. otoplasty
    4. ophthalmoplasty
    5. dermatoplasty

14. 1. appendectomy
    2. encephalotome
    3. ophthalmoscope
    4. otic
    5. tonsillectomy
    6. colopexy
    7. angiorrhaphy
    8. otoscopy

15. 1. E
    2. J
    3. C
    4. I
    5. H
    6. B
    7. F
    8. A
    9. G
    10. D

16. 1. deficiency
    2. rupture
    3. resembling
    4. abnormal fear
    5. prolapse
    6. -oma
    7. -pathy
    8. -rrhea
    9. spasm

10. -rrhage
17. 1. phlebitis
    2. appendicitis
    3. otitis
    4. ophthalmitis
    5. dermatitis
18. 1. chirospasm
    2. angiectasis
    3. pyromania
    4. ophthalmorrhagia
    5. encephalocele
    6. gastrocele
    7. dermatosis
    8. neuralgia
    9. ophthalmalgia
    10. blepharoptosis
    11. cardiorrhexis
    12. hematemesis
19. 1. capable of, able to
    2. pertaining to
    3. sugar
    4. enzyme
    5. specialist; one who studies
    6. pertaining to
    7. membrane
    8. condition or theory
    9. one who
    10. pertaining to
20. 1. D
    2. A
    3. I
    4. E
    5. G

6. H
7. B
8. F
9. C

Self-Test

A. 1. amyl/o (starch) + -lysis (destruction)
   2. appendic/o (appendix) + -itis (inflammation)
   3. blephar/o (eyelid) + -ptosis (drooping)
   4. dermat/o (skin) + -logist (specialist)
   5. lip/o (lipid) + -ase (enzyme)
   6. muc/o (mucus) + -oid (resembling)
   7. neur/o (nerve) + -plasty (repair)
   8. ophthalm/o (eye) + -rrhagia (hemorrhage)
   9. ot/o (ear) + -ic (pertaining to)
   10. tonsill/o (tonsil) + -ectomy (excision)
B. 1. gland
   2. skin
   3. study of
   4. hand
   5. surgical fixation
   6. sugar
   7. breast

8. nerve
9. eye
10. abnormal softening
C. 1. B
   2. K
   3. F
   4. J
   5. E
   6. H
   7. L
   8. D
   9. C
   10. A
   11. G
   12. I
D. 1. dermatitis
   2. otoscopy
   3. mammoplasty
   4. anesthetic
E. 1. amylase
   2. ophthalmoscopy
   3. tracheotomy
   4. appendicitis
   5. otitis
   6. neural
   7. tonsillectomy
   8. dermatologist
   9. lithotripsy
   10. mastectomy
F. 1. B
   2. B
   3. C
   4. D
   5. B

6. C
7. A
8. B
9. A
10. A
11. A
12. B
13. D
14. C
15. A
16. D
17. B
18. A
G. 1. gerontologist
   2. skin
   3. kidney function
   4. lungs
   5. kidneys
H. chirospasm, incision an-jē-**or**-uh-fē, **kī**-rō-spaz-um, in-**sizh**-un, **mam**-ō-plas-tē, roo-muh-**tol**-uh-jē
I. 1. (endocrinologist) obstetrician
   2. (dermatome) dermatoplasty
   3. (Angiectomy) Angiorrhaphy
   4. (stasis) spasm
   5. (Sucrose) Sucrase

Chapter 3
Exercises

1. 1. B
   2. B
   3. E
   4. F
   5. A
   6. D
   7. C
   8. A
2. 1. diplo-, double
   2. hyper-, excessive, more than normal
   3. hemi-, half
   4. hypo-, beneath
   5. pan-, all
   6. poly-, many
   7. primi-, first
   8. quadri-, four
   9. semi-, partly
   10. super-, excessive

11. tetra-, four
12. ultra-, excessive
3. 1. away from, toward
   2. behind
   3. inside, outside
   4. between, within
   5. above
   6. within
   7. against
   8. beneath
   9. same
   10. middle
   11. near
   12. within
   13. away
   14. outside
   15. inside
4. 1. circum-, around
   2. dia-, through
   3. exo-, outside
   4. endo-, inside

5. epi-, on
6. hypo-, beneath or under
7. meso-, middle
8. peri-, around
9. per-, through
10. pre-, in front of (before)
11. retro-, behind or backward
12. sub-, beneath or under
13. super-, above or beyond
14. syn-, together
15. trans-, across (through)
5. 1. C
   2. E
   3. J
   4. B

5. I
6. C
7. I
8. B
9. G
10. I
11. F
12. D
13. A
14. H
6. 1. C
   2. A
7. 1. brady-, slow
   2. tachy-, fast
   3. hypo-, less than normal
   4. hyper-, more than normal
   5. in-, not
   6. mal-, bad (poor)
   7. anti-, against

8. in-, not
9. dys-, difficult
10. contra-, against
11. anti-, against
12. para-, near
13. para-, near
14. hypo-, less than normal
15. hyper-, more than normal
16. eu-, normal
17. hypo-, less than normal
18. hyper-, more than normal

8.
1. one
2. first
3. part (or half)
4. three
5. two
6. no (or zero)
7. partly (or partially)
8. many
9. many
10. four
11. one
12. below normal
13. large
14. excessive
15. many
16. small

9.
1. three
2. toward
3. transdermal
4. difficulty
5. bradykinesia
6. oxygen
7. anesthesia
8. without
9. water
10. without

10.
1. red; condition

2. yellow; condition
3. black; tumor
4. white; skin
5. green; vision
6. white; condition
7. blue; pertaining to

11.
1. against
2. without (lacking)
3. black
4. woman
5. excessive
6. green
7. yellow
8. white
9. cyanosis
10. erythrocytes
11. leukemia
12. jaundice

12.
1. process; instrument
2. process
3. hemolysin
4. cephalometer
5. carcinogenesis; cancer
6. disease
7. nutrition
8. eat
9. movement (or motion)
10. cell

13.
1. movement
2. softening
3. eating
4. enlarged
5. hardening
6. eat
7. speech
8. paralysis
9. split
10. movement
11. large
12. split

14.
1. aer/o, air
2. phon/o, voice
3. carcin/o, cancer; gen/o, origin
4. cry/o, cold
5. electr/o, electricity
6. erythr/o, red
7. lith/o, stone
8. myc/o, fungus; dermat/o, skin
9. necr/o, dead
10. psych/o, mind; gen/o, origin
11. py/o, pus; gen/o, origin
12. scler/o, hard

Self-Test

A.
1. F
2. D
3. H
4. J
5. E
6. I
7. B
8. A
9. C
10. G

B.
1. E
2. C
3. B
4. D
5. A
6. F

C.
1. albino
2. electrocardiography
3. contralateral
4. ipsilateral

D.
1. C
2. C
3. B
4. D
5. B

6. C
7. B
8. B
9. D
10. C

E.
1. breasts
2. sides
3. drooping
4. eyelid
5. blood sugar

F.
1. dysphonia
2. melanoma
3. hyperlipemia (hyperlipidemia)
4. multicellular
5. polydipsia
6. tachycardia
7. endotracheal
8. cephalometry
9. hemiplegia
10. bradykinesia

G. dystrophy, pyoderma, syndrome *(in-truh-**mus**-kū -lur, **dis**-truh-fē, of-thul-**mop**-uh-thē, pī -ō -**dur** -muh, **sin**-drōm)*

H.
1. paralysis of one side of the body
2. difficulty or impairment in speech
3. difficulty in swallowing
4. sudden attacks of drowsiness and stupor, or sleep
5. malignant skin cancer that is composed of melanocytes

. . . .

Chapter 4
Exercises

1.
1. acute
2. chronic
3. diagnosis
4. prognosis

2.
1. A
2. A
3. B
4. B
5. A

3.
1. systolic
2. diastolic

4.
1. pulse
2. respiration
3. thermometer
4. systolic
5. palpation
6. percussion
7. auscultation

5.
1. A
2. B
3. F
4. D
5. E
6. C

6.
1. electrocardiograph
2. electrocardiography
3. electrocardiogram
4. cephalometry
5. ophthalmoscope
6. ophthalmoscopy
7. microscope
8. otoscopy

7.
1. endoscopy
2. catheterization
3. catheterize
4. cannula

7. G

8.
1. ech/o; sound
2. fluor/o; emitting or reflecting light
3. radi/o; radiant energy
4. tom/o; to cut
5. son/o; sound

9.
1. E
2. D
3. A
4. B
5. C

10. 1. algesi/o; sensitivity to pain
    2. chem/o; chemical
    3. pharmaceut/i; drugs or medicine
    4. therapeut/o; treatment
    5. tox/o; poison
11. 1. analgesic
    2. antineoplastic
    3. chemotherapy
    4. cryotherapy
    5. cytotoxic
    6. pharmacotherapy
    7. radiotherapy
    8. thermotherapy
12. 1. BP, P, T
    2. CT (computed tomography)

3. diagnosis
4. no

Self-Test
A. 1. B
   2. A
   3. A
   4. A
   5. B
   6. C
   7. D
   8. A
   9. B
B. (no particular order)
   1. pulse rate
   2. respiration rate
   3. body temperature
C. 1. B
   2. A
   3. B

4. B
5. D
D. 1. palpation
   2. percussion
   3. auscultation
   4. thermometer
   5. cephalometry
   6. ophthalmoscopy
E. 1. sound waves
   2. pain
   3. magnetic
   4. ultrasound imaging
F. fluoroscopy, neoplasm, symptom, stethoscope (*floo-**ros**-kuh-pē, **nē**-ō-plaz-um, **simp**-tum, **steth**-ō-skōp, thur-mō-**ther**-uh-pē*)
G. 1. narcotic

2. analgesic
3. sign
4. therapeutic
5. chemotherapy
6. acute
7. radiolucent
8. radiopaque
9. chronic
10. specimen
H. 1. (Narcoleptic) Narcotic
   2. (Tomography) Radiotherapy
   3. (Invasive) Radiolucent
   4. (palpation) percussion
   5. (catheter) cannula

Chapter 5
Exercises
1. 1. cell
   2. tissue
   3. organ
   4. body system
   5. organelle
2. 1. D
   2. C
   3. B
   4. A
3. 1. B
   2. C
   3. A
   4. D
4. 1. front, anterior
   2. tail or inferior, caudal (caudad)
   3. head, cephalad
   4. far or distant, distal
   5. back side, dorsal
   6. lowermost or below, inferior
   7. side, lateral
   8. middle, medial or median
   9. back, posterior
   10. nearer the origin, proximal
   11. uppermost or above, superior
   12. belly, ventral
5. 1. anter/o, front; medi/o, middle
   2. poster/o, back; extern/o, outside

3. poster/o, back; medi/o, middle
4. dors/o, back; later/o, side
5. poster/o, back; later/o, side
6. anter/o, front; later/o, side
7. medi/o, middle; later/o, side
8. anter/o, front; super/o, above
9. poster/o, behind; super/o, above
10. infer/o, under; medi/o, middle
6. 1. posterior
   2. superior
   3. distal
   4. dorsal
7. 1. C
   2. A
   3. B
   4. F
   5. E
   6. D
8. 1. B
   2. A
   3. A
   4. B
9. (any order)
   1. head
   2. neck
   3. torso (or trunk)
   4. extremities
10. 1. lapar/o

2. som/a, somat/o
3. dactyl/o
4. acr/o
5. blephar/o
6. onych/o
7. thorac/o
8. omphal/o, umbilic/o
11. 1. acr/o, extremities; -al, pertaining to
   2. blephar/o, eyelid; -al, pertaining to
   3. blephar/o, eyelid; -plasty, surgical repair
   4. blephar/o, eyelid; -plegia, paralysis
   5. blephar/o, eyelid; -spasm, twitching
   6. blephar/o, eyelid; -tomy, incision
   7. cephal/o, head; -algia, -dynia, pain
   8. cephal/o, head; -metry, measurement
   9. lapar/o, abdominal wall; -tomy, incision
   10. lapar/o, abdominal wall; -scopy, examination
   11. lapar/o, abdominal wall; -scope, instrument used for viewing

12. omphal/o, umbilic/o, umbilicus; -ic, -al, pertaining to
13. omphal/o, umbilicus; -itis, inflammation
14. omphal/o, umbilicus; -rrhagia, hemorrhage
15. omphal/o, umbilicus; -rrhexis, rupture
12. 1. posteroanterior
   2. left lateral
13. 1. acrocyanosis
   2. laparoscopy
   3. peritonitis
   4. cephalometry
   5. abdominothoracic
   6. acral
   7. blepharoplasty
   8. omphalorrhexis
   9. thoracentesis
   10. thoracotomy
   11. cephalopelvic
   12. ascites
   13. omphalocele
   14. acrohypothermy
14. 1. blephar/o, eyelid; -edema, swelling
   2. blephar/o, eyelid; -itis, inflammation
   3. blephar/o, eyelid; -ptosis, sagging (prolapse)

4. onych/o, nail;
   -malacia, softening
5. thorac/o, chest;
   -dynia, pain
6. thorac/o, chest;
   -stomy, formation of
   an opening
7. thorac/o, chest;
   -tomy, incision
8. thorac/o, chest;
   -plasty, surgical
   repair
9. thorac/o, chest;
   -scopy, visual
   examination

15. 1. E
    2. G
    3. A
    4. H
    5. B
    6. F
    7. C
    8. D
16. 1. cyt/o (sometimes
       cellul/o)
    2. thromb/o
    3. coagul/o
    4. erythr/o
    5. leuk/o (also leuc/o
       and alb/o)
17. 1. B
    2. A
    3. D
    4. C
    5. E

18. 1. thrombocytes
    2. erythrocytes
    3. leukocytes
19. 1. B
    2. C
    3. B
    4. C
    5. A
20. 1. plasma
    2. hematoma
    3. hemolysis
    4. hemodialysis
    5. coagulation
    6. anticoagulant
    7. thrombosis
    8. thrombopenia
    9. anemia
    10. phagocytes
    11. hematopoiesis
    12. leukocytosis
    13. leukopenia
    14. erythrocytosis
21. 1. A
    2. B
    3. B
    4. A
    5. B
22. 1. A
    2. A
    3. B
    4. B
23. 1. antigen
    2. susceptible
    3. nonspecific
    4. specific

    5. Active (or Specific)
    6. immunodeficiency
24. (no particular order):
    bacteria, fungi, protozoa,
    viruses
25. 1. weapons
    2. Disease
    3. bioterrorism
    4. disseminated

Self-Test
A. 1. sagittal
   2. transverse
   3. frontal
   4. superior
   5. inferior
   6. lateral
B. 1. G
   2. J
   3. H
   4. C
   5. F
   6. B
   7. I
   8. D
   9. E
   10. A
C. 1. hypertrophy
   2. hyperplasia
D. 1. A
   2. C
   3. C
   4. C
   5. B
   6. A
   7. D

   8. D
   9. C
   10. A
E. (no particular order)
   1. connective
   2. epithelial
   3. muscle
   4. nervous
F. anaphylaxis,
   fibrin, hypertrophy,
   immunosuppressant
   (an-uh-fuh-**lak**-sis,
   fī-brin, hī **pur**-truh-fē,
   im- ū-nō-suh-**pres**-unt,
   soo-pi-**nā**-shun)
G. 1. antigen
   2. anticoagulant
   3. hematopoiesis
   4. anterolateral
   5. aplasia
   6. abdominothoracic
   7. thrombosis
   8. bioterrorism
   9. leukocytes
      (leucocytes)
   10. intracellular
H. 1. (Homeostasis)
      Hydrotherapy
   2. (metastasize)
      metastasis
   3. (Infection)
      Inflammation
   4. (omphalocele)
      abscess
   5. (artificial) natural

PART TWO

Chapter 6
Exercises
1. 1. protection
   2. support
   3. movement
   4. formation
   5. fat
   6. minerals
2. 1. J
   2. D
   3. H
   4. I
   5. E
   6. E
   7. F
   8. B
   9. E
   10. G

   11. C
   12. A
3. 1. clavicle
   2. humerus
   3. ulna
   4. femur
   5. fibula
   6. tarsus
4. 1. carpal
   2. cranial
   3. femoral
   4. humeral
   5. vertebral
   6. lumbar
   7. pelvic
   8. spinal
   9. costal
   10. thoracic

   11. radial
   12. ulnar
5. 1. E
   2. D
   3. F
   4. A
   5. C
   6. B
6. 1. chondr/o, cartilage
   2. vertebr/o, vertebra;
      chondr/o, cartilage
   3. cost/o, rib;
      chondr/o, cartilage
7. 1. fascia
   2. destruction
   3. disease
   4. muscle
   5. pain

8. 1. myofibrosis
   2. myasthenia
   3. paraplegia
   4. quadriplegia
   5. myocele
9. 1. B
   2. D
   3. A
   4. C
10. 1. cellulitis
    2. osteomyelitis
    3. osteochondritis
    4. chondrosarcoma
    5. fibrosarcoma
    6. leukemia
    7. osteoporosis
    8. osteomalacia
11. 1. spondylarthritis

2. polyarthritis
3. ankylosis
4. bursitis
5. arthroscopy
12. 1. bifida
2. scoliosis
3. dystrophy
4. arthritis
5. osteoarthritis
6. rheumatoid
7. arthrodynia
8. erythematosus
9. gout
10. hyperuricemia
13. 1. a fracture in which the bone is broken into two pieces, but does not protrude through the skin
2. the smaller bone of the lower leg
3. joint pain
4. examination of the interior of a joint with an endoscope
5. inflammation of a bone and joint
6. lateral curvature of the spine
14. 1. C
2. D

3. B
4. A
15. 1. diskectomy
2. myelosuppression
3. antiinflammatories
4. arthrocentesis
5. myoplasty
16. 1. craniotomy
2. cranium
3. craniectomy

Self-Test
A. 1. N
2. F
3. J
4. L
5. C
6. M
7. G
8. G
9. H
10. D
11. G
12. B
13. I
14. E
15. A
16. B
17. K
B. ankylosis, coccyx femoral, flexion, laminectomy (*ang-*

kuh-lō-sis, **kok**-siks, **fem**-uh-rul, **flek** -shun, lam-i-**nek**-tuh-mē
C. 1. G
2. B
3. E
4. D
5. A
6. C
7. F
D. 1. cervical
2. thoracic
3. lumbar
4. sacral
5. coccygeal
E. 1. C
2. A
3. B
F. 1. B
2. A
3. C
4. B
5. C
6. C
7. D
8. B
9. C
10. C
G. 1. extension
2. arthroscopy
3. vertebroplasty

4. scoliosis
5. wrist
H. 1. myolysis
2. osteochondritis
3. myelosuppression
4. antiinflammatories
5. anti-osteoporotics
6. clavicular
7. cervical
8. humeral
9. tarsoptosis
10. reduction
I. 1. rheumatoid
2. arthroplasty
3. osteoarthritis
4. extremity
J. 1. gout
2. joint
3. joints
4. bone
5. wrist
K. 1. (Adductors) Abductors
2. (extension) circumduction
3. (Hypouricemia) Hyperuricemia
4. (kyphosis) fibrosarcoma
5. (Antiosteoporotics) Antiarthritics

....

Chapter 7
Exercises
1. (no particular order): lymphatic, cardiovascular
2. (no particular order)
   1. arteries
   2. arterioles
   3. capillaries
   4. veins
   5. venules
3. 1. B
2. A
3. C
4. 1. C
2. B
3. A
4. F
5. D
6. C
7. C
8. E
5. 1. aort/o, aorta
2. arteri/o, artery

3. arteri/o, artery; ven/o vein
4. vascul/o, vessel
5. ven/o, vein
6. 1. F
2. J
3. I
4. B
5. G
6. D
7. C
8. A
9. H
10. E
7. 1. increased pulse rate
2. low blood pressure
3. irregularity or loss of rhythm of the heart beat
4. the record produced in electrocardiography
5. enlargement of the heart

8. 1. arteriosclerosis
2. aortitis
3. cerebrovascular
4. thrombophlebitis
5. polyarteritis
9. 1. A
2. F
3. C
4. E
10. 1. antiarrhythmic
2. open
3. cardiopulmonary
4. beta
5. pacemaker
11. 1. E
2. C
3. D
4. B
5. A
12. 1. CABG
2. aortoplasty
3. angioplasty
4. phlebectomy
5. antihypertensives

6. antilipidemics
13. 1. D
2. E
3. C
4. B
5. A
Self-Test
A. 1. lymphangi/o
2. arter/o *or* arteri/o
3. arteriol/o
4. phleb/o *or* ven/o
5. venul/o
B. 1. B
2. B
3. B
4. D
5. C
6. A
7. A
8. C
9. A
10. D
C. 1. aorta
2. arterioles

3. oxygen
4. veins
5. atrium
6. lymphatic
7. coronary
8. endocardium
9. myocardium
10. epicardium

D. adenoidectomy, cholesterol, defibrillator, infarction (ad-uh-noid-**ek**-tuh-mē, kuh-**les**-tur-ol, kahr-dē-ō-**vas**-kū-lur, dē-**fib**-ri-l-tur, in-**fahrk**-shun)

E.
1. necrosis of a portion of cardiac muscle
2. increased blood pressure
3. increased levels of lipids in the blood
4. introduction of a catheter into the heart
5. chest pain caused by insufficient oxygen to the heart

F.
1. asystole
2. tachycardic

3. cardiac
4. systolic
5. pulse

G.
1. outer layer
2. high blood pressure
3. pericardial

H.
1. hypotension
2. antihypertensive
3. splenomegaly
4. lymphadenopathy
5. tonsillectomy
6. tachycardia
7. lipids
8. angiocardiography

9. endocardium
10. capillaries

I.
1. arteriogram
2. aneurysm

J.
1. (Electrocardiography) Echocardiography
2. (Cardiomegaly) Cardiomyopathy
3. (vasodilation) ischemia
4. (thrombus) embolus
5. (Antihypertensives) Vasodilators

Chapter 8
Exercises

1.
1. homeostasis
2. inspiration
3. expiration
4. oxygen

2.
1. A
2. B
3. G
4. E
5. C
6. F
7. D
8. D
9. E
10. H

3.
1. alveol/o, alveolus
2. bronchi/o, bronchus
3. laryng/o, larynx
4. nas/o, nose
5. nas/o, nose; pharyng/o, pharynx
6. pharyng/o, pharynx
7. pneum/o, lung or air
8. pneum/o, lungs; cardi/o, heart
9. pulmon/o, lungs
10. trache/o, trachea

4.
1. E
2. D
3. B
4. A
5. F
6. C

5.
1. increased pulse rate
2. increased respiratory rate

3. labored or difficult breathing
4. acute inflammation of the lungs and bronchioles
5. a physician who specializes in the lungs and respiratory disorders

6.
1. polyp
2. pharyngeal
3. laryngeal
4. laryngalgia
5. aphonia
6. aphasia
7. alveolar
8. rhinitis
9. sinusitis
10. sputum

7.
1. coni/o
2. atel/o
3. ox/o
4. home/o
5. silic/o
6. spir/o

8.
1. pneumonitis
2. bronchopneumonia
3. atelectasis
4. aphasia
5. syndrome
6. emphysema
7. asthma
8. pneumoconiosis

9.
1. C
2. B
3. E
4. D
5. A

10.
1. rhinoplasty
2. thoracocentesis
3. tracheotomy
4. pneumectomy
5. bronchodilator
6. mucolytic

Self-Test

A.
1. G
2. A
3. B
4. F
5. E
6. C
7. D

B.
1. mucolytic
2. antitussive
3. dysphonia
4. bronchoscopy
5. tracheotomy
6. pharyngitis
7. alveolar
8. bronchogram
9. rhinoplasty
10. endotracheal

C.
1. B
2. A
3. B
4. D
5. C
6. A
7. C
8. C
9. D
10. A

D.
1. bronchoscopy
2. hemothorax

E.
1. effusion or pleural effusion

2. bronchiectasis
3. emphysema
4. bronchitis
5. pneumonia
6. dyspnea
7. sputum
8. pulmonary embolism
9. pneumothorax
10. bronchodilator

F. asphyxiation, embolus, laryngitis, pneumocardial, pulmonic (as-fik-sē-**ā**-shun, **em**-bō-lus, lar-in-**jī**-tis, noo mō-**kahr**-dē-ul, pul-**mon**-ik)

G.
1. bronchospasm
2. dyspnea
3. bronchodilation
4. paroxysmal
5. hypoventilation
6. hypoxemia

H.
1. fluid
2. surgically removed
3. emphysema

I.
1. (antihistamines) decongestants
2. (expiration) paracentesis
3. (Bronchogenic) Bronchopulmonary
4. (Dysphonia) Paroxysmal
5. (hypoxia) effusion

Chapter 9
Exercises

1. 1. ingestion
   2. digestion
   3. absorption
   4. elimination
2. (no particular order)
   1. carbohydrates
   2. proteins
   3. lipids (fats)
3. 1. lactase
   2. lipase
   3. protease or proteinase
   4. amylase
4. 1. B
   2. B
   3. D
   4. E
   5. F
   6. A
   7. C
   8. G
5. 1. D
   2. C
   3. E
   4. B
   5. G
   6. G
   7. F
   8. A
6. 1. an/o, anus
   2. duoden/o, duodenum
   3. gastr/o, stomach
   4. enter/o, small intestine
   5. esophag/o, esophagus
   6. gloss/o, tongue
   7. rect/o, rectum
7. 1. choledoch/o
   2. pancreat/o
   3. hepat/o

4. cholecyst/o
5. sial/o
8. 1. esophagogram
   2. cholelithiasis
   3. choledocholithiasis
   4. pancreatolithiasis
   5. sialography
   6. esophagoscopy
   7. colonoscopy
   8. sigmoidoscopy
9. 1. mellitus
   2. hyperglycemia
   3. polyuria
   4. polydipsia
   5. glycosuria
   6. gestational
   7. hypoglycemia
   8. lipids (fats)
   9. hyperemesis
   10. emaciation
   11. anorexia
   12. bulimia
   13. polyphagia
   14. malnutrition
10. 1. cholelithiasis
    2. cirrhosis
    3. an ulcer
    4. gastrocele
    5. glossitis
    6. hemorrhoids
11. 1. esophagitis
    2. gastroenteritis
    3. enterostasis
    4. gastroscopy
    5. cholecystitis
    6. cirrhosis
12. 1. F
    2. C
    3. A
    4. D
    5. H
    6. G
    7. E
    8. B

13. 1. a physician specializing in diseases of the GI tract
    2. inflammation of the colon
    3. herniation of the stomach
    4. a disease characterized by resistance to insulin or lack of insulin secretion

Self-Test

A. 1. A
   2. B
   3. E
   4. C
   5. D
B. 1. C
   2. A
   3. D
   4. B
C. 1. B
   2. D
   3. A
   4. C
   5. D
   6. B
   7. B
   8. B
   9. B
   10. C
D. 1. jejunostomy
   2. anorexiant
   3. amylase
   4. hyperemesis
   5. pancreatolithectomy
   6. vagotomy
   7. gastritis
   8. esophageal
   9. dyspepsia
   10. cholelithiasis

E. cholangiography, enteral, hepatic, nasojejunal, proctoscope (kō-lan-jē-**og**-ruh-fē, **en**-tur-ul, huh-**pat**-ik, nā-zō-juh-**joo**-nul, **prok**-tō-skōp)
F. (no particular order)
   1. carbohydrates (lactose, lactase, starch, amylase)
   2. proteins (protein, protease or proteinase)
   3. lipids (fats) (lipids, lipase)
G. 1. B
   2. A
   3. B
   4. A
   5. A
   6. A
   7. B
   8. B
H. 1. C
   2. A
   3. D
   4. D
   5. B
   6. B
   7. A
   8. B
I. 1. cholelithiasis
   2. gastroduodenostomy
   3. jaundice
J. 1. (alimentation) digestion
   2. (lipid) lipase
   3. (glossal) gingival
   4. (hypoglycemia) hyperlipidemia
   5. (peritonitis) cirrhosis

Chapter 10
Exercises

1. 1. water
   2. blood
   3. hydrogen
   4. waste
   5. pressure
   6. erythropoietin
2. 1. C
   2. A
   3. D

4. B
5. F
6. E
3. 1. A
   2. B
   3. C
   4. B
   5. D
   6. E
4. 1. B
   2. A

3. C
4. D
5. (no particular order)
   1. glomerular filtration
   2. tubular reabsorption
   3. tubular secretion
6. 1. albuminuria
   2. hematuria
   3. ketonuria
   4. pyuria
   5. glycosuria

6. nephrotomography
7. catheterization
8. urinalysis
7. 1. cystoscopy
   2. polyuria
   3. anuria
   4. oliguria
   5. nephromegaly
   6. glomerulonephritis
   7. pyelitis
   8. nephroptosis

9. nephromalacia
10. nephrolithiasis
11. uremia
12. nephrosonography

8. 1. abnormal presence of sugar, especially glucose, in the urine
   2. presence of protein in the urine
   3. presence of blood in the urine
   4. end products of lipid metabolism

9. 1. A
   2. D
   3. B
   4. C
   5. A

10. 1. diuretic
    2. nephrectomy

3. cystitis
4. hemodialysis
5. pyelostomy

Self-Test

A. 1. E
   2. D
   3. A
   4. C
   5. B

B. 1. B
   2. B
   3. B
   4. B
   5. A

C. 1. C
   2. B
   3. A
   4. C
   5. D

D. 1. C

2. C
3. D
4. A
5. C

E. 1. polyuria
   2. nephron
   3. cystoscopy
   4. pyelitis
   5. hemodialysis
   6. pyelostomy
   7. urethral
   8. nephrolithiasis
   9. nephropexy
   10. ureteroplasty

F. cystocele, nephrectomy, oliguria, suprapubic, urinary (*sis*-tō-*sēl*, nuh-**frek**-tuh-mē, ol-i-**g**-rē-uh, soo-pruh-**pū**-bik, **ū**-ri-nar-ē)

G. 1. C
   2. B
   3. A
   4. C
   5. A
   6. A
   7. B
   8. B
   9. C
   10. B

H. 1. cystolithiasis
   2. polycystic

I. 1. (pyelitis) uremia
   2. (polyuria) oliguria
   3. (reabsorption) filtration
   4. (nephrotoxic) polycystic
   5. (Lithotripsy) Nephrectomy

Chapter 11
Exercises

1. 1. genitalia
   2. gonads
   3. ovum
   4. spermatozoon
   5. ovary
   6. testis or testicle
   7. reproduction

2. 1. B
   2. H
   3. G
   4. C
   5. E
   6. D
   7. F
   8. A

3. 1. D
   2. B
   3. E
   4. C
   5. A

4. 1. A
   2. D
   3. E
   4. B
   5. C

5. 1. uter/o, uterus
   2. uter/o, uterus
   3. ovar/o, ovary
   4. vagin/o, vagina
   5. vulv/o, vulva

6. 1. cervical
   2. uterine
   3. endometrium

4. perimetrium
5. myometrium
6. ovulation
7. menstruation
8. climacteric
9. fetus
10. progesterone

7. 1. speculum
   2. Pap
   3. dysplasia
   4. colposcopy
   5. hysteroscopy
   6. hysterosalpingogram

8. 1. B
   2. C
   3. A
   4. D

9. 1. B
   2. A
   3. D
   4. C

10. 1. colpitis
    2. endometriosis
    3. colposcopy
    4. hysteroptosis
    5. endometritis

11. 1. abstinence
    2. intrauterine
    3. spermicides
    4. coitus
    5. rhythm

12. 1. hysterectomy
    2. colpoplasty
    3. colporrhaphy

4. oophorectomy (ovariectomy)
5. salpingorrhaphy
6. ligation
7. laparoscopy
8. curettage
9. laparotomy
10. conization

13. 1. pertaining to the period of life after normal cessation of menstruation
    2. removal of both ovaries and uterine tubes
    3. examination of the external and internal female genitalia
    4. herniation of the urinary bladder through the wall of the vagina

14. 1. amni/o
    2. nat/i
    3. fet/o
    4. par/o

15. 1. C
    2. A
    3. B
    4. D

16. 1. a woman who is pregnant for the third time

2. a physician specializing in pregnancy and childbirth
3. intrauterine position in which the buttocks or feet of the fetus are presented
4. incision through the walls of the abdomen and uterus for fetal delivery

17. 1. secundipara
    2. fetus
    3. ectopic pregnancy
    4. neonatal
    5. cephalic
    6. amnion
    7. Down syndrome
    8. amniotomy
    9. placenta
    10. abruptio placentae

18. 1. A
    2. D
    3. B
    4. C

19. 1. gon/o
    2. pen/o
    3. prostat/o
    4. scrot/o
    5. semin/o
    6. spermat/o
    7. orchi/o, orchid/o, test/o, testicul/o
    8. vas/o

20. 1. penis
    2. prostate
    3. scrotum
    4. semen
    5. testis (testicle)
21. 1. cryptorchidism
    2. hyperplasia
    3. prostatitis
    4. orchitis
    5. hydrocele
    6. anorchism
    7. hydrocele
    8. intersexuality or hermaphrodism
    9. prostatic
    10. torsion
22. 1. orchiopexy (orchidopexy)
    2. circumcision
    3. vasectomy
    4. orchiectomy (orchidectomy)
    5. prostatectomy
    6. ablation
23. 1. D
    2. B
    3. A
    4. D
    5. D
    6. A

    7. D
    8. A
    9. C
24. 1. gonorrhea
    2. within
    3. chancre
    4. chlamydial
    5. immunodeficiency
    6. Kaposi
    7. herpes
    8. warts
    9. hepatitis
    10. trichomoniasis
    11. candidiasis
    12. lice

Self-Test
A. 1. oophor/o
    2. salping/o
    3. hyster/o
    4. cervic/o
    5. colp/o
    6. vas/o
    7. urethr/o
    8. pen/o
    9. prostat/o
    10. orchi/o
    11. scrot/o
B. 1. D
    2. A
    3. B

    4. E
    5. C
    6. F
C. 1. hysterosalpingogram
    2. vasectomy
D. 1. B
    2. C
    3. A
    4. D
    5. B
    6. D
    7. C
    8. C
    9. A
    10. A
    11. B
    12. D
    13. C
    14. D
    15. C
    16. C
    17. B
    18. C
    19. B
    20. B
E. 1. neonate
    2. implantation
    3. amniotomy
    4. episiotomy
    5. climacteric

    6. dysmenorrhea
    7. cervical
    8. hysteroptosis
    9. amniocentesis
    10. ovulation
F. cervicocolpitis, chorionic, cystocele, syphilis (*sur-vi-kō-kol-**pī**-tis, kor-ē-**on**-ik, **sis**-tō-sēl, **sif**-i-lis*)
G. 1. (pelvis) breast
    2. (Metrorrhagia) Menorrhagia
    3. (vasotomy) vasovasostomy
    4. (secundipara) primigravida
    5. (endometriosis) oophorosalpingitis
H. 1. spherical bacteria in pairs located both within and outside cells
    2. gonorrhea
    3. gonococcus
I. 1. placenta
    2. cervix
    3. after birth
    4. cesarean
    5. antenatal

Chapter 12
Exercises
1. 1. integument
    2. microbes (microorganisms)
    3. brain
    4. salts (or salt or waste)
2. 1. B
    2. C
    3. A
3. 1. xer/o
    2. erythemat/o
    3. adip/o or lip/o
    4. ichthy/o
    5. follicul/o
    6. pil/o or trich/o
    7. kerat/o
    8. seps/o or sept/o
    9. onych/o or ungu/o
    10. seb/o
4. 1. accessory
    2. axillary
    3. sudoriferous
    4. perspiration

    5. sebaceous
    6. ungual
5. 1. A
    2. C
    3. D
    4. E
    5. B
6. 1. B
    2. A
    3. C
    4. D
    5. E
7. 1. cysts
    2. wheals
    3. keloid
    4. urticaria
    5. laceration
8. 1. superficial
    2. dermis
    3. deep
9. 1. D
    2. E
    3. C
    4. A
    5. F

    6. B
    7. I
    8. H
    9. J
    10. G
10. 1. D
    2. C
    3. A
    4. B

Self-Test
A. (no particular order)
    1. covers and protects the body
    2. helps control body temperature
    3. has receptors that receive stimuli
    4. has sweat glands that excrete water and salt
    5. vitamin D synthesis
B. (no particular order)
    1. epidermis
    2. dermis

    3. subcutaneous adipose tissue
C. antiperspirant, axillary, follicle, integument, petechia or petechiae (*an-tē-**pur**-spur-unt, **ak**-si-lar-ē, **fol**-i-kul, in-**teg**-ū-ment, puh-**tē**-kē-ē*)
D. 1. keloid
    2. skin graft
    3. sepsis
    4. full- and partial-thickness
    5. onychomycosis
E. 1. hypopigmentation
    2. second-degree
    3. xerosis
    4. urticaria
    5. petechiae
F. 1. ichthyosis
    2. onychomycosis
G. 1. A
    2. F
    3. C

4. D
5. G
6. E
7. B
H. 1. A
2. D
3. A
4. A
5. B

6. A
7. C
8. C
9. D
10. B
I. 1. furuncle
2. laceration
3. albinism
4. contusion

5. onychopathy
6. lipoma
7. scleroderma
8. xerosis or xeroderma
9. hidradenitis
10. ungual
J. 1. (bullae) vesicles
2. (Psoriatic) Pilomotor

3. (Necrotic) Circumscribed
4. (pediculosis) frostbite
5. (antimicrobial) topical

- -

Chapter 13
Exercises
1. 1. information (data)
2. movement
3. changes
4. homeostasis
5. afferent
6. efferent
7. somatic
8. autonomic
2. (no particular order)
1. central nervous system
2. peripheral nervous system
3. 1. central
2. peripheral
3. neuron
4. glial or neuroglial
4. 1. E
2. A
3. D
4. F
5. H
6. B
7. G
8. C
5. 1. cerebellum
2. coccyx
3. dura mater
4. brain
5. neuroglia or sticky substance
6. mind
7. nature
8. spine
6. 1. cranium

2. meninges
3. cerebrum
4. hemispheres
5. cortex
6. spinal
7. 1. stroke
2. hydrocephalus
3. electroencephalography
4. subdural
5. epidural
6. intracerebral
8. 1. F
2. D
3. H
4. A
5. I
6. B
7. E
8. C
9. J
10. G
9. 1. zo/o
2. -orexia
3. claustr/o
4. pseud/o
5. agora-
6. -esthesia
7. arachn/o
8. -asthenia
9. -lexia
10. 1. F
2. I
3. D
4. G
5. B
6. A
7. C

8. H
9. E
10. J
11. 1. dysphagia
2. cephalgia
3. dyskinesia
4. dyslexia
5. narcolepsy
12. 1. B
2. F
3. C
4. A
5. D
6. E
7. G

Self-Test
A. 1. central
2. peripheral
3. central
4. neuron
5. glial or neuroglial
6. meninges
7. anxiety
8. analgesics
B. 1. pyromania
2. craniotomy
3. encephalopathy
4. neurolysis
5. kleptomania
6. arachnophobia
7. phobia
8. dyslexia
9. cranioplasty
10. neurorrhaphy
C. 1. C
2. B
3. D

4. D
5. B
6. B
7. A
8. A
9. A
10. A
D. 1. hemiplegia
2. paraplegia
3. meningocele
E. 1. ischemic
2. transient
3. speech
4. CVA
5. hydrocephalus
F. 1. dysphasia
2. hyperkinesia
3. Alzheimer disease
4. anorexia
5. multiple sclerosis
G. 1. acrophobia, peripheral, pseudoplegia, thalamus (a*k-rō-fō-bē-uh, puh-rif-ur-ul, soo-dō-plē-juh, sub-doo-rul, thal-uh-mus)*
H. 1. (coccygeal) ventriculoperitoneal
2. (pseudoplegia) psychosomatic
3. (epidural) intracerebral
4. (cervical) sciatic
5. (aphasic) ischemic

Chapter 14

Exercises

1. 1. peripheral
   2. receptors
   3. (no particular order): eyes, ears, skin, mouth, nose
2. 1. H
   2. E
   3. I
   4. C
   5. F
   6. B
   7. A
   8. G
   9. D
   10. J
3. 1. conjunctiva
   2. tear
   3. cornea
   4. iris
   5. cornea, hard, horny
   6. tear
   7. eye
   8. retina
4. 1. conjunctiv/o, conjunctiva
   2. choroid/o, choroid
   3. corne/o, cornea
   4. irid/o, iris
   5. lacrim/o, tear
   6. ocul/o, ophthalm/o, eye; opt/o, vision
   7. pupill/o, pupil
   8. retin/o, retina
5. 1. B
   2. E
   3. A

4. C
5. D
6. F
6. 1. retinopathy
   2. ptosis
   3. nyctalopia
   4. conjunctivitis
   5. glaucoma
   6. blepharitis
   7. amblyopia
   8. photophobia
   9. hordeolum or stye
   10. achromatopsia
7. 1. E
   2. F
   3. C
   4. D
   5. A
8. 1. accommodation reflex
   2. glaucoma
   3. tonometry
   4. visual field
   5. nyctalopia
9. 1. acoust/o; hearing
   2. audi/o; hearing
   3. audi/o; hearing
   4. aur/o, auricul/o, ot/o; ear
   5. cochle/o; cochlea
10. 1. B
    2. E
    3. C
    4. A
    5. F
    6. D
11. 1. tympanostomy
    2. otoplasty

3. cerumen or earwax
4. cochlear, cochlea
12. 1. photoreceptors
    2. thermoreceptors
    3. nociceptors
    4. mechanoreceptors
13. 1. B
    2. C
    3. A
    4. D

Self-Test

A. 1. D
   2. F
   3. A
   4. C
   5. E
   6. B
B. 1. myopia
   2. cochlear
   3. tonometry
   4. cochlear
C. 1. D
   2. A
   3. B
   4. B
   5. A
   6. B
   7. D
   8. A
D. 1. cerumen
   2. hyperopia
   3. anosmia
   4. olfactory
   5. nociceptor
   6. mechanoreceptor
   7. cryoextraction
   8. tympanostomy
   9. blepharoptosis

10. malleus
E. 1. retinopathy
   2. lacrimation
   3. nyctalopia
   4. tinnitus
   5. sclera
F. 1. ear pain
   2. hearing
   3. eardrum
   4. noise in the ears
   5. dizziness
G. cataract, eustachian, ocular, ceruminolytics (**kat**-uh-rakt, ū-**stā**-kē-un, **ok**-ū-lur, **kat**-uh-rakt, ol-**fak**-tuh-rē, suh-roo-mi-nō-**lit**-iks)
H. 1. eyes
   2. achromatopsia
   3. tonometry
   4. cochlea
   5. eustachian
   6. audiologist
   7. media
   8. tympanostomy
   9. skin
   10. tongue
I. 1. (tinnitus) Meniere
   2. (amblyopia) conjunctivitis
   3. (olfaction) anosmia
   4. (aural) acoustic
   5. (presbyopia) astigmatism

Chapter 15

Exercises

1. 1. coordinates with the nervous system to regulate the body's activities
   2. insufficient secretion
   3. excessive secretion
2. 1. glands (endocrine glands)
   2. hormones
   3. endocrine glands are ductless and secrete their hormones into the bloodstream.

Exocrine glands open into a body surface and discharge their hormones through ducts.
4. endocrine
5. target organ
6. hormones are released in response to nervous system; or, endocrine glands respond to hormones produced by the pituitary gland.

3. 1. B
   2. D
   3. A
   4. E
   5. G
   6. C
   7. F
   8. H
4. 1. -gen

7. pituitary (hypophysis)
8. (no particular order): pancreas, pineal gland, thyroid, parathyroid, adrenal, ovaries, testes

3. 1. B
   2. D
   3. A
   4. E
   5. G
   6. C
   7. F
   8. H
4. 1. -gen

2. -physis
3. -gen
4. -tropic
5. -tropin
6. -uria
5. 1. C
   2. D
   3. E
   4. B
   5. A
6. 1. diabetes insipidus
   2. diabetes mellitus
   3. hypothyroidism
   4. polyuria
   5. hyperglycemia
   6. polydipsia
   7. exophthalmos

8. glycosuria

7. 1. A
2. C
3. E
4. D
5. G
6. B
7. F

8. 1. hypoglycemia
2. thyroxine
3. hyperinsulinism
4. euthyroid
5. adenoma

9. 1. hyperglycemia
2. polyphagia
3. polyuria
4. antidiuretic
5. glycosuria

10. 1. hypophysectomy
2. insulin
3. glucose
4. adenectomy
5. thyroidectomy
6. parathyroidectomy

11. 1. exenteration
2. radioresistant
3. fractionation
4. linear

5. brachytherapy
6. immunotherapy

Self-Test

A. (no particular order): pineal gland, thyroid, parathyroids, adrenals, pancreas, ovaries, testes

B. 1. coordinates with the nervous system to regulate body activities
2. a gland is a structure that is specialized to secrete or excrete hormones. Hormones are chemical substances that have a specific effect on cells or organs.
3. pituitary (hypophysis)
4. organ or structure toward which a hormone is directed.
5. deficiency (hyposecretion)

or excess (hypersecretion)

C. 1. D
2. A
3. B
4. B
5. A
6. B
7. C
8. B
9. B
10. D
11. B
12. D
13. A
14. C

D. 1. gigantism
2. hypoglycemia
3. hypoparathyroidism
4. hypophysectomy
5. polydipsia
6. polyuria
7. adenoma
8. adenectomy
9. thyroidectomy
10. thyrotoxicosis

E. 1. bulging outward of the eyes

2. enlarged thyroid
3. increased activity of the thyroid
4. excision of the thyroid

F. 1. T
2. F
3. T
4. F
5. F

G. 1. hypophysectomy
2. goiter

H. adrenaline, cretinism, goiter, hypersecretion, myxedema (*uh-**dren**-uh-lin*, ***krē**-tin-iz-um*, ***goi**-tur*, *hī-pur-sē-**krē**-shun*, *mik-suh-**dē**-muh*)

I. 1. (thyrotoxicosis) cretinism
2. (adrenal) insulin
3. (extremities) eyeballs
4. (adrenal) pineal
5. (Two) Four

Illustration Credits

© AlexRaths/iStock/thinkstock.com. **Unnumbered Figure 12.1, Unnumbered Figure 15.1**

© Andrei310/iStock.com. Figure **5.21**

© andresr/iStock.com. Figure **2.7**

© Barbara Penoyar/Photodisc/thinkstock.com. **Unnumbered Figure 7.7, Unnumbered Figure 8.7**

© Bluesing media/istock.com. Figure **13.7B**

© Bojan89/iStock/thinkstock.com. **Unnumbered Figure 6.2**

© BorupFoto/iStock/Thinkstock.com. Figure **4.12**

© bowdenimages/iStock/thinkstock.com. **Unnumbered Figure 14.2**

© Cameron Whitman/iStock.com. **Unnumbered Figure 11.8**

© choja/iStock.com. Figure **4.3F**

© Comstock/Stockbyte/thinkstock.com. **Unnumbered Figure 13.1**

© cthoman/iStock/Thinkstock.com. **Unnumbered Figure 1.10**

© David Ahn/iStock.com. **Unnumbered Figure 3.10**

© dblight/iStock.com. Figure **13.12A**

© dene398/iStock/Thinkstock.com. **Unnumbered Figure 1.11**

© DME Photography/iStock/Thinkstock.com. **Unnumbered Figure 1.5**

© Digital Vision/DigitalVision/thinkstock.com. **Unnumbered Figure 10.5**

© doomu/iStock/Thinkstock.com. **Unnumbered Figure 1.9, Unnumbered Figure 2.9**

© DragonImages/iStock/thinkstock.com. **Unnumbered Figure 8.1, Unnumbered Figure 14.7**

© drduey/iStock/Thinkstock.com. **Unnumbered Figure 2.10**

© ELizabethHoffmann/iStock/thinkstock.com. Figure **14.19B**

© Faysal Ahamed/iStock/Thinkstock.com. **Unnumbered Figure 4.3**

© franciscodiazpagador/iStock/thinkstock.com. Figure **12.4**

© Hlib Shabashnyi/iStock.com. Figure **5.20B**

© images by barbara/iStock.com. Figure **14.18**

© itsmejust/iStock.com. Figure **6.10A**

© jarun011/iStock/Thinkstock.com. **Unnumbered Figure 3.1**

© JCPJR/iStock/thinkstock.com. Figure **15.17**

© johavel/iStock/Thinkstock.com. **Unnumbered Figure 4.4**

© John Foxx/Stockbyte/thinkstock.com. **Unnumbered Figure 10.2**

© Jose Luis Pelaez Inc./Blend Images/thinkstock.com. **Unnumbered Figure 12.2**

© Juanmonino/iStock.com. **Unnumbered Figure 9.4, Unnumbered Figure 10.3**

© Jupiterimages/PhotoObjects.net/thinkstock.com. **Unnumbered Figure 13.7**

© jurgenfr/iStock/Thinkstock.com. **Unnumbered Figure 1.8, Unnumbered Figure 2.8**

© KatarzynaBialasiewicz/iStock/thinkstock.com. Figure **15.14**

© kchungtw/iStock/Thinkstock.com. **Unnumbered Figure 1.7**

© Brofsky/Photodisc/Keith thinkstock.com. **Unnumbered Figure 5.4**

© Keithfrith/iStock/thinkstock.com. Figure **2.4**

© KiwiRob/iStock/thinkstock.com. Figure **15.7**

© kzenon/iStock/thinkstock.com. **Unnumbered Figure 6.1**

© lawcain/iStock/thinkstock.com. Figure **6.6B**

© Lazar Cvjetkovic/iStock/Thinkstock.com. Figure **2.12**

© lisafx/iStock/thinkstock.com. **Unnumbered Figure 6.8, Unnumbered Figure 8.3**

© Lucian3D/iStock/Thinkstock.com. **Unnumbered Figure 1.2**

© luckyraccoon/iStock.com. **Unnumbered Figure 15.2**

© maclifethai/iStock.com. **Unnumbered Figure 4.6**

© Maksim Tkachenko/iStock.com. Figure **5.35**

© masterzphotois/iStock/Thinkstock.com. **Unnumbered Figure 1.4**

© Michael Blann/Photodisc/thinkstock.com. **Unnumbered Figure 15.6**

© MichaelJay/iStock/thinkstock.com. **Unnumbered Figure 13.9**

© Milenko Bokan/iStock.com. **Unnumbered Figure 14.5**

© monkeybusinessimages/iStock/thinkstock.com. **Unnumbered Figure 4.1, Unnumbered Figure 11.1, Unnumbered Figure 11.3**

© monkeybusinessimages/iStock/thinkstock.com. **Unnumbered Figure 7.2**

© naumoid/iStock.com

© neicebird/iStock.com. **Unnumbered Figure 9.1**

© Neustockimages/iStock.com. Figure **2.8, 15.17**

© Ondine32/iStock/thinkstock.com. **Unnumbered Figure 11.10**

© pagadesign/iStock.com. Figure **2.3**

© Panptys/iStock/Thinkstock.com. **Unnumbered Figure 3.6**

© Photodisc/Photodisc/thinkstock.com. **Unnumbered Figure 9.6, Unnumbered Figure 12.4**

© PSNJua/iStock/Thinkstock.com. **Unnumbered Figure 4.5**

© Purestock/thinkstock.com. **Unnumbered Figure 12.6**

© Quarta_/iStock/Thinkstock.com. **Unnumbered Figure 1.6**

© Ranta Images/iStock/thinkstock.com. **Unnumbered Figure 8.9**

© Ronnie_21/iStock/thinkstock.com. **Unnumbered Figures 4.2, 4.3**

© Rutchapong/iStock/Thinkstock.com. **Unnumbered Figure 1.3**

© sale 123/iStock.com. **Unnumbered Figure 2.1**

© Sashkinw/iStock.com. Figure **5.2A**

© shawshot/iStock.com. Figure **11.16**

© Steve Debenport/iStock.com. Figure **2.14, Unnumbered Figure 1.12**

© Stockbyte/Stockbyte/Thinkstock.com. **Unnumbered Figure 4.7**

© StudioM1/iStock/Thinkstock.com. **Unnumbered Figure 1.1**

© Thinkstock Images/Stockbyte/thinkstock.com. **Unnumbered Figure 10.1**

© TommL/iStock.com. Figure **4.10A**

© TommyIX/iStock.com. Figure **3.4**

© Trish233/iStock/Thinkstock.com. Figure **4.11A**

© WILLSIE/istock.com. Figure **11-15B**

© vgajic/iStock.com. Figure **2.6**

© violet-blue/iStock/thinkstock.com. **Unnumbered Figure 9.3**

© Wavebreakmedia/iStock/thinkstock.com. Figure **14.6, Unnumbered Figure 7.1**

© XiXinXing/iStock/thinkstock.com. **Unnumbered Figure 6.6, Unnumbered Figure 7.5, Unnumbered Figure 15.4**

© YakobchukOlena/iStock/thinkstock.com. Figure **14.9**

Abrahams, P. H., Boon, J., & Spratt, J. D. (2008). *McMinn's clinical atlas of human anatomy* (ed. 6). St Louis: Mosby. Figure **5.1** (photo)

Abrahams, P. H., Spratt, J. D., Loukas, M., & van Schoor, A.-N. (2014). *McMinn and Abrahams' clinical atlas of human anatomy* (ed. 7). St Louis: Mosby. Figures **2.2** (modified), **5.13** (modified), **6.6A, 6.7**

Adam, A., Dixon, A. K., Grainger, R. G., & Allison, D. J. (2008). *Grainger and Allison's diagnostic radiology* (ed. 5). New York: Churchill Livingstone. Figure **4.10B**

Applegate, E. (2011). *The anatomy and physiology learning system* (ed. 4). St Louis: Saunders. Figures **5.27, 5.32**

Aspinall, R. J., & Taylor-Robinson, S. D. (2002). *Mosby's color atlas and text of gastroenterology and liver disease*. St Louis: Mosby. Figure **9.8B, 9.9BC**

Athanasoulis, C. A., Pfister, R. C., Greene, R., & Robeson, G. H. (1982). *Interventional radiology*. Philadelphia: Saunders. Figure **10.18**

Atlas, R. M. (1995). *Principles of microbiology*. St Louis: Mosby. Figure **5.34F**

Ball, J. W., Dains, J. E., Flynn, J. A., et al. (2019). *Seidel's guide to physical examination* (ed. 9). St Louis: Mosby. Figures **2.18, 2.19, 3.7, 3.11, 4.5, 5.20A, 6.5A, Unnumbered Figures 2.12, 4.8**

Ballinger, P. W., & Frank, E. D. (1999). *Merrill's atlas of radiographic positions and radiologic procedures* (ed. 9, Vol. 1). St Louis: Mosby. Figure **4.9A**

Ballinger, P. W., & Frank, E. D. (2003). *Merrill's atlas of radiographic positions and radiologic procedures* (ed. 10). St Louis: Mosby. Figures **4.15, 6.20**

Ballinger, P. W., & Frank, E. D. (2012). *Merrill's atlas of radiographic procedures* (ed. 12). St Louis: Mosby. Figure **4.7B**

Barkauskas, V., et al. (2002). *Health and physical assessment* (ed. 3). St Louis: Mosby. Figures **5.15, 6.16**

Barrett, J. P., & Herndon, D. N. (2001). *Color atlas of burn care*. Philadelphia: Saunders. Figure **12.11D**

Beare, P. G., & Myers, J. L. (1998). *Adult health nursing* (ed. 3). Mosby. Figures **9.7, 15.15**

Behrman, R., Kliegman, R., & Jenson, H. B. (2004). *Nelson textbook of pediatrics* (ed. 17). Philadelphia: Saunders. Figure **7.25**

Belchetz, P. E., & Hammond, P. (2003). *Mosby's color atlas and text of diabetes and endocrinology*. London: Mosby. Figure **10.7B**

Bernstein, E. F. (2006). Laser treatment of tattoos. *Clinics in Dermatology*, 24(1), 43. Figure **12.28**

Black, J. M., Hawks, J. H., & Keene, A. M. (2001). *Medical-surgical nursing: Clinical management for continuity of care* (ed. 6). Philadelphia: Saunders. **Unnumbered Figure 13.2**

Black, J. M., & Hawks, J. H. (2005). *Medical-surgical nursing: Clinical management for positive outcomes* (ed. 7). Philadelphia: Saunders. Figure **4.16**

Black, J. M., & Hawks, J. H. (2009). *Medical surgical nursing: Clinical management for positive outcomes* (ed. 8). Philadelphia: Saunders. Figures **6.30A, 11.8, 15.13** and **Unnumbered Figure 15.7**

Bonewit-West, K. (2015). *Clinical procedures for medical assistants* (ed. 9). St Louis: Saunders. Figures **3.15, 10.7C, 11.21** and **Unnumbered Figure 3.12**

Bontrager, K. L., & Lampignano, J. (2010).*Textbook of radiographic positioning and related anatomy* (ed. 7). St Louis: Mosby. Figure **10.10**

Bontrager, K. L., & Lampingnano, J. (2014). *Textbook of radiographic positioning and related anatomy* (ed. 8). St Louis: Mosby. Figure **6.12C**

Bork, K., & Brauninger, W. (1998). *Skin disorders in clinical practice* (ed. 2). Philadelphia: Saunders. Figure **12.3A**

Boyle, A. C., & Shipley, M. (1993). *A colour atlas of rheumatology* (ed. 3). London: Mosby. Figure **6.23A**

Braunwald, E., Zipes, D. P., & Libby, P. (2001). *Heart disease: A textbook of cardiovascular medicine* (ed. 6). Philadelphia: Saunders. Figure **7.12** and **Unnumbered Figure 7.8**

Brunzel, N. A. (2018). *Fundamentals of urine and body fluid analysis* (ed. 4). St Louis: Saunders. Figure **10.8**

Callen, J. P., Greer, K. E., Paller, A. S., & Swinyer, L. J. (2000). *Color atlas of dermatology* (ed. 2). Philadelphia: Saunders. Figures **2.8B**

Cameron, J. L., & Cameron, A. M. (2017). *Current surgical therapy* (ed. 12). Philadelphia: Elsevier. Figure **12.14**

Canale, S. T. (1998). *Operative orthopaedics* (ed. 9). St Louis: Mosby. Figure **6.18**

Canby, C. (2007). *Problem-based anatomy*. St Louis: Saunders. Figure **11.14**

Chipps, E. M., Clanin, N. J., & Campbell, V. G. (1992). *Neurologic disorders*. St Louis: Mosby. Figure **3.16A**

Conlon, C. P., & Snydman, D. R. (2000). *Mosby's color atlas and text of infectious diseases*. St Louis: Mosby. Figure **12.21** and **Unnumbered Figure 12.8**

Copyright Dennis Kunkel Microscopy, Inc., 1994. Figure **5.28**

Cotran, R. S., Kumar, V., & Collins, T. (2004). *Robbin's pathologic basis of disease* (ed. 7). Philadelphia: Saunders. Figure **11.39**

Coté, C. J., Lerman, J., & Anderson, B. J. (2019). *Coté and Lerman's a practice of anesthesia for infants and children* (ed. 6). Philadelphia: Elsevier. Figure **14.12**

Courtesy Cory J. Bosanko, OD, FAAO; Eye Centers of Tennessee, Crossville, Tenn. Figure **14.7**

Courtesy Department of Neurological Surgery, Vanderbilt University Medical Center, Nashville, Tenn. Figure **13.20A**

Courtesy Department of Pathology, Duke University Medical Center, Durham, NC. Figure **10.11**

Courtesy Dr. Jeffrey P. Callen. Figure **12.15** and **Unnumbered Figure 12.7**

Courtesy E. Tessa Hedley-Whyte. Figure **13.11**

Courtesy Kruse H, photographer. Figure **3.14A**

Courtesy PresMark Publishing. Figure **8.14**

Courtesy the Department of Human Anatomy and Cell Science, University of Manitoba, Winnipeg, Manitoba, Canada. Figure **13.14** and **Unnumbered Figure 13.5**

Courtesy the Royal College of Obstetricians and Gynaecologists. Figure **11.13A**

Courtesy Zimmer, Inc. Warsaw, Ind. Figure **6.27B**

Curry, R. A., & Tempkin, B. B. (2004). *Sonography: Introduction to normal structure and function*. Philadelphia: Saunders. Figure **11.22A**

Custalow, C. (2005). *Color atlas of emergency department procedures*. Philadelphia: Saunders. Figure **5.23**

Dalrymple, N. C., Leyendecker, J. R., & Oliphant, M. (2009). *Problem solving in abdominal imaging*. St Louis: Mosby. Figure **11.9** and **Unnumbered Figure 11.6**

Damjanov, I., & Linder, J. (2000). *Pathology: A color atlas*. St Louis: Mosby. Figure, **5.29, 7.6, 7.11, 9.6** and **Unnumbered Figure 9.7**

Damjanov, I. (2012). *Pathology for the health professions* (ed. 4). St Louis: Saunders. Figure **3.14B, 9.11B, Unnumbered Figure 11.2**

Damjanov, I. (2017). *Pathology for the health professions* (ed. 5). St Louis: Saunders. Figure **9.11, 10.12** and **10.16**

Dorland's illustrated medical dictionary (ed. 30). (2004). Philadelphia: Saunders. Figure **15.8B** and **Unnumbered Figure 15.8**

Dorland's illustrated medical dictionary (ed. 32). (2012). Philadelphia: Saunders. Figures **5.25, 12.12**

Drake, R., Vogl, W., & Mitchell, A. W. M. (2015). *Gray's anatomy for students* (ed. 3). New York: Churchill Livingstone. Figure **7.21, 8.9B, 11.6C**

Draper, B. K., Robbins, J. R., & Stricklin, G. P. (2005). *Bullous Sweet's syndrome in congenital neutropenia: Association with pegfilgrastim. J Am Acad Dermatol*. Elsevier. Figure **12.6** (bullae)

Elkin, M. K., Perry, A. G., & Potter, P. A. (2003). *Nursing interventions and clinical skills* (ed. 3). St Louis: Mosby. Figure **9.18**

Falcone, T., & Goldberg, J. M. (2010). *Basic, advanced, and robotic laparoscopic surgery: Female pelvic surgery video atlas series*. Philadelphia: Saunders. Figures **2.9, 11.7B, 11.17B, 11.18, 11.19**

Finkbeiner, W. E., Ursell, P. C., & Davis, R. L. (2009). *Autopsy pathology: A manual and atlas* (ed. 2). Philadelphia: Saunders. Figure **12.9B**

Forbes, B. A., Sahm, D. F., & Weissfeld, A. S. (2007). *Bailey & Scott's diagnostic microbiology* (ed. 12). St Louis: Mosby. Figures **5.34D, 11.34**

Frank, E. D., Long, B. W., & Smith, B. J. (2012). *Merrill's atlas of radiographic positions and radiologic procedures* (ed. 12). St Louis: Mosby. Figures **11.27B** (modified), **15.16, 15.18**

Fuller, J.K. (2022). *Surgical technology*, (ed.8), St Louis: Mosby. Figure **6.26B, 12.28**

Gartner, L. P. (2017). *Textbook of histology* (ed. 4). Philadelphia: Elsevier. Figure **5.4**

Getty Images: Photodisc CD: health and medicine 2, vol 40, Seattle, Wash. Figure **2.5**

Goldman, L., et al. (2008). *Cecil textbook of medicine* (ed. 23). Philadelphia: Saunders. Figure **8.15**

Goldstein, B. J., & Goldstein, A. O. (1997). *Practical dermatology* (ed. 2). St Louis: Mosby. Figure **7.24**

Greer, I., Cameron, I., Kitchner, H., & Prentice, A. (2001). *Mosby's color atlas and text of obstetrics and gynecology*. St Louis: Mosby. Figure **5.2A**

Habif, T. P., Campbell, J. L., Chapman, M. S., et al. (2011). *Skin disease: Diagnosis and treatment* (ed. 3). Philadelphia: Saunders. Figure **6.21**

Habif, T. P. (2010). *Clinical dermatology: A color atlas guide to diagnosis and therapy* (ed. 5). St Louis: Mosby. Figures **12.19, 12.27**

Harkreader, H., Hogan, M. A., & Thobaben, M. (2007). *Fundamentals of nursing: Caring and clinical judgement* (ed. 3). Philadelphia: Saunders. Figures **4.8B, 5.12B, 8.19A**

Hart, C. A., & Broadhead, R. L. (1992). *Color atlas of pediatric infectious diseases*. London: Mosby. Figure **5.26**

Hockenberry, M. J., Rodgers, C. C., & Wilson, D. (2017). *Wong's essentials of pediatric nursing* (ed. 10). St Louis: Mosby. Figures **6.5B, 11.25**

Ignatavicius, D. D., Workman, M. L., & Mischler, M. A. (1999). *Medical-surgical nursing across the health care continuum* (ed. 3). Philadelphia: Saunders. Figures **12.22B, 15.10**

Ignatavicius, D. D., & Workman, M. L. (2002). *Medical-surgical nursing: Critical thinking for collaborative care* (ed. 4). Philadelphia: Saunders. Figure **14.17A**

Ignatavicius, D. D., & Workman, M. L. (2006). *Medical-surgical nursing: Critical thinking for collaborative care* (ed. 5). Philadelphia: Saunders. Figures **8.7, 12.18**

Ignatavicius, D. D., & Workman, M. L. (2010). *Medical-surgical nursing: Critical thinking for collaborative care* (ed. 6). Philadelphia: Saunders. Figure **13.20B**

Ignatavicius, D. D., & Workman, M. L. (2013). *Medical-surgical nursing: Critical thinking for collaborative care* (ed. 7). St Louis: Saunders. Figures **11.31** (redrawn), **13.19**

Ignatavicius, M. S., & Workman, M. L. (2016). *Medical-surgical nursing: Patient-centered collaborative care* (ed. 8). St Louis: Saunders. Figure **5.6** and **Unnumbered Figures 5.6, 5.7, 5.8**

Ignatavicius, D. D., & Workman, M. L. (2018). *Medical-surgical nursing: Critical thinking for collaborative care* (ed. 9). St Louis: Saunders. Figures **2.7, 4.6, 6.30B, 8.3, 12.11C, 14.17B**

Ishihara, J. (1920). *Tests for color blindness*. Tokyo: Kanehara. Figure **14.4**

Jacob, S. (2008). *Human anatomy: A clinically orientated approach*. St Louis: Churchill Livingstone. Figures **7.3C, 10.3A**

James, W. D., Berger, T., & Elston, T. (2016). *Andrews' Diseases of the skin: Clinical Dermatology*. Elsevier. Figure **12.17**

Kamal, A., & Brockelhurst, J. C. (1991). *Color atlas of geriatric medicine* (ed. 2). St Louis: Mosby. Figure **3.13**

Kelley, L. L., & Petersen, C. (2019). *Sectional anatomy for imaging professionals* (ed. 4). St Louis: Mosby. Figure **4.11B**

Keohane, E., Smith, L., & Walenga, J. (2016). *Rodak's Hematology: Clinical principles and applications* (ed. 5). Philadelphia: Saunders. Figures **5.5** (modified), **5.31, 6.22B**

Kliegman, R. M., Bonita, M. D., Stanton, M. D., et al. (2016). *Nelson's textbook of pediatrics* (ed. 20). Philadelphia: Saunders. Figure **12.13**

Kowalczyk, N., & Mace, J. D. (2014). *Radiographic pathology for technologists* (ed. 6). Mosby. Figure **7.13B** and **Unnumbered Figure 7.9**

Kumar, P., & Clark, M. (2017). *Kumar & Clark's Clinical Medicine* (ed. 9). Edinburgh: Elsevier. Figure **12.9A**

Kumar, V., Abbas, A. K., & Aster, J. C. (2015). *Robbins & Cotran pathologic basis of disease* (ed. 9). Philadelphia: Saunders. Figure **8.13**

Lemmi, F. O., & Lemmi, C. A. E. (2000). *Physical assessment findings CD-ROM*. Philadelphia: Saunders. Figures **6.24A, 11.35, 11.38**

Leonard, P. C. (2012). *Building a medical vocabulary: With Spanish translations* (ed. 8). St Louis Mosby. Figure **1.2**

Leonard, P. (2022). *Building a Medical Vocabulary with Spanish translations* (ed. 11). St Louis: Elsevier, Inc. **1.3, 2.20, 5.6, 8.10, 11.31B, Unnumbered Figure 10.4** (modified)

Lewis, S., Heitkemper, M. M., & Dirksen, S. R. (2004). *Medical surgical nursing, assessment and management of clinical problems* (ed. 6). St Louis: Mosby. Figure **10.13**

Lewis, S. M., Heitkemper, M. M., Dirksen, S. R., et al. (2011). *Medical-surgical nursing: Assessment and management of clinical problems* (ed. 8). St Louis: Mosby. Figures **5.18, 7.15A**

Lewis, S. M., Bucher, L., Heitkemper, M. M., & Dirksen, S. R. (2014). *Medical-surgical nursing: Assessment and management of clinical problems* (ed. 9). St Louis: Mosby. Figure **12.11E**

Lewis, S. L., Bucher, L., Heitkemper, M. M., Harding, M. M., Kwong, J., & Roberts, D. (2017). *Medical-surgical nursing, assessment and management of clinical problems* (ed. 10). St Louis: Mosby. Figures **6.17, 7.17AB**

Liebgott, B. (2011). *The anatomical basis of dentistry* (ed. 3). St Louis: Mosby. Figure **9.2** (adapted)

Long, B. W., Rollins, J. H., & Smith, B. J. (2016). *Merrill's atlas of radiographic procedures* (ed. 13). St Louis: Mosby. Figures **4.13, 4.14, 4.17, 5.10, 6.9A&B, 6.11, 6.27A, 7.7, 11.26A, 15.17**

Male, D., Brostoff, J., Roth, D., & Roitt, I. (2013). *Immunology* (ed. 8). Philadelphia: Saunders. Figure **5.30**

Marks, J. G., Jr., & Miller, J. J. (2019). *Lookingbill and Marks' principles of dermatology* (ed. 6). Philadelphia: Saunders. Figures **2.21, 12.7**

Mendeloff, A. I., & Smith, D. E. (1956). Acromegaly, diabetes, hypermetabolism, proteinuria and heart failure. *Clin Pathol Conf Am J Med*, 20, 133. Figure **15.9**

Miller, M. D., Howard, R. F., & Plancher, K. D. (2003). *Surgical atlas of sports medicine*. Philadelphia: Saunders. Figure **6.26A**

Monahan, F. D., & Neighbors, M. (1998). *Medical surgical nursing: Foundations for clinical practice* (ed. 2). Philadelphia: Saunders. Figure **12.25**

Morse, S., Moreland, A., & Holmes, K., eds. (1996). *Atlas of sexually transmitted diseases and AIDS* (ed. 2). London: Mosby-Wolfe. Figure **11.37**

Murray, P. R., Rosenthal, K. S., Kobayashi, G. S., & Pfaller, M. A. (1994). *Medical microbiology* (ed. 3). St Louis: Mosby. Figure **5.34B**

Murray, P. R., Rosenthal, K. S., Kobayashi, G. S., & Pfaller, M. A. (1994). *Medical microbiology* (ed. 3). St Louis: Mosby. Figure **5.34E**

Murray, P. R., Rosenthal, K. S., & Pfaller, M. A. (2016). *Medical microbiology* (ed. 8). Philadelphia: Saunders. Figure **11.40**

Murray, S. S., & McKinney, E. S. (2006). *Foundations of maternal-newborn nursing* (ed. 4). Philadelphia: Saunders. Figure **11.24**

National Library of Medicine, National Institutes of Health. Figure **6.1**

Noble, J. (Ed.), (2001). *Textbook of primary care medicine* (ed. 3). St Louis: Mosby. Figures **11.36, 12.6** (macules, papules, plaques, vesicles, pustules), **12.8**

Palay, D. A., & Krachmer, J. H. (Eds.), (2005). *Ophthalmology for the primary care physician* (ed. 2). St Louis: Mosby. Figure **14.1B**

Patton, K. T., & Thibodeau, G. A. (2010). *Anatomy and physiology* (ed. 7). St Louis: Mosby. Figure **15.2** (modified)

Patton, K. T., & Thibodeau, G. A. (2013). *Anatomy and physiology* (ed. 8). St Louis: Mosby. Figures **13.3A, 14.21B**

Patton, K. T., & Thibodeau, G. A. (2016). *Anatomy and physiology* (ed. 9). Mosby. Figures **12.2, 13.12B** (modified), **14.21A**

Patton, K. T., & Thibodeau, G. A. (2014). *The human body in health and disease* (ed. 6). St Louis: Mosby. Figure **5.7**

Patton, K. T., & Thibodeau, G. A. (2018). *The human body in health & disease* (ed. 7). St Louis: Elsevier/Mosby. Figures **11.5B&C, 15.4**

Perry, A. G., Potter, P. A., & Ostendorf, W. (2018). *Clinical nursing skills and techniques* (ed. 9). St Louis: Mosby. Figures **4.1A, 4.2A, 4.2C, 4.4C**

Polaski, A. L., & Tatro, S. E. (1996). *Luckmann's core principles and practice of medical-surgical nursing*. Philadelphia: Saunders. Figures **1.1, 3.16B**

Polaski, A. L., & Tatro, S. E. (1996). *Luckmann's core principles and practice of medical-surgical nursing*. Philadelphia: Saunders. Figure **13.9**

Potter, P. A., Perry, A. G., Stockert, P., & Hall, A. (2013). *Fundamentals of Nursing* (ed. 8). St Louis: Mosby. Figures **4.2B** and **4.3E**

Potter, P. A., Perry, A. G., Stockert, P., & Hall, A. (2017). *Fundamentals of Nursing* (ed. 9). St Louis: Mosby. Figures **4.1B, 4.2D, 4.4C, 8.4, 8.6**

Price, S., & Wilson, L. (2003). *Pathophysiology: Clinical concepts of disease processes* (ed. 6). St Louis: Mosby. Figure **10.9**

Proctor, D. B., Niedzwiecki, B., Pepper, J., Garrels, M., & Mills, H. (2017). *Kinn's the medical assistant: An applied learning approach* (ed. 13). St Louis: Saunders. Figure **3.8**

Rakel, R. E., & Rakel, D. P. (2016). *Textbook of family medicine* (ed. 9). Philadelphia: Saunders. Figure **14.15**

Rumack, C. M., & Levine, D. (2018). *Diagnostic ultrasound* (ed. 5). St Louis: Mosby. Figure **11.22B**

Schoenwolf, G. C., Bleyl, S. B., Brauer, P. R., & Francis-West, P. H. (2008). *Larsen's human embryology* (ed. 4). London: Churchill Livingstone. Figure **5.2B** photo, **11.20B**

Seidel, H. M., Ball, J. W., Dains, J. E., et al. (2003). *Mosby's guide to physical examination* (ed. 5). St Louis: Mosby. Figures **2.8A, 2.10, 4.4A, Unnumbered Figure 4.10**

Shiland, B. J. (2016). *Mastering Healthcare Terminology* (ed. 6). St Louis: Mosby. Figure **4.16, 12.26, 14.13**

Sorrentino, S. A. (2000). *Mosby's textbook for nursing assistants* (ed. 5). St Louis: Mosby. Figure **4.3D**

Stevens, A., Lowe, J. S., & Scott, I. (2009). *Core pathology* (ed. 3). St Louis: Mosby. Figure **6.2** Abrahams, P. H., Boon, J., & Spratt, J. D. (2008). *McMinn's clinical atlas of human anatomy* (ed. 6). St Louis: Mosby. Figure **6.3**

Stevens, A., & Lowe, J. S. (2005). *Human histology* (ed. 3). Philadelphia: Elsevier. Figure **11.20B**

Stone, D. R., & Gorbach, S. L. (2000). *Atlas of infectious diseases*. Philadelphia: Saunders. Figures **7.23, 12.16**

Swartz, M. H. (2014). *Textbook of physical diagnosis, history, and examination* (ed. 7). Philadelphia: Saunders. Figures **5.22, 6.25, 11.6B, 14.20**

Symonds, E. M., & MacPherson, M. B. A. (1994). *Color atlas of obstetrics and gynecology*. London: Mosby. Figure **11.13B**

Talbot, L. A., & Myers-Marquardt, M. (1997). *Pocket guide to critical care assessment* (ed. 3). St Louis: Mosby. Figure **8.8**

Thibodeau, G. A., & Patton, K. T. (2010). *The human body in health & disease* (ed. 5). St Louis: Mosby. Figures **14.19A, 15.12; Unnumbered Figure 14.4**

Vidic, B., & Suarez, F. R. (1984). *Photographic atlas of the human body*. St Louis: Mosby. Figure **8.2**

Weston, W. L., Lane, A. T., & Morelli, J. F. (2007). *Color textbook of pediatric dermatology* (ed. 4). St Louis: Mosby. Figure **12.20**

Weston, W. L., & Lane, A. T. (1991). *Color textbook of pediatric dermatology*. St Louis: Mosby. Figure **2.22** and **Unnumbered Figure 2.11**

Wilson, S. F., & Giddens, J. F. (2017). *Health assessment for nursing practice* (ed. 6). St Louis: Mosby. Figures **3.18, 4.4B, 5.16, 15.8A, Unnumbered Figure 4.9**

Zakus, S. (2001). *Mosby's clinical skills for medical assistants* (ed. 4). St Louis: Mosby. Figure **10.7A**

Zitelli, B. J., McIntire, M. D., & Nowalk, A. J. (2012). *Zitelli and Davis' atlas of pediatric physical diagnosis* (ed. 6). St Louis: Mosby. Figure **6.24B**

Zitelli, B. J., McIntire, S., & Nowalk, A. J. (2018). *Zitelli and Davis' Atlas of pediatric physical diagnosis* (ed. 7). St Louis: Mosby. Figures **2.17, 3.12, 9.10, 12.22A, 14.10, 14.11, 15.11, Unnumbered Figures 3.11, 14.1**

Index

Page numbers followed by "*f*" indicate figures, "*t*" indicate tables, and "*b*" indicate boxes.

465